Myofascial Trigger Points

Senior Content Strategist: Alison Taylor
Senior Content Development Specialist: Ailsa Laing
Senior Project Manager: Sukanthi Sukumar
Designer: Charles Gray
Illustration Manager: Gillian Richards

Myofascial Trigger Points

Comprehensive diagnosis and treatment

Edited by

Priv. Doz. Dr. med. Dominik Irnich

Interdisciplinary Pain Management Centre,
Department of Anaesthesiology,
Munich University Hospital – City Centre,
Munich, Germany

Translated by

Jackie K Jones

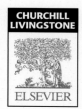

CHURCHILL
LIVINGSTONE

ELSEVIER

Edinburgh London New York Oxford Philadelphia St Louis Sydney Toronto 2013

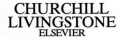

First edition published in English © 2013, Elsevier Limited. All rights reserved.
First edition published in German under the title *Leitfaden Triggerpunkte* in 2009.
First Edition 2009, © Elsevier GmbH, Urban & Fischer, Munchen.

ISBN 978-0-7020-4312-3

British Library Cataloguing in Publication Data
A catalogue record for this book is available from the British Library

Library of Congress Cataloging in Publication Data
A catalog record for this book is available from the Library of Congress

Notices
Knowledge and best practice in this field are constantly changing. As new research and experience broaden our understanding, changes in research methods, professional practices, or medical treatment may become necessary.

Practitioners and researchers must always rely on their own experience and knowledge in evaluating and using any information, methods, compounds, or experiments described herein. In using such information or methods they should be mindful of their own safety and the safety of others, including parties for whom they have a professional responsibility.

With respect to any drug or pharmaceutical products identified, readers are advised to check the most current information provided (i) on procedures featured or (ii) by the manufacturer of each product to be administered, to verify the recommended dose or formula, the method and duration of administration, and contraindications. It is the responsibility of practitioners, relying on their own experience and knowledge of their patients, to make diagnoses, to determine dosages and the best treatment for each individual patient, and to take all appropriate safety precautions.

To the fullest extent of the law, neither the Publisher nor the authors, contributors, or editors, assume any liability for any injury and/or damage to persons or property as a matter of products liability, negligence or otherwise, or from any use or operation of any methods, products, instructions, or ideas contained in the material herein.

your source for books, journals and multimedia in the health sciences
www.elsevierhealth.com

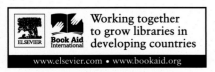

Working together to grow libraries in developing countries
www.elsevier.com • www.bookaid.org

The Publisher's policy is to use **paper manufactured from sustainable forests**

Printed in China

Preface

It has taken more than 5 years for this book to come to fruition, from concept to completion. The reason for this length of time is simple: all the authors are practitioners and are daily involved with patients with myofascial trigger points; in their remaining free time they are educating themselves or training other colleagues. There is little time left for writing. This is a book by practitioners for practitioners.

However, in the end modern medicine and doctors and therapists demand the best evidence from research results, personal experiences and available skills for individually successful treatment, so experience alone is not enough. Current scientific evidence from basic and clinical research must be presented and the necessary skills must be made graphically accessible to the potential user. This book tries to fulfil this requirement.

However, if we ask the patient what they want from their therapist and what constitutes successful treatment from their point of view, other factors play a much greater role: Communication and partnership, understanding of the worries and expectations of the patient and the illness, the personal relationship with the doctor or therapist, the fostering of health, a positive attitude and an interest in the effects of the symptoms on daily life are scientifically proven factors of influence on the result. This requires from the therapist a comprehensive understanding of disease and health. This book tries to fulfil this requirement as well.

Therefore, the doctor–patient relationship, the 'holistic' view of the muscles, and also unconventional therapies, get plenty of space in this book. Some of this is drawn from the authors' experience and must remain anecdotal. There is still insufficient research with suitable methods for some procedures. There is also a lack of finance.

But what if I just want to find and treat the muscle trigger points? It's a good question. The practitioner can quickly get to the (trigger) point with the aid of the pain charts, function tables and muscle descriptions. This book is therefore a channel for rapid diagnosis and treatment of myofascial trigger points in everyday life. We cannot go into the significance of the muscles or trigger points here. That is what the book is for.

The book would not exist without the commitment of the contributors, some of whom are good friends, especially Nicolas Behrens and Jochen Gleditsch.

Most of all, however, it could not exist without the incredibly committed and extremely competent support of Christl Kiener and the whole team at Elsevier.

Nor without the support and patience of my wonderful wife and our children, my family!

Dominik Irnich
Munich, October 2008

Contents

Contents

Contents

Contributors

Joseph F. Audette, MA MD
Assistant Professor
Harvard Medical School
Department of Physical Medicine & Rehabilitation
Boston
Massachusetts, USA

Dr. med. Jürgen Bachmann
Specialist in Orthopaedics – Rheumatology
amc – augusta-medical-clinic Hattingen/Ruhr

Prof. Dr. med. Dr Phil Winfried Banzer
Director of the Department of Sports Medicine
Goethe-University Frankfurt am Main
Germany

Dr. med. Nicolas Behrens
Doctor of Physical Medicine and Rehabilitation
Acupuncture
Naturopathic Treatments
Munich, Germany

Dr. med. Beat Dejung
Specialist FMH (Swiss Medical Association) for
Rheumatology
Physical Medicine and Rehabilitation
Winterthur
Zurich, Switzerland

Peter T. Dorsher, MS MD
Mayo Clinic Jacksonville
Florida, USA

David Euler, L Ac
Course Director
Structural Acupuncture for Physicians
Harvard Medical School
Boston
Massachusetts, USA

Dr. med. Johannes Fleckenstein
Interdisciplinary Pain Management Centre
Department of Anaesthesiology
Munich University Hospital – City Centre
Munich, Germany

Roland Gautschi, MA PT
Senior Instructor in Trigger Point Therapy IMTT®
Baden, Switzerland

Dr. med. Jochen Gleditsch
Lecturer in Acupuncture
Ludwig-Maximilians-University
Munich, Germany

Dr. phil. Markus Hübscher
Department of Sports Medicine
Goethe-University Frankfurt am Main
Germany

Christine Irnich, Dip
Sports Instructor for Prevention and Rehabilitation
Landsberg, Germany

Priv. Doz. Dr. med. Dominik Irnich
Interdisciplinary Pain Management Centre
Department of Anaesthesiology
Munich University Hospital – City Centre
Munich, Germany

Dr. med. Martin Kosub
Orthopaedic Practice
Hattingen, Germany

Dr. med. Philip Lang
Department of Anaesthesiology
Munich University Hospital – City Centre
Munich, Germany

Prof. Dr. med. Karel Lewit
Rehabilitation Department of Medical Faculty 2
Karls University
Praha-Motol
Czech Republic

Dr. med. Gunnar Licht
Specialist in Orthopaedics
Trigger Point Therapist®
Superintendant of Dörenberg Hospital
Bad Iburg, Germany

Priv. Doz. Dr. med. Markus Maier
Orthopaedic Practice
Starnberg, Germany

Dr. med. Martin Offenbächer
Doctor of Physical and Rehabilitative Medicine
Munich, Germany

Dr. med. Francisco Pedrosa Gil
Inn Valley Hospital Dr. med. Rother
Simbach am Inn, Germany

Dr. med. Florian Pfab
Hospital and Health Centre for Dermatology and Allergy
Munich University of Technology
Lecturer in Acupuncture at Regensburg University
Germany

Dr. med. dent. Jean-Marc Pho Duc
Dental Prosthetics Centre
Ludwig-Maximilians-University
Munich, Germany

Dr. med. Raymund Pothmann
Centre for Integrative Paediatric Therapy and Palliative Medicine
Hamburg, Germany

Dr. biol. hum. Dipl. Psych. Robert Schleip
Research Director of the European Rolfing Association e.V.
Munich, Germany

Dr. med. Hans-Joachim Schmitt
Johannesbad Hospital
Bad Füssing
Germany

Jay P. Shah, MD
Rehabilitation Medicine Department
National Institutes of Health
Bethesda
Maryland, USA

Armin Slugocki
Physiotherapist
Kaufering
Germany

Dr. med. Michael Späth
Internist/Rheumatology
Gräfelfing, Germany

Dr. med. dent. Kathrin Spiegl
Dental Prosthetics Centre
Ludwig-Maximilians-University
Munich, Germany

Dr. med. Andreas Winkelmann
Interdisciplinary Pain Management Centre
Department of Anaesthesiology
Munich University Hospital – City Centre
Munich, Germany

Section | 1 |

Introductory overview

Chapter | 1 |

Guide to the book

Dominik Irnich

Pain and limited function of the locomotor (or musculo-skeletal) system are two of the most common reasons for consulting a doctor or therapist. The muscles have a key role in this, because of their anatomical and functional properties (see Ch. 5). The importance of the muscles is frequently underestimated in practice, however, although muscular imbalances, muscle tension and painful disorders of muscle function play a large part in both acute and chronic locomotor system symptoms, according to current knowledge. The clinical correlate is the myofascial trigger point (mTrP).

The problem is the extraordinarily wide range and differentiated form of these functional muscle pathologies. The natural course of muscle pain is very variable in the individual and ranges from spontaneous remission to persistence without progression to chronification with increasing pain and definite limitation of function (Fig. 1.1).

The clinical significance in individual cases relies on the subjective description of the condition by the patient, and the exact diagnosis (see Ch. 13) can only be assessed by means of a unified, i.e. biopsychosocial, patient-centred approach (see Ch. 12). Psychosocial factors should be considered at an early stage. Overlooking these associations is a professional error!

For this reason, this book comprehensively examines the muscles and their (dys)function as part of the human system, in terms of: a compensatory mechanism and an expression of a functional disorder of the whole locomotor system (see Ch. 7); the parallels to the views and knowledge in traditional Chinese medicine (TCM; see Ch. 8); connections with the muscular fascia network (see Ch. 9); the difficult problem of pain in multiple locations, fibromyalgia (see Ch. 10); psychosomatic pain (see Ch. 11); and a human sensory organ and organ of expression (see Ch. 12).

However, initially, we need to explain the anatomical and physiological prerequisites for the occurrence of mTrP. There is a great deal of scientific knowledge available about this (see Chs 5 and 6). To facilitate the use of consistent language in communication with and about patients, knowledge of the definitions is essential (see Ch. 2). In this book, we rely for the most part on the guidelines of the pioneers in the field of trigger point research, Janet Travell and David Simons (Travell, Simons 2002).

We understand the mTrP to be a site or band that is hypersensitive and palpably tense compared to the surrounding area in a muscle that is often shortened, and which demonstrates changes in tone and consistency ('taut band'). It is painful when palpated and from it pain and autonomic disorders may be caused in an area that cannot usually be attributed to a particular segment ('referred pain'). We describe the resulting muscle pain as myofascial pain syndrome (MPS).

Diagnostic criteria are:

- a localised, dull, pressing, dragging, occasionally burning spontaneous pain associated with acute or chronic muscular strain,
- tenderness with typical pain reproduction within a palpable 'taut band' of muscle,
- a pain which predominantly radiates in a distal direction after mechanical stimulation,
- painful limitation of movement,
- muscular weakness without atrophy.

As these are not 'hard', evidence-based criteria but subjective information and findings, an appropriate findings-oriented medical differential diagnosis is an indispensable prerequisite for making the diagnosis of 'myofascial pain' with or without limitation of movement (see Ch. 14).

http://dx.doi.org/10.1016/B978-0-7020-4312-3.00001-5

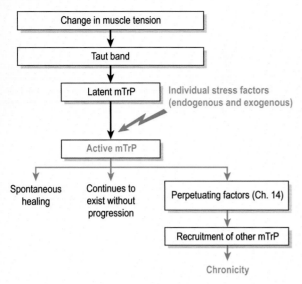

Fig. 1.1 Course of myofascial pain.
(Modified from Simons 1996)

If other causes can be ruled out, we recommend making a comprehensive and function-related diagnosis for producing a clear treatment plan (see Ch. 13).

Various therapeutic procedures for the treatment of myofascial pain have been described: in the treatment of acute muscle pain (e.g. following trauma, acute strain, etc.) analgesics, physical therapies, manual techniques, acupuncture and therapeutic local anaesthetic (LA) frequently bring sufficient pain relief, either individually or in combination. The main aim of treatment of acute muscle pain is the rapid and effective relief of pain, as there is evidence that insufficient pain relief for an acute event can be a factor in the pain becoming chronic.

The treatment of chronic myofascial pain is often a therapeutic problem. This is because the cause of chronic myofascial pain can be complex. The attitude and cooperation of the patient play a crucial role in recovery. Long-term results can only be achieved with a motivated patient in an individually compiled multimodal overall therapy concept. The keystones of such a concept can be manual medical and physiotherapy procedures (see Ch. 18), physical procedures (see Ch. 20), infiltration techniques (see Ch. 21), acupuncture and related techniques (see Ch. 22). Naturopathic treatments, specific relaxation techniques (see Ch. 24) and psychotherapeutic methods can also be modules in a long-term treatment concept.

For many patients the motivation for self-help following instruction (extension, muscle coordination) is necessary and sensible. This helps not only to avoid recurrence but also gives the patient the chance to make their own contribution to their recovery and to take responsibility for the disease.

The prescription of analgesics, muscle relaxants and non-steroidal anti-inflammatory drugs (NSAIDs) fades into the background when it comes to long-term treatment, as they are frequently only effective for a short time and if taken for longer are associated with a high rate of undesirable side effects.

To assess the efficacy of the selected procedures a close examination of the findings and an evaluation of the effects of the therapy by the patient are necessary (see Ch. 13).

> The main purpose of the treatment of chronic myofascial symptoms is pain relief. This avoids the negative consequences of persistent protective and incorrect posture and increases the patient's capacity for physical function.

This book is a plea to give muscle pain the status of a disease that should be taken seriously; the disease can restrict all areas of the life and existence as a human being if it becomes chronic and these areas of life can, in turn, also influence the disease. Terms such as 'a little bit of muscle tension' or 'insignificant additional findings' will then disappear from medical communication (see Fig. 1.2).

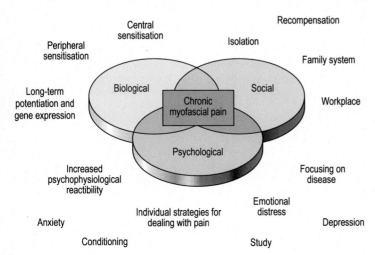

Fig. 1.2 Biopsychosocial model for chronic pain.

Chapter | 2 |

Terminology

Dominik Irnich, Roland Gautschi, Nicolas Behrens

The following is a brief explanation of the terms used in this book. Most expressions can be defined clearly, thanks predominantly to the work of Travell and Simons. Nevertheless, in everyday speech the key term 'trigger point' is used with a wide variety of meanings. Value is frequently not given to the affected structure. Terms such as 'tenderpoint', 'myelogelosis', 'gelosis', 'tendomyosis' and 'taut muscle' are also often used as synonyms for mTrPs. The use of these terms implies, however, various causes and points of view, leaving the door open to misunderstanding. We therefore consider it necessary to identify and name the structure underlying the trigger point to avoid inaccuracies (see Table 2.1).

> The term 'tenderpoint' should be reserved as a criterion for classification of fibromyalgia (see Table 2.2). However, fibromyalgia patients often have additional mTrPs!

Trigger point

A trigger point is a site of increased irritability in a tissue that demonstrates a hypersensitive reaction to mechanical stimulation (pressure or traction) and causes ('triggers') an additional (pathological) physiological reaction. The symptoms caused can be local or regional; however, additional symptoms in areas of the body far removed from the site of provocation are frequently reported (*referred pain, transferred phenomenon*).

Myofascial trigger point (mTrP)

Compared to the surrounding area, the mTrP is a particularly sensitive, overexcitable, tender area within a cord-like shortened skeletal muscle fibre bundle (taut band), which is frequently palpable as a thickened section. Pain, strange sensations and autonomic phenomena can be caused with mechanical stimulation (pressure, traction or needling).

The mTrP is the morphological correlate of myofascial pain syndrome (MPS). An mTrP can be distinguished from the trigger points of other structures named in Table 2.1. The mTrP can have various levels of sensitivity (active, latent).

Active mTrP

An active mTrP is an mTrP which is already symptomatic at rest and/or during physiological strain (spontaneous activity) and feels tender as well as having sensory, motor function and/or autonomic phenomena in its related transfer zones (see Table 2.2).

Latent mTrP

A latent mTrP is not symptomatic at rest and/or during physiological strain but still demonstrates localised tenderness as well as causing regional sensory, motor function and/or autonomic phenomena in its related transfer zones. A latent mTrP can turn into an active trigger point (see Table 2.2).

Primary (initial) trigger point

A primary (initial) trigger point is an mTrP activated by acute or chronic strain, traumatic overextension or direct trauma to the affected muscle. Primary mTrPs do not occur in another muscle of the body as a result of mTrP activity.

Related trigger point

A related trigger point is a small mTrP in the immediate neighbourhood of the primary mTrP, which is located in the same muscle.

http://dx.doi.org/10.1016/B978-0-7020-4312-3.00002-7

Table 2.1 Trigger point terminology

TYPE OF TRIGGER POINT	AFFECTED STRUCTURE	CHARACTERISTICS	EXAMPLE
Cutaneous	Cutaneous nerve ending	Electrifying, hyperaesthetic	Primary hyperaesthesia
Connective tissue, subcutaneous	Connective tissue	Swelling of connective tissue	Panniculitis
Involving ligaments, tendons	Ligaments, tendons	Frequently inflammatory components	Epicondylopathy
Myofascial	Muscles	Dull, pressing	Myofascial pain syndrome
Periosteal, bony	Bones and periosteum	Deep pain	'Periostitis'
Visceral	Visceral organs (frequently via the fascia)	Dull, diffuse	McBurney's point

Table 2.2 Differentiation of active and latent mTrPs and tenderpoints

FINDING	ACTIVE mTrP	LATENT mTrP	TENDER POINT (FIBROMYALGIA)
Palpable thickening	Common	Possible	Rare
Taut band	Yes	Yes	No
Spontaneous pain	Yes	No	Possible
Tenderness	Yes	Yes	Yes
Restricted movement	Common	Possible	Possible
Referred pain	Common	Possible	No
Clinically known symptoms can be reproduced	Yes	No	Possible

Associated trigger point

Associated trigger points occur as a result of trigger point activity in another muscle. Associated trigger points fall into two categories: secondary and satellite trigger points.

Secondary trigger point

An mTrP is described as secondary if it has developed secondarily in a muscle that is an antagonist or synergist of the muscle affected by the primary mTrP. A secondary mTrP arises from strain because the muscle must either excessively support the muscle affected by the primary mTrP as a synergist or counteract its increased tension as an antagonist. A secondary mTrP can thus be caused by mTrP in another muscle and is an example of an associated mTrP; these should be differentiated from satellite mTrPs.

Satellite trigger points

An mTrP that has formed in the referred pain zone of a primary mTrP is described as a satellite mTrP. A satellite mTrP can be caused by mTrP activity in another muscle and is therefore an example of an associated mTrP; these should be differentiated from secondary mTrPs.

Taut band

Taut bands are rope-like bundles of shortened muscle fibres within a muscle that can contain an mTrP (see Fig. 2.1a).

Local twitch response

The local muscle twitch response is a microcontraction within a taut band of muscle and is caused by mechanical stimulation of an mTrP within the taut band. This phenomenon is caused relatively regularly if the precise spot of an mTrP is touched by an acupuncture needle or an injection cannula. It is also occasionally caused by very frequent irritation of the fascia surrounding the mTrP or by snapping palpation or pressure of the superficial muscles (see Fig. 2.1b and c).

Referred pain

Referred pain means radiation of pain from a pathologically changed structure into the surrounding area or even into other regions of the body. The pattern of spread cannot

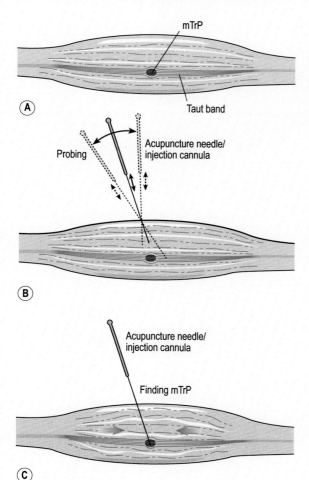

Fig. 2.1 Diagram of a taut band and a trigger point (a). Probing the mTrP with an acupuncture needle (b) by lifting and lowering, and causing a local twitch response when it meets the mTrP exactly (c).

be explained by a radicular segmental innervation pattern (dermatome, myotome) nor by the innervation area of the peripheral nerves. The most common phenomenon of this type is the referral of pain from an active mTrP.

Referred phenomena

Referred phenomena are sensory (pain, dysaesthesia), motor function (weakness, poor coordination) and autonomic (vasodilation, vasoconstriction, sweating, nausea, dizziness) symptoms, which are referred by a pathologically changed structure into the surrounding area or even into other regions of the body. Pain referred from an mTrP is the most commonly occurring form of a referred phenomenon.

Myofascial syndrome (MFS)

MFS refers to all of the symptoms caused by mTrPs. MFS occurs regionally and can be distinguished from generalised disorders. The morphological correlate of MFS is the mTrP.

Myofascial pain syndrome (MPS)

MPS refers to a MFS where the main symptom is pain and can represent a complex psychological and physiological event in the sense of a chronic pain syndrome. The morphological correlate of MFS is the mTrP.

Primary MPS

The term should be used when the muscles are pathologically changed and mTrP has been demonstrated.

Secondary MPS

Secondary MPS can arise as a result of various diseases of the visceral organs and non-muscular parts of the locomotor system. Reflex mechanisms from the spine are involved, caused by pain from the internal organs or as a result of protective or incorrect posture originating from diseases of the locomotor system of non-muscular cause, such as arthritis or following trauma. An mTrP can make pain worse, but in some cases pain transmitted by the mTrP can be superimposed on pain caused by an underlying disease.

Chapter 3

Epidemiology

Johannes Fleckenstein

3.1 AETIOLOGY OF DISEASE

The term 'aetiology' does not just describe the theory of the causes and the clinical psychology of disease in medicine (see Ch. 4), but all the factors that contribute to the occurrence of a disease, particularly in epidemiology.

Causative factors: the pathogenesis of mTrPs is controversial (see Ch. 6). A specific factor that causes mTrP is not yet known.

Contributive factors: possible causes under discussion for the occurrence of mTrPs are joint dysfunction, afferent pain from spondylosis, arthritis and disorders of the internal organs, lack of exercise, influence of the weather, nerve lesions (e.g. radiculopathy), psychological factors (anxiety, stress), hormonal disorders and vitamin and nutrient deficiencies (e.g. iron, folic acid, vitamin B12 deficiency, etc.) as well as anatomical variants (difference in leg length, incorrect tooth position or bite). These factors play an important role in the activation and the persistence of mTrPs.

Correlative factors: in a Danish work there was evidence of a connection between musculoskeletal pain and social status and smoking. Single mothers who smoke and who have little support from their social milieu demonstrate more frequent contractions of the muscles of the neck and throat. In another Danish work there was evidence of a connection between the place of work, specifically working at a sewing machine, and the development of musculoskeletal symptoms. Other correlations have been described but still await confirmation from scientific studies.

3.2 EPIDEMIOLOGICAL INDICATORS

There is currently no generally applicable evidence for the incidence and prevalence of mTrPs in the population. There is a lack of comprehensive representative studies and exact comprehensive evidence for the epidemiology in the population is not available. However, individual studies have provided some information on the risk of possible disease and the distribution of mTrPs.

People aged between 30 and 49 in particular frequently suffer from a pain syndrome caused by an activated mTrP; this is often a time of life when the greatest physical demands are made on the body. A latent mTrP with no detectable, disturbing influence on the patient is differentiated from an active mTrP which may be part of an MPS or be involved with it in the form of a myofascial pain component in other complex pain syndromes (see Ch. 2).

The frequency of mTrP is as follows: among healthy recruits in the US Air Force, approximately 50% of every 100 male or female recruits had active or latent mTrPs in the muscles of the pectoral girdle. In another investigation of 269 nursing auxiliaries, a frequency of up to 54% of active and latent trigger points in the muscles of the head and neck was described.

Observations of healthy volunteers showed an occurrence of up to 50% for latent trigger points in the lumbo-gluteal muscles and also in the rest of the skeletal muscles (see Table 3.1).

http://dx.doi.org/10.1016/B978-0-7020-4312-3.00003-9

Table 3.1 Prevalence of mTrPs in various muscle groups in unselected patients

MUSCLE GROUP	PREVALENCE OF mTrPs	NUMBER OF CASES	SOURCE
Pectoral girdle	54% f, 45% m	$n=200$	Sola et al. 1955
Muscles of mastication and pectoral muscles	28–54% f	$n=269$	Schiffman et al. 1990
Lumbogluteal muscles	5–45%	$n=100$	Fröhlich, Fröhlich 1995
Musculoskeletal system	37% f, 65% m	$n=1504$	Drewes, Jennum 1995
f, female; m, male.			

If patients report pain symptoms, an mTrP is often the only clinical finding to be found. Depending on the profession, an mTrP was found in 85–93% of patients in outpatient departments specialising in pain therapy. In a dental department, 55% of patients showed evidence of trigger points, as did 30% of patients in a medical practice. In an orthopaedic department, almost all patients were diagnosed with a latent mTrP, although only about one-fifth of patients were diagnosed with an active mTrP (see Table 3.2).

One investigation of the occurrence of trigger points in specific pain syndromes talked of a frequency of 68 up to 100% (see Table 3.3). According to one study, the prevalence of tension headaches was 78% over a lifetime whereas 3% of the general population suffers from tension headaches.

Table 3.2 Prevalence of mTrPs in selected patient groups

MUSCLE GROUP	PREVALENCE OF mTrPs	NUMBER OF CASES	SOURCE
Medical practice	30% of pain patients	$n=54$	Skootsky et al. 1989
Pain centre	93% myofascial symptoms, 74% main cause	$n=96$	Gerwin, Gevirtz 1995
Specialist pain centre	85%, two investigators	$n=283$	Fishbain et al. 1986
Dental clinic for head and face pain	55% main cause	$n=164$	Fricton et al. 1985
Orthopaedic department	94% latent mTrP, 21% active mTrP	$n=97$	Fröhlich, Fröhlich 1995

Table 3.3 Prevalence of mTrPs in specific pain syndromes

PAIN SYNDROME	PREVALENCE OF mTrPs	NUMBER OF CASES	SOURCE
Fibromyalgia	68%	$n=60$	Granges, Littlejohn 1993
	100%	$n=19$	Finestone et al. 1995
	72%	$n=25$	Gerwin, Gevirtz 1995
RSD	82%	$n=84$	Lin et al. 1995
Cervicogenic headache	100%	$n=80$	Lin et al. 1995
Tension headache	38%	$n=40$	Langemark, Olesen 1987
		$n=1000$	Rasmussen 1991, Jensen et al. 1993
		$n=25$	Fernández-de-las-Peñas et al. 2007c
RSD, reflex sympathetic dystrophia (complex regional pain syndrome).			

The occurrence of mTrPs was up to 38% higher in this group compared to a headache-free control (see Table 3.3). This leads to high costs for the whole welfare system. If tension headaches do not respond to standard therapy, there may be at least a partial connection with mTrPs, and they should be investigated, because symptoms that are similar to a tension headache frequently occur as part of an MPS.

Note, however, that the study results on the prevalence of mTrP crucially depend on the diagnostic capability of the therapist and the diagnostic criteria used and cannot therefore be generalised in all cases.

mTrPs are widespread in the population. However, there are wide variations in the information on trigger points in relation to location, frequency, duration or even symptoms. If we look at it from the angle of health economics in particular, unrecognised chronic MPS may represent a serious cost factor in our welfare system.

Chapter | 4 |

Aetiology of myofascial pain syndrome

Dominik Irnich, Hans-Joachim Schmitt

4.1 CAUSATIVE FACTORS

Hans-Joachim Schmitt

Voluntarily controlled skeletal muscle represents the biggest organ complex of the human body, in terms of total volume. It is accepted that it has a high clinical relevance to mTrP, and this is partially confirmed in the literature.

The pathophysiological details of trigger points are described in Chapter 6. In summary, the underlying integrated trigger point hypothesis assumes that there is an energy crisis in the muscle, the muscle fibres or the sarcomere in each case. An increase in calcium outside the sarcoplasmic reticulum (possibly as a result of a muscle lesion or due to a biochemical or electrophysiological cause) produces increased contractility. The process is maintained by a dysfunctional nerve ending with continued release of acetylcholine (possibly sympathetically provided). The permanent contraction produces local ischaemia and hypoxia as a result of vascular compression in the muscle caused by increased energy requirements. The release of neuroactive substances irritates the sensory and autonomic nerve endings and nociceptors (see Fig. 6.5).

This is the reason for tenderness on palpation, referred pain, the twitch response and malfunction, as well as for disorders of autonomic function (e.g. skin temperature, sweat secretion). This leads to advanced mechanical, biochemical and/or electrophysiological irritation of neighbouring muscle fibres and their sarcomeres (a chain reaction), so that the symptoms become chronic. Persistent strain factors favour the perpetuation of this process (Fig. 4.1).

The causative factors are extremely varied. For the sake of simplification, we try in the following to differentiate between acute and delayed myofascial pain.

Even if there is a single cause, psychosocial factors must always be included in the assessment, particularly when it comes to the development of chronic myofascial symptoms. These must be recognised promptly, as they can represent a hindrance to treatment.

4.1.1 Causative factors of acute myofascial pain

Blunt muscle trauma (contusion)

- Hit or bump as may occur in sport, on a door frame or on the corner of a table.
- Fall (the muscles absorb the bump, but if they fail, e.g. in the elderly, there is an increased risk of hip fracture at the neck of the femur).
- Pressure, as may be caused by a wallet kept in a trouser pocket, or clothes that are too tight (e.g. wearing a bra).
- Interstitial increase in pressure (oedema/haematoma).

Pulled muscle (usually eccentric muscle strain)

- Sudden stop in movement ('stop and go' – sports like tennis, volleyball, badminton, etc.) or interruption of movement, e.g. opponent grasping the throwing arm.
- Rapid overextension of the muscles when lifting heavy loads, unaccustomed lever strain (e.g. when moving house), reaching out suddenly after a fall or when catching an object.
- Long-term persistent incorrect posture, e.g. working in a kitchen.

http://dx.doi.org/10.1016/B978-0-7020-4312-3.00004-0

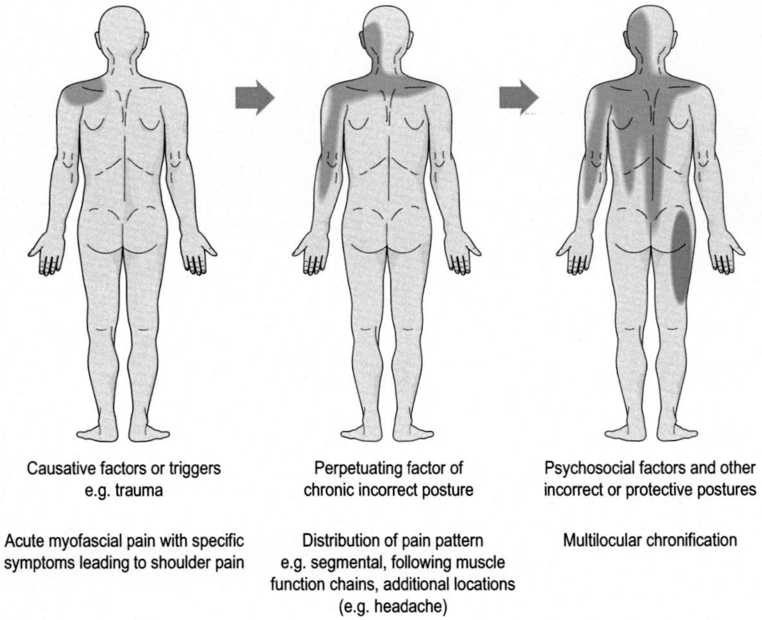

Fig. 4.1 Causative and perpetuating factors for myofascial pain.

Causative factors or triggers e.g. trauma

Perpetuating factor of chronic incorrect posture

Psychosocial factors and other incorrect or protective postures

Acute myofascial pain with specific symptoms leading to shoulder pain

Distribution of pain pattern e.g. segmental, following muscle function chains, additional locations (e.g. headache)

Multilocular chronification

Torn muscles (complete or incomplete, usually caused by eccentric muscle strain)

- Sudden increase in muscle tension, e.g. sport and exercise without warming up. Uncoordinated stress, stress that exceeds the flexibility or stamina of the muscles involved such as at the end of training or the competitive phase.
- Trauma caused by crushed muscle and subsequent necrosis, or cutting injury or fracture and tear.

Sprain or dislocation of joints

- As a result of wrenching, e.g. of the arm when fixing an object against the power of a machine (e.g. when using a drill, saw, grinder, etc.), or of the leg when skiing (rotation with a long lever).
- As a result of wrenching of segments of the vertebral column, such as from rear-end automobile collisions (first or second degree) or riding on a carousel, bumper car, etc.
- By straining the capsular ligaments, e.g. at the knee or ankle, playing football (straddle position) or going over on the ankle on the kerb of the pavement.

Increased isometric muscle contractions

- When carrying bags on the wrist with the joint in a slightly extended or volar position (strain of the extensors or flexors).
- When carrying bags over the shoulder (shoulder elevation).

- When holding sports equipment (tennis racquet), writing equipment (ballpoint pen).
- When using a computer keyboard or mouse.
- When sitting, e.g. in the neck or the lumbar or thoracic spine.

Shortening of the muscles

- As a result of posture, e.g. knee roll, pillow, etc.
- As a result of being in the same position for a long time, e.g. sitting position (breakfast, car, bus, train, office work, seated hobby), lying down as a result of a requirement for bed rest (after an operation, serious infectious disease, etc.).
- Poor posture with muscular imbalance (head and shoulder protraction, lateral deviation of the vertebral column, hunched back, hyperlordosis, etc.).
- As a result of functional disorders of the joints (iliosacral joint, blockades at segments of the vertebral column).
- As a result of poor posture or deformity such as different leg lengths (relative or absolute), scoliosis of the vertebral column, deformity of the arch of the foot (spread foot or flat foot).

Increase in muscle tension caused by climate

- In cold weather.
- In a draught.
- When it is hot.

Change in muscle tension of psychogenic cause

- During stress caused by sympathetic effects.
- With anxiety and tension in reaction to the expectation of the event.
- Anger and annoyance without the required offloading of emotion.
- Depressive mood with loss of muscle tension and strain.

Slight muscular strain due to prior conditions

- Type 1 diabetes or hypoglycaemia.
- With hypothyroidism.
- With asthma and high tension in the accessory respiratory muscles (pectoral girdle, neck, chest).
- Myopathy and myositis.
- Neuromuscular diseases (hemiplegia, entrapment of peripheral nerves, nerve root compression in the region supplied by the nerve).
- Vascular diseases.
- Vitamin deficiencies (B, C).
- Reduced physical condition.

4.1.2 Causative factors of delayed myofascial pain

Chronic strain

- Continued use of the muscles on one side.
- Too many demands made on the muscle.
- Being forced into an awkward position.
- Advanced functional disorders (blockade of segments of vertebral column).
- Lack of coordination/poor exercise technique.
- Poor posture.
- Deformity of vertebral column or joints.
- Irritation of the roots of peripheral nerves.
- Entrapment of peripheral nerves.

Psychogenic factors

- Depression.
- Anxiety.
- Stress.

4.2 PERPETUATING FACTORS OF MYOFASCIAL PAIN

Hans-Joachim Schmitt

Some of the causative factors can also become perpetuating or maintaining factors for myofascial pain. However, factors from other medical areas can also play a role here. Even if some of these factors cannot be eliminated as the cause, it is always sensible to treat myofascial pain to achieve at least short- or medium-term pain relief. Perpetuating factors can be:

- poor posture or deformity or incorrect position (segments of the vertebral column) of the skeletal system or the locomotor apparatus,
- constant functional disorders of the locomotor apparatus,
- poor diet (alcohol, minerals, vitamins, smoking),
- anaemia and hypoxia affecting the muscles (hyperuricaemia, hypoglycaemia, thyroid disorders),
- underlying medical, urological or gynaecological diseases via the reflex arcs,
- sleep disorders, irritations caused by lifestyle (stress, relaxation),
- psychogenic factors such as inability to express one's own feelings, stress, depression, anger/annoyance, lack of challenge and anxiety.

4.3 CHRONIFICATION OF MYOFASCIAL PAIN

Dominik Irnich

The route to pain becoming chronic is a complex event, which may be different in each individual case, and depends on various physical, psychological and social factors. At the same time, the pain itself also has an effect on the patient's coping strategies.

Among the biological factors are peripheral and central sensitising mechanisms. These can lead to neurogenic inflammatory self-perpetuating cascades, neuronal reconstruction processes and the expression of transcription factor genes with resulting new receptors and ion channels (neuronal plasticity) at the level of the spinal cord and changed neuronal pain processing in the brain. An insufficient pain defence system, as well as genetic factors, seems to have an influence on chronification.

Dysfunctional coping strategies are among the psychological chronification factors. These include a lack of internal conviction, feelings of helplessness and impending catastrophe, excessive protective and avoidance behaviour, or rigidly carrying on without considering the personal stress. Other factors are an excessive amount of primary, secondary or tertiary illness, conditioning, learning, and inadequately dealing with feelings and psychological tension. Poor processing of stress and an increased likelihood of psychological or physiological reactions can also play a part in an illness becoming chronic.

Social factors should in no way be underestimated: these can include stress or dissatisfaction at work, bullying, the negative influence of long-term proceedings for damage claims, surveys and reports, retirement, family conflict, social isolation, low level of education, a feeling of insufficient recompense for performance, including a lack of recognition, and elements in the health system that can promote illness. With many chronic pain diseases there is also a poor quality of life or a lack of a life plan and this may be an expression of only a simple spirituality.

All these factors can pave the way to chronic pain disease, depending on their significance for the individual or the extent of their development. A muscle is a highly sensitive, innervated organ and is a potential target for attack by all these factors of influence. Myofascial pain based on a relevant mTrP as the physical bearer or biological basis of the pain can easily be sufficient to maintain the most severe chronic pain.

This knowledge is largely scientific and can produce a definite indication for therapy: treatment should be supportive at all levels, including the way a person feels inside. If this does not happen, there will be no reduction in the huge number of chronic pain diseases.

Chapter | 5 |

The anatomy and physiology of the muscles

Joseph F. Audette, Jay P. Shah

5.1 MACROSCOPIC STRUCTURE

5.1.1 Development

The embryonic origin of the transverse skeletal muscles is in the mesoderm. The muscles of the scalp and eyes originate in the ectoderm of the branchial arches. Myofibrils arise from the fusion of individual myoblasts (muscle stem cells). Muscle fibres arise from the bundling of these myofibrils.

The first muscle movements by the fetus take place between the 14th and 16th weeks of pregnancy. Postnatal growth of the muscles is enabled by hypertrophy and lengthening of the fibres.

5.1.2 Structure and fine structure

Muscle fibres: the length of the muscle fibres can be up to 40 cm, although they are usually shorter than 10 cm. Each muscle fibre is surrounded by an endomysium, a delicate membrane of connective tissue. Muscle fibre bundles are enclosed by more connective tissue septa, the perimysium, and divided into fascicles (fibre bundles). The external muscle cover is again formed from thick connective tissue: the epimysium (muscle sheath) forms the outer fascia.

The muscle fibres are arranged as follows:

- Fusiform (spindle-shaped): these have a parallel arrangement of fibres from the origin to the insertion.
- Pennate: fibres attach diagonally to the tendon, either on one side of the muscle or along the centre of the muscle belly (majority of muscles).
- Fan-shaped: the fibres are arranged in the shape of a fan.

Contraction of the muscle fibres within the tube-shaped fascia occurs without movement of the neighbouring structures or skin. The vascular and nerve supply lies within the muscular connective tissue fascia. The blood vessels form a thick capillary network around each muscle fibre running parallel to the surface of the fibre.

Fascicles: fascicles are bundles of muscle fibre surrounded by connective tissue. They consist of 10^2–10^3 myofibrils and reach a diameter of 10–100 μm.

Myofibrils: myofibrils are the contractile units of the muscle fibres. They are created by the fusion of myoblasts and consist of chains of sarcomeres. The length of a sarcomere is about 1.5–2.2 μm. These sarcomeres comprise more than 1500 thick myosin and 3000 thin actin filaments. The interconnection of these filaments gives rise to the characteristic transverse striation of the myofibrils. The individual myofibrils are surrounded by sarcoplasm. This contains important components for contraction processes and providing energy: the sarcoplasmic reticulum, T-tubuli and mitochondria.

Myosin or thick filaments: the diameter of a myosin filament is about 11–12 nm. The filaments consist of 200–300 individual myosin molecules. These are extremely heavy (molecular weight approximately 500 000 Da) hexamer molecules in the form of a thin rod. Proteolytic splitting then separates the myosin into its two fragments, light meromyosin and heavy meromyosin. Two heavy peptide chains pass into the shaft in the form of a double helix and end in spherical heads where ATPase activity is bound. There is also a binding site for actin. The light chains form the biggest part of the molecule shaft. The myosin molecules associate parallel to each other in several hundreds and lie in bundles. The molecules are arranged so that the myosin heads project out sideways.

http://dx.doi.org/10.1016/B978-0-7020-4312-3.00005-2

Actin or thin filaments: G-actin monomers polymerise into double helices and form polymeric F-actin filaments. Each actin monomer has a precise binding site for myosin. G-actin is also joined to an ADP molecule. Precisely seven actin monomers are each wound around long tropomyosin molecules. Along all seven monomers a globular troponin molecule is arranged for the tropomyosin, the molecules of which consist of three subunits (T, I and C). They predominantly regulate the interactions of actin and myosin.

Connection: in the sarcomeres, the actin filaments bind to so-called Z-plates/layers. The meshing together of actin and myosin molecules leads to the characteristic striation of the sarcomeres:

- the A-striation is formed by the myosin filaments arranged in parallel,
- the Z-striation is the linking zone of the actin filaments,
- the H-striation is the area in the middle of the A-striation, which consists only of myosin filaments; right in the middle it is therefore also called M-striation,
- The I-striation consists of actin filaments and borders on the Z-striation.

The arrangement of the striation in the sarcomere always takes place in the sequence Z-I-A-H-A-I-Z.

5.2 FUNCTION

5.2.1 Muscle contraction

Course of muscle contraction

Action potentials reach the motor end plates of the α-motoneuron of an individual fibre. This opens Ca^{2+} channels which are sensitive to tension. Acetylcholine (ACh) is released from vesicles in the synaptic cleft (approximately 10 000 ACh molecules per vesicle = 1 quantum). In the resting condition, the spontaneous release of small quantities of ACh takes place continuously. This leads to a miniature end-plate potential (or MEPP), which is not associated with a muscle contraction.

One hundred to 200 ACh quanta lead to the release of the end-plate potential (or EPP). The 'all or nothing' rule applies: exceeding a specific stimulus threshold always causes a strong individual twitch. The binding of ACh to the muscle membrane receptor leads to the opening of Na^+ channels and depolarisation of the muscle cells. The action potential spreads throughout the muscle. Released ACh is very quickly deactivated again by acetylcholinesterases in the synaptic cleft. The resulting choline is then taken up by the presynaptic nerve ending and resynthesised to ACh.

The postsynaptic EPP leads to opening of the intracellular Ca^{2+} channels in the sarcoplasmic reticulum. In 1–2 ms more than 250 nmol of Ca^{2+} is released per gram of muscle. The increase in Ca^{2+} concentration leads to a conformational change in the tropomyosin with release of myosin-binding sites on the actin molecule, which in low-calcium conditions are blocked by tropomyosin. The myosin heads then bind to the actin fibres in a rudder-like movement. This head movement leads to a shift of the actin in relation to the myosin filament by about 2 nm (see Fig. 6.1), which corresponds to 1% of the length of the sarcomere.

With isotonic contraction, the thin (actin) and thick (myosin) filaments slide together with each other (Huxley's sliding filament theory); with isometric contraction the same interaction sites keep reacting between myosin heads and actin filament.

Ca^{2+} ions are pumped back again into the sarcoplasmic reticulum by means of a calcium pump. When the intracellular Ca^{2+} concentration drops to about 10^{-7} mol/l a myosin-associated ATPase is activated in the absence of Mg^{2+}. The ATPase splits the energy-rich ATP and the energy released is used to separate the myosin heads from the actin again.

The complete muscle contraction is achieved by many successive actin–myosin binding processes and dissolutions (approximately 10–100 per second) through the consumption of ATP.

ATP sources for muscle contraction include the following.

- A creatinine kinase (or CK) bound to the myofilaments continuously rephosphorylates the ADP molecules formed by the actin–myosin binding to ATP. This aims for a high ATP/ADP ratio in the muscle.
- Anaerobic glycolysis (Embden–Meyerhof pathway) produces pyruvic acid and ATP: glucose + 2 ADP + 2 P → 2 pyruvic acid + 2 ATP. This energy is made available 2.5 times faster than by the aerobic route.
- Energy preparation is carried out in aerobic glycolysis in the citrate cycle: 36 ATPs are gained by oxidation of glucose. Myoglobin has an important role. It stores oxygen and speeds up the diffusion of energy into the muscles.
- Glycogen degradation is an abundant source of energy for continuous contraction. Glycogen is the first energy source during muscle contraction. Under anaerobic conditions, glycogen catabolism ends with the formation of lactic acid (lactate). The ratio of aerobic to anaerobic energy production is 12:1.

The contraction ends when the Ca^{2+} concentration falls to normal values as a result of an ATP-dependent pump which brings the Ca^{2+} back into the sarcoplasmic reticulum. Continuous tension is maintained by a small quantity of myosin heads that remain in contact with the actin filaments. The rigor mortis that follows death is caused by an absence of ATP, which means that all of the available actin–myosin bonds remain.

Muscle fibre types (see Fig. 5.1)

- **Type I fibres ('red fibres')** are rich in myoglobin. Functionally, they are capable of persistent contractile activity. On activation there is a slow twitch of 75 ms duration (slow-twitch fibres). The high level of oxidative enzymes, low level of phosphorylases, small amount of glycogen storage and capacity for resistance to tiredness are remarkable. Type I fibres are numerous in postural muscles.
- **Type IIB fibres ('white fibres')** contain less myoglobin than type I fibres. Functionally they are designed for rapid contractions. On activation there is a fast twitch of 25 ms duration (fast-twitch glycolytic fibres). Type II fibres are rich in phosphorylase and glycogen. The very high number of mitochondria is histologically remarkable. As glycolysis is the main route for energy production, they tend to get tired quickly. They participate in short, fast movements.
- **Type IIA fibres (mixed type)** favour aerobic oxidative energy metabolism as well as glycolysis (fast-twitch oxidative glycolytic); they possess a moderate resistance to tiredness.

Very intensive interval training increases type I fibres and reduces type IIB fibres.

Types of muscle contraction

- Concentric contraction by muscle shortening with an increase in strength (e.g. activity of the quadriceps while playing football).

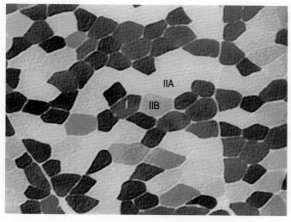

Fig. 5.1 Muscle fibre types. Microscopic uptake of the M. vastus medialis lateralis, using an indicator for ATPase at pH 4.6. Type I or red fibres are rich in myoglobin and tire slowly. Type IIB or white fibres are rich in phosphorylases and glycogen and tire quickly. Type IIA fibres are an intermediate form, between type I and type IIB fibres. (From Liebermann et al. 1994)

- Eccentric contraction by muscle extension with an increase in strength (e.g. activity of the quadriceps while landing after a jump).
- Isometric contraction without changing the length with an increase in power (e.g. activity of the quadriceps while crouching for a long time).
- Isotonic contraction with changes of length without a change in power (bicycle ergometry test of the quadriceps with constant resistance from the pedals).

5.2.2 Muscle healing after injury

Types of injury

- Cutting injury: the fibres and covering fascia of the muscle rupture as a result of direct trauma or tear.
- Closed injury: only the fibres are damaged; this injury frequently occurs after repeated eccentric strain or after injection of LA.

Muscle regeneration after injury

Muscle regeneration after injury occurs:

- inconsistently as a result of the formation of new fibres,
- continuously as a result of repair and regeneration processes on available fibres.

Satellite small mononuclear cells with myogenic potential, which lie under the basal layers that surround the muscle fibres, are activated in response to an injury. An intact basal layer is a prerequisite for this. If this is not the case, the damaged region is replaced by connective tissue and a scar forms. The satellite cells proliferate and later fuse to so-called myotubes. The concentration of satellite cells is elevated in type I muscles. Their concentration is lower in older people. Their concentration remains the same, even after repeated injury.

The recovery phases are as follows.

- **Non-inflammatory degenerative phase:** the Z-layers react most sensitively to injury caused by exercise. Autolysis occurs as a result of the interruption of Ca^{2+} homeostasis. The first regeneraton processes have been observed 4–8 h after injury.
- **Inflammatory degenerative phase:** start of phagocytosis due to immigrating macrophages. These eliminate damaged fibre residues. Introduced by increased proteolysis of the extracellular matrix, an increase in neutrophil concentration takes place within 1–6 h. Collagenase is thus secreted by fibroblasts as an important proteolytic enzyme. Other inflammatory cells secrete cytokines and growth factors. The administration of non-steroidal anti-inflammatory drugs (NSAIDs) affects the repair processes in the damaged muscles.
- **Regenerative phase:** takes place quicker with closed injuries. It begins with the activation of the satellite cells if the basal lamina are intact. Growth factors originating from fibroblasts and blood platelets are involved.

- **Maturation phase:** the differentiation of the satellite cells is stimulated by somatomedin (insulin-like growth factor (IGF) I). Gene expression is altered in the meantime by the fusion of the cells so that formation of muscle-specific proteins begins. Myogenesis goes through the stages of embryonic development. Fast-twitch filaments are formed from undifferentiated embryonic myosin filaments. Slow-twitch myosin is produced from innervation that leads to slow-twitch muscle; creatinine kinase activity also increases.

Hypothyroidism inhibits the formation of fast-twitch myosin filaments from undifferentiated myosin. Reduced mechanical loading of the muscle also decreases regeneration.

5.2.3 Consequences of reduced muscle training

Muscle fibre distribution

- Ending stamina training leads to a shift from IIA to IIB fibres.
- Ending strength training leads to an increase in type I fibres.

Muscle diameter

- Stopping short-term training causes a reduction in muscle diameter, which is mainly due to a reduction in the diameter of IIA fibres. This results mostly in a loss of muscle strength compared to stamina.
- A long-term pause of training in athletes causes a reduction in the diameter of fast- and slow-twitch fibres. There is also a reduction in the ratio of fast- to slow-twitch fibres.
- Stopping training decreases enzyme activity in athletes: reduction in oxygen capacity by 30–40%, daily loss of aerobic capacity (VO_{2max}) of 0.9%.
- Decrease in muscle strength as a result of immobilisation. Loss of 25–50% muscle strength can occur with an immobilisation of 3–8 weeks. The muscle diameter decreases by about 20%. This leads to a reduction in the rest frequency of the motor neurons. Motor areas in the cerebral cortex are reorganised. A reduction in the size of the areas associated with muscle activity takes place.

5.3 NEUROPHYSIOLOGY

5.3.1 Motor function

It is predominantly the distal muscle groups responsible for fine motor control that define voluntary motor function. The control of voluntary motor function is carried out via the pyramidal tract system, the direct connection between the pyramidal cells in the motor cortex (upper motoneurons) and the α-motoneurons in the cerebral cortex and the spinal cord (lower motoneurons).

The support motor function is responsible for phylogenetically older movements rather than voluntary motor function. This includes the upright posture of the body, movement processes (e.g. walking, sitting, chewing) and learned automatic movements. These are predominantly carried out by the skeletal and axial muscles. Involuntary (reflex) processes play a main part in this. This is why support motor functions are also described as reflex motor functions. Control of this system is also carried out in the motor cortex, by subcortical structures and by the cerebral cortex. Switching is carried out by multi-limbed chains that descend into the spinal cord.

5.3.2 The lower motoneurons

The common destination of all motor function tracts are the lower motoneurons. This is the terms for all the neurons whose axons leave the spinal cord to innervate the muscles. Control of these motoneurons is segmental and vertical in exhibition as well as inhibition:

- α-motoneurons innervate the work muscles (extrafusal fibres),
- γ-motoneurons innervate the muscle spindles (intrafusal fibres),
- Renshaw cells are inhibitory interneurons which are activated by recurrent collaterals of axons from the α-motoneurons. Their task is self-limitation of the activity of the α-motoneurons.

5.3.3 Muscle afference

Group I fibres: large medullary fibres (Aα-fibres); Ia fibres lead afferences from muscle spindles, Ib fibres create the connection to the Golgi tendon receptors.
Group II fibres: medium-sized medullary fibres (Aβ-fibres); secondary muscle spindle endings and Pacini bodies run through these.
Group III fibres: thin medullary fibres; analogous to the Aδ-fibres of the skin (conduction of warmth, cold, pain). They conduct afferences of free nerve endings and Pacini bodies.
Group IV fibres: thin non-medullary fibres; analogous to the C-fibres of the skin (pain fibres). Afferent connections of free nerve endings are passed on (see Fig. 5.2, Fig. 5.3).

5.3.4 Neuromuscular synapses

The neuromuscular synapse is a 50 nm cleft between a nerve ending and a muscle.

Presynaptic ending: the axon endings have a high number of mitochondria. In high concentrations, the synaptic blisters that appear contain not only ACh but also calcitonin gene-related peptide (CGRP), nitric oxide (NO),

Fig. 5.2 Nerve fibre types. Aα- and β-fibres or group-I and -II fibres contain bone marrow and supply the muscle spindles and tendons, Aδ-fibres or group-III fibres are thin fibres containing bone marrow; C-fibres or group-IV fibres do not contain marrow.

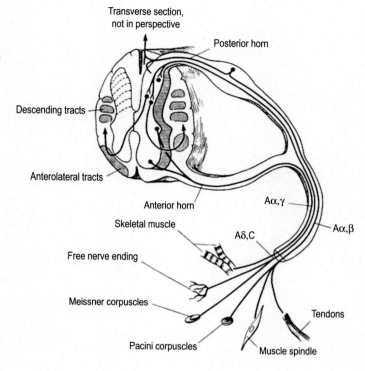

Fig. 5.3 Muscle innervation. Diagram of the nerve supply of a muscle (supply area in brackets) with group Ia fibres (muscle spindles), group Ib fibres (Golgi apparatus), group II fibres (spindles and Pacini bodies), group III fibres (Pacini bodies and free nerve endings) and group IV fibres (free nerve endings). The free nerve endings are embedded in the fascia bordering the vessels.

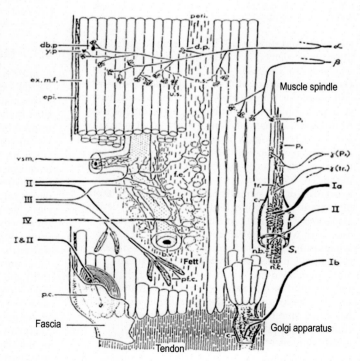

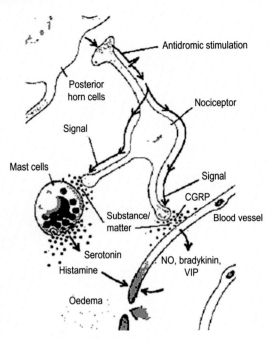

Fig. 5.4 The neurosecretory function of the group IV or nociceptor fibres can lead to a cascade of events which cause neurogenic inflammation. SP and CGRP can lead to vasodilation and the distribution of histamine and serotonin from the mast cells, and bradykinin, NO and vasoactive intestinal polypeptide (VIP) from the endothelium, with an effect on the nociceptor and consecutive peripheral sensitisation.

adenosine and substance P (SP). The release of ACh into the synaptic cleft is Ca^{2+}-dependent and is dynamically regulated (see Fig. 5.4).

Dynamic regulation of the Ca^{2+} channels at the motor end plate: this is influenced by the sympathetic nervous system. Stimulation of α-adrenergic receptors increases ACh release, and stimulation of β-adrenergic receptors reduces ACh release. Depending on the type of activated adenosine receptor, adenosine can inhibit or strengthen the release of ACh (by reducing or increasing the activity of the Ca^{2+} channels).

Exocytosis of the synaptic blisters on the presynaptic membrane: this requires a number of proteins: vesicle-associated membrane protein (VAMP), the protein associated with the presynaptic membrane (25 kDa synaptosome associated protein, SNAP 25), syntaxin, synaptobrevin (associated with VAMP), neurexin and synaptotagmin.

Postsynaptic membrane: there is a strongly invaginated sarcolemma for enlarging the postsynaptic surface, which has a high number of ACh receptors. In the immediate surrounding area is the ACh-degrading acetylcholinesterase.

Factors that influence the excitability of the postsynaptic membrane are described below.

- CGRP improves the contraction of the transversely striated muscle as well as the spontaneous release of ACh from the neuromuscular end plate; the synthesis of ACh receptors at the neuromuscular synapse is increased and the acetylcholinesterase is regulated to a low level.
- Postsynaptic recoupling following presynaptic ACh release: there is a link mechanism from the muscle cells back to the nerve endings. With increased Ca^{2+} release from the sarcoplasmic reticulum the inflow of Ca^{2+} in the tension-dependent Ca^{2+} channels of the nerve ending is inhibited. This leads to a reduction in ACh release from the presynaptic blisters.
- Ca^{2+} release from the sarcoplasmic reticulum is autonomically regulated. $β_2$-Adrenoceptors make Ca^{2+} release from the sarcoplasmic reticulum easier by activation of so-called ryanodine receptors (as shown in rats). Cyclic AMP (cAMP) is another sympathetically mediated messenger material which makes it easier for Ca^{2+} release from the sarcoplasmic reticulum (without causing motor action potentials, without changing the neuronal Na^+/K^+ concentration).

CLINICAL SIGNIFICANCE

These factors strengthen the contraction of muscle fibres (without an action potential at the motor unit) and may contribute to the formation of tension, the most common characteristic of trigger points and myofascial pain.

5.3.5 Muscle spindles

A muscle spindle is a fusiform end organ arranged in parallel between the fibres of skeletal muscle, and which acts as a mechanoreceptor. They can be found in high densities in the muscle fibres and act as receptors for impulses responsible for stretching, which means that they control fine motor function and body posture.

Sheath structure: the muscle spindle measures the length of the muscle and controls the length via the so-called stretch/extension reflex. It consists of muscle fibres which are contractile only at the end pieces (infrafusal muscles). The non-contractile middle piece represents a receptor sensitive to stretching and extension. Intrafusal muscle fibres are ensheathed in a parallel manner by extrafusal fibres (the surrounding working muscles). The intrafusal fibres are very elastic. They are divided into nuclear bag (NB) and nuclear chain (NC) fibres. The NC fibre group guides the information on the absolute length of the muscle to the central nervous system (CNS), while the NB fibre group provides information on the speed of extension.

Primary (Ia) and secondary (II) afferent nerve endings end in the central part of the spindle. The afferent fibres are sensitive to extension. The contractile muscle spindle poles are innervated by γ-motoneurons. Contractions change the impulse loading rate or the sensitivity of the central afferent fibres.

Function: during activation of the muscle spindles by muscle extension, the impulse loading rate of the tendon organs does not increase. With muscle contraction, the impulse loading rate of the muscle spindles drops and the loading rate of the tendon organs increases.

The α- and γ-motorneurons are activated simultaneously during voluntary movements. This is described as α–γ-co-activation or as α–γ-bonding. γ-Activation maintains the extension in the spindle. The impulse loading rate of the muscle spindle is maintained during the muscle contraction. This enables recording of small changes in length during contraction.

A delayed nociceptive (painful) influence on the muscle reduces the γ-activation and the motor activity and slightly increases the motor activity of the antagonists. This may lead to persistent spasm, but the exact mechanism is unclear. A delayed nociceptive influence from the joints and connective tissue increases the γ-activation, increases motor activity and lowers the activity again over time. The activation of mechanoreceptors in joint swelling causes inhibition of the motor activity.

Static γ-motoneurons increase the loading rate of the afferences during static extension and are active during slow planned movement.

Dynamic γ-motoneurons increase the loading rate of afferences during dynamic extension. They increase the muscle response during rapid changes of length and are active during rapid involuntary movements.

In the extension reflex, Ia afferent fibres respond to sudden extension. Monosynaptic bondings exist with all α-motoneurons of the muscle, and Ia collateral fibres activate synergistic muscles less strongly and also activate inhibitory interneurons which affect the antagonistic muscles. Reflex activation is made possible facilitiation.

CLINICAL SIGNIFICANCE: CINDERELLA HYPOTHESIS

Muscle power during submaximum loading uses only part of the available motor units. These motor units (predominantly small type I fibres) are called Cinderella fibres because they are continuously overloaded actively and metabolically while surrounding fibres remain inactive and are not included. This leads to local muscle pain and tension. Less strenuous activities lead to the inclusion of the muscle while using the same motor-unit stereotype patterns.

Hypothesis: even small efforts, such as computer work, can lead to chronic overloading of exclusively Cinderella fibres and may be susceptible to injury. This is substantiated by a higher percentage of damaged red fibres ('moth-eaten fibres'). As an indicator of muscle membrane damage there is an increase in intracellular Ca^{2+} release and a loss of muscular lactate dehydrogenase.

5.3.6 Low-threshold mechanoreceptors

The low-threshold mechanosensitive fibres represent a subgroup of group III and IV fibres. They respond to active muscle contractions and there is a linear relationship between muscle strength and discharge rate. They allow indirectly systemic circulatory responses to muscle activity. Activation by acupuncture needles, for example, can cause similar responses.

5.3.7 Nociceptors of group III and IV fibres

Analysis of the structure of the locomotor nerves of the gastrocnemius muscle in cats revealed 67% non-myelinised and 33% myelinised fibres; 25% of the myelinised fibres and 43% of the non-myelinised fibres were nociceptive.

Morphology: the nerve endings lie in the adventitia of arterioles, sheathed in Schwann cells. In small blank areas between the Schwann cells the endings lie in direct contact with the interstitial fluid. At these exposed sites there is a high density of specific receptors and a high frequency of neurotransmitter blisters.

Physiology: the stimulation threshold is well under that which causes tissue damage, so a warning is provided about approaching tissue damage. There is no stimulation response to physiological stretching and contraction processes. There is usually a response to damaging pressure or chemical stimuli. This limits the spatial termination of nociception (pain perception), which lies in the distribution of the afferences in different axons for muscle, joints and skin.

The nociceptors of the muscle can be sensitised and/or activated and receptor-mediated by a number of algesic substances: by bradykinin (or BK), which occurs as a result of splitting from the plasma protein kallidin; by serotonin (5-hydroxytryptamine, 5-HT), which is released from platelets; by an increased concentration of H^+ or a reduction in pH value; by an increase in K^+ concentration; a distribution of prostaglandins from endothelial cells; by ATP from damaged muscle cells; by interleukin 6 (IL 6), which is formed from myocytes; and by nerve growth factor (NGF).

Neurosecretory function: secretion of neuropeptides, SP (the SP concentration is lower than in the skin, the SP concentration in red fibres is higher than in white ones; SP leads to the release of histamine from mast cells), CGRP (CGRP influences ACh receptor synthesis at the end plate, an increase in vessel permeability is under debate, thus a countereffect on the vasoconstrictor effect of the sympathic fibres is conceivable) and somatostatin (SRIH) (see Fig. 5.4).

Neurogenic inflammation: distribution of SP, CGRP and SRIH at the nociceptor leads to a release of bradykinin from the blood plasma, 5-HT from the platelets, prostaglandin (including prostaglandin E_2, or PGE_2) from the endothelial cells and tumour necrosis factor (TNF-α) and interleukin 1β (IL 1β) from activated macrophages (see Fig. 5.4).

Sensitised peripheral nociceptors: the threshold for mechanical stimulation is lower; bradykinin, 5-HT and prostaglandin lead to increased sensitivity of the nociceptors. This leads to potentiation of bradykinin through serotonin or PGE_2. A higher ion flow is made possible by a change in the conformation of the Na^+ channels. The absence of prostaglandin causes a phosphorylation cascade which leads to a change in conformation. This results in a change in the bradykinin receptor from B2 to B1, the density of Na^+ channels increases and new Na^+ channels with shortened refractory time are formed.

Clinical signs: mechanical allodynia or increased stimulation response with low stimulation thresholds, hyperalgesia or high-frequency irritation response to noxious substances.

5.3.8 The spinal cord

The spinal cord (or the medulla spinalis) is part of the CNS from where the extremities, the trunk and a large part of the neck are supplied via the spinal nerves. In adults it extends from the exit point of the first spinal nerve to the level of the first or second lumbar vertebral body. From there it exits into the conus medullaris and continues as fibrous glial tissue (filum terminale) into the sacral canal.

The spinal cord is linked to each section of the vertebral column and is named according to the on the exiting spinal nerves: cervical, thoracic, lumbar, sacral and coccygeal cord.

As it grows more slowly than the vertebral canal, the position of each section of the spinal cord is not at the level of the vertebral body. This means that the nerve roots that leave the spinal cord must first run downwards before they leave the relevant intervertebral foramina. From L1 this causes a bundle of nerve fibres known as the cauda equina.

In cross-section, the spinal cord is divided into grey and white parts (matter).

Grey matter

Grey matter typically has a butterfly-shaped configuration. The wider part of the butterfly's wing is at the front and the narrower part at the back. The anterior part is known as the anterior horn and is responsible for motor function. The posterior part, the posterior horn, receives sensory information. In accordance with this division the anterior motor function roots arise from the anterior horn and the posterior sensory roots from the posterior horn. These nerve roots unite at a segmental level to the relevant spinal nerves.

Histologically, the grey matter can be divided into differently constructed cell layers (laminae) which are numbered I–X dorsal to ventral.

White matter

The white matter is divided into the anterior cord (between the anterior horns of the grey matter), the lateral cord (between the anterior and posterior horns) and the posterior cord (between the posterior horns). Both the anterior and posterior cords are separated into two halves by a fissure anterior or posterior to the spinal cord. This division does not have any functional assignment: in the cords both motor function and sensory tracts run up and down. In front of the grey matter remains a narrow seam (commissura alba anterior and posterior), in which criss-crossing tracts pass from one half to the other.

5.3.9 Posterior horn

Fibres that lead sensitive afferences from the periphery end in the posterior horn. From there they proceed to the thalamus and are projected further into the cerebrum. Almost all afferences are switched from the first neuron to a second neuron in the posterior horn; the third neuron is usually in the thalamus.

Histologically, the posterior horn is constructed from laminae I–VI, in which lie important nerve nuclei:

- **dorsal nucleus (Stilling Clarke):** the most anterior in laminae V–VI of the thoracolumbar cord. It receives predominantly proprioceptive afferences from muscle spindles, joint and tendon receptors (so-called deep sensitivity);
- **nucleus proprius:** more or less in the middle of the posterior horn. Besides impulses of deep sensitivity, it also receives afferences from the skin;
- **substantia gelatinosa:** functionally a very important key complex of laminae II–III, which contain proprioceptive and exteroceptive afferences. These run over the tractus spinothalamicus to the thalamus.

It is very significant that the synaptic switches in these key regions can be influenced by the brain. The key areas of the rhombencephalon (hindbrain) project into the posterior horn and inhibit the pain impulse transfer with the serotonin and noradrenaline (norepinephrine) transmitters. Endorphinergic interim neurons play an important part in this. These also receive afferences from somatosensitive cutaneous fibres and can thus inhibit pain continuation into the brain. This mechanism is known as the 'gate control theory' of pain referral.

5.3.10 Activation of the posterior horn

The first synapses of the muscle afferences are in laminae I, IV or V. There, the muscle afference is switched to the second neuron. Second-order neurons rarely respond only to muscle afferences. Activation of specific brain regions (anterior gyrus cinguli) takes place; this area is involved in the emotional, affective components of pain.

Principle of convergence: wide dynamic range (WDR) neurons

Most second-order neurons activated by muscles are known as WDR neurons and receive convergent signals from the skin, the joints and the viscera.

By contrast, nociceptors of the skin are more commonly synaptically associated with skin-specific second-order neurons. The output of WDR neurons depends on the intensity of the stimulation.

Clinical signs: this convergence of various stimuli leads to poor localisation of muscle pain. Convergences can cause cutaneous hypoaesthesia or hyperaesthesia associated with muscle pain. Articular or visceral dysfunction or inflammation can be expressed as muscle pain.

Principle of divergence

The persistent high-frequency afferent input to WDR neurons leads to activation of 'sleeping' synapses. Superior and inferior branches extend for seven to eight segments. Partial opening of these synapses is produced by SP and CGRP release. Involvement of activated glial cells has been debated. This leads to release of proteinases and cytokines. The threshold for pain and stretching reflexes is reduced. Nerve nuclei on the other side of the midline of the spinal cord are involved in continuing the stimulation.

This enlarges the receptive field (or RF) so second-order neurons can now be stimulated by previously ineffective afferent associations of the skin, muscles, joints and viscera, which lie far from the place of origin. Places far from the injured tissue can demonstrate an excessive response to weak stimuli.

Clinical signs: a multisegmental relationship pattern develops. Development no longer follows cutaneous segmental innervation. The relationship pattern demonstrates an agreement with the acupuncture meridians.

Neuroplasticity and neuromodulation

Persistent nociceptive input leads to sensitisation of WDR neurons, caused by a cascade of various processes at a molecular level. Processes of decreasing neuromodulation also play a key role.

The complex processes in the tract segment and potential influences of the decreasing nerve modulation, which can lead to pronounced allodynia and hyperalgesia, are demonstrated in Fig. 5.5.

Clinical signs: mechanical allodynia and hyperalgesia.

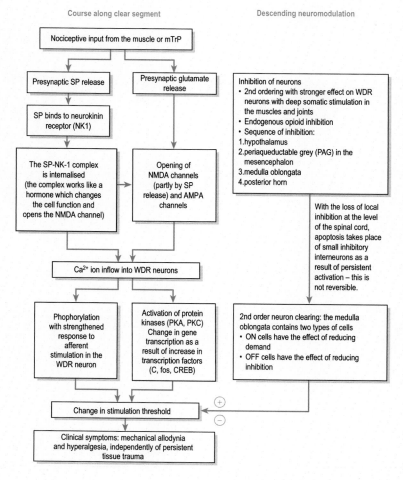

Fig. 5.5 Neuroplasticity and neuromodulation as a consequence of nociceptive input from the muscle. AMPA, α-amino-3-hydroxy-5-methyl-4-isoxazolepropionic acid; NMDA, N-methyl-D-aspartate.

Course along clear segment

Descending neuromodulation

Nociceptive input from the muscle or mTrP

Presynaptic SP release

Presynaptic glutamate release

SP binds to neurokinin receptor (NK1)

Inhibition of neurons
• 2nd ordering with stronger effect on WDR neurons with deep somatic stimulation in the muscles and joints
• Endogenous opioid inhibition
• Sequence of inhibition:
1. hypothalamus
2. periaqueductable grey (PAG) in the mesencephalon
3. medulla oblongata
4. posterior horn

The SP-NK-1 complex is internalised (the complex works like a hormone which changes the cell function and opens the NMDA channel)

Opening of NMDA channels (partly by SP release) and AMPA channels

With the loss of local inhibition at the level of the spinal cord, apoptosis takes place of small inhibitory interneurons as a result of persistent activation – this is not reversible.

Ca²⁺ ion inflow into WDR neurons

Phophorylation with strengthened response to afferent stimulation in the WDR neuron

Activation of protein kinases (PKA, PKC) Change in gene transcription as a result of increase in transcription factors (C, fos, CREB)

2nd order neuron clearing: the medulla oblongata contains two types of cells
• ON cells have the effect of reducing demand
• OFF cells have the effect of reducing inhibition

Change in stimulation threshold

Clinical symptoms: mechanical allodynia and hyperalgesia, independently of persistent tissue trauma

Chapter | 6 |

Pathophysiology

Johannes Fleckenstein, Dominik Irnich

6.1 HISTORICAL DEVELOPMENT

The so-called taut bands were first described in 1843 by Robert Froriep (he called them 'muscle calluses'), and they later became synonymous in English with the term 'myelogelosis'. They refer to a palpable knot in a bundle of contracted muscle fibres. The term mTrP arose in connection with the phenomenon since myelogelosis can demonstrate typical pain referral (referred pain pattern).

The pathogenesis of mTrP is still not fully understood today. From a pathological point of view various mechanisms have been described over the years.

- Elliot published a report on the increased activity of motor function units in 1944. The pain–spasm–pain theory first developed on the basis of this.
- In 1981 for the first time, Simon and Travell described how mTrP demonstrates a shortening of the sarcomeres. They introduce the theory of a basal contraction energy crisis as a causative factor.
- In 1986, Sessle et al. referred to a connection between generalised pain and a neuronal convergence of nociceptive fibres (including those of the muscles), which gather in the CNS.
- In 1990 Brückle reported on a local hypoxia which leads to the sensitisation of surrounding nociceptors.
- In 1993 Hubbard and Berkoff described spontaneous electromyographic (EMG) activity in some areas of trigger points. This preliminary work led to the later development of the hypothesis of dysfunction of the end plates as a cause of trigger points.
- In 1996 Hong described the increased occurrence of small nerve fibres at trigger points. These are classified as nociceptive fibres as an expression of the close relationship between trigger point and pain receptor.

- Since the 1990s Mense (see Bibliography) has been carrying out comprehensive research in the field of the pathophysiology of mTrPs. Molecular biology investigations in particular have led to a definite deepening of the understanding of muscle nociceptors and their activation of the substances involved. In particular Mense describes the central processing, especially at the level of the spinal cord, and contributes to the understanding of the origin and maintenance of mTrPs.

6.2 UNDERLYING THEORIES OF PATHOPHYSIOLOGY

6.2.1 Energy crisis theory

The energy crisis theory is based on three key properties of contractile muscle fibre bundles:

- there are no other action potentials,
- the fibre bundles are locally sensitive to pressure,
- if the trigger point is inactivated there is an immediate relaxation and decrease in tenderness.

A local physiological contracture, without the effect of the electrical activity of motoneurons, causes an increased metabolic rate. Ischaemically induced hypoxia also occurs. This is caused by continuous maximum activity and an increased energy requirement. In terms of an energy crisis the cited pathomechanisms lead to the distribution of neuroreactive substances (e.g. bradykinin, serotonin (5-hydroxytryptamine, 5-HT), prostaglandin) and the sensitisation of surrounding nociceptors.

According to the energy crisis theory this local hypoxia does not just result in a release of neuroreactive substances

http://dx.doi.org/10.1016/B978-0-7020-4312-3.00006-4

but also in an increase in vasoneuroactive messengers, which leads to venous stasis through local oedema and further promotes local ischaemia or hypoxia. Local hypoxia then causes a lack of ATP, which leads to dysfunction of the muscular Ca^{2+} pump (see Fig. 6.1). The sarcomeres are no longer able to free themselves and remain hooked up to each other. This intensifies the formation of taut bands. The Cinderella hypothesis should also be mentioned in connection with this (see Section 5.3.5).

6.2.2 End-plate hypothesis

In 1993 Hubbard and Berkoff described spontaneous EMG activity in some areas of trigger points. This activity was attributed to dysfunctional muscle spindles. There is also evidence of an involvement of the sympathetic nervous system. Histochemically, it is possible to measure highly increased quantities of released ACh in these areas as a result of increased depolarisation.

There is also EMG evidence of high-frequency, similar components with low amplitude. Spontaneous interference of this noise and an action potential are only found at some neuromuscular junctions. This effect can be emphasised by the fact that administration of the ACh blocker botulinum toxin can reduce the occurrence of neuromuscular junction noise.

These active locations of abnormal activity are distributed in pressure-sensitive trigger points between 'normal' neuromuscular junctions. Hubbard and Berkoff postulate a key role for them in the malfunction of muscular trigger points (see Fig. 6.2).

6.2.3 Pain–spasm–pain theory

The pain–spasm–pain theory arose before there was complete understanding of muscle reflexes. The cause of trigger points was explained by the increased activity of motor function units. Pain increases the γ-motoneuron activity,

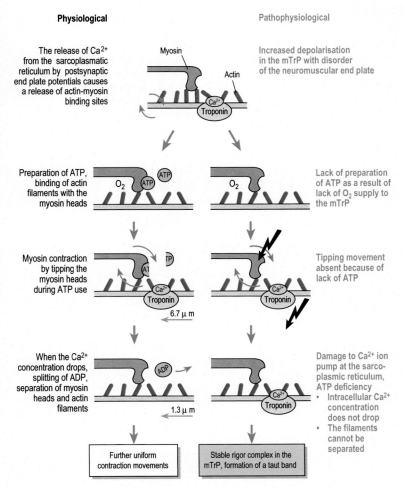

Physiological — **Pathophysiological**

The release of Ca^{2+} from the sarcoplasmatic reticulum by postsynaptic end plate potentials causes a release of actin-myosin binding sites

Myosin — Actin — Troponin

Increased depolarisation in the mTrP with disorder of the neuromuscular end plate

Preparation of ATP, binding of actin filaments with the myosin heads

O_2 — ATP — O_2

Lack of preparation of ATP as a result of lack of O_2 supply to the mTrP

Myosin contraction by tipping the myosin heads during ATP use

TP — Ca^{2+} Troponin — 6.7 μm — Ca^{2+} Troponin

Tipping movement absent because of lack of ATP

When the Ca^{2+} concentration drops, splitting of ADP, separation of myosin heads and actin filaments

ADP — 1.3 μm — Ca^{2+} Troponin

Damage to Ca^{2+} ion pump at the sarcoplasmic reticulum, ATP deficiency
- Intracellular Ca^{2+} concentration does not drop
- The filaments cannot be separated

Further uniform contraction movements

Stable rigor complex in the mTrP, formation of a taut band

Fig. 6.1 Muscle rigidity in the mTrP as a result of ATP deficiency because of local ischaemia (energy crisis theory).

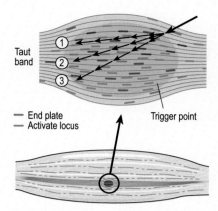

Taut band

1
2
3

— End plate
— Activate locus

Trigger point

Fig. 6.2 Diagramatic representation of an mTrP region with normal end plates alternating with so-called active loci, the dysfunctional end-plate regions. The EMG therefore shows a changing pattern.

this causes an increase in α-motoneuron activity, which is responsible for the resulting spasm. However, it has long been accepted that this does not lead primarily to muscle spasms. Spastic α-motoneuron activity could also not be demonstrated in EMG leads to be correlated with the pain. Indeed, it was shown that particularly visceral stimulation leads immediately to a spastic muscle response, but the ensuing pain only occurs later, with a latency of about an hour.

There is no evidence of other somatic stimulation in this connection. Nevertheless, a muscle spasm can be induced by stimulation of the tendons, dysfunction of the joints or even directly by muscular trigger points. However, these spasms are not immediately involved in the pain event. Nevertheless, it is possible, of course, that there is a juxtaposition of pain and spasm. In the pain–spasm–pain theory, these connections should be associated, but this theory is not enough to explain the phenomenon.

6.3 SPECIFIC PATHOPHYSIOLOGY

6.3.1 Changes in the nociceptive system

Peripheral sensitisation: the nociceptors are not just passive receptors. They also influence the biochemical milieu around them while secreting neuropeptides such as SP and CGRP. These neuropeptides, together with other substances already mentioned, can sensitise the nociceptors. The pronounced hyperalgesia in the area of the mTrP can only partially be explained, however, by the peripheral sensitisation of nociceptors.
Central sensitisation: tests mostly by Mense showed that the persistent irritation of sensory afferences from muscles

leads to neuroplastic changes in the posterior horn of the spinal cord. The various findings have produced various explanatory models; it explains, for example, the allodynia frequently associated with active mTrPs.

The nociceptors in the muscles involve free nerve endings. These are linked to the posterior horn via type III and type IV fibres. The posterior horn contains high-threshold mechanosensitive (HTM) neurons, low-threshold mechanosensitive (LTM) neurons, neurons that respond to both strong and weak stimuli (WDR) and interneurons. By the release of SP, CGRP and glutamate, which can be distributed from the primary afferent fibres on activation of the nociceptors both at the receptive and the spinal ends, all these neurons can be both sensitised (hyperalgesia) and enter into new synaptic associations with other posterior horn neurons. The distribution of SP and CGRP in the posterior horn is caused by severe and persistently painful stimuli, as is the case with an mTrP. The resulting association between LTM and HTM neurons has as a consequence, for example, that now not just HTM neurons spread pain but so too do LTM neurons. This leads to a mechano–nociceptor coupling in the posterior horn. Hyperalgesia and allodynia are possible consequences.

Mense in particular was able to show that the long-term presence of muscle pain can lead to an extension of the spinal region of influence (secondary activation of additional neurons) of impulses from the muscle (see Fig. 6.3).

This is how Mense supplies an explanation of the clinical phenomenon that patients have a diffuse sense of pain in spite of localised muscle pathology.

6.3.2 Pain modulation at the level of the spinal cord

Other investigations indicate pain modulation involving the nerve nucleus complex of the posterior horn (see Fig. 6.4). Both ascending and descending fibres there experience inhibitory influences via endorphinergic interneurons. The therapeutic effect of trigger point injections can be weakened in both subjective (e.g. intensity of pain) and objective (e.g. range of movement) parameters by the administration of naloxone.

Two key explanations for this have been discussed.

- The descending antinociceptive tracts represent an especially important pain-inhibiting system. The originating neurons of the system lie in the mesencephalon, which is linked to the nucleus of the nucleus raphe magnus in the medulla oblongata. From there descend multiple tracts, which run all the way along the spinal cord and here inhibit nociceptive posterior horn neurons. It is conceivable that a

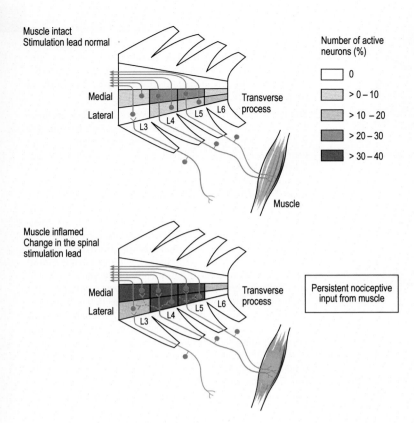

Fig. 6.3 Spread of the spinal area of influence by persistent nociceptive input. (Mense 1999)

Muscle intact
Stimulation lead normal

Medial
Lateral
L3 L4 L5 L6
Transverse process

Number of active neurons (%)

☐	0
☐	> 0 – 10
☐	> 10 – 20
☐	> 20 – 30
■	> 30 – 40

Muscle

Muscle inflamed
Change in the spinal stimulation lead

Medial
Lateral
L3 L4 L5 L6
Transverse process

Persistent nociceptive input from muscle

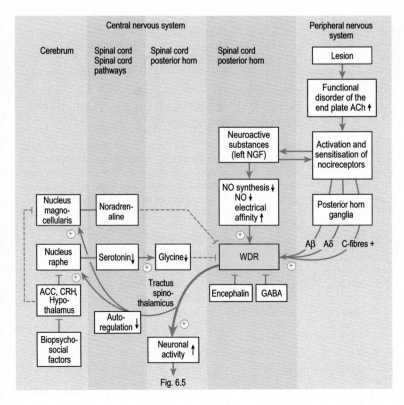

Fig. 6.4 Nociceptive and antinociceptive influences on the WDR posterior horn neuron. ACC, anterior cingulate cortex; CRH, corticotropin-releasing hormone; GABA, γ-aminobutyric acid; WDR, wide-dynamic-range neuron.

Central nervous system

Peripheral nervous system

Cerebrum | Spinal cord Spinal cord pathways | Spinal cord posterior horn | Spinal cord posterior horn

Lesion

Functional disorder of the end plate ACh ↑

Neuroactive substances (left NGF)

Activation and sensitisation of nocireceptors

NO synthesis ↓ NO ↓ electrical affinity ↑

Posterior horn ganglia

Nucleus magno-cellularis

Noradren-aline

Aβ Aδ C-fibres +

Nucleus raphe

Serotonin↓

Glycine↓

WDR

ACC, CRH, Hypo-thalamus

Tractus spino-thalamicus

Encephalin GABA

Biopsycho-social factors

Auto-regulation ↓

Neuronal activity ↑

Fig. 6.5

30

malfunction of the descending antinociceptive system could lead to chronic generalised spontaneous pain and hyperalgesia in deep tissues (muscles, tendons, fascia, joints) without the presence of a lesion there.

- Another attempt at explanation of this peripheral central reflex arc lies in the so-called WDR neurons (see Section 5.3.10). If these neurons are sensitised, they can also react to other subliminal stimulus saccades (e.g. pressure, isotonic tension, stretching). The convergence of various stimuli leads to poor localisation of the muscle pain. Divergence greatly enlarges the receptive field of pain perception.

6.3.3 Pain modulation in the CNS

Measurements of human cortical activity using imaging techniques have shown that different cortical areas are stimulated during painful stimulation of a skeletal muscle than during painful stimulation of the overlying skin. The pattern of activity distribution in the cortex shows definite differences in muscle and skin pain. During painful stimulation of the muscle there is definitely stronger activation in the anterior gyrus cinguli. The gyrus cinguli is connected to affective-emotional pain components, with increased attentiveness during pain stimuli.

> The transfer of muscle pain is indicated as an incorrect localisation of the pain, caused by neuroplastic conversion processes in the spinal cord and brain.

6.3.4 Current research results

Mense et al. showed in 2001 that inhibition of nitric oxide (NO) synthesis leads to a significant increase in frequency of firing exclusively in nociceptive neurons. As there is a fall in the number of NO-synthesising neurons under chronic pain conditions, the resulting lack of NO could cause spontaneous pain in patients.

Kuan et al. reported in 2007 on spinal cord association with muscular trigger points. Trigger points do not differ in their sensory afferences and motor function efferences from other tissue. However, the small diameter of the motoneurons running to the trigger points is conspicuous.

Chen et al. (2007) developed a procedure for identifying and diagnosing trigger points with magnetic resonance imaging. The stiffness of the taut band in patients with myofascial pain was about 9.0 kPa and therefore 50% greater than the stiffness of the surrounding tissue. It is thus possible to measure the differences in muscle tension.

Work published by Shah et al. in 2005 and 2008 determined the pH value and the electrolyte concentration in trigger points. Using a micropipette, the biochemical milieu was compared in active and passive trigger points and in non-specific control points. Shah et al. determined a significant increase in inflammatory mediators (see above) and a lowering of pH value in the active trigger points compared to the two control groups.

6.4 THE EXTENDED INTEGRATED HYPOTHESIS

The theories put forward are generally associated with each other by a so-called integrated hypothesis (see Fig. 6.5).

Any muscular tissue damage can cause activation of both a peripheral and a central pathomechanism. The peripheral cell damage causes distribution of active mediators (neuroactive, inflammatory, vasoactive), which in their turn are accompanied by local inflammation, with the formation of oedema and cellular loss of function. This also leads to a functional disorder of the peripheral neuromuscular junction, with excessive ACh release. This means the muscle cell membrane is continuously depolarised. The ACh causes high-frequency discharges at the postsynaptic membrane, which are demonstrated as end-plate noise. Myofibrillary contractures arise as a result, without activation of the neuromuscular end plate. The damage to functional cellular units (e.g. of the sarcoplasmic reticulum) leads to dysfunction of the Ca^{2+} ion pump, which increases cytoplasmic Ca^{2+} concentration in the muscle cells, the sarcomeres are shortened and no action potentials are passed on. According to current pathophysiological models, this condition leads to local ischaemia with increased metabolism. These processes get continuously stronger, in a 'vicious circle'. The result is a local energy crisis, as mentioned at the start of this chapter, with lowered pO_2 values (hypoxia), lowered ATP concentration and a failure of Na^+/K^+-ATPase. The muscular tissue is acidified and the pH value is lowered. This leads to the release of further inflammatory mediators (bradykinin, SP, prostaglandins), which in their turn stimulate peripheral nociceptors, possibly leading to the sensation of pain.

This release of neuroactive substances activates spinal cord cells via decreasing motor function and sensorimotor nerve tracts; of particular significance in this is the divergent distribution of the WDR neuron. The neuronal NO concentration drops and electrical activity increases. The autonomic nervous system, particularly sympathetic activity, is stimulated and a further reduction in the pain threshold is conceivable. Sympathetic stimulation causes further muscle tension. This could provide an explanation for the frequent additional autonomic symptoms of mTrP patients.

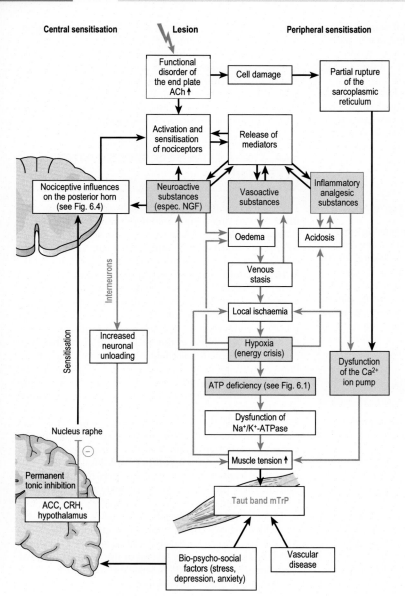

Central sensitisation

Lesion

Peripheral sensitisation

Fig. 6.5 Extended integrated hypothesis of the occurrence of myofascial trigger points.

Functional disorder of the end plate ACh↑

Cell damage

Partial rupture of the sarcoplasmic reticulum

Activation and sensitisation of nociceptors

Release of mediators

Nociceptive influences on the posterior horn (see Fig. 6.4)

Neuroactive substances (espec. NGF)

Vasoactive substances

Inflammatory analgesic substances

Oedema

Acidosis

Venous stasis

Interneurons

Local ischaemia

Sensitisation

Increased neuronal unloading

Hypoxia (energy crisis)

Dysfunction of the Ca²⁺ ion pump

ATP deficiency (see Fig. 6.1)

Dysfunction of Na⁺/K⁺-ATPase

Nucleus raphe

⊖

Muscle tension ↑

Permanent tonic inhibition

ACC, CRH, hypothalamus

Taut band mTrP

Bio-psycho-social factors (stress, depression, anxiety)

Vascular disease

Chapter | 7 |

The trigger point as expression of a functional disorder of the locomotor system

Karel Lewit

Despite all efforts to explain the cause of pain in the locomotor system, we are unable to successfully identify a definite pathological anatomical lesion in 85–90% of affected patients. These pains are therefore still described as non-specific (i.e. without a recognisable cause or appropriate diagnosis). The experienced clinician, and particularly one experienced in manual therapy or physiotherapy, is in a position to determine a number of symptoms that are evidently connected with the problems. This frequently involves muscle, joint or soft tissue findings, which characteristically affect function and disappear again after normal function is restored.

Muscle, joint and soft tissue findings are frequently functionally reversible and for this reason are not ascertainable in terms of pathological anatomy. They are, however, no less real than the changes that can be anatomically or histologically verified. Consequently, even diagnosed function disorders are no less specific than those that are supposedly objectively demonstrated, such as by imaging procedures.

Conversely, the presence of structural changes to the locomotor system is not by itself evidence that these changes are the cause of the problems.

> Functional disorders usually correlate better with the patient's symptoms than most anatomical findings. It is frequently seen that anatomical changes only cause pain when they affect function (Lewit 1993).

Of all the functionally reversible changes, the mTrP may be cited as the best researched and from many viewpoints the most significant finding (Simons 2004). It is the one that is involved in the direct cause of the pain. Because of the histological findings and the information gained elsewhere from the empirical knowledge that mTrPs can be functionally reversible, it can be accepted that both reversible and irreversible mTrPs exist. This is also based on the experience that many mTrPs can be made to disappear after postisometric relaxation (PIR) combined with reciprocal inhibition (RI) and as a result of chain reactions.

On the other hand, however, there are chronic mTrPs that can no longer be influenced through reflectory paths but which must be treated in our experience with the aid of needling or traumatising massage (i.e. 'destroyed'). The transition from reversible to irreversible disorders is given here as this must also be recognised as a differential diagnosis.

7.1 THE FUNCTION OF THE LOCOMOTOR SYSTEM IN ASSOCIATION WITH MEMORY

The function of the locomotor system involves not just a reflectory mechanism under the control of the CNS. It is rather more to do with programming of the memory so that it is available when needed and can be adjusted to the conditions.

There are essentially two underlying programmes:

- the upright human posture,
- acquired skills.

http://dx.doi.org/10.1016/B978-0-7020-4312-3.00007-6

33

7.1.1 Upright posture

Upright posture develops automatically in infancy. The neonate is initially in flexion with the head reclined (see Fig. 7.1a), incapable of adopting an active posture. As soon as it looks around for its mother for the first time, it begins to lift its head, which is enabled by the concomitant activity of the extensors of the neck and trunk. At about the end of the fourth month (see Fig. 7.1b) it takes on a balanced posture, supported on its forearms and knees. Not only the flexors and extensors of the trunk are involved in this posture, but also the adductors and abductors, the lateral and medial rotators and the flexors and extensors of the extremities.

The upright posture is therefore the result of a coordinated cocontraction of antagonists. The model developed in the 4-month-old infant is essentially the same as that demonstrated by the weight lifter (see Fig. 7.1c) (Kolár 2006).

The cocontraction pattern described here goes from the long muscle chains of the feet, which maintain the extremely labile balance of the legs above the round heel, to the pelvis above the head of the femur, then further to the thorax, which is supported on the labile lumbar spine, and finally to the head, which balances on the atlas joint with the round occipital condyle (see Fig. 7.2).

The upright posture can only happen by means of coordinated muscle activity. This means that the upright posture of this extremely labile balance of the skeleton is only possible by means of coordinated muscle activity. A particular problem is the so-called 'mast bracing' of the vertebral column. Something similar also applies to the arch of the foot. This involves chains of mostly long muscles radiating from the feet, a muscle which forms a fixed point. The more superior muscles are attached here (Lewit 2003).

Because the vertebral column is divided into sections, unlike a rigid mast, and according to Panjabi (1992), Cholewicki et al. (1997) and others, because the connection between two neighbouring vertebrae is unstable, the individual vertebrae would buckle (similarly for the ankle) if there was not also a 'deep stabilisation system'. This is found dorsally in the short Mm. multifidi (Hides et al. 1996) and ventrally in the abdominal space, where stability is dependent on its walls (i.e. the diaphragm), M. transversus and M. obliquus abdominis, and the pelvic floor. This system also develops automatically, even before the infant stands up (see Fig. 7.3).

7.1.2 Acquired skills

Specific, individually differentiated skills then develop during childhood. The game of tennis is a good example of this: at first, you throw a ball to a small child and it catches the ball with both hands. It takes some time before the child can catch the ball, first with both hands and then with one hand. One day, the child is given a tennis racquet and learns to catch the ball on that and return it.

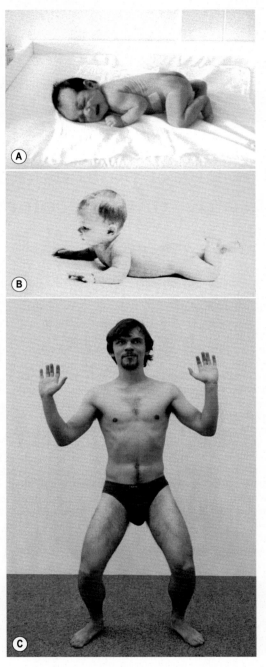

Fig. 7.1 Development of upright posture. (a) The neonate is in a predominantly flexed position. (b) Posture after the third month, supported on the elbow symphysis and knee with balanced cocontraction of the flexors and extensors of the trunk and extremities, by the abductors and adductors and the lateromedial rotators of the extremities. (c) This position leads to straightening up: the best balanced cocontraction can be seen in weightlifters (concentration of the joints and facilitation of the muscles).

What happens here? Traditional neurology would interpret it thus: the player sees the ball, and the information goes from the eye via the optic pathway to the occipital area. The process via parietal areas of the cerebral cortex, motor function cortex, spinal cord, peripheral neurons and afferent response via the cerebellum to the cerebral cortex is the result of a complex chain of signals. In the meantime, the ball has long fallen to the ground. What has changed? A programme develops over the years: in the moment when the player sees the ball, the body reacts holistically.

If one section is incorrect – neck, foot or arm – it must be reprogrammed. The function thus normally includes the whole locomotor system and holistic thinking is essential for making associations.

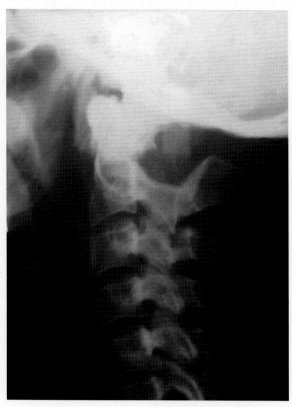

Fig. 7.2 The precarious balance of the head with the round condyles in the joint socket of the atlas is definitely illustrated if the arch of the atlas is missing.

> Characteristic chain reactions (Lewit 2003) result from a locoregional disorder, which can be established in patients with chronic pain if examination is adequate and these reactions include the whole system or at least a significant part. mTrPs and the blockages associated with them play a crucial role in this.

It is no accident that the most common chain reactions are closely associated with disorders of the deep stabilisers of the trunk, feet, shoulder blades and the (upper) neck.

7.2 PATHOPHYSIOLOGICAL ROLE OF mTrP

We know that mTrPs restrict mobility (Dejung 2003). This provides stability where it is in disorder or is insufficient. Thus there is a close connection with the blocking phenomenon which itself is not fully understood. The great osteopathic physiologist, Irvin M. Korr, brought it to our attention:

> *The same contractile powers which create movement also serve to work against movement.*

> (Korr 1975)

After explaining the role of the muscle spindle he continues: 'The high gain hypothesis is consistent with and offers an explanation for the steeply rising resistance to motion (bind) in one direction', which corresponds precisely to the effect of an mTrP and blocking. It is not by chance that it is neuromuscular mobilisation techniques which can be used most effectively to treat these blockages physiologically. These are essentially aimed at the mTrP. That is how these functional disorders are associated with pain.

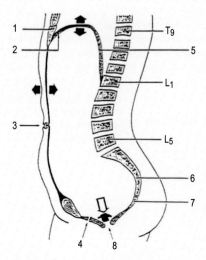

Fig. 7.3 Diagram of abdominal space with its walls.

7.2.1 Agonists and antagonists

The following laws can be derived from mTrPs: mTrPs occur in antagonists to immobilise a joint or a motion segment of the vertebral column. If an mTrP is in the M. biceps brachii, mTrPs are also regularly found in the triceps. The result is limited movement (stabilisation) of the elbow. Other examples are:

- ischiocrural muscles: M. biceps femoris; M. quadriceps femoris;
- M. triceps, a section of the fan-shaped M. pectoralis: M. erector spinae in the relevant segment.

However, if it involves stabilisation of the upright posture, then chains are formed by the long muscles, which allow the vertebral column to be tensioned like a mast and stabilise the legs over the feet. The more inferiorly positioned muscle forms a fixed point that stabilises the more superior attachments. These chains usually run down one side so it is possible for an experienced therapist to distinguish between 'right-sided' and 'left-sided' patients. Contralateral intersecting functional chains on the other side tend to be the exception. Chains can run from the occiput or even the muscles of mastication to the feet. However, they are frequently not continuous.

> mTrPs in agonists and antagonists can be in balance. However, the ontogenetically older system often prevails, i.e. the flexors, while the extensors, i.e. the antagonists, tend to demonstrate some weakness.

The predominance of the flexors, adductors and medial rotators correspond to the 'muscular dysbalance' (see Janda 2000) which is associated with 'stooped posture'. The most common cause of chains is a functional disorder in the area of the deep stabilisers of the trunk and the feet and in the area of the upper cervical region. Particularly easy to palpate are mTrPs in the area of the diaphragm (see Fig. 7.4a), the pelvic floor (see Fig. 7.4b) and the soles

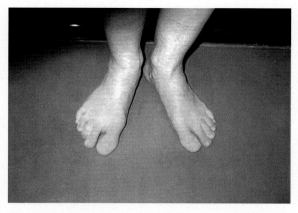

Fig. 7.5 Vele's test: automatic toe flexion at the end of the range of movement when leaning forwards in the upright position. This is missing on the right.

of the feet, back of the foot and the lower leg, although it is more difficult in the Mm. multifidii (see Fig. 7.5). The deep stabilisers are also linked to each other (i.e. the diaphragm, the M. transversus and M. obliquus abdominis, the M. coccygeus and the Mm. multifidi), and these in their turn with the muscles of the foot. It is the long muscles which then have to compensate for the function of the deep stabilisers with the aid of mTrPs, thus causing pain (Lewit 2006a).

7.2.2 The stabilisers in the pathogenesis of mTrP

The deep stabilisers in particular have a special significance in the pathogenesis of mTrP. Studies by Hodges indicated this (Hodges et al. 1995): they showed that if healthy volunteers raised their arms and the muscle activity in the deltoid and deep stabilisers (M. transversus abdominis or diaphragm) was recorded at the same time, the activity in the deep stabilisers preceded the activity in the deltoid.

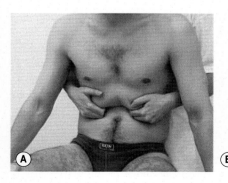

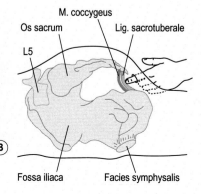

M. coccygeus

Os sacrum   Lig. sacrotuberale

L5

Fossa iliaca   Facies symphysalis

Fig. 7.4 Palpation of mTrPs (a) in the diaphragm and (b) in the M. coccygeus via the Lig. sacrotuberale.

In patients with functional disorders, e.g. lumbago, there is no longer any essential interplay between stabilising muscles and muscles performing movement. This means that voluntary movement is insufficiently assured if the stabilisers are not functioning properly.

This reveals another property of the deep stabilisers: although this is transversely striated muscle, we cannot access it with willpower. This was shown in another Hodges study: a volunteer carried out voluntary movement with the aid of the deltoid. But he was unaware of the contraction of the M. transversus, the muscles of the pelvic floor, the Mm. multifidii and the diaphragm. He had to learn the conscious contraction of the deep stabilisers, including in the foot, which is still under discussion (see Section 18.2).

The interplay of the diaphragm and the M. transversus abdominis takes on a key role among the trunk stabilisers according to P. Kolár (Kolár 2006). The diaphragm is not just the main respiratory muscle but is also significantly involved in the stability of upright posture. J. Skládal, the physiologist, formulated the observation for the first time in 1970:

The diaphragm is a respiratory muscle with a postural function and the abdominal muscles are postural muscles with a respiratory function.

(Skládal et al. 1970)

If functioning correctly during inspiration, the diaphragm contracts concentrically and the M. transversus abdominis excentrically. This can be palpated at the side of the waist if functioning correctly.

7.2.3 The role of feet and toes

The toe flexors play a similar role with the feet (Lewit 2006a). It is illustrated here how voluntary movement differs from automatic postural function.

- If you lean forwards (Vele's test, see Fig. 7.5) this automatically leads in the end phase to flexion of the toes, a reflex which obviously prevents falling forwards. This postural reflex can be missing and the patient then has great difficulty learning it, although the toes can voluntarily be flexed with normal strength.
- Another example of the complex interplay of voluntary movement and postural function can be observed with the big toe: the M. abductor hallucis also supports the arch of the foot and its weakness is often associated with hallux valgus. Voluntary abduction of the big toe is not easy, however, and must first be learnt.

The typical chain reaction with dysfunction of the feet (most commonly a blockage in the Lisfranc joint with mTrP deep in the sole of the foot and also on the back of the foot) is a forward posture (see Fig. 7.6) with mTrP – especially in the abdominal and back muscles – and definite tension of the neck muscles. If the patient now straightens up, the neck tension is suddenly reduced. At the same time, you often find a blockage of the head of the fibula with mTrP in the M. biceps femoris. This in turn results in insufficient fixation of the pelvis as a result of dysfunction of the ischiocrural muscles. This leads to tension in the M. rectus abdominis, which indeed fixes the pelvis. The consequence is numerous mTrPs in this muscle (on one side, sometimes on both sides), which (usually) causes a forward posture. The most important clinical signs are – as described above – the sudden relaxation of the neck muscles which are tense when standing if the patient straightens up with the head upright.

7.2.4 The role of the shoulders

The shoulder blades play a key role for the arms and here again it is mostly the ascending (lower) part of the M. trapezius, which has a stabilising effect with the M. serratus. This is clearly shown when the very common tension of the upper part of the trapezius is momentarily relaxed and the patient learns to intentionally tense the lower part.

7.2.5 The role of trunk rotation

A short but clinically very important chain concerns trunk rotation. This is a function which ontogenetically develops later (after the sixth month) and is only associated with people who use great power in movements such as throwing a discus, golf, shot put, etc. Limited trunk rotation is usually attributed to a blockage in the thoracolumbar transition, because anatomy teaches us that the rib cage and the ribs inhibit rotation and the joints of the lumbar spine do not allow rotation. Trunk rotation can therefore only take place in the area of the free ribs, i.e. in the thoracolumbar transition.

Any scoliosis, even in the lumbar spine, is associated with rotation. Lewit (1997) showed that scoliosis with rotation takes place on trunk rotation while seated with a fixed pelvis (see Fig. 7.7).

Clinically, it has now been shown that limited trunk rotation is regularly associated with mTrPs of the thoracolumbar M. erector spinae, the M. quadratus lumborum and the M. psoas on the opposite side. It is sufficient to relax the mTrP of only one of the three muscles in order to achieve symmetrical trunk rotation. It has also been shown that limited trunk rotation is often linked with limited neck rotation. Then the trunk rotation is usually

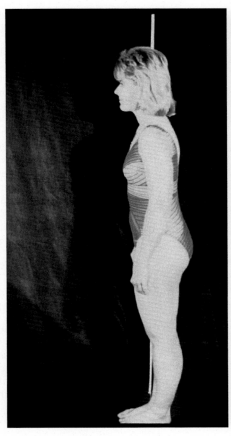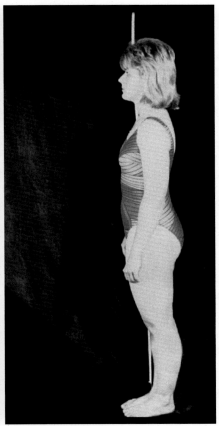

Fig. 7.6 Forward posture before and after treatment.

given precedence to the neck rotation so that after treatment of one of the mTrPs cervical rotation is also normalised.

7.2.6 The role of the elbow

Another important chain exists in radial epicondylalgia. This is tendinitis due to strain at the insertion sites of the following three muscles, with limitation of concomitant finger and wrist flexion:

- the wrist and finger extensors,
- the supinator,
- the biceps muscle.

This can be seen by an increased distance of the fingers from the forearm with concomitant flexion in the wrist and fingers. Pronation and elbow extension are also limited compared to the non-painful side. In this case, it is necessary to treat each of these muscles where mTrPs can be found.

Epicondylalgia is also frequently associated with limited movement in the area of the cervical spine and deficient fixation of the shoulder blades, especially with insufficiency of the ascending part of the lower M. trapezius (Kolár 2006; Lewit 2006b).

7.2.7 Soft tissue changes, fascia and internal organs

If the situation is chronic, mTrPs and blockages are often associated with changes in soft tissue. The fascia are of special significance here, as they can slide insufficiently over the underlying medium (usually bone). 'Active' scars are of particular significance here. These are scars where the soft tissue has become changed: it is difficult to stretch them and their movement against bone or each other is limited, and frequently painful.

The significance of soft tissue changes is obviously that soft tissue must be able to move during all movements

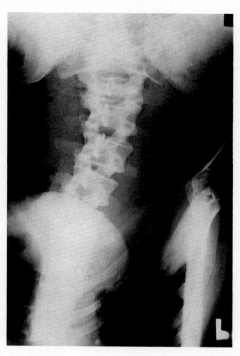

Fig. 7.7 Trunk rotation to the right with right-sided scoliosis and rotation of the lumbar spine.

of the (real) locomotor apparatus; that is, it must be able to stretch and slide. If this is not the case, we diagnose pathological barriers here too.

This also applies to the internal organs, which must be able to move freely during exercise and respiration. If this is not the case, pathological barriers occur here too and we treat them with light pressure in that direction. After a short period of latency, release occurs whether we are dealing with skin, fascia or internal organs. The muscles involved here also typically react with mTrPs.

Finally, we must not forget that with painful disease of the internal organs reflex blockages can occur in the relevant muscle segment. It is even possible to state that as long as there are no mTrPs in the area of the locomotor system, visceral disease produces hardly any pain. These findings are so characteristic for most internal organs that they are called 'disorder patterns of the internal organs' (see Fig. 7.8).

> The locomotor system is to some extent a mirror of what is happening in the body.

Fig. 7.8 The nociceptive stimulation of skin, joint, periosteum, tendon, muscle and internal organs regularly produces an autonomic and somatic (muscular) reaction via the spinal ganglion and spinal cord.

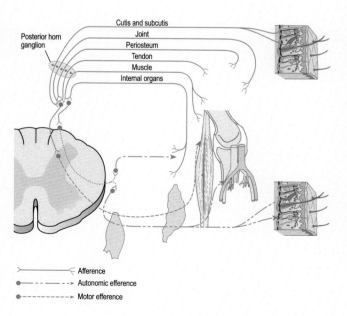

Chapter | 8 |

Trigger points and myofascial pain: acupuncture points and the meridian system

Peter T. Dorsher, with the assistance of Johannes Fleckenstein

8.1 TRIGGER POINTS AND ACUPUNCTURE POINTS

The teaching of acupuncture was systematically compiled for the first time in the *Nei Jing* (approx. 200 BCE) (Unschuld 2003). Although only about 30% of the application of acupuncture deals with the treatment of pain, this is its most well-known indication in Western medicine. The main indication for most classical acupuncture points is actually the treatment of non-painful 'internal' diseases, although it is recorded in current literature (Deadman et al. 1998; O'Connor, Bensky 1981) that practically all these acupuncture points also have a pain indication. Only two acupuncture points have no pain indication attributed to them: BL 8 and ST 17.

Melzack et al. compared acupuncture and myofascial pain for the first time in 1977 in a study of their anatomical and clinical similarities. A 100% correspondence between trigger points and acupuncture points and a 71% correspondence between the clinical pain indications was described in this study. However, the meaningfulness of this study is limited for the following reasons.

- First, only 48 defined trigger points of the 255 described in the *Trigger Point Manual* (Travell, Simons 1983, 1992) were investigated.
- Second, no investigation was carried out as to whether the acupuncture points could be attributed to the same muscles as their anatomically relevant trigger points.
- Third, only a limited number of classical acupuncture points were studied which are used in pronounced pain syndromes or discrete pain locations; as already mentioned, practically every classical acupuncture point is also used for pain, in addition to its clinical indications.

8.2 REFERRED PAIN PATTERNS AND MERIDIANS

Almost 30 years later, trigger points and acupuncture points were studied with regard to their similarities in anatomy, pain pattern and somatovisceral correspondence and referred pain pattern and meridians (Dorsher 2006). In this study, all 255 trigger point locations described in the *Trigger Point Manual* were compared with the 361 classical acupuncture points and the 386 'new' and 'different' acupuncture points described by the Shanghai College of Traditional Medicine (O'Connor, Bensky 1981).

A prerequisite for an anatomical correlation between acupuncture points and trigger points was that the two points were no more than 2 cm from each other and that each acupuncture point was attributed to the muscle of the relevant trigger point.

The anatomical correspondence was confirmed by the anatomical atlases of Clemente (1981), Netter (1989) and Chen (1995) using functional anatomy software (Hillman 2002). Further studies were conducted as to whether the pain indications of the correlating acupuncture points included similar local pain indications, like the relevant trigger points. The flow of the acupuncture meridians was also compared with the myofascially referred pain patterns of the anatomically relevant points.

Dorsher's study showed that with the above prerequisites 92% of the 255 trigger points related to the anatomically appropriate acupuncture points and that 79.5% of these trigger points demonstrated similar local pain indications to the relevant acupuncture points. Furthermore, 76% of the relevant acupuncture and trigger points showed a correlation of the meridians and the myofascially referred pain distribution. Another 14% of the point parallels

http://dx.doi.org/10.1016/B978-0-7020-4312-3.00008-8

demonstrated an at least partially local or distal correlation of the meridians to the referred pain patterns.

Critics maintain that the above study results should be regarded skeptically because of the following three theoretical considerations: most acupuncture points are not used primarily for the treatment of pain, nor are acupuncture points tender to touch (White 2007) and in the end trigger points can occur anywhere in a muscle according to current myofascial theories and do not have a discrete localisation (in the *Trigger Point Manual* the most commonly used trigger points are marked with a cross).

Our response to this is that trigger points are used predominantly for the treatment of myofascial pain so any comparison of these points with acupuncture points should concentrate on their use in the treatment of pain. Although most classical acupuncture points, as already mentioned above, are used mainly for the treatment of non-painful symptoms, all 361 classical acupuncture points are indicated for the treatment of local pain with the exception of two points.

The second argument, according to which acupuncture points are not tender, can be refuted with quotations from standard works. In their textbook, O'Connor and Bensky (1981) reported:

> *...the main criterion for the exact location of an acupuncture point is that of tenderness (pain when pressed).*

Acupuncturists have always carefully examined the body surface to find any tender sites, heated areas, changes in the skin or subcutaneous hardening. These phenomena are then connected with the pathology of the neighbouring meridian in each case. Similar statements which say how important it is to find and treat local and distal tender acupuncture points can be found in other acupuncture textbooks, including Deadman et al. (1998), Wiseman and Ellis (1991) and Helms (1995). The underlying significance – especially in the treatment of pain – of seeking tender local and distal acupuncture points in clinical practice is definitely described as an underlying principle of acupuncture practice.

The latter argument means that stating the exact location of trigger points is not possible but that they can occur anywhere in a muscle or a muscle region. It is postulated that myofascially referred pain is characteristic of a muscle or muscle group, but this is not the case for trigger points (Dommerholt, Simons 2007). Nevertheless, the *Trigger Point Manual* (Travell, Simons 1983) shows that different trigger points of a muscle possess different referral patterns as well. Two pronounced trigger point subregions are indicated there e.g. for the descending part of the trapezius muscle, three more trigger point subregions for the transverse part and two trigger point subregions for the ascending part, which all demonstrate differently referred pain patterns (see Fig. 8.1). The same applies to the sternocleidomastoid, pectoralis major and paraspinal muscles, which also demonstrate three or more anatomical regions, each of which contains several trigger point subregions with different pain referral patterns.

These trigger point-specific referrals are also found in other descriptions, that have all found similar predilection sites for the usually described trigger points in the muscles.

Figs 8.1–8.6 show that the referred pain pattern can be predicted by the flow of a meridian in a muscle region.

8.3 OTHER STUDY RESULTS

Other studies have been carried out for the further investigation and possible refutation of the concept that referred pain originates from regional muscle parts instead of relatively regularly localised trigger points. As Dorsher's study of 2006 dealt with almost two-thirds of the point correlations of classical acupuncture points, only a partial repeat of the analysis was necessary.

8.3.1 Anatomical correlations

By means of extended regional consideration of myofascial pain the analysis of the trigger point locations (regions) could be limited to anatomical comparison with the classical acupuncture points. To define these correlations of trigger points and classical acupuncture points the question was posed as to whether the classical acupuncture point is to be found in the relevant muscle region. No defined distances have been established; on the other hand, previous studies in 2006 established that points are no more distant than 2 cm from one another.

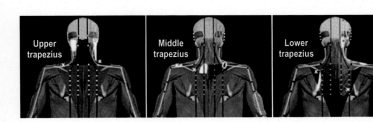

Upper trapezius   Middle trapezius   Lower trapezius

Fig. 8.1 M. trapezius, pars descendens, traversa and ascendens: trigger point subregions and attributed referred pain patterns.

It must also be stressed that in the remainder of this chapter the term 'trigger point' relates to the muscle regions which in the *Trigger Point Manual* contain the classical 255 trigger point locations. This theory postulates that trigger points do not occur regularly but may vary in their location in a particular muscle area.

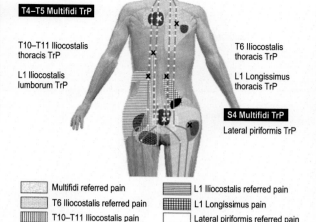

Multifidi referred pain	L1 Iliocostalis referred pain
T6 Iliocostalis referred pain	L1 Longissimus pain
T10–T11 Iliocostalis pain	Lateral piriformis referred pain

Fig. 8.4 Posterior view of torso, gluteal muscles and proximal thigh: relationships between the trigger points on the iliocostalis thoracis muscle (TP6 and TP10–TP11), iliocostalis lumborum muscle (L1), longissimus thoracis muscle (L1), multifidi muscles (TP4–TP5 and S4) and on the lateral piriformis muscle and their referred pain patterns on the bladder meridian (darker areas represent areas with more strongly concentrated pain).

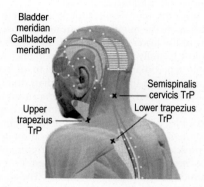

Fig. 8.2 Posterolateral view of head, neck and upper back: relationships between trigger points on the descending or ascending parts of the trapezius muscle and semispinalis cervicis muscle and their referred pain patterns on the gallbladder and bladder meridians (darker areas represent areas with more strongly concentrated pain).

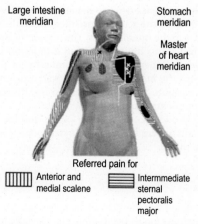

Referred pain for

| Anterior and medial scalene | Intermmediate sternal pectoralis major |

Fig. 8.3 Anterior view of head, neck and torso: relationships between the trigger points on the anterior or posterior scalene muscle and the pectoralis major muscle and their referred pain patterns on the large intestine, stomach and pericardial meridians (darker areas represent areas with more strongly concentrated pain).

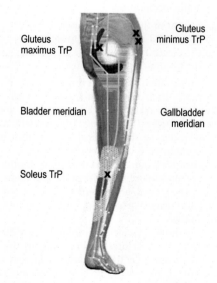

Fig. 8.5 Posterolateral view of the lower extremity: relationships between the trigger points on the gluteus maximus, gluteus minimus and soleus muscles and their referred pain patterns on the bladder and gallbladder meridian (darker areas represent areas with more strongly concentrated pain).

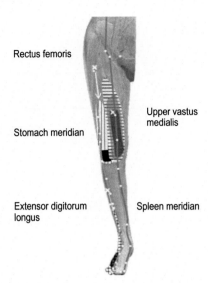

Rectus femoris

Upper vastus
medialis

Stomach meridian

Extensor digitorum
longus

Spleen meridian

Fig. 8.6 Anterior view of the lower extremity: relationships between the trigger points on the rectus femoris, proximal vastus medialis and extensor digitorum longus muscles and their referred pain patterns on the stomach and spleen meridian (darker areas represent areas with more strongly concentrated pain).

The renewed comparison of trigger point location defined in this way with the classical acupuncture points increased the correlation between the two to 97.7%. Only six trigger points could not be attributed to anatomically relevant classical acupuncture points:

- a trigger point in the pterygoideus muscle,
- two in the medial subscapularis muscle,
- one in the iliacus muscle,
- two in the obturator internus muscle.

Figs 8.2–8.6 illustrate why such an improvement in the results took place. Each illustration shows for each of the tested muscles the usually used trigger point location according to the *Trigger Point Manual* (marked with a cross) and their relations to the classical acupuncture points, which are represented on the relevant meridians.

The posterior neck muscles and the thoracolumbar back muscles are predominantly parallel to the axis of the vertebral column. The gluteal, posterior thigh and posterior calf muscles are also usually arranged parallel to the axis of the lower extremities.

Figs 8.2, 8.4 and 8.5 show that the bladder meridian also runs parallel to the vertebral column and on the lower extremity and directly over these muscles. Likewise, the lateral pelvic and leg muscles on the lateral thigh and calf are oriented parallel to the axis of the lower extremity. The gall-bladder meridian runs there as well, and is found over these muscles (gluteus minimus in Fig. 8.5 and the peroneus). As the muscles lie parallel to the acupuncture meridians, which run over these muscles, the large number of trigger

point locations in all these muscles compared to the locations described in the *Trigger Point Manual* has no effect on the anatomical relation between the trigger points and the acupuncture points on the relevant muscle or the meridian lying on the relevant muscle region. This means that a trigger point remains anatomically close to the bladder or gall-bladder meridian (and the acupuncture points here), no matter where in the muscle the trigger point is located. A more inaccurately located/described trigger point location within the muscle also allows that a correlation to any classical acupuncture on this muscle is possible. This in its turn leads to a higher level of anatomical correlation between trigger points and acupuncture points.

The same results were obtained for the anterior thigh and calf (see Fig. 8.6). The muscles here are also almost parallel to the axis of the lower extremity, with the rectus femoris running more laterally than the vastus medialis. The stomach and spleen meridians also run parallel to the axis of the lower extremity, with the stomach meridian running over the rectus femoris and the spleen meridian running over the vastus medialis (see Fig. 8.6). Analogous to the back and posterior leg muscles already mentioned, a more inaccurately located/described trigger point location in the anterior leg muscles means that the affected trigger points still always lie near the meridians (and their acupuncture points), which run through these muscles. The anatomical correlations of the trigger points and acupuncture points are therefore strengthened to the same extent.

The same results were developed for the facial and anterior neck muscles, whereby the individual muscles and the acupuncture meridians that run through them are largely vertically oriented.

The muscles of the thorax and the lateral abdomen on the other hand are more or less transversely arranged (i.e. more or less at right angles to the axis of the vertebral column). However, the acupuncture meridians run almost at right angles to the muscle fibres. The reason for this should be investigated in a future study, but is probably related to the segmental innervations of the muscles of the trunk. Nevertheless the more inaccurately located/described trigger point locations in these muscles increase the correlation to the acupuncture points and meridians.

Fig. 8.3 shows the usual trigger points and myofascially referred pain pattern for the middle sternocostal part of the pectoralis major.

It is interesting that the stomach meridian runs directly medial to these trigger points in the sternocostal part of the pectoralis major, while the pericardial meridian lies directly lateral to these points. The referred pain pattern from these trigger points concentrates on the anterior thorax on the flow of the stomach meridian, the anteroproximal anterior upper arm, i.e. on the area of the pericardial meridian.

It is therefore possible to predict that a trigger point situated medially to the usual points would refer pain over the front of the chest to the area of the stomach meridian. A trigger point lateral to the usual trigger point locations would, on the other hand, fall in the region of the pericardial meridian. This strengthens possible anatomical correlations of trigger points and acupuncture meridians and points in certain muscle parts.

The situation of the abdominal muscles is more complex, as many of the trigger points situated here possess either no or only locally referred pain patterns near the trigger points. It should be sufficient here to establish that the more inaccurately located/described handling of the trigger point locations in this area also strengthens their correlation to the classical acupuncture points.

In summary, the more generous handling of the anatomical trigger point locations (muscle regions instead of defined, 'X'-oriented trigger point location), shows that 97.7% of trigger points can be attributed to an anatomically relevant acupuncture point.

In a separate analysis, the estimated distances were determined between the usual trigger point locations described in the *Trigger Point Manual* and the anatomically relevant classical acupuncture points. Some 89 (36%) of the 249 correlating trigger and acupuncture point pairs are found at an estimated distance of less than 1 cm from one another, 107 point pairs (43%) are 1–2 cm distant from each other and another 32 point pairs (13%) are 2–3 cm from each other.

8.4 PAIN AND SOMATOVISCERAL CORRELATIONS BETWEEN TRIGGER POINTS AND ACUPUNCTURE POINTS

In this section, too, the term trigger point refers to the muscle regions in which the 255 usually used trigger locations described in the *Trigger Point Manual* are found. These locations, which are marked with a cross in the muscle trigger point handbook, anatomically fix the location of the points.

Of the 249 usual points with an anatomically relevant classical acupuncture point, 17 (7%) do not have any pain indications and only somatovisceral functions are described. These include the 'arrhythmia' point in the pectoralis major muscle, the 'eructation' point in the obliquus externus abdominis muscle and 15 'diarrhoea' points in the lower transverse abdominal muscles. Of the remaining 232 acupuncture points, 220 (95%) have local musculoskeletal or neurological pain indications which are comparable with the anatomically relevant trigger points. Another 2% of these acupuncture points are indicated for painful symptoms which tally with the pain patterns referred by trigger points (see Table 8.1). Only 3.5% (8/232) of trigger

Table 8.1 Acupuncture points with clinical pain indications in the distribution area of referred pain from the anatomically relevant trigger points

mTrP NO.	ACUPUNCTURE POINT	PAIN INDICATION
30 M. digastricus (anterior part)	Ren 23	Mouth ulcers, trismus (lockjaw)
78 M. brachialis (proximal part)	LU 4	Pain in the area of the medial upper arm
99 M. flexor carpi ulnaris	HT 3	Numbness in the upper extremity, elbow pain
101 M. flexor digitorum superficialis (humeral head)	HT 3	Numbness in the upper extremity, elbow pain

points have clinical pain indications which differ from those of the anatomically relevant acupuncture points. These involve only five definite classical acupuncture points (PC 4, SP 8, SP 11, LR 9 and LR 10).

In the *Trigger Point Manual* somatovisceral effects are described for 61 mTrP regions or trigger points, where for 17 of these points only non-painful somatovisceral indications are recorded (Travell, Simons 1983, 1992). Forty-eight (79%) of the anatomically relevant acupuncture points had identical somatovisceral indications and another 10 acupuncture points (16%) had possible somatovisceral indications (see Table 8.2).

It should be noted here that according to acupuncture teaching, depending on the type of needle manipulation, the opposite clinical effect to that described can theoretically be provoked at a certain point. For example, replenishing (supplying energy to) ST 28 would ease constipation, while depleting (taking energy away from) this point would lead to worsening of the constipation. At only three trigger points did the somatovisceral effects not show any correlation to the effects of the anatomically relevant classical acupuncture points in each case. Two of these trigger points are close to the clavicular part of the sternocleidomastoideus muscle, and the third point is the 'arrhythmia' trigger point.

Other musculoskeletal effects of trigger points are described for 15 usually non-painful points (see Table 8.3). For 12 (80%) of these points there is evidence of probable or certain correspondence of the indications to the anatomically relevant acupuncture points in each case.

Table 8.2 'Probable' correlation between trigger points and acupuncture points with regard to their somatovisceral indications

mTrP NO.	VISCERAL INDICATION	ACUPUNCTURE POINT	ACUPUNCTURE INDICATION
24 M. temporalis	Pain in the posterior upper jaw	GB 7	Caries (together with ST 42)
27 M. pterygoideus lateralis	'Sinusitis'	ST 7	Pain/swelling of the cheeks
28 M. pterygoideus lateralis	'Sinusitis'	ST 7	Pain/swelling of the cheeks
142 Lower abdominal muscles	'Causes diarrhoea'	ST 28	Flatulence in the lower abdomen, retained stool
145 Lower abdominal muscles	'Causes diarrhoea'	ST 28	Flatulence in the lower abdomen, retained stool
146 Lower abdominal muscles	'Causes diarrhoea'	ST 28	Flatulence in the lower abdomen, retained stool
150 Lower abdominal muscles	'Causes diarrhoea'	ST 28	Flatulence in the lower abdomen, retained stool
153 Lower abdominal muscles	'Causes diarrhoea'	SP 13	Constipation, fullness and pain in the lower abdomen
207 M. adductor magnus	Pain in the pelvis	BL 36	Difficult bowel movement and micturition, pain in the genitalia, cold in the uterus
255 M. soleus	Pain in the jaw and cheek	GB 35	Facial or eye swelling, painful blockage of the throat

8.4.1 Correspondence of acupuncture meridians and myofascially referred pain

The 249 trigger and acupuncture point pairs were then examined to see whether the meridian distribution of these acupuncture points correlated with the distribution of the myofascially referred pain patterns of the anatomically relevant trigger points. Remember that for 17 trigger points only somatovisceral effects and no myofascially referred pain patterns were described. Therefore 232 anatomically relevant trigger point and acupuncture point pairs remain for analysis. Of these, 187 pairs (81%) demonstrated complete or almost complete agreement and for another 9% of pairs partial agreement of the distribution of myofascially referred pain patterns and the associated acupuncture point meridians were observed. Only 10% of pairs showed little or no agreement of the referred pain patterns and the acupuncture point meridians.

Figs 8.2–8.6 illustrate this correlation. Essentially, the myofascially referred pain patterns of the vertebral column are predominantly aligned parallel to the axis of the vertebral column, while the myofascially referred pain patterns at the extremities are also aligned parallel to the axes of the limbs. The cause of this is probably the linear development of the vertebral column and the extremities during the first few weeks of embryonic development. Figs 8.2, 8.4 and 8.5 illustrate the anatomy of the nuchal, thoracolumbar, gluteal, femoral and crural muscles, where the pain pattern largely follows the flow of the bladder meridian. This also applies to the pain pattern of the occipitalis and frontalis muscles (not shown). The whole flow of the bladder meridian can therefore be interpreted as the referred pain pattern of the above muscles.

However, in the area of the thoracolumbar muscles, a small part of the myofascially referred pain pattern follows the course of the spinal nerves at the level of the trigger points and not the bladder meridian. The more lateral gluteal and crural muscles (e.g. peronei muscles) possess referred pain patterns to the same extent parallel to the limb axes, but on the lateral body surface of the lower extremity, which corresponds well to the flow of the gallbladder meridian (see Fig. 8.3). This also applies to the anterior side of the leg (see Fig. 8.6), where the referred pain pattern of the rectus femoris muscle and the extensor digitorum longus muscle at the anterolateral leg parallel to the limb axis runs

Table 8.3 Comparison of trigger points and acupuncture points with regard to their indications for symptoms of the locomotor apparatus

mTrP NO.	MUSCULOSKELETAL INDICATION	ACUPUNCTURE POINT	ACUPUNCTURE INDICATION
6 M. levator scapulae	Torticollis	SI 15	Pain in the shoulder and shoulder blade, stiff neck
47 M. levator scapulae	Torticollis	SI 14	Fixed neck, stiffness
56 M. infraspinatus	Shoulder joint pain	SI 11	Pain and heavy feeling in shoulder
57 M. infraspinatus	Shoulder joint pain	SI 11	Pain and heavy feeling in shoulder
54 M. subscapularis	Frozen shoulder	HT 1	Inability to lift the shoulders
93 M. extensor digitorum	Stiff fingers	LI 10	Pain and limited mobility in the arm
94 M. extensor digitorum	Stiff fingers	TH 9	Pain in the forearm, paresis of the upper extremity
96 M. supinator	Tennis elbow	LU 5	Elbow pain, limited mobility in the elbow
97 M. palmaris longus	Dupuytren's contracture	PC 4	Chest pain, heart pain, state of arousal, sleep disorders
193 M. rectus femoris	Hypermobile hips	ST 31	Atrophy of blockage in the thigh or gluteal muscles
194 M. vastus medialis	Hypermobile knee	SP 11	Symptoms in the inguinal area and the outer genitalia
195 M. vastus medialis	Hypermobile knee	SP 10	Pain in the medial thigh, menstrual and micturition disorders
196 M. vastus intermedius	Hypermobile hips	ST 31	Contraction of the thigh muscles, hemiplegia
197 M. vastus lateralis	Hypermobile patella	ST 34	Knee pain, knee flexion or extension difficult
198 M. vastus lateralis	Locked patella syndrome	GB 33	Knee flexion or extension not possible

in a flow that corresponds well with the flow of the stomach meridian. The referred pain pattern of the vastus medialis muscle which anatomically lies medially to the rectus femoris muscle also runs parallel to the limb axis and thus lies medially to the referred pain pattern of the rectus femoris muscle, a distribution which corresponds extremely well with the spleen meridian (see Fig. 8.6).

Fig. 8.3 shows the pain referral pattern of the anterior and medial scalene muscle at the anterior side of the neck and trunk. This is distributed over the shoulder to the lateral upper arm and forearm distally as far as the metacarpal bones I and II and the index finger. The scalene trigger point region lies anatomically close to the acupuncture points LI 17 and LI 18. The myofascially referred pain pattern of the sternocostal part of the pectoralis major muscle is also represented in Fig. 8.3. The referred pain pattern of this muscle region is concentrated very much on the chest but also spreads along the medial part of the upper arm; another part of the referred pain radiates into the anteromedial part of the proximal forearm. The pain referral pattern runs along the arm parallel to its axis, but medially. The pain of these trigger points that is referred to the chest agrees well with the flow of the stomach meridian, while the pain referred to the arm is aligned with the pericardium meridian. One might therefore predict that a trigger point region on the sternocostal part of the pectoralis major muscle, which lies medial to the usual trigger point locations in Fig. 8.3, provokes referred pain patterns on the chest in the area of the stomach meridian (see Fig. 8.3). A trigger point region lateral to the usual trigger point locations would on the other hand lead to a referred pain pattern in the area of the pericardial meridian.

In summary, the referred pain patterns of all muscle regions almost always correspond to the flows of the acupuncture meridians which run through each region. This even applies to complex muscles such as the trapezius (see Fig. 8.1), for which a total of seven referred pain patterns for the various muscle areas are described in the *Trigger Point Manual*. Fig. 8.1 illustrates that the flows of the large intestine, gallbladder, triple warmer and bladder meridians, which run through the various trigger point regions to the trapezius muscle, accurately predicts the distribution of the myofascially referred pain pattern for each of the trapezius trigger point areas. The referred pain pattern of the 232 trigger point regions described in the *Trigger Point Manual* demonstrate in 81% of cases a complete or almost complete correlation with the flows of the meridians that run through these trigger point regions. Another 9% show at least a certain level of overlapping. Only 10% of the trigger point regions did not show any correlation between myofascially referred pain patterns and the flow of the meridian.

8.5 SUMMARY

Depending on point of view and the assumptions made, there are definite correlations to be found between the myofascial trigger point regions and the classical acupuncture points. There are correlations with regard to their anatomical positions in up to 97.7% of cases and with regard to their clinical pain manifestation in more than 95%. The myofascially referred pain patterns and the flow of the acupuncture meridians match in 81% and another 9% they show a partial match.

The investigations introduced here tell us that the characteristics of myofascial pain were set down in the *Nei Jing* 2000 years before the appearance of the *Trigger Point Manual*. The myofascial concept could therefore be a sort of rediscovery of the classical meridians.

Nothing is new.

(John Edward Everett, *Quillings in Verse*)

Chapter | 9 |

Myofascial trigger points and fascia

Robert Schleip

9.1 ANATOMY: DEFINITIONS

For several decades the fascia played a type of 'Cinderella' role in musculoskeletal research, but today they are increasingly moving into the foreground of medical attention (Findley, Schleip 2007). Conventionally the fascia are that omnipresent tissue, which used to be regarded as 'white packaging material'. Frequently, attention is only paid to a few important parts of this white, fibrous tissue, such as the fascia lata or the fascia lumbodorsalis.

As the fascial tissue represents a particularly large interlinked architecture, it is reflected in an extraordinary number of divided concepts and descriptions in anatomical texts, which are often confusing. Many authors, for example, label only collagen fibre connective tissue as fascia, and this has a firm, irregular structure which covers a large flat area, delimited by ligaments, tendons, tendon plates and loose subdermal connective tissue, although the latter is explicitly described in most standard works as the fascia superficialis.

However, more precise anatomical investigations make it clear that even with the classical, tough, superficial fascia such as the fascia lata or the fascia lumbodorsalis, there is no predominance of 'irregular' fibre alignment, but a clearly describable architecture of differently arranged layers (Barker, Briggs 1999; Barker et al. 2006; Fourie 1997; Stecco et al. 2007). Furthermore, these investigations also showed that even with the cited classical fascia, a clear delimitation of the other seamlessly joined fibrous connective tissue in the real body (as opposed to that shown in an anatomy book) makes only little sense; for example, their transitions to joint capsules, tendon plates, retinacula,

muscle septa, rotator cuffs, nuchal ligaments, intramuscular perimysium, periosteum, etc.

Against this background and with regard to the tensegrity architecture described in the next section, the term fascia has been increasingly used in a more comprehensive manner since the First International Fascia Research Congress in 2007. In congruence with the Latin origin of the word (*fascia*: alliance, bundle, association, merging) all fibrous collagenous connective tissue is described as coherent fascial tissue. This forms a network surrounding and penetrating the whole body and all the organs which is distinguished by a complex branching 'bag in bag' packaging structure (Myers 2005). The manifold septa, surrounding tangle of fibres, the ligamental or capsular bands, the superficially strengthened tendon plates, etc. are nothing more, according to this model, than local adjustments of a connected network for specific local traction loading. Even the thinner intramuscular connective tissue sacs (such as the endomysium surrounding each individual muscle fibre) and the meninges and the perineurium belong to this fascial network just as much as the visceral specialisations of the peritoneum, mesenterium, mediastinum or pleura.

In the following, therefore, all collagenous, fibrous connective tissue structure are described as fascial tissue (First International Fascia Research Congress 2007, Glossary of terms, http://fasciacongress.org/2007/glossary.htm). This comprehensive definition of the term fascia covers as far as possible what lay people understand by 'connective tissue', while in medicine all tissue originating from embryonic mesenchyma belongs to connective tissue, including bones, cartilage and fatty tissue.

http://dx.doi.org/10.1016/B978-0-7020-4312-3.00009-X

9.2 BIOMECHANICAL FUNCTION

In the conventional kinesiological model, it is accepted that contracting muscle fibres transfer their power to the bones directly via their tendons. However, as the research by Huijing and colleagues shows, a significant transfer of power also takes place via the intra- and extramuscular fascial sac (Huijing et al. 2007). This explains how very different traction strengths in a muscle can often be measured at the same time at its origin and insertion and that a mechanical transfer of power also takes place on antagonistic muscle groups. The contribution of the fascia to biomechanics is further reflected in current biomechanical model calculations which attribute a significant role in the stabilisation of the back and in the human gait to the fascia lumbodorsalis (Barker et al. 2007; Zorn 2007).

According to the tensegrity concept popularised by Buckminster-Fuller, fixed struts are attached and harnessed in a complex harness network so that these strut elements do not touch each other anywhere and the connections are made only by the harnessing elements (Myers 2005) (Fig. 9.1). As such tensegrity models show a large dynamic malleability and a relative independence from gravity in contrast to classical stone-on-stone architecture, in biology the presence of tensegrity-similar models is used for the understanding of biomechanical structures to an increasing extent (Chen, Ingber 1999). The fascia network as a global tensioning network evidently appears to support a stability of the human body similar to tensegrity. Instead of defining

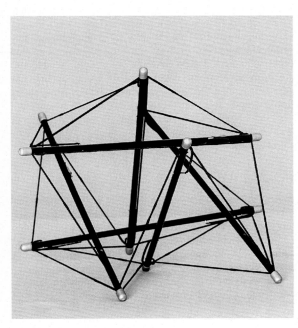

Fig. 9.1 Tensegrity model.

the skeleton as a piece of support apparatus (which, like a clothes stand, bears the rest of the body and serves as a support that remains stable under compression), the bones are increasingly seen in recent concepts as islands floating in the ocean that is the global tension network (Levin 2002; Myers 2005). In this, the global fascia network specialising in tensile strength therefore plays a supportive role for the body structure (Rolf 1997b).

Interestingly, there are no limited local changes in such a tensegrity network. Each change of an individual element also works continuously on the positioning of all other elements. This architectonic correlation possibly offers itself as a suitable explanation for the frequent clinical observation according to which local disorders and local therapeutic interventions often lead to changes in distant body areas.

9.3 MUSCLE HARDENING (TAUT BANDS)

Fascia contain contractile connective tissue cells (myofibroblasts) which may contribute to stiffening of the tissue similar to smooth muscle (Schleip et al. 2006). In the medically described conditions Dupuytren's contracture (palmar fibromatosis) and frozen shoulder, a large proliferation of these cells can in the long term also cause fascial contractures, which can lead to chronic taut bands with the aid of matrix remodelling. This tendency to contraction of the fascia is evidently strengthened in an acidic tissue milieu and by messenger material associated with inflammation in the body (Pipelzadeh, Naylor 1998).

According to the unanimous opinion of almost all medical researchers, the muscles are inactive and electrically 'silent' when people are resting (Basmajian 1978). Nevertheless, local muscle hardening can often be found. This is primarily observed in the so-called tonic muscle groups, as in the upper trapezius, the calf muscles or on the back of the thigh (Janda 2000). Taut bands are also to be found in trigger points.

It is accepted that resting muscle tone (passive stiffness) is primarily determined by the viscoelastic properties of the myofascial tissue (Simons, Mense 1998). Titin protein plays a significant role in this intramuscularly, although – as recent research has shown – mainly only in the phasic and less in the tonic muscle fibres (Linke, Leake 2005). It is therefore supposed that the tendency of tonic muscles to increased passive stiffness is associated predominantly with their fascial elements. Interestingly, increased myofibroblast density has been found in the perimysium (i.e. in the intramuscular fascia layer which surrounds the muscle fibre bundles, in which most of the intramuscular nerves and blood vessels run as well). As the tonic muscles have available an especially pronounced perimysium, this gives rise to the supposition that the increased resting stiffness of tonic muscles stems primarily from their perimysial fascia. A similar mechanism could possibly play a role in areas of taut bands around the trigger points as well. Both suppositions have however not been confirmed at the present time.

9.4 FASCIA AS A SENSORY ORGAN

Starting from the number of sensory nerve endings, the fascia network is our most extensive sensory organ on the basis of the above definition of fascia (perimysium, endomysium, subcutis, periosteum, etc.) (Mitchel, Schmidt 1977). There are a number of mechanosensory receptors within the fascia, which are used for proprioception and interoception. These fascial receptors are usually divided into four types: Golgi receptors, Ruffini endings, Paccini receptors and free nerve endings. Among the numerous free nerve endings there are about the same number with a low inflammatory threshold as with a high mechanical inflammatory threshold.

Not all free nerve endings are considered as nociceptors these days; a considerable percentage are non-nociceptive mechanoreceptors. With inflammatory processes and chronic pain, cytokines are distributed in the activated peripheral region (e.g. SP, CGRP, NGF), which leads to sensitisation of the nociceptors. This can lead to the same mechanical stimulation previously not experienced as painful and afterwards to definite pain distribution in the bone marrow and a definite pain reaction.

As on the one hand the muscle spindles are the only muscle receptors that are located within muscle fibre tissue and not in the intramuscular fascia network, and on the other hand stimulation of muscle spindles does not lead directly to pain, it should be accepted that a local cause of muscle pain is distributed predominantly by free fascial nerve endings. An examination of the lumbar fascia in 24 people with chronic back pain showed – contrary to expectations – that these fascia had virtually no sensory receptors, in contrast to the situation in people with healthy backs (Bednar et al. 1995). There are possibly parallels here to phantom pain and tinnitus for which a connection has been shown between a lack of real peripheral sensory stimulation and an associated erroneous process in the associated cortical area.

If that is the case, the presence of an interaction between fascial proprioceptive impoverishment and cortical malprocessing fits well with the recorded findings of reduced lumbar proprioception in patients with back pain. This would also support the supposition that manual therapy (or needle-induced) stimulation of the fascial mechanoreceptors leads to a reorganisation of pathologically changed central pain perception and is therefore suitable for avoiding or reducing chronic muscle pain.

9.5 RELATION TO TRIGGER POINTS: THERAPEUTIC CONSIDERATIONS

These findings on the muscular fascial network suggest the following applications in relation to trigger points: pain sensations caused by trigger points supposedly originate mostly from fascial receptors which have undergone sensitisation. A possible treatment plan is the therapeutic stimulation and proprioceptive sensitisation of other fascial receptors (preferably in the area belonging to the same cortical area). Fascial changes supposedly also play a key role in changed muscle stiffness in the area around a trigger point as well. For acupuncture at least it has been shown that fascial connective tissue cells can also be structurally influenced with this method (Langevin et al. 2006). It suggests that such a chain of effect between therapeutic stimulation and fascial cell function can also be sought around a trigger point with regard to changed passive muscle stiffness as well.

Chapter | 10 |

Fibromyalgia syndrome

Martin Offenbächer

10.1 EPIDEMIOLOGY

Fibromyalgia syndrome and mTrP frequently exist together. The principles, diagnosis and therapy of fibromyalgia syndrome are also known to any trigger point therapist.

- Population studies have shown that 20–25% of the population suffers from regional musculoskeletal pain.
- Chronic widespread pain (or chronic multilocular musculoskeletal pain) has a frequency of 10–11%.
- Both forms of pain are more commonly found in women (ratio 1.5:1).
- The prevalence of fibromyalgia according to the criteria (chronic widespread pain plus 11 out of 18 positive tenderpoints) of the American College of Rheumatology (ACR) of 1990 is reported to be about 2% of the population.
- Fibromyalgia affects mainly women (ratio about 8:1).
- In general medical practice up to 4% are fibromyalgia patients, in rheumatological practices almost one in five patients suffers from fibromyalgia.

Fibromyalgia and chronic widespread pain have an effect on capacity to function, state of health and a patient's capacity for work, as well as making high demands on the health services.

10.2 THE PATIENT'S PATTERN OF SYMPTOMS

Symptoms of fibromyalgia are:

- pain,
- sleep disorder,
- tiredness,
- muscle stiffness,
- psychological symptoms.

Other commonly occurring symptoms are:

- sensory disorders such as a burning sensation,
- tingling or the feeling that the limbs are swollen (differential diagnosis of neuropathy),
- problems with concentration or capacity for awareness,
- headaches (differential diagnosis of tension headaches/migraine),
- irritable bowel (differential diagnosis of irritable colon),
- irritable bladder,
- tendency to hypertension,
- high resting pulse,
- reduced ability to withstand stress.

10.2.1 Investigation

- **Pain:** changing location throughout the locomotor apparatus; made worse by physical exercise,

http://dx.doi.org/10.1016/B978-0-7020-4312-3.00010-6

monotonous or forced postures (even sitting, lying down, standing) and other factors (e.g. stress, cold weather); relieved by warmth and a good night's sleep.

- **Sleep disorder:** difficulty getting to sleep or sleeping through (waking several times because of pain and restlessness), not refreshed in the morning.
- **Tiredness:** tiredness during the day, state of exhaustion (is often felt to be more stressful than pain).
- **Muscle stiffness:** persisting for minutes up to hours (also after sitting for a long time).
- **Psychological symptoms:** depressive mood, anxiety, stressful life events, psychosocial stress factors.

10.2.2 Inspection and physical examination

- The inspection is unproductive.
- The clinical evaluation should include the whole locomotor apparatus and a basic medical and neurological examination.
- Patients with fibromyalgia exhibit positive, i.e. painful, tenderpoints on palpation of typical sites (according to the ACR criteria) (see Fig. 10.1, Table 10.1).
- Muscle shortening and incorrect posture as well as excessive dermographism/dermatographic urticaria are frequent clinical findings.

> Besides the positive tenderpoints, fibromyalgia patients usually have a lowered tenderness threshold, i.e. patients report pain as a result of light pressure on palpation even away from the tenderpoints. This phenomenon does not rule out the diagnosis of fibromyalgia.

10.2.3 Laboratory tests

A standard medical rheumatological laboratory test will give the first indications of the presence of possible differential diagnoses (erythrocyte sedimentation rate (ESR), blood count, thyroid hormones, electrolytes, parathormones, antinuclear antibodies, C-reactive protein, rheumatoid factor and creatinine kinase).

The laboratory chemistry and machine-aided diagnosis is normal if fibromyalgia syndrome is present. At the beginning of the disease this serves for further investigation of a differential diagnosis or to rule out or find comorbidities in later stages of fibromyalgia as well.

Peripheral pain generators should be identified both clinically and from the history. These include arthritis (e.g. coxarthritis and gonarthritis), vertebral column syndrome (e.g. scoliosis, spinal canal stenosis, lumbar spine syndrome with or without radiculopathy), mTrP, inflammatory joint disease, neuropathy, hypermobility, migraine, enthesopathy, irritable colon.

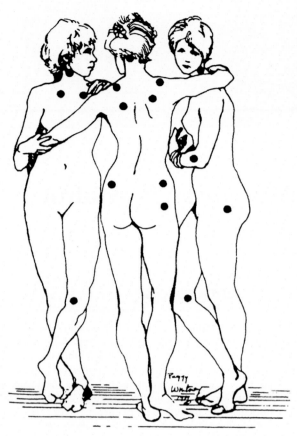

Fig. 10.1 Localisation of tenderpoints in fibromyalgia according to the criteria of the ACR (from Wolfe et al. 1992) visualised by using 'The Three Graces' by Jean Baptiste Reynault (1793), Louvre, Paris.

Some 15–25% of patients have sleep apnoea syndrome. An even higher percentage exhibit restless leg syndrome. If there is any suspicion, appropriate investigations and therapy should be carried out.

10.3 DIAGNOSIS

The diagnosis of fibromyalgia is based on the ACR criteria of 1990. These are as follows.

- **History of generalised pain.** Definition: spontaneous pain in the muscles, along the tendons and tendon insertions typically located on the trunk and/or the extremities or the jaw region which have been present for at least 3 months at three or more different parts of the body above and below the waist.
- **Evidence of pain at 11 out of 18 tenderpoints on manual palpation.** Definition: palpation with the

Table 10.1 Tenderpoints in fibromyalgia	
Occiput	Insertion sites of the suboccipital muscles
Lower neck	Intertransversal spaces C5–C7
M. trapezius	In the middle between the insertion of the neck and the acromion
M. supraspinatus	Middle part over the spina scapulae
Second rib	Cartilage bone border
Lateral epicondyle	2 cm distal from the epicondyle
Gluteal region	Upper lateral quadrant of the gluteal region (over the lateral margin of the gluteus maximus muscle)
Greater trochanter	Posterior to the trochanteric prominence
Knee	Medial fat pad proximal to the medial knee joint space

fingers should be performed with a strength of about 4 kg/cm^2. A tenderpoint is assessed as positive if the patient reports that palpation is painful. 'Sensitive' does not necessarily mean painful. The tenderpoints can be found at defined symmetrical anatomical locations (see Table 10.1).

10.3.1 Differential diagnosis

If there is any clinical suspicion of a number of other diseases, these must be ruled out to exclude any differential diagnoses. These include:

- inflammatory diseases caused by pathogens (particularly hepatitis, borreliosis (Lyme disease), human immunodeficiency virus),
- inflammatory rheumatic disease (e.g. chronic polyarthritis, seronegative spondyloarthropathy, collagenosis, myositis, vasculitis, polymyalgia rheumatica),
- non-inflammatory diseases, particularly thyroid function disorders, neoplasia or myopathy.

Overlapping/features in common with fibromyalgia: symptoms with depression, chronic fatigue syndrome, somatoform pain disorders, irritable colon and multiple chemical sensitivity. The demarcation is often difficult.

10.4 TREATMENT

10.4.1 General

The guidelines for fibromyalgia syndrome were adopted in 2008 with the cooperation of some of the authors of this book (M. Offenbächer, D. Irnich, A. Winkelmann) and accepted by the Association of the Scientific Medical Societies (AWMF) in Germany. They can be found on the AWMF website (www.awmf.org/).

Effective treatment of patients with fibromyalgia requires a biopsychosocial approach. It is the physician's job to arrange management with the patient based on this approach.

Successful long-term management of this chronic disease requires:

- building a workable partnership between patient and physician/therapist,
- support for the patient in becoming an expert in the daily management of his/her symptoms,
- support for the patient in understanding his/her symptoms. Symptoms often have several causes so the therapy is variable as well.

Another important factor is that both patient and doctor agree on a therapeutic course of action (shared decision-making).

There are general guidelines which should be taken into account in the treatment of fibromyalgia:

- safe diagnosis and identification of concomitant diseases,
- the disease must be explained to the patient and his/her family,
- individual treatment of each patient as there is no specific therapy which will help each person to the same extent,
- avoidance of unnecessary diagnostic measures or operations.

Advice for the patient plays an important role in treatment. Important aspects of an education programme are:

- explanation about the non-destructive nature of the disease,
- focus on improvement of function and not on healing,
- formulation of realistic treatment aims as patients often have expectations that are too high,
- discussion of medical and non-medical therapeutic options,
- introduction to self-help (e.g. instructions on the use of physical measures),
- evidence of a significant connection between soma psyche (e.g. instruction in meditation and/or relaxation techniques),
- instruction on sleep hygiene,
- explanation of the need for lifelong gentle physical stamina training,

- emphasis on the importance of the active role of the patient in the management of treatment,
- advice on planning a balanced day (alternating phases of exercise and relaxation).

10.4.2 Medical treatment

The medical treatment possibilities for fibromyalgia are limited.

- Low-dose tricyclic antidepressants (e.g. amitriptyline 25 mg at night); aim: improved sleep and influence on the pain threshold, side effects even at low dosage; the effect is often lost after a year.
- Analgesics: simple analgesics (favourable risk–benefit profile); NSAIDs are of limited clinical benefit.

10.4.3 Non-medical treatment

Stamina training

Eighty per cent of fibromyalgia patients are physically unfit, 83% do not carry out any regular physical exercise, 29% do not reach the anaerobic threshold. It is a vicious circle of pain–inactivity–deconditioning. Regular endurance/stamina training is associated with a positive outcome for fibromyalgia.

Practical considerations/instructions on performing endurance training:

- the aim should be to improve function, not to reduce pain,
- at the beginning, there is often an increase in pain and tiredness as possible evidence of training too hard,
- begin with gentle interval training in order to keep the increase in pain low after training, the patient should feel: 'I could have done more,'
- patients should increase training slowly up to three to four times a week; the aim should be achieved in 6–12 months,
- training should involve little stress on the joints (e.g. ergometer training, walking or aquarobics),
- minimisation of eccentric muscle work during training in order to reduce microtrauma in the muscles and nociceptive stimulation,
- group training stimulates compliance and provides positive feedback,
- additional regular exercise programme at home is necessary, including muscle extension/stretching, light strength and endurance training,
- regular training should become part of life.

Physiotherapy

Practical instruction/aspects of physiotherapy

- avoid strain at work and in everyday life,
- look out for incorrect posture and hypermobility; this leads to muscle strain, increase in tiredness and myofascial pain,

- a strained muscle system leads to further pain and stiffness,
- economic sitting–standing–lying down,
- poor sleeping position (e.g. hyperflexion of the neck) can trigger pain in the shoulder and neck girdle; recommendation: anatomically shaped neck pillow,
- strengthen deconditioned muscles: ideally as part of cardiovascular fitness training,
- instructing the patient with regard to eccentric and concentrated muscle work,
- muscle extension: daily programme for all large muscle groups and particularly shortened muscles, 5–15 min,
- use of heat application when necessary (tense muscles) using, e.g., hot bath, shower, volcanic mud,
- avoidance of inactivity and planning of regular rest breaks in the course of the day.

Physical measures

- Massage and underwater massage: some patients react with an increase in pain at too high an intensity (lymph drainage is then better).
- Heat therapy in any form (e.g. mudpacks, sauna, steam bath).
- Other procedures: Stanger (hydroelectric) bath, carbonated baths and Kneipp (cold water) drench.
- Cold chamber exposure: some patients feel some pain reduction in the short term.

> The patient can carry out many of these procedures by himself/herself. **Warning:** avoid creating a passive role for the patient!

Psychotherapeutic procedures/relaxation techniques

- Psychotherapeutic procedures for overcoming pain and disease with appropriate stress.
- Use of relaxation techniques (e.g. autogenic training or progressive Jacobsen relaxation); see also Ch. 24.

10.4.4 Other possibilities for treatment

Acupuncture

- There is a lack of quality studies.
- However, it appears that acupuncture has a significant effect on pain and the pain threshold.
- The long-term effect and type of optimum treatment (point combination and frequency) are unclear.

Tai chi and Qigong

- Tai chi or Qigong with the aim of increasing body awareness.

Trigger point injections

- Fibromyalgia patients have a number of predominantly 'inactive' mTrPs.
- Few have symptomatic mTrPs requiring treatment.
- The reaction to an mTrP injection is delayed in fibromyalgia patients and pronounced and more persistent than in patients with MPS, especially with dry needling.
- No more than three to four trigger points should be treated per session.
- Follow-up treatment programme (e.g. muscle extension, heat applications, massage) is important.

Transcutaneous electrical nerve stimulation (TENS)

- An attempt at treatment is sensible for localised pain.

Multidisciplinary therapy integrating the above measures in a balanced programme is most likely to be successful in the treatment of fibromyalgia.

Chapter | 11 |

Myofascial trigger points and somatoform pain

Francisco Pedrosa Gil

11.1 INTRODUCTION AND CLINICAL SIGNS

For many centuries, 'somatic disorders' have received a number of overlapping diagnoses. For example, 'generalised syndromes' have been described using the terms 'autonomic dystonia', 'neurasthenia', 'Briquet syndrome' and 'nervous symptoms', among others, in association with a number of differing and varying organ symptoms, exhaustion and sleep disorders. Other terms such as 'functional syndrome' (so-called organ neurosis with functional respiratory, cardiac, joint and muscle pain, among others) and 'pain syndrome' (for example, psychogenic head and back pain) are of significance here.

These disorders are listed as follows in the *International Classification of Diseases*, 10th edition (ICD-10, ch. V (F); Dilling et al. 1991):

- F45.0 Somatisation disorder,
- F45.1 Undifferentiated somatoform disorder,
- F45.3 Somatoform autonomic dysfunction,
- F45.4 Persistent somatoform pain disorder.

For all these disorders there is repeated presentation of physical symptoms together with persistent requests for medical tests, in spite of negative test results and assurance by the physician that the physical symptoms are not the result of an underlying physical disease (see ICD-10, Dilling et al. 1991). An inclusion criterion for somatoform pain disorder (F45.4) in the ICD-10 is the presence of continuous and persistent severe and stressful pain in one part of the body which has lasted for a minimum of 6 months (chronicity criterion), which cannot be adequately explained by evidence of a physical disorder. This remains the main focus of the patient's attention.

Psychosocial stress factors (emotional stress, psychological conflict) must also be diagnosed if they occurred close to the time the pain symptoms began. This evidence often emerges only in the course of psychotherapy. This is why a patient's statement that 'everything is fine' should always be questioned when taking a psychosocial history.

These 'pain diseases' also demonstrate a series of additional complications: secondary physical damage can occur as a result of pharmacological and surgical treatment, increased physical inactivity, and conflict with medical and nursing staff and subsequent discontinuation of treatment. In addition, there is an effect on the patient's feeling of self-worth, which may resolve into depressive–affective symptoms.

11.2 EPIDEMIOLOGY

According to studies, prevalence is approximately 5–7% in general medical practice and up to 25–30% in interdisciplinary pain clinics in university hospitals; 'persistent somatoform pain disorder' can occur in up to 40% of patients with chronic pain. Women are more frequently affected, in a ratio of 2–3:1. The most common locations are the extremities, the face area and the lower abdomen.

11.3 AETIOLOGY AND PATHOGENESIS

Evidently, psychosocial stress factors in childhood and adolescence predispose to the later development of somatoform pain disorder (Egle et al. 1998). From a psychodynamic point of view, disorders of early bonding behaviour

http://dx.doi.org/10.1016/B978-0-7020-4312-3.00011-8

are encountered where the infant's/small child's primary need to bond is inadequately met by the primary person to whom they relate emotionally (such as the mother). This can happen in the form of emotional disinterest or in the sense of excessive restriction of curiosity, but physical or sexual mistreatment are also significant risk factors which are empirically well covered elsewhere (Egle et al. 2000). Scarinci et al. (1997) showed, for example, that the pain threshold in the childhoods of traumatised women with various gastrointestinal disorders was definitely lower than that of non-traumatised patients.

In the aetiopathogenesis the combination of physical pain experiences and affective conditions in childhood and adolescence is usually therefore of great significance. For example, the patient reaches back unconsciously to the 'pain model' from childhood and the primary family when locating pain symptoms. However, current psychosocial stress situations (such as accidents) and/or 'inner conflict situations' in adults are also important factors of influence (see Fig. 11.1). These so-called life events (stressful life events) can then be the cause of the pain; real or imaginary loss or illness are possible causes.

mTrP can be asymptomatic or can be found in patients with somatoform disorders as well as 'pain carriers'. In the end, we cannot explain to what extent patients with somatoform disorders suffer from myofascial pain. In fibromyalgia syndrome – depending on the test – mTrPs can be identified in up to 100% of patients (see Ch. 13).

As this pain is predominantly chronic, it is often difficult to work out when it started. However, we can usually assume that mTrP as a symptom comes to the fore slowly and gradually, particularly if the patient complains of pain in the locomotor system.

It is certainly difficult to regard mTrPs and particularly persistent symptoms as an expression of a mental disorder. A key piece of evidence is whether mTrPs frequently change locality and severity.

11.4 DIFFERENTIAL DIAGNOSIS

There is evidence of a somatoform pain disorder if:

- the anatomical margins of sensory supply are not met (for example, with intervertebral disc pain of a radicular character),
- the location and type and intensity of pain vary or sometimes the description of the pain is vague,
- the pain begins in a specific locality and spreads widely,
- the pain is intense and there are no intervals free of pain.

Carrying out a differential diagnosis of a somatoform pain disorder is recommended as part of a close interdisciplinary cooperation between the individual specialisms. The biopsychosocial model of pain understanding serves as the basis

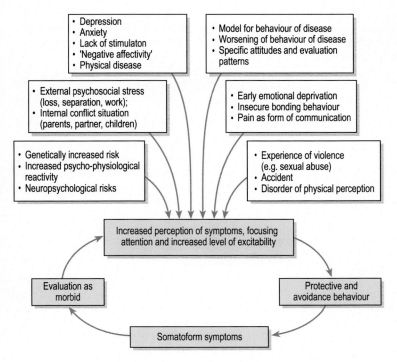

Fig. 11.1 Model for the occurrence of somatoform disorders. *(Modified from Rief, Hiller 1992)*

for all those involved (Uexküll et al. 1986). It is of great importance not to convey to the patient specific (chance) findings and deviations from the norm as the cause. The psychosomatic diagnostic investigation should be given the same standing as a medical or neurological investigation. A careful psychosomatic diagnosis should also made as quickly as possible, particularly with patients who have had pain for a long time (3–6 months).

11.5 THERAPY

When dealing with this patient group, it is important to be sympathetic and to take the pain seriously, as with those patients where an organic cause can be found. Avoid a reproduction of the parent–child relationship in the physician–patient one, and especially avoid placing further emphasis on the physical symptoms. This can frequently lead to often far-reaching indications for operations (sometimes repeated invasive tests as well) with subsequent iatrogenic 'physical damage' (Egle et al. 2000). If the patient's lifestyle is largely determined by the restrictions caused by the pain, it is important that the primary medical intervention avoids at least further spread of these restrictions. For the above reasons, a psychotherapy route is the first choice, particularly in view of the frequently present bonding difficulties with psychological trauma. Further recommendations are:

- relaxation techniques should also serve as part of the multimodal inpatient therapy programme to promote the motivation for psychotherapy (see Ch. 24),
- good treatment results can be covered in symptom-related therapy groups (Egle et al. 1992),
- individual psychotherapy should be used for patients who are not suitable for group therapy.

Indications for inpatient treatment in a psychosomatic department can be:

- significant misuse of analgesics or other drugs,
- frequent absence from work or inability to work,
- where there seems little point in sending the patient for outpatient psychotherapy, as the patient cannot perceive the link between psychological problems and pain symptoms.

There is evidence of mTrPs in many patients with somatoform pain disorder. Effective treatment of the myofascial pain should not be withheld from the patient. However, it is a prerequisite that you make clear to the patient that this may be only a concomitant symptom and that the underlying somatoform disorder is the priority.

Medical treatment (antidepressants, particularly amitriptyline and clomipramine) is really only indicated if the criteria of a depressive disorder are also fulfilled. On the other hand, in the last few years there has also been occasional positive evidence from meta-analyses of placebo-controlled studies on the efficacy of antidepressive medication for somatoform pain disorders (O'Malley et al. 1999). There is no indication for analgesic use.

mTrPs should always be treated as well, as they may be the structure which gives expression to the pain. Non-invasive procedures can be offered here (particularly manual therapies), as well as methods which influence the overall regulation of the autonomic system (for classical natural remedies see Ch. 23; for acupuncture see Ch. 22; for relaxation techniques see Ch. 24).

11.6 ASSESSMENT OF ABILITY TO WORK

The medical examination to diagnose inability to work or examination of somatoform (pain) disorders includes not only the diagnostic classification but rather crucially the manner and extent of the concrete symptoms and the progress with the question of chronification, psychiatric co-morbidity and course of the disease over several years, or failed rehabilitation measures. The psychological or psychopathological symptoms and the resulting actual concrete effects can then be assessed (Schneider et al. 2001), for example by using the Schepank (1995) impairment score. The effects on social communicative associations are also described as well as the level of physical and psychological suffering and/or impairment.

Chapter | 12 |

Integrated holistic consideration of the muscles

Nicolas Behrens

12.1 INTRODUCTION

The aim of this chapter is to provide a comprehensive, in-depth understanding of the nature of muscles and people with muscular disorders and symptoms.

> The muscles are not just necessary for posture and movement; they are also an important sensory organ and an organ of expression. They therefore also help with (self) awareness and behaviour.

We almost never use one muscle in isolation. It is not until we form an intention to act that a complex pattern of motor function is activated in the premotor cortex. We are unconscious of the ways in which agonistic, cocontracting muscles up to whole muscle function chains and antagonistic muscles work together. Bigger movements affect the whole body – basic tone, autonomic function, cardiovascular system, respiration, etc. – and can influence 'mood' and attitude to life. We try to describe this comprehensive view of humans with terms such as 'biological', 'psychological' and 'social'. The categories used suggest, however, that they are easily separated, which is does not do justice to the simultaneousness and unity of the physical and spiritual reality of a human being. The body is not 'a thing of itself' (Buytendijk 1957). We are moved by 'spiritual stirrings'. Feelings and meanings which we attribute to things and events lead to intentions that are the origin of all movements. These movements 'move' us mentally or spiritually at the same time. One example is the improvement in depressive mood resulting from

exercise or successful acupuncture and the fact that our outer bearing reflects our current and basic mental attitudes.

A predominantly mechanistic manner of looking at the muscles can be sensible and helpful for the treatment of acute problems in otherwise healthy people; such as sports injuries or after a simple strain.

With therapy-resistant symptoms we must understand that spiritual problems and relationship and behavioural disorders are also reflected in muscle disorders and pain. Such disorders are also accessible to therapy via the muscles. The type and distribution of muscular disorders can provide valuable guidelines for somatopsychological access to the whole person.

If persistent muscular disorders or chronic pain are an expression of a disturbed attitude to oneself, to others or to life, it is sensible for the long-term success of the treatment to address and treat this attitude. This requires a therapist (in the team) who is also capable of and prepared for 'relationship medicine', to meet and treat the patient on a relationship level. The feeling of being accepted, considered and understood does not happen just as a result of verbal contact; it also requires careful touch and movement. This direct, physical approach is not just more immediate and genuine; it also corresponds to our first experiences of handling and healing from early childhood. It can help patients to recover from stress, high tension, overexertion or 'flight' from oneself or from reality and form new, 'real' experiences.

> For such a somatopsychological procedure, however, the patient must be prepared to agree to being physically 'touched' and mentally 'affected'. As generally applies to pain therapy, the patient must want to get better.

For severely traumatised patients, a great deal of trust is also required from the patient and experience on the part of the therapist. Even then strong or paradoxical reactions can occur.

In the muscle descriptions given later in this volume (see Chs 26–34) there is also advice on the possible significance of associations with individual muscles and muscle groups. These are the first experiences which must be added to other empirical and scientific investigations. An overall view of the patient at rest and in motion is essential.

12.2 FUNCTION AND PURPOSE OF THE MUSCLES

The skeletal muscles are a significant component of the human body by themselves. As a key component of the locomotor system, they should be regarded in functional connection with:

- bones: structure/stability,
- nerves: control/coordination,
- connective tissue:
  - transfer of power/connection (fixed connective tissue: tendons and capsules),
  - metabolism (soft connective tissue, the system of basic regulation together with the vessels and the autonomic nervous system).

Muscle is the element of the locomotor system which is capable of producing power: this means concentric contraction, but also eccentric loosening in the sense of stretching or giving way. It fulfils the following interconnecting and mutually interdependent functions or functional aspects.

12.2.1 Motor function

In complex movements, the following functional aspects engage closely with each other:

- (loco)motion: movement of body parts including moving forward/locomotion,
- dynamic control: centring of moved joints,
- static and dynamic stabilisation: safeguarding of joints or body regions that provide resistance during active movement.

The body always strives for optimally coordinated, whole-body cooperation of motion and postural functions which are as economic as possible. In a healthy person, movements are visibly harmonious, and the person finds it easy.

In the sick person, on the other hand, disorderly, disharmonious, 'tight' movements quickly become evident. They are felt as strenuous, unpleasant or even painful.

Harmonious, naturally flowing movements and relaxed muscles correlate with good health.

In humans, movement is not so much conquering the environment, fighting a battle or finding the energy, but more getting on with work, creating the environment, sport and play, as well as essential contact and relationships with other people. Correspondingly, other movement and stress patterns have developed.

Modern working patterns and daily life lead to a large number of non-physiological stresses. For example, working at a computer often makes little demand on or provides little exercise for the lower part of the body, while excessive demands are made on the shoulder and neck area. Add to this poor posture or a cramped position caused by external forces or the excessive demands which one might make on oneself, and taut bands with mTrPs are bound to occur.

12.2.2 Expression: communication

We can soon find parallels in everyday language between body tension and resulting attitude (to life): feeling washed out, being a bit lethargic, 'feeling tense' or being a bit slack. Body language forms an essential component of interpersonal communication. It goes beyond facial expressions or gestures; the whole body is used. We signal by means of our posture and our muscle tone whether, if, where and how we would like to be touched. Facing the person you are talking to with relaxed muscles is an invitation, while tense muscles or defensive actions are a dismissal.

By activating mirror cells in the premotor cortex (Bauer 2006) we are in a position to empathise using our own body with the person we are talking to. As these non-verbal signals both in the sender and in the receiver take place at an unconscious level, this is direct, genuine communication which is essential for forming relationships and for psychotherapy.

We can use the body language of our patient to unlock the available knowledge (e.g. Molcho 1983). However, we can also consciously imitate and reflect their posture and tension. Changing our own attitude and feelings can help us to feel 'from the inside' what is probably 'motivating' our patients.

12.2.3 Feelings

For our body perception (sensory perception, proprioception) the feedback from the many muscle spindles (and tendon receptors) is a key input. All in all, we can regard the latter as an almost whole-body sensory organ. It supplies us (that is, our CNS) with information on the length and tension of the individual muscles and their changes. This is how we perceive the position of individual body parts of themselves and in relation to each other and their movements (sense of position, strength and movement). We also consciously perceive our current body shape and the condition of our muscles (relaxed or tense).

> The joint muscles and the muscles close to the vertebral column in particular have many receptors which inform the brain of the position of the moving segments of the joint/vertebral column and the tension of the relevant muscles. This is important for efficient treatment: untreated trigger points in these 'sensor muscles' easily lead to recurrence. We must therefore ensure thorough, deep treatment, assuming we have sufficient anatomical knowledge.

12.2.4 Perception of ourselves in relation to the environment

The 'body image' held by the muscle sensors is, together with information from the vestibular organ, a prerequisite for remaining stable (upright) in the field of gravity and safely orientating ourselves and moving: our perception of ourselves in relation to the environment. The afferences (close to the atlanto-occipital joint) from the short neck muscles are of particular significance here, as they demonstrate an extreme abundance of proprioceptors. Scherer (1997) describes these neck receptors as an accessory sensory organ without which a person is incapable of life. Their purpose is not to maintain balance. In the interplay with the other neck muscles, they mainly allow us to keep our head and eye level horizontal and still, to enable us to see properly (see Ch. 27).

> Practical consequence: if the patient is suffering from dizziness, poor balance or visual disorders, examine and possibly treat the short muscles of the neck (atlanto-occipital joint region)!

There are numerous expressions which show us how essential the information from our muscles is for our perception of ourselves and the way our body feels: 'I feel so listless today', '. . .so tense', 'everything is such an effort', 'that makes me feel hemmed in, 'my heart is open'. We are conscious of this, whether it is pleasant or disturbing, when we are attentive but at rest, for example when meditating or during acupuncture treatment, but during pain as well.

Our feelings influence basic muscle tension directly or via a change in the sympathetic nervous system: an increase in the concentration of noradrenaline (norepinephrine) directly increases basic muscle tension. Anxiety (with the reaction 'I'm running away or protecting myself and holding out') as well as annoyance and brooding tend to lead to an increase in tension, while anxiety in the sense of a playing dead reflex or grief tend to lead to a reduction in tension. At the same time, these feelings can also be perceived via current muscle tension and changed feelings in the body.

Example: The widely reduced muscle activity of the lower trunk as a result of working at a desk leads to reduced perception of this area. According to Glaser® psychotonics, this represents grounded vitality or lust for life – the opposite to exaggerated thinking, pondering/brooding or even a depressive attitude. Back pain can therefore be more comprehensively treated for 'brain-workers' – after adequate pain therapy with loosening of hardened muscles throughout the trunk – by activating the underworked, little perceived lumbar spine region, and introducing an appropriate topic such as joy or pleasure into actions. Perception and attitude can be changed: pleasure in one's own strength and body instead of rest and anxiety. A similar procedure has been shown to be very effective in integrative back therapy programmes.

> According to Keidel (1994), people experience best through movement, with emotional perception of self and self-experience via exercise and appropriate changes in muscle tone.

In summary, we sense and express ourselves strongly via our locomotor system, especially the muscles, and this is quite different from the internal organs.

> *Man does not have a sense of the individual organs nor the individual muscles. Our experience of ourselves is neither through our organs nor through individual muscles, but through the body, particularly the outer layer, where disorders of the internal organs project themselves and emotions are perceived. (Body = living, animated body.) The so-called 'language of the organs' is therefore not a natural fact but a [voluntary] classification based on our [Western] mental approach. In this respect, using the body to find the person inside, especially if immediate therapy is possible, is a sensible part of a comprehensive treatment plan.'*
>
> (T. Ots, personal communication)

In acupuncture, trigger point and physical therapy, where the emotions and the basic attitudes to life are taken into account (see below), we therefore have a sensible, practicable 'somatopsychological' approach to psychosomatic symptoms, indeed the whole person, via our access from outside through the body, particularly through muscle tone.

The consideration of the meridians and emotions and basic attitudes to life embodied in acupuncture adds a helpful diagnostic and therapeutic aspect.

Experience shows that muscles are both a reservoir of emotions and experiences and a means of access to them. mTrPs can be regarded as the 'memory points' of the muscles, the peak of a 'peripheral' consciousness (see Gleditsch 2007).

12.2.5 Narrowing and widening

We can basically differentiate two poles of muscle tone: constriction correlates with unpleasant feelings, particularly anxiety, while relaxation is generally sensed as pleasant ('open-hearted').

Anxiety or fear can cause a life-saving flight reflex. In humans, unfortunately, this flight/escape reflex is often directed inwards. The resulting constriction is usually associated with withdrawal from surroundings and relationships. With internal escape – not wanting to be there – muscle tone tends to be slack. With a need for protection, our muscles can become rigid and strained like a suit of armour. This condition might be understood as withheld aggression as a result of or as compensation for an earlier injury (physical and/or mental), or even fear.

To distinguish between the emotions, it is worthwhile asking about feelings of fullness or tightness in the chest and the direction of pressure. Tightness, oppression, i.e. feeling of pressure from the outside in ('as if something is crushing me') correlates with anxiety/fear (angst; Latin: *angustus* = tight, narrow). A feeling of pressure from inside out ('bursting out of the skin') equates more with annoyance and repressed rage (Ots 2002).

Such restricted feelings, correlating with restrained feelings felt to be unpleasant or even threatening, can be regarded as a lack of trust, a negation of self and others and a resistance to life, or at least can result in this in the long term. Then life no longer 'flows'; nor does Qi feel as if it flows in the body.

Negative basic attitudes gained as a result of our upbringing or from (valued) observation and experience in the past often have a massive effect on our lives, putting them in 'context' or providing a 'set of beliefs' – loosely interpreted from Benjamin Franklin: 'We are not in reality prisoners, but we are imprisoned by our imagination and our values' – a self-constructed protection system which is physically manifested in tension and withdrawal and can lead to even more obdurate imprisonment. This applies particularly to pain. We can regard pain as a cry from the body for us to pay more attention to it, as a deficiency of life. This may be found in extreme form in borderline patients who scratch or cut themselves to feel better (as well as punishing themselves or getting rid of auto-aggressive feelings). Openness, on the other hand, is associated with being true to oneself, trust, being related, contributing, and accepting what is real: in the end a 'yes' to oneself, others, the world around you and life (= love).

The experience-based term sensorimotor amnesia (Hanna 2003) is interesting here in connection with the phenomenology of pain and the association of sensory and motor function. Hanna describes how there is often a reduced ability to perceive temperature (which can be extreme in fibromyalgia patients) or touch. At the same time, there is limited mobility – whether it is in the form of unused movement possibilities or caused by reduced perception (protection from criticism or pain?) – as a protective posture and/or the resulting tension and contraction.

Clinically, it is often difficult to say which came first (the pain and the protection or the muscle hardening?), just like the question of which came first: the chicken or the egg.

Consciousness of the body, even when induced by control of body sensation by handling, touching and exercising, acupuncture/dry needling or infiltration can be very helpful in making people who feel bad feel better, both in the sense of somatic awareness and mental sensation. This 'finding one's way back to physical reality' (in pleasant surroundings or contact) often immediately causes shortened ('pulled back'), hardened muscles with resulting better mobility.

12.3 APPROACH USING ACUPUNCTURE

Reflex-like muscle tension can be released in acupuncture treatment, allowing the Qi of traditional Chinese medicine (TCM) to flow freely again. This attitude explains the often surprising immediate effects of acupuncture, even via distal points, which is hard to understand using the usual neurophysiological views such as activation of gate control and descending inhibition. The essence of acupuncture is the 'Dao Qi', the control of the Qi, here understood as consciousness or awareness of the body and the resulting feeling of liveliness. By treating (healthy) points on the extremities, for example the hand for shoulder pain, the patient is invited to trace the area of the shoulder, where perception is reduced, back to the hand. Acupuncture (and trigger point therapy) can thus also be understood as body awareness training. Then if the patient is able to regain quality of life again after this loss of body awareness, the risk of recurrence is less. A prerequisite for the success of acupuncture or any mTrP therapy is a preparedness and capacity on the part of the patient to connect with the reality of the body and to be 'in the zone'.

Muscle hardening can often correspond to inner hardening, usually as a result of injury (depending on the patient's evaluation). At one stage this was a physical protection mechanism but now it restricts our physical and mental mobility, halts the flow of life and can even be visible in withdrawal postures (e.g. neck and chest), disrupted or tight movements which take up little space.

During the treatment of muscle hardening (taut bands), patients may find they make contact with previously suppressed feelings. It is as if these have been stored in the muscles (in their 'body therapy' Wilhelm Reich and Alexander Löwen spoke of 'feelings frozen in the muscles' or 'guarding postures') and can be released during treatment, within a suitable framework with a feeling of being safely and securely uplifted. Patients often shed tears, sometimes with, or sometimes without, specific memories. You could say that trigger points/acupuncture points function like a peripheral memory – 'the tissue remembers' (Gleditsch 2007) – and the experiences of decades can be stored in the muscles.

For the therapist lacking in psychotherapeutic experience, it is sensible to remain as quiet and calm as possible without touching the patient the first time that there is a deep reaction, to give the person space and, if possible, time to deal with the event without trying to control or influence it too much; possibly asking but not pushing too hard, 'just letting it flow'. Of course, patients who regularly react histrionically without a real change are an exception: other approaches are required here.

Practical tip: if a patient reports feeling cold (despite the room being warm enough), or is even shivering, and has a tight feeling as if experiencing pressure from outside, the patient is most probably suffering from anxiety/fear. It can be helpful to address this specifically.

The patient often feels better after such a cathartic reaction, as if relieved. If this is not the case, a further course of action should be discussed (in the team and with the patient). With old dreams and difficult relationships, it may be necessary to reappraise the past with the aim of changing attitudes and behaviour in the present. It would be sensible to arrange a consultation with a psychotherapist who is experienced with pain patients, and to integrate this into the treatment plan.

The aim of the treatment, if we are not dealing with a current physical or mental protection mechanism, is to loosen any tension and its implications. The visible and palpable findings here are also a good indicator for the course and success of the treatment. The ongoing course of treatment also indicates whether some protection may be required. A person needs to be more mellow, more active, looser, more in flow; to shape their life and become more capable of relationships; to be able to regulate their own quality of contact in terms of closeness and distance, and just be more alive to oneself and to reality.

If you treat pain patients more intensively and are confronted by appropriate mental aspects, you may need the support, for example, of a supervision group.

Chapter | 13 |

Diagnosis of myofascial pain

Nicolas Behrens, Dominik Irnich, Gunnar Licht, Hans-Joachim Schmitt

13.1 PRINCIPLES

Dominik Irnich

Recognising myofascial pain can be both very simple and very complex. One approach is the diagnostic procedure depending on the acuteness of the symptoms. If the pain in the locomotor system is acute with a definite pathomechanism in an otherwise healthy patient, such as an athlete with an accidental strain, it is sufficient to look for the mTrP. After taking a short history (see Questioning, Section 13.2) proceed with the diagnostic criteria described in Section 13.4 and commence treatment of any relevant mTrPs.

If the symptoms are chronic or recur frequently with pain and/or restricted mobility of the locomotor system, the above procedure is not enough. Right from the first contact, information must be gathered on any psychosocial chronification factors and matched to the individual model of the disease, and the doctor and patient work together to pursue further diagnosis and therapy.

> Overlooking any relevant psychosocial chronification factors is a professional error on the part of the doctor.

Reduction to the physical findings tends to lead to iatrogenic chronification (see Ch. 16). Under these conditions, detailed questioning at the first consultation (see Section 13.2) and a comprehensive physical examination (see Section 13.3) are essential. As this process is often not possible in everyday practice, questioning and physical examination can either be carried out in stages (e.g. several short 15 min appointments) or the patient can be seen at the end of consulting hours when the time pressure is not so great.

> Time invested at the initial appointment is repaid several times over.

Usually, the history alone provides valuable evidence for the presence of myofascial pain. Pay particular attention to how the problem started (e.g. strain), the quality of the pain (e.g. dull, throbbing), when the pain occurs (e.g. pain on exercise) and its location (e.g. pattern of radiation).

The detailed physical examination then represents the next important step. Initially, pay attention to the neuromusculo-articular unit; only after appropriate information has been gained should a differentiated examination of the muscles and their chains of function should be carried out.

The effect of a comprehensive physical examination on the formation of trust (building of a workable doctor–patient relationship) and as part of the therapy should not be underestimated. Frequently, the physical examination is sufficient to allay the patient's fears of a severe illness, which may even require an operation. In a time of increasing technical tests, the findings are often overvalued as the limits of pathology are ever more closely defined, so therapy through talking is an essential quality characteristic of good medicine.

Technical examinations (see Section 13.5) are only indicated if there is a definite query after the history has been

http://dx.doi.org/10.1016/B978-0-7020-4312-3.00013-1

taken and the physical examination has been performed. Even if it sometimes seems difficult, the wishes of the patient for further tests should only be met under these conditions, because studies show that the patient may well be more satisfied at first, but does not benefit in the long term from the non-selective use of technical tests. You may need to explain this to the patient.

Of course, an appropriate differential diagnosis for the findings and symptoms should be considered. Both an overestimation and an undervaluing of the myofascial findings can have long-term negative consequences for the course of the disease. This is why we recommend a procedure relating to both structure (see Section 14.1) and location (see Section 14.2) in case this should produce a differential diagnosis.

Making the diagnosis and drawing up an individual treatment plan (see Section 13.6) forms the preliminary conclusion of the first examination. If the diagnosis is related to structure and function, this produces not only clear advice for co-therapists, referrals, etc., but a clear treatment plan and at the same time a basis for taking an interim history and checking the findings.

13.2 QUESTIONING

Nicolas Behrens, Dominik Irnich

13.2.1 General instructions on history

The history can provide valuable information on the presence of MFS or at least a myofascial component of the symptoms; it may even limit the muscles which come into question. However, in the presence of varied symptoms it is hard to rule out MFS from the history. The history can also provide information leading to the consideration of a somatoform pain disorder or a neurological or systemic disease (see Ch. 14). Pain can usually be separated into acute, subacute or chronic. A distinction based solely on the duration of the pain is not reliable. The following question is helpful.

> Does the patient have pain (acute pain) or does the pain have the patient (chronic pain)?

It is all about understanding the pain. Acute pain has a physical warning and protection function, whereas chronic pain is usually the expression of a complex event and can have a warning function on another level from that of 'biological'. It can also be a symptom of a relationship problem (with oneself, with other people) or a life crisis. It is important to try to understand the patient fully (see Ch. 16). The Mainz study model of pain chronification provides important information on the extent of the chronification (Mainz Pain Staging System (MPSS) from Gerbershagen) (see Fig. 13.1).

The distinction between acute and chronic is important for the decision as to whether interventional therapy is sufficient or whether longer and more comprehensive biopsychosociomentally oriented treatment is required.

13.2.2 Practical tips

- Ask an open question to begin with ('What has brought you to me?') and allow the patient to talk for at least 2 min. After the examinations, time is needed to give the patient the feeling that the physician is taking the time to listen.
- When taking the history make sure that the situation is relaxed, undisturbed and comfortable (for the patient and for yourself).
- Try to gain an overall impression of the patient.
- Structure what has been said, if necessary; listen attentively without making a judgement.
- If the patient talks endlessly ('like a record') as if they cannot stop, and you are becoming restless or aggressive (counter transference), you should interrupt immediately and if possible change the level of the relationship. One possibility is to tell the probably latently aggressive patient that you yourself are becoming restless or annoyed, even though the patient is still calm. Then you could ask the patient whether they recognise this from other situations.
- Observe how the patient describes the symptoms: do pain and emotionality go together? What is the posture like? How does the patient seem: anxious, helpless, tense, restless or relaxed?
- Try to imitate the patient's posture as normally as possible. How do you feel? This can lead to a better understanding of the patient by means of your own body.
- The use of questionnaires and pain diaries can save time and improve understanding of the patient and their pain (some questionnaires can be found on the homepage of the DRK Pain Centre Mainz: www.dknp.de/cb/www/mediapool/pdf/gerbershagen.pdf) (see Fig. 13.1).
- Models or diagrams of the body in which the patient can draw their pain also help to make the diagnosis more accurate, especially if communication is difficult (see Fig. 13.2).
- Diagrams showing the main trigger points and their areas of radiation (e.g. trigger point tables in the *Trigger Point Manual*; Travell, Simons 2002) can be hung in the waiting room and may spark the patient's interest to look at them for themselves and save time by contributing essential information.

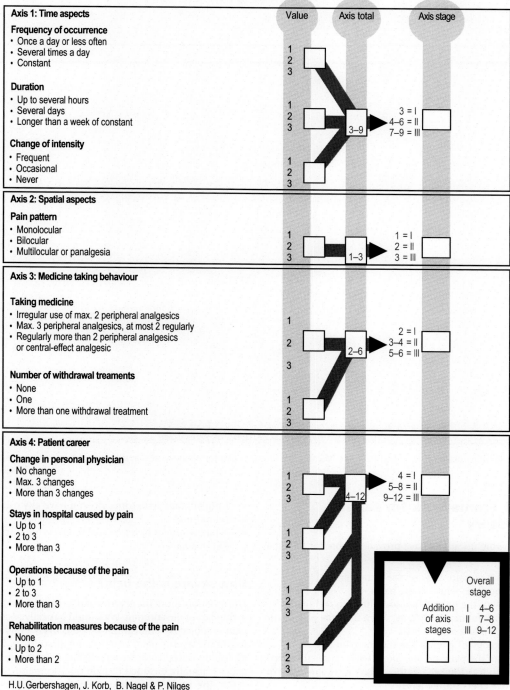

Fig. 13.1 The Gerbershagen pain questionnaire.

Please colour in **all** the areas of the following body diagrams where you have pain.

Please mark the whole pain area (by shading in with a pencil or ball point pen, or by colouring with a felt tip pen or text marker, etc) so that we know **all** the areas where you have pain.

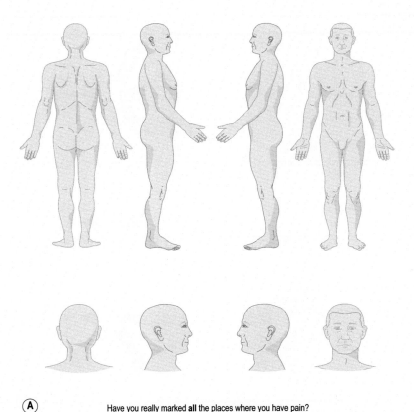

(A)   Have you really marked **all** the places where you have pain?

Fig. 13.2 (a) Body diagram, modified from the Mainz pain questionnaire for patients, also available to download (see text).

Continued

13.2.3 Framework for taking the history

The following questions have proved reliable for taking a comprehensive history:

- Intensity of pain: how severe is the pain?
- Pain location: where is the pain?
- Quality of the pain: what does the pain feel like?
- Times when the pain occurs: when does the pain occur and when is it at its worst?
- Chronology of pain: when did the pain first occur?
- Cause of the pain: do you know what causes the pain?
- Pain modulation: what is there that causes a negative or positive effect on the pain?
- Painful movements and movement restrictions: which movements are painful and which are difficult?

- Concomitant symptoms: do you have any other symptoms?
- What treatment have you had so far? What sort of effect did this have?

How severe is the pain?

The question about the severity of the pain should be asked at the start of questioning. We should basically assume that pain is subjective and cannot be objectively evaluated. To record the level of pain, visual analogue scales and numerical rating scales have proved reliable. At least one of these scales is usually included in pain questionnaires.

On the visual analogue scale the pain intensity is encoded using a length measurement (e.g. 10 cm: 0–10) with a slider (see Fig. 13.3). With numerical scales, the

Please colour in **all** the areas of the following body diagrams where you have pain.

Please mark the whole pain area (by shading in with a pencil or ball point pen, or by colouring with a felt tip pen or text marker, etc) so that we know **all** the areas where you have pain.

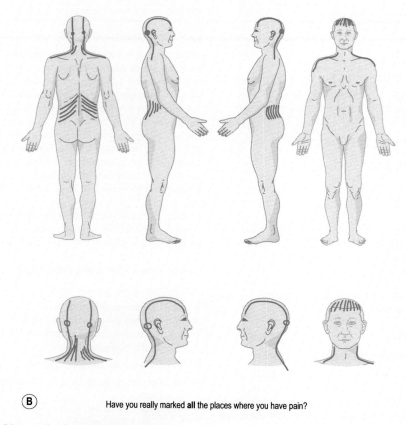

(B)   Have you really marked **all** the places where you have pain?

Fig. 13.2 cont'd—(b) Example of a body diagram filled in by a patient.

intensity can be directly read from the scale. A range of 0–10 has proved reliable. The value 0 corresponds to no pain while the value 10 is the maximum bearable pain.

Pain intensity should usually be tested as:

- pain at rest,
- pain on provocation (e.g. certain movements, cough),
- maximum pain strength,
- lowest pain strength,
- average pain strength.

Your own measurement of the strength of the pain – even in relation to supposed causes – must never be conveyed to the patient.

In some cases, the pain intensity should also be tested by the patient's use of a diary for a specified period of time. A diary is indispensable for the diagnosis and assessment of the progress of headaches in particular.

There should then be few further questions about the intensity of the pain during the course of treatment, as the aim of treatment is relief from pain, not to focus on it. A question about the percentage of pain improvement is sensible.

When it comes to patients with chronic pain we also recommend questioning to establish the extent to which the

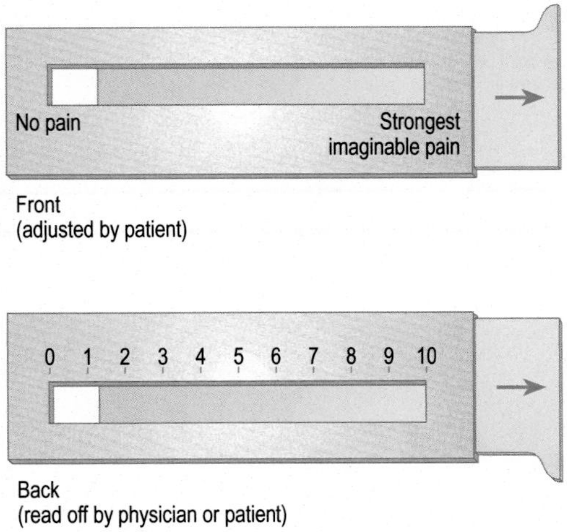

Front
(adjusted by patient)

Back
(read off by physician or patient)

Fig. 13.3 Visual analogue scale.
(From Bäcker, Hammes 2004)

patient accepts the pain. This is the level of pain which the patient is able to accept and tolerate and which can also be used to agree the aim of treatment. The definition of acceptance is helpful, especially with demanding patients, in order to counter any unrealistic expectations (e.g. freedom from pain after decades of back pain) and lessen pressure on the treatment situation.

Where is the pain?

Find out exactly where the pain is located

The location of the pain can give direct information on the affected muscles by following the typical pattern of distribution (see Chs 26–34). The pain areas drawn on the body diagram by the patient can be made more precise if necessary and it should be possible to attribute them to the anatomical landmarks.

Is a point or an area indicated?

This can indicate information for treatment.

- Points of pain are more easily treated at the point of the pain or at a defined trigger point, or by using Gross' contralateral technique (needling or infiltration on the exactly symmetrical other half of the body). The use of consensual reactions is often effective here as well.
- If there are several zones, it is helpful to enumerate these in order to clarify them: do you think for example pain 1 is associated with pain 2? Later on in the history you can then ask about the different pains.

Has the pain topography changed during the course of the disease?

It is possible that the pain has been spread by recruiting other mTrPs along their preferred muscle function chains.

It can also be caused by secondary disorders (such as poor posture) or by other separate disorders. A change in location can also be caused by an improvement in the underlying segmental function disorder, a prolapsed intervertebral disc or a nerve stimulation so that the remaining myofascial symptoms are then isolated.

Does the pain radiate into the extremities?

If the pain does radiate into the extremities, ask about the precise pattern of distribution and any possible neurological symptoms (changed sensitivity or motor function). The classification of sensory disorders (it is only possible for this to be precise if there is hypoalgesia; you must test peak sensation) is carried out according to the pattern of the dermatomes or the peripheral sensory innervations. If pain can be sensed both in the dermatome and in the associated myotome (dermatome and myotome of a spinal nerve can usually be distinguished by the location) it is often difficult to make a definite classification from the pain topography.

If the pain reaches as far as the fingers or toes, and especially if there are negative symptoms, a nerve compression or entrapment should be considered (see Section 14.2.2).

What does the pain feel like?

The following are typical of MPS:

- dull, pressing, dragging pain,
- deep-seated pain (rarely felt subcutaneously, usually muscular, sometimes even in the bones/joints or even inside the abdomen).

The following pain qualities can also occur:

- cramp-like pain, ranging from mild to strong or even agonising,
- burning, due to extremely severe cramping of the associated muscles,
- mTrPs of the muscles of mastication can project into the teeth, with pain as if the neck of the tooth has been exposed,
- less commonly trigger point pain can be felt in the form of neuralgia: sharp, stabbing or shooting pains, like a lightning flash. Very rarely, it can also occur in a form of dysaesthesia; sometimes with paraesthesia, or even in the form of allodynia (pain sensation on normal touch). If the patient reports this sort of pain, further questioning and a neurological examination are essential.

If the sensations resemble paraesthesia, dysaesthesia or numbness the extent of any neuropathic pain should be urgently investigated, so as not to delay any possibly required neurolysis.

When asking about the pain quality, include questions about the sensations and feelings associated with the pain. Examples of sensations include adjectives such as cramp-like, dragging, etc. Set against these must be the feelings used to evaluate the pain (tormenting, wearing down, dreadful, devastating, etc.). If the descriptions are predominantly affective (high affective pain evaluation), this is evidence of a severely emotional pain experience. If these components are in the forefront, this can indicate a somatoform pain component. The Geissler Pain Scale (Geissler 1992) helps to describe the ratio of sensation to affection.

When does the pain occur and when is it at its worst?

Does the pain come and go or is it there all the time? Is it always bad, or is it sometimes less painful? If the pain is there all the time at the same intensity, one must consider chronic pain with a high resistance to treatment. If it only occurs from time to time it is helpful to ask directly about the course of the pain during a typical day or week or to ask the patient to keep a diary. Ask about the pain on holiday as well.

If the pain is dependent on movement, ask the patient to demonstrate any movements which typically trigger the pain. It is also possible to differentiate between pain, weakness or strain which occurs during certain movements (strained agonists, typically in contracture) or whether the symptoms occur at the end of the range of movement with or without restricted movement (antagonist pain on extension). The precise reconstruction allows one to narrow down the muscles in question; more precise differentiation is then carried out by manual examination (see Section 13.3).

If symptoms are dependent on weight-bearing, it may be worth asking for a description of the place of work (e.g. with a photograph of patient at work; are the seating position and desk suitable?). Do symptoms occur at rest, such as at night, or in certain positions? Are the muscles affected those which frequently help to maintain posture?

If symptoms occur at night or in the morning in particular, ask about sleep quality and preferred sleeping position as well. You can also ask about the condition of the mattress and the pillows used. This can usually produce practical information for supportive measures. Is the patient known to bite hard or grind his teeth (it may be necessary to ask the partner), as this can be one of the causes of the symptoms and represents craniomandibular dysfunction (CMD); it can also be a cause of cervical spine problems.

When did the pain first occur?

In terms of both diagnosis and treatment, a pain which has only recently occurred for the first time is different from a pain which has existed for longer. It is worth questioning the patient very closely. Patients often report an acute start to the pain, but it is not uncommon for closer questioning to reveal that there have been several episodes of pain

already or that the problem has existed for longer than first reported. For problems in the area of the vertebral column, patients report pains that are associated with each other as unrelated and evaluate them separately (e.g. recent cervical spine symptoms, but lumbar spine symptoms for years). If this happens, you should ask why the patient has come to you now. This provides information on the disease model (how the patient explains the disease; see below) and the expectations of the patient.

If the pain starts as acute the patient will usually describe the cause (e.g. trauma such as a pulled muscle or strain) or at least the trigger (sometimes a relatively small injury to existing hardened or strained muscles).

If the pain began gradually, this indicates a chronic strain of the muscles (and the whole being) (see Ch. 12).

Do you know what causes the pain?

Ask about possible and supposed triggers. Depending on the location and the muscles that might be affected it may be possible to ask about specific triggers (see Chs 26–34). The following circumstances can often be found for the occurrence of mTrP:

- **Physical:**
  - strain while pursuing work, sport, a hobby, gardening, etc. (especially unaccustomed or unbalanced exercise or a long period of awkward posture),
  - a long period of immobilisation, such as after an operation or an accident,
  - illnesses (particularly viral infections), giving birth,
  - changes in habits (e.g. sleeping in a different place),
  - dental treatment (CMD),
  - change of medicine or hormones.
- **Psychological:** withheld feelings or trauma felt to be overwhelming such as fear, anger, grief caused by loss or death, attacks, phobia, depression, stress, demand (e.g. as a result of professional/financial situation), etc. How did the patient react?
- **Social:** workplace situation, relationship with family, partner, friends (watch out for systemic associations).
- **Mental:** life crisis, new phase of life, etc.

Division into these areas is artificial and didactic as it corresponds to what we are used to. In reality there are no borders and the areas interact. This is how, for example, physical stress immediately affects our mental and emotional life and vice versa. There is often a long period of time between mental injury and the start of physical symptoms. It is often only the addition of various triggers/injuries over a long period of time that becomes the last straw.

Ask about the pattern of the disease; that is, the supposed cause of the disease (patient's pathogenetic makeup). The patient's disease pattern can also be shaped by previous therapists. It can be important to take such ideas into account. For example, if someone thinks they have a 'slipped disc' or something wrong with a disc, these restrictive ideas may have to be consciously solved. It is not uncommon for patients to be convinced by X-ray images that their symptoms are the result of degenerative (bone) changes so cannot be resolved ('nocebo' or 'voodoo' effect). If you look at the X-ray images together with the patient you can point out that the vertebrae are in a nice straight row. This may be helpful in allaying their fears. It may not be until after successful treatment that the patient comes out of this restricted trance-like awareness (dehypnotising effect).

What is there that causes a negative or positive effect on the pain?

Modulation of the pain not only provides diagnostic information; the patient's experiences can often be used directly for therapy as well and indicate possibilities for self-treatment. We recommend asking detailed questions about some modalities, as these have sometimes not occurred to the patient or have been forgotten during consultation. Don't forget to ask about the effect of heat and cold.

Characteristic information on the presence of myofascial pain or myofascial pain components is listed below.

Improvement resulting from:

- short rest pauses,
- slow, constant passive extension of the affected muscle, particularly with the application of heat (see below),
- (moist) heat where the effect of the application on the mTrP is definitely greater than if the referral zone is warmed,
- loose movement (without effort or strain),
- mTrP-specific therapy.

Deterioration as a result of:

- effort,
- pressure on the mTrP,
- start-up symptoms in the sense of periarthropathy (stiffness and pain, including in the morning, improved by movement) after a long period of rest, particularly if the affected muscle has been contracted,
- persistent or very often repeated contraction of the affected muscle (repetitive strain injury (RSI) syndrome); e.g. muscles of the forearm/fingers through working on a computer with a mouse,
- cold environmental conditions, particularly in combination with damp or draughts (air conditioning),
- tension, stress, anger or other internal factors (although this is rarely consciously perceived),
- cold packs on the affected muscle or directly on the mTrP. In the referred pain zone, however, cold can provide a certain amount of relief.

In order to investigate any differential diagnosis, look at the history of the modalities:

- changing location of the symptoms suggests a relevant emotional (stress) component (in acupuncture: liver Qi disorder). These patients also report sensitivity to draughts,
- if cooling produces an improvement (ask how this has affected the patient, not what has been recommended) then inflammation should also be considered,
- long-term pain after relatively small strain suggests irritation (e.g. as a result of osteochondrosis or aseptic spondylodiscitis); proceed particularly cautiously with locoregional treatment, as it may be better to use the distal points of acupuncture at first.

Which movements are painful and which are difficult?

Allow the patient to demonstrate which movements are painful. Pain with certain movements indicates a problem with the relevant agonist muscle, while pain at the end of the range of movement, and especially limited movement, is more likely to be caused by shortened antagonists.

A precise reconstruction makes it easier to identify the muscles in question; more precise differentiation can then be performed by active/passive examination (see Section 13.3); the tables listing the muscle regions in the introductory chapters of this volume are a further aid to differentiation.

Do you have any other symptoms?

Are there any autonomic or other symptoms? Ask about these, as patients do not often volunteer this information because they do not consider it relevant:

- headaches,
- toothache,
- tinnitus,
- crepitations (which joints?),
- sensory deficits,
- abdominal symptoms including dysmenorrhoea, recurrent diarrhoea or cystitis, or dysuria (mTrP of the abdominal muscles),
- sleep disorders,
- cold extremities,
- sensitivity to changes of weather or draught,
- reduced resistance,
- increased sweating, possibly only in certain areas (consider segmental reflex complex or fibromyalgia syndrome; see Ch. 10).

Sleep disorders (caused by depression, stress, overexertion, sleep apnoea, asthma, etc.) and vitamin deficiencies can cause myofascial symptoms to develop.

What treatment have you had so far?

What treatment has been carried out so far and what has been the outcome? Consider the patient's medical history. These questions provide both information for a diagnosis and help to avoid unnecessary treatment and identify sensible approaches. It is often worth asking closely how the therapy was carried out; for example, were there any significant differences in acupuncture treatment? If the patient has been given any medicine it will often be considered as ineffective even if it has only been taken once or the dose was not sufficient.

Further questions

Questions can be asked more or less openly about any psychological associations, depending on the level of trust, the patient's openness and the situation. It is sufficient to start at whatever level the patient is currently at. If you ask the wrong questions or ask them too soon, the relationship of trust can be permanently marred; on the other hand, the physician should not be afraid. Many patients are grateful if these topics are approached.

- What is the overall attitude to life? What relationships does the patient have and what are they like?
- What physical and mental injuries have there been? Separations, bereavements, setbacks?
- How intact is the family system or family support? What resources are there? What possibilities for stabilisation are there; e.g. learning relaxation techniques or physical or breathing and exercise therapies such as Qigong.
- Of what use could the symptom be to the patient? (Ask about the work situation or even a desire to retire, but do not reproach.)
- How would it be if all the pain went away tomorrow? (This is the DeShazer miracle question, which may give hints about underlying psychology.)

Psychometric questionnaires, e.g. on tendency to depression or somatisation, are also sensible here.

At the end of the consultation, ask an open question: is there anything I have not asked about but which could be important in connection with your symptoms?

13.3 PHYSICAL EXAMINATION

Nicolas Behrens

The basic principles of a physical examination are dealt with in this section. A comprehensive examination and history (see Section 13.2) can in many cases provide an explanation of the cause, particularly:

- the presence of a purely myofascial pain or dysfunction syndrome,
- whether the patient's symptoms are caused by another, non-myofascial pathology or if one of these other pathologies correlates with myofascial findings (primary or secondary) (see Ch. 14).

13.3.1 Aims of the physical examination

The objectives of the physical examination are summarised in Table 13.1.

Structural differentiation and exclusion of diagnoses

As close an identification as possible of the structures from which the patient's symptoms are referred enables treatment to be closely targeted. In practice, it is not always possible to make an exact structural differentiation in view of the limited means available (in terms of finances, time, specialism), and also in view of a basic limitation of diagnostic possibilities. A brief test treatment can be sensible here in simple cases, if there is no (acute) danger of irreversible lesions.

Note: simple disorders (e.g. mTrP of the paravertebral muscles) are common; serious clinical pictures are rare (spondylodiscitis, vertebral-column metastases). A single X-ray is usually sufficient, while a computed tomography (CT)/magnetic resonance imaging (MRI) scan is only required for a specific query.

The correlation between objective findings (arthritis, prolapsed intervertebral disc, etc.) and subjective findings or symptoms is often slight, especially when symptoms are chronic.

Location of the muscles and mTrPs to be treated

A key aim of the physical examination is to find the exact muscles affected and the mTrPs requiring treatment (muscle examination; see Table 13.3). This enables treatment to be targeted and is at the same time a prerequisite for further treatment (e.g. stretching, etc.).

Specific examination with more complex disorders

With complex clinical pictures, it is sensible to record as many of the possible associations and aspects as possible and to approach these with a clear plan, usually multimodal (see Section 13.5). However, the complexity is often

Table 13.1 Aims of physical examination

Aims of first examination	• Structural differentiation and diagnosis exclusion (see Section 14.1) • Location of the mTrP to be treated
	• Specifically for more complex disorders: – recording the whole clinical picture – understanding the patient Then make a comprehensive diagnosis and an individual treatment plan (see Section 13.6).
Before and during each treatment	Checking findings, including location of the mTrP to be treated this time
After each treatment and in the final examination	Checking the effect of therapy

not revealed until a series of treatment is being undertaken; for example, as a result of resistance to treatment. A follow-up examination is then required.

Understanding the clinical picture and identifying pathogenic mechanisms

To understand the disease as completely as possible in complex disorders the physical examination should provide answers to the following questions.

- What is the primarily affected structure or function?
- Are several structures affected or are there several functional disorders, which add up or reinforce each other? This may correspond to the pattern of the straw that broke the camel's back. For example, slight hip dysplasia can be compensated for over a long period. However, if for example a gait disorder caused by flattening of the arch of the foot with the formation of a hallux valgus and a failed operation occurs, the already defective system can 'give way' as a result of a relatively minor additional injury or strain.
- Are there chains of effect? For example, impingement of the shoulder with strain of the shoulder elevators (M. trapezius descendens and M. levator scapulae) and subsequent strain of the cervical spine with development of restricted movement and/or headaches.
- Is there a vicious circle? For example, arthritis with strain; often one-sided hardening of the muscles that span and/or stabilise the joint with the consequence of further deterioration of the arthritis caused by increased strain on the joint surfaces.

- What cannot be corrected and what can be compensated for? Where is there any useful movement potential? For example, fixed kyphosis of the thoracic spine due to osteoporosis with the development of myofascial pain along the whole of the spine, particularly in the area of the cervical and lumbar spine where there is compensating lordosis; it may be possible to relieve the pain by improving mobility of the pelvis (particularly extension into the hip joints).

Understanding the patient

As the therapist you can use touch during the examination to empathise with and understand the patient better. The following steps are helpful.

- Try to copy the patient's body position, including imitating posture and tension. What does this cause? Where is there too much/too little tension?
- Check the patient's state (see below).
- Monitor the patient's breathing (process/rate/level). High-level breathing, pronounced in the upper part of the chest, can be a sign stressed thoughts, and (with high tension in the pelvis/abdominal area) in the sense of control due to anxiety; overall flat breathing can be caused by feeling uncomfortable in a situation, but can also be caused by restrained feelings; rapid breathing expresses internal unrest.
- Monitor and trace the muscle tension (easily possible using passive movement of the extremities).
- Establish the temperature of the different regions. Cold areas can correspond to a lack of perfusion or a tendency to retreat; apart from inflammation, overheated regions can be caused by a sense of shame or almost 'exploding' feelings.
- Note any heavy sweating. With autonomic disorders this generally correlates with excessive demands, particularly if these cannot be adequately expressed, a discrepancy between inner experience and that which is indicated on the outside.
- Watch movement processes. Are these flowing and harmonious, (excessively) broad or narrow; which spaces – to the back, the side or in front – are restricted (there may be a correlation with the axes of acupuncture meridians); what is contact like downwards and upwards?
- Observe where the patient finds the sensation of touch comfortable and they react guardedly or draw back. The patient's avoidance pattern, such as guarding or drawing back, and also narrowing of the space feels around themselves, can often correlate with regions of the body or with meridians (see Ch. 22) and can be used diagnostically and therapeutically with psychosomatic anomalies of the muscle regions and as evidence of a disturbed behaviour pattern or a reduced capacity for relationships (pain as relationship disorder).

- Check whether the history, mood, gestures and facial expressions, body language, movements, touch findings and other impressions are consistent. What is your impression? What could do the patient good straight away?

A thorough examination usually makes the patient feel you have understood them properly. Establishing a good rapport can improve compliance considerably (the examination has the effect of supporting the therapy). It is particularly important for the therapist to have a good approach, as patients consciously and certainly unconsciously perceive a great deal from the therapist's touch and attitude. You can actively improve this.

Making a comprehensive diagnosis and an individual treatment plan

The aim of the detailed physical examination is to create a comprehensive, functionally based diagnosis. It should explain as far as possible which pathomechanisms are affecting each other, how the body compensates and which resources are available, including compliance, and how a realistic course of action could look (see Section 13.6).

Examination to check the effect of therapy

In more than 80% of all indicated mTrP treatments there is an immediate effect, usually on both movement-dependent pain and range of movement. These checks on the success of treatment immediately after therapy are key for both therapist and patient. They allow the therapist the opportunity to check the efficacy of the chosen approach to treatment straight away and at the same time convince the patient that the course of action is correct. Besides optimising motivation, non-specific effects can be activated (e.g. positive expectation of overall success).

A regular check on the findings enables the therapist to learn from each treatment. It may be that other mTrPs are found for the next treatment or another differential diagnosis may arise, if the therapy has not produced sufficient improvement.

13.3.2 Progress and the principles of examination, findings and consequences

We basically recommend proceeding in a standardised manner, always in the same order.

- Inspection.
- Testing active mobility, possibly including isometric tests.

- Testing passive mobility.
- Basic neurological examination if there is any referred pain.
- Palpation.
- Specific tests.
- Possibly interdisciplinary testing.

Instruct the patient before examination that they should immediately report any symptoms caused by the examination (particularly radiated pain). If the pain provocation is too intense, the patient should clearly say 'stop'.

For notes on inspection see Table 13.2.

Testing active mobility

The examination of active mobility is performed using complex movements and then the isolated movement of individual joints or regions of the vertebral column, and finally (as far as possible) isolated testing of individual muscles (see Table 13.3, Chs 26–34). Disorders of passive and active mobility often occur in combination. Due to reciprocal innervation of agonists and antagonists and their close cooperation in contracting at the same time to produce harmonic movement and centred control of the joints, it is always sensible to investigate the antagonists as well for hardening and shortening if there is pain and functional disorder (see Chs 26–34).

Testing passive mobility

The examination of passive mobility (comparing the sides) is always sensible for precise differentiation if there is pain and limited movement (see Table 13.4).

The term 'capsular pattern' describes how characteristic patterns of restriction in the various directions of movement can be found where there are arthritic contractures, depending on the joint. For the shoulder, for example, *lateral rotation > abduction > medial rotation* are affected (> means affected relatively more strongly or earlier). This is phenomenologically correct. The underlying concept should be analysed, as contractures are (predominantly) caused by adhesions or shrinkage of the joint capsule. Capsular adhesions can definitely be a cause of contractures. However, there are capsular patterns even after joint replacements where the capsule has been removed or cut open. Sometimes there is a pronounced capsular pattern again immediately after mobilisation under anaesthetic or debridement with free mobility under anaesthetic. Many years of limited mobility can be improved or made almost normal as a result of targeted intensive needling of shortened muscles with soft or soft elastic feeling at the end of

Table 13.2 Findings on inspection of the patient

FINDINGS	DIFFERENTIATION	EVIDENCE OF
Asymmetry of posture in the frontal plane: surplus or shift, scoliosis or scoliotic posture, e.g. due to standing with pelvis inclined and/or poor posture or deformity in the sagittal plane: flat, round or hollow back	History	Habit, leaning on one side (e.g. sport, work), pain, structural damage (e.g. deformed vertebral body posttraumatic, traumatic or due to osteoporosis, Scheuermann muscle)
	Correction not possible	Fixed deformity (scoliosis, Scheurmann muscle, etc.)
	Increase in pain due to correction	Protective posture, e.g. due to intervertebral disc prolapse
	Correction possible but unusual	Abnormal body shape
	Passive resistance to correction	e.g. Asymmetric muscle tone, muscle shortening
	Active resistance to correction	Fear of causing pain
	Genuine/variable difference in leg-length overtake phenomenon	Post-traumatic/postoperative leg shortening or pelvic congestion with iliosacral joint-function disorder
	Muscle palpation	Muscle tone disorder, mental attitude
	X-ray	Structural damage (see Section 14.1)
Atrophy	History	Immobilisation, trauma, operation, neurological disease
	Examination of movement processes	Protection, reduction of functional strain
	Testing of strength and painfulness	Paresis caused by nerve compression or nerve lesion or by reduced innervation due to pain
	Neurological examination (see below)	Neurological disease
Hypertrophy	History	Strain (on one side) (e.g. sport, work)
	Palpation	e.g. Permanently increased or taut tone
Trophic disorder	Taking temperature, hair growth, nail trophism, oedema, livid discoloration, glossy skin (leiodermia), ninhydrin assay (sweating) quantitative sensory testing	Complex regional pain syndrome (CRPS or Sudeck's disease) Involvement of sympathetic segmental reflex symptoms

the range of movement. The above capsular pattern of the shoulder can also be explained by shortening of the subscapularis muscle to the latissimus dorsi and teres major/minor muscles and the infraspinatus muscle.

If the therapist is sufficiently qualified, it is worth supplementing this with a manual medical examination of joint play.

Basic neurological examination if there is any pain referred into the extremities

This is a test for ruling out a particular diagnosis. The first diagnostic evidence of neuropathic pain is the burning character and/or sudden attack of shooting pains or a feeling like an electric shock.

Table 13.3 Testing active mobility

FINDINGS	EVIDENCE OF	FURTHER EXAMINATION
Restricted ROM with pain (and 'soft' feeling at end of ROM)[1], improvement with assisted examination[2]		Precise palpation, trial therapy; manual examination
	Partial rupture of accessory tendons	Ultrasound, possibly therapeutic local anaesthesic at the tendon
	Protection due to joint disorder (bone/cartilage) or bursitis	Manual examination, X-ray, ultrasound
Restricted ROM without pain with soft (elastic) feeling at end of ROM	Pain-free shortening (with latent mTrP)	Precise palpation, trial therapy
Restricted ROM without pain with hard or firm elastic feeling at end of ROM	Congenital or post-traumatic bony or capsular contracture	History, possibly X-ray, manual examination
Pain on movement without reduced ROM	mTrP agonistic muscles/overloaded structure (joint, vertebral column segment, tendon, bursa, etc.)	Assisted examination, movement with targeted relief of passive structures
Movement deviations and inharmonious process (with/ without reduced ROM)	mTrP of agonistic muscles mechanical problem with referred pain reaction (e.g. arthrosis, shortened antagonists) disturbing influences movement modulating muscles	Assisted examination, trial therapy joint examination more precise examinations of all the structures surrounding the joint, particularly the muscles for extension and mTrP
	Stereotypical faults	History, correction possible?
	Reduced or changed physical sensation	Check physical perception[3]
	Strain	Move loosely together[4]
	Neurological disorder (weakness, rigidity, spasms, etc.)	Neurological examination
Weakness, paresis, plegia or pain	Protection	Examination of the muscles; mTrP?
	Complete tendon rupture	Palpation, ultrasound
	Neurological disorder	Neurological examination, possibly EMG
(Isometric) tension	mTrP agonistic muscles strained joint structure	Apply as targeted/isolated exertion as possible, ideally differentiating with/ without joint distraction

ROM, range of motion/movement.
[1]End feeling: how does it feel when the joint to be examined is passively moved a bit further at the end of the active movement as far as it will go: soft elastic or hard? A hard end feeling (= hard motion stop) indicates involvement of the bone (imaging investigation of the joint), a firm elastic stop is evidence of capsular restriction (see nest section, on capsular pattern); a soft or soft elastic end feeling is usually of muscular cause. In the last case, it makes sense to distinguish the affected muscle (see Chs 26–34). During this examination, the joint must be tested in isolation (firm resistance), otherwise a hard end feeling in particular can be overlooked as a result of continued (deviant) movement.
[2]During assisted movement (the effect of gravity is reduced by the therapist), if the pain or disorder disappears or is definitely eased, the symptoms are partially or wholly from actively used structures, i.e. the agonistically active muscles, the accessory tendons or other overloaded/damaged parts of the locomotor system as a result of muscular disorders of motion (tendon sheaths, bursae, joints, etc.).
[3]The examination of body perception is best performed by touching and questioning, testing the sense of position, comparing the sides with each other and from body markings.
[4]Any conscious or unconscious effort (attitude: 'I must' – typically due to depression or anxiety – see Ch. 12) leads to uneconomical, cramped use of the muscles and thus to inharmonious movements which strain the passive structures, particularly the joints.

Table 13.4 Testing passive mobility

FINDINGS: RESTRICTED MOVEMENT	EVIDENCE OF (SEVERAL COMBINATIONS POSSIBLE)	FURTHER EXAMINATION*
End feeling soft elastic, with or without pain	Muscle contraction	Muscle palpation, trial therapy
End feeling firm elastic, with or without pain at the end of the ROM	Capsule involvement	Testing of capsular pattern testing of joint play
End feeling bony and hard, with or without pain at the end of the ROM	Bone involvement, e.g. post-traumatic arthritic joint deformity	Imaging, e.g. X-ray
Pain during movement	Painful antagonist joint or vertebral column segment disorder, e.g. instability	Joint or segmental examination, trial therapy
'Crepitation'	Incorrect movement or loading of joints as a result of asymmetrical muscle traction or capsule-ligament apparatus disorder	Trial therapy
	Arthritis	Imaging, e.g. X-ray
Instability	Post-traumatic or inflammatory lesion of the capsule-ligament apparatus	History, functional imaging (X-ray), possibly scintigraphy or MRI

*Trial therapy: TrP treatment and/or 'decontraction': eccentric muscle tension of the antagonists of the muscle to be tested (i.e. slowly exerting pressure on the antagonists to cause them to give way) can lead to the release of the shortened agonist, which may be causing the restricted movement.

Because of the poor regeneration capacity of neurons, which often requires a rapid therapeutic or surgical intervention, neurological damage should not be overlooked (see Table 13.5).

If any palpation findings are abnormal, always check them on the other side as well for comparison.

Palpation of the soft tissue

Palpation serves to further distinguish the structures and the precise location of the parts of the locomotor system that have changed in consistency, have become pathologically taut or 'stuck together' and/or tender to touch. This allows a very targeted approach to treatment.

Palpate laterally to medially the skin and subcutis, connective tissue, muscles, tendons and tendon insertions, possible bursae/tendon sheaths and accessible bony structures. Commence palpation with light, superficial pressure. Progress in stages to the next deeper layer, increasing pressure slightly each time. Types of palpation are demonstrated in Figs 13.4 to 13.6.

It is sensible to always palpate a large area around the area of pain so that no key findings are missed. Ideally, several segments should be palpated all around the whole trunk and the whole extremity along the anterior branches of the spinal nerves.

There are several different types of palpation.

- Palpation at rest: the body area to be examined remains motionless; the palpating finger moves gently to determine and differentiate each structure. To examine the tension and consistency of muscles and tendons they are first palpated across the direction of their course (taut bands where mTrPs lie). With stronger pressure, a local twitch response (of the taut band) can sometimes be triggered. For more precise location of the mTrP, palpate along the taut band.

Table 13.5 Neurological damage

EXAMINATION	CHARACTERISTIC FINDINGS	PLACE OF DAMAGE
Testing of • reflexes • muscle strength • sensitivity	'Minus symptoms': weakness or loss of function, paresis, reduced sensitivity, particularly hypalgia[1] Further differentiation: • Complex distribution pattern • Relatively precise attribution to the nerve root • Depending on the nerve (part) motor function and/or sensory deficits	'Peripheral' compression (nerve root or distally from it) • Fascicle or plexus affected • Nerve root • Peripheral nerve
Detailed neurological examination including pathological reflexes, coordination test	Mostly hypersymptoms[2] with a non-unified pattern: spasticity, coordination disorders, possibly different sensory qualities locally differently affected	Disorder of central structures (above, distal motor neuron)
Deep sensitivity • vibration sensation (tuning fork) • sense of position	Mostly no pain but possible strain of compensating structures	Polyneuropathy (toxic damage, diabetes, etc.)

[1]Hypalgia is easily examined with a sterile needle; it remains the only sensory deficit with known dermatome limits and so can be most certainly diagnosed.
[2]A mild hypersymptom (or 'plus symptom') with muscular hypertension or formation of mTrPs and hyperalgesia (very rarely as far as allodynia) can occur and there can also be irritation of peripheral nerve structures. Such referred pain caused by irritation of nerve structures in the sense of entrapment (see Section 14.2.2) can often be treated via mTrPs (e.g. thoracic outlet syndrome). If it leads to excessive autonomic reactions, a complex referred segmental event or trophic disorders of the complex regional pain syndrome (CRPS) should be considered (Sudeck's disease, reflex dystrophy).

• During palpation of the muscles for mTrPs (Table 13.6) the pressure should be held for 10 s. It is often only then that the patient feels the referred pain. Sometimes this can be better and more precise if the muscle is lifted by folding it in a pinch grip (e.g. for the Mm. trapezius descendens, sternocleidomastoideus, masseter; for the posterior and anterior armpit, the arm, the calf, etc.), especially if there is no bony buffer.
• With palpation during movement (dynamic palpation) the structure to be examined is moved with one hand while the palpating hand remains still so as not to disturb perception with the palpating hand. This can be carried out, for example, on the shoulder in order to palpate the greater and lesser tubercle below the acromion during medial and lateral rotation of the arm and definitely identify the long biceps tendon.
• During dry needling, 'palpation with the needle' is always carried out as well: it is worth paying attention to the consistency of the tissue being needled in each case. This can vary from quite soft to very firm (fatty tissue, relaxed muscle, fascia, skin, hardened muscle (it can go so far as to be of the consistency of a rubber eraser), tendons, tough ligaments, aponeuroses, bones). Apart from a good needle technique, a prerequisite is a high-quality needle with a good sharp finish and an abrasion-resistant coating.
• The palpation of key acupuncture points provides evidence of the patient's current constitution and mental and emotional state.

Segmental diagnosis

In order to attribute the findings to segments, note any increasing inferior shift from the cervical to the lumbar spine if there are any changes to the skin or subcutis (dermatome).

In the interpretation of the findings in relation to interactions between the abdominal organs and the segments, the authors concentrate primarily on the correlative acupuncture points (see Section 22.2). After these have been needled about 2–3 cm deep, they work more via the central myotome (innervated by the dorsal branch in each case). There are still other systems or patterns, such as connective tissue massage (see Fig. 13.7) or cupping zones (see Fig. 13.8). Their greater relationship to the dermatome is explained by sometimes supplementary but also sometimes rather differing location information (Table 13.7).

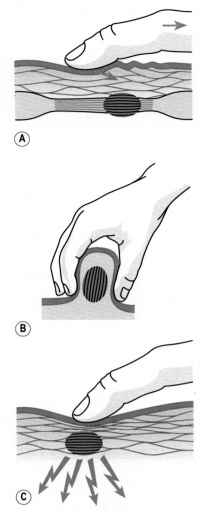

Fig. 13.4 Types of palpation: stroking palpation (a), pinch palpation (b), pressure palpation (c).

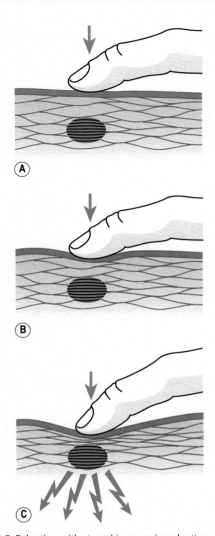

Fig. 13.5 Palpation with staged increase in palpation pressure. Skin (a), subcutis (b), muscle node painful with increased pressure (c).

Fig. 13.6 Dynamic palpation.

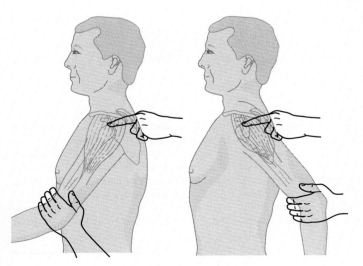

Table 13.6 Typical palpation findings and affected structures

STRUCTURE	FINDINGS	EVIDENCE OF
Checking consistency		
Skin	Thickening	• Skin diseases • Referral involvement (e.g. cutivisceral reflex) in the sense of a head zone
Subcutis, connective tissue	Swellings	• Connective tissue disorder, gelosis (usually referred) • Local inflammation
Muscles	Isolated thickening	• Taut band with mTrP • (previous) Muscle fibre tear
	Taut band	• Longstanding multiple taut bands with mTrPs
Tendons	Structural inhomogeneity	• (Partial) rupture • Inflammatory or post-inflammatory condition (ultrasound)
Tendon sheath	Thickening and pain	• Tendovaginitis (ultrasound)
Bones	Exostosis, periarticular swelling or change	• Previous trauma, chronic overload, arthritis
Checking tenderness		
Skin	Skin sensitive	• Allodynia • Neuropathic pain
Subcutis, connective tissue	Normal consistency, tenderpoints sensitive	• Fibromyalgia
	Swollen, thickened as with panniculitis	• Connective tissue zone (see Fig. 13.11) • Segmental reflex complex • Visceral disruption input • Trophic changes
Muscles (first transverse then lengthwise palpation)	Referred pain (known to patient?)	• Active mTrP

	Local pain	• With shortening: latent mTrP
		• Without shortening
		  – Previous trauma
		  – Tenderpoint
		  – Other causes (e.g. polymyalgia)

Tendons, insertions	Tendinitis, insertion tendinopathy	• Strain, abnormal consistency and metabolism of the accessory muscles
Lig. supraspinalia or interspinalia	Sensitive to light pressure (positive Maigne's test)	• Segmental function disorder • Segmental reflex complex
Bones	Inflammation of the periosteum	• Mechanical strain
Testing of movement of tissues against each other		
Skin, connective tissue and tendon/muscle	Adhesions post-traumatically or inflammatory, scars, swellings	• With scars think of potential area of disorder • Test and therapy using Very Point technique® (see Fig. 13.10)
Palpation of peripheral pulses		
Arteries	Pulsation?	• Peripheral artery occlusive disorder

Continued

Table 13.6 Typical palpation findings and affected structures—cont'd

STRUCTURE	FINDINGS	EVIDENCE OF
Tenderness of acupuncture points (see Fig. 13.9)		
CV 17, location: sternal periosteum at the level of the nipples	Tenderness*, reaction of patient Large area very tender	Mental stress situation Suspected fibromyalgia
LR 3, localisation: interosseus muscles in the proximal angle between metatarsals I and II	Tenderness*, reaction of patient	Emotional stress situation, stifled anger

*Specific statement only if a neighbouring area of comparable tissue is definitely less sensitive.

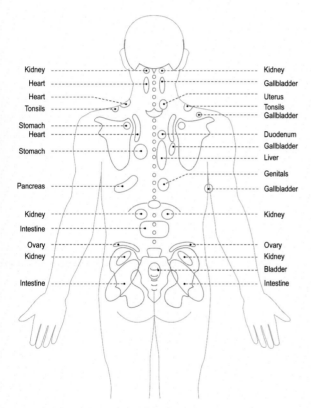

Fig. 13.7 Point- and area-related organ associations developed from connective tissue massage.
(From Gleditsch 2005)

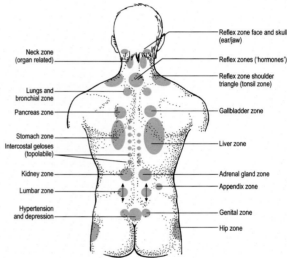

Fig. 13.8 Cupping zones.
(Redrawn from Abele 1999)

Specific tests

Specific tests and a differentiated neurological examination should be carried out if indicated by the findings. If the findings are confirmed, it would now be sensible, if you have not already done so, to arrange for the patient to see a specialist in the relevant discipline.

If sensible for the diagnosis of myofascial disorders, specific tests can be carried out on the individual regions and muscles. Please refer to the literature for the multitude of orthopaedic tests.

Interdisciplinary cooperation in diagnosis and therapy

Differing points of view, exchange of ideas, increase in competence and optimisation of therapy can all arise from interdisciplinary working. Depending on your own competence, it can make sense to work together with the following disciplines (we do not claim that the list is comprehensive).

DENTIST, ORTHODONTIST	CMD
Manual medicine, osteopath	Segmental movement disorders or 'blockages', disorders of abdominal function or craniosacral system, detailed functional examination and treatment if necessary
Neurologist	Exclusion of neurological diseases
Radiologist, orthopaedist	Structural diagnosis
Psychotherapist	Life history associations, somatoform disorders, etc.
Doctor of physical medicine	Overall plan for physiotherapy, detailed functional examination
Physiotherapist	Targeted stretching, massage, manual trigger point treatment, mobilisation, instruction on exercises with training in harmonious sequence of movement
Pain therapist	Overall treatment plan, drug treatment, pain therapy, nerve block
Doctor with additional acupuncture qualification	Far-point access (body acupuncture and somatopia; Gleditsch) supplementary treatment of the 'inner' (the abdominal and psychosomatic aspects)
Qigong or Tai chi instructor	Combination of breathing and exercise therapy, meditative approach, body awareness training
Breathing therapist	Somatopsychological approach, improvement in body awareness and capacity to relate, sensory-oriented exercises
Doctor with additional qualification in naturopathic treatment	Supplementary diagnosis (fields of interference, acid-base disorders, basic regulatory system, etc.) and possibly treatment (neural therapy, fasting/F.X. Mayr therapy, homeopathy, etc.)
Sports instructor fitness studio	Targeted training of weakened muscles (after sufficient pain/trigger point therapy)

Table 13.7 Methods for segmental diagnosis

METHOD	STRUCTURE EXAMINED	TYPICAL FINDINGS	ADVANTAGE
Kibler fold (see Fig. 13.11)	Subcutis	Reduced folding, pain during Kibler fold test	Easy
Connective tissue massage, stroking	Skin, subcutis	Fingers lose their 'bow wave' due to swollen areas	Easy, pain free
Maigne key test	Lig. supra- and interspinalia	Sensitive to light pressure	Easy, more precise attribution of segment (in the ligament no shift in relation to the vertebral bodies)
Gleditsch Very Point method® (see Fig. 13.10)*	Skin and subcutis	Due to even, saccade-shaped slipping and 'needling' over the paramedian area of the skin with a needle painfulness and reduced resistance in the area of the swellings	Diagnosis = treatment instrument, fast and efficient segmental therapy

Continued

Table 13.7 Methods for segmental diagnosis—cont'd

METHOD	STRUCTURE EXAMINED	TYPICAL FINDINGS	ADVANTAGE
Posterior–anterior stress in prone position, testing at the level of the thoracic and lumbar spine	Movement of the vertebral bodies against each other	Provocation of patient's symptoms when the spinous process of the vertebral body being examined is pushed from dorsal to ventral (posterior–anterior), testing of the relevant motion segment parts (intervertebral discs, vertebral joints, ligaments, relevant muscles, etc.)	Easy, good for checking success of therapy
Examination of segment motion ('joint play') (manual medicine)	Mobility of the vertebral bodies against each other	Reduced (hypomobility or blockage) or increased extent of movement (hypermobility to instability)	Differentiated statement, note the direction of movement
Attribution table muscles to segments	Affected or abnormal tone of the muscles (extremities)	With deep needling (3–5 cm) 1–2 finger widths lateral to the line of the spinous process at the level of the disordered segments A. Gunn's 'invisible sign': difficult penetration of the needle into the deep paravertebral muscles	Approach via the central myotome part

*Also very sensible for precise acupuncture point location.

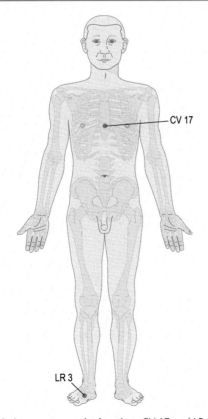

Fig. 13.9 Acupuncture point locations CV 17 and LR 3.

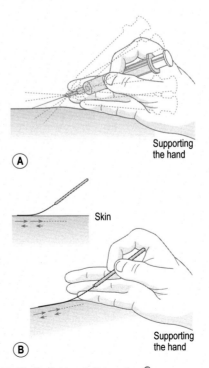

Fig. 13.10 Gleditsch Very Point method®.

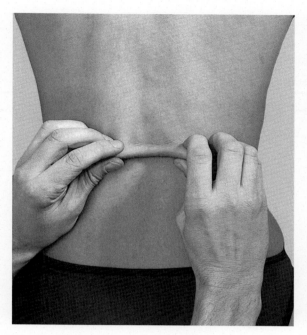

Fig. 13.11 Kibler fold segment examination.

Table 13.8 Criteria for diagnosis of mTrPs

ENGLISH	GERMAN
Taut band	*Hartspannstrang*
Tender spot in taut band	*Schmerzpunkt entlang des Hartspannstrangs*
Recognition of pain	*Wiedererkennen des Schmerzes als den spezifischen Problemen zugehörig*
Restricted range of stretch	*Eingeschränkte Verlängerungsfähigkeit des Muskels (meist Schmerz am Ende der Bewegung)*
Nodule in taut band	*Knötchenstruktur entlang des Hartspannstrangs*
Local twitch response	*Lokale Zuckungsreaktion des palpierten Hartspannstrangs*
Specific referred pain pattern	*Übertragungsschmerz (-muster) spezifisch für jeden Muskel*
Muscle weakness	*Muskelschwäche (keine Atrophie)*
Painful contraction	*Schmerzen bei kräftiger Kontraktion*
Autonomic phenomena	*Autonome Phänomene (kalte Haut, Schweiß, Piloreaktion, . . .)*

13.4 SPECIFIC DIAGNOSIS OF mTrPs

Gunnar Licht

13.4.1 Diagnostic criteria for mTrPs

mTrPs are now part of the internationally active vocabulary of locomotory system medicine. The credit for this is due essentially to Janet Travell and David Simons, who have demonstrated the immense significance of the dynamic locomotor apparatus in numerous publications over the last decade. Their medical legacy, the *Trigger Point Manual* (Travell, Simons 2002), has become the undisputed standard work on the subject and is now one of the most purchased medical books in the world. Travell and Simons clearly define the MPS and especially its clinical manifestation: mTrPs. The diagnosis criteria for finding an mTrP are demonstrated in Table 13.8.

13.4.2 Manual mTrP diagnosis

The following represents the standard established by the society for mTrP therapy and adopted by the *Medizinischen Gesellschaft für Myofasziale Schmerzen MGMS e.V.* (Medical Society for Myofascial Pain) for manual mTrP diagnosis. For a better overview, the individual stages of palpation are cited one after the other, although some of these take place concurrently (see Fig. 13.12).

Identification of a painful region in the general examination

- Indications as to which muscles should be examined more closely are produced from the history in the knowledge of referred pain patterns and from a general examination to check mobility, extension and strain.

Making contact with the muscle structure

- Contact is first made with the skin in the region above the selected muscles. Pressure is increased. Look for tension and pain. Movements should be still largely large scale for this. Experience has shown that palpation across the muscles has proved reliable in improving orientation.
- After finding a painful site with increased tension, the therapist does not seek further but increases pressure on the detected site. (This pressure should not be standardised as the consistency of the soft tissue to be

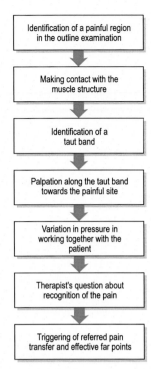

Fig. 13.12 Standard established by the Society for Myofascial Trigger Point Therapy and adopted by the *Medizinischen Gesellschaft für Myofasziale Schmerzen MGMS e.V.* (Medical Society for Myofascial Pain) for manual mTrP diagnosis.

examined is much too heterogeneous. Predefined pressure can lead to a violent guarding reaction and counter-resistance from one patient, whereas with another patient the same pressure may not overcome skin resistance.)

- This phase is described as 'sinking in' as far as the muscles. After some time, the therapist actually perceives the rope-like structures of the muscles.
- It is not until now that the taut bands can be identified.
- This last stage of the examination is probably the most important step in finding an mTrP. It often takes some time until the described phenomenon occurs.
- If you are not quite sure whether the muscles are under the palpating finger, you can ask the patient to tense the appropriate muscles. This can allay any remaining uncertainties.

Identification of a taut band

- The taut band can now be palpated in the muscle. Only minimal movements with the examining finger are now needed (across the course of the fibres) to identify the taut band.

- Plucking at this taut band can often trigger a twitch reaction.

Palpation along the taut band depending on the most painful site

- Pressure is maintained at a relatively constant level. Do not release this pressure or further information may be lost.
- Use minimal movements to search the taut band for the most painful point, which is sometimes firmer or thicker.

Variation of pressure in teamwork with the patient: if the therapist has found the most painful point, pressure is increased on the identified site.

The therapist should ask the patient whether they recognise the pain: it is often not until now that a crucial diagnosis criterion is seen. The patient recognises the pain caused by the examination as being a pain that is part of the symptoms.

Causing referred pain

- Other diagnostic criteria are usually also only recognised now.
- The referred pain is sometimes sensed by the patient in very distant areas, as described by Travell and Simons.

The therapist may now vary the pressure. This is the point where diagnosis can lead directly to treatment. This is carried out in accordance with the model of ischaemic compression at the patient's pain limit. Signs of too much pressure on the mTrP are an increase in muscle tension under the palpating finger and active guarding and evasion by the patient.

13.4.3 Interpretation of the diagnosis criteria

With the help of the diagnosis criteria, a differentiation may be made between latent and active mTrPs.

To diagnose a **latent mTrP**, key criteria must be fulfilled. The taut band and the painful spot on the taut band define the latent mTrP. A latent mTrP usually remains clinically silent. The patient is not familiar with the pain provoked by the examination. A latent mTrP occurs from the same pathophysiological mechanism as an active mTrP and is combined with the functionally changed properties of the muscles such as reduced extension capacity or premature response of the muscles to the demands made on it. As a result of the changed static and dynamic properties of the affected muscles there is a tendency for the MPS to spread along functionally and neurophysiologically determined muscle chains. New mTrPs form which may be active or latent. An active mTrP can develop at any time from a latent mTrP.

An **active mTrP** is identified from the interaction with the patient. Recognition of the pain by the patient as 'his' or 'her' pain defines the active mTrP. An active mTrP is therefore directly involved in the pain sensed by the patient.

Table 13.8 lists the criteria that confirm the diagnosis of an mTrP.

A **local twitch reaction** here has a high diagnostic value. It is not always triggered by palpation with the hands. A 'local twitch' is more likely to be triggered with an acupuncture needle or an extracorporeal shock wave therapy (ESWT) device. The local twitch response is a strong criterion for an mTrP but is not an essential criterion.

A history of **referred pain** can be a useful criterion to guide the focus to certain muscles, as it is specific for each muscle. Referred pain is not an essential criterion for an mTrP, but it is a confirmatory criterion. The patient may not be aware of any referred pain at all.

The other criteria, such as a knot structure along the taut band, autonomic phenomena, muscle weakness or pain on muscle contraction should be regarded as optional and only confirm the diagnosis of an mTrP based on the essential criteria (see Table 13.8).

After the examination of active and latent mTrPs it is worth addressing another important question. Are there any signs of a serious disease which has caused the activation of an mTrP? This must be ruled out in the patient's mind by excluding the diagnosis of structural disease (see Section 14.1). Once the therapist has appraised the clinical picture, he must find out whether the mTrP should be evaluated as the dominant or non-dominant disease factor.

Attempted treatment of an active mTrP using suitable methods of treatment usually answers this question by itself. If a recurrence occurs very soon afterwards, either the key trigger point was not treated or a disease has quickly 'triggered' the symptoms again.

13.4.4 Reliability of the clinical examination of mTrPs

The International Federation of Manual Medicine (FIMM) decided in 2001 that 'The examination techniques of manual medicine are not reliable.'

However, this statement should be made more specific, as follows.

- The examination techniques of manual medicine to differentiate pain in the locomotor system, e.g. the segmental examination techniques of the vertebral column, may not produce reliable results in scientific tests.

- Furthermore, in a meta-analysis (Conradi, Smolenski 2005) the lack of sufficient scientific data on the quality of the test criteria used in manual medicine was pointed out and a high-quality debate on this topic was requested.

- The FIMM has been asking for years for an investigation of the reliability of the different examination techniques in manual medicine in order to work out the principles of a sound 'specific' clinical assessment of the patient on the basis of a scientifically meaningful statement.

- The muscles are easily accessible to clinical examination and the manual examination technique makes less complex demands on the therapist and the patient than the examination of segmental function disorders of the vertebral column.

- Scientific tests on the reliability of the clinical examination of mTrP have been carried out for years with heterogeneous results.

- The scientific quality of a clinical test is determined by its reliability. Statistically, the reliability of a clinical test which cannot be measured against a gold standard is expressed in tersm of its reproducibility or precision. Reproducibility can be calculated by using Kappa statistics where the chance agreement of the therapists is removed from the calculation.

- A pilot study on this topic was carried out by Gerwin (1997b) with good results for the shoulder girdle and neck muscles.

- Clear definitions and treatment instructions are necessary to achieve reliable examination results. With the *Trigger Pont Manual*, Travell and Simons (2002) have succeeded in producing a precise standard work which gives interested parties clear treatment instructions and definitions.

- Experienced therapists are a prerequisite for reliable diagnosis of mTrPs. Gerwin (1997b) also attributes the poor results of the reliability studies by Wolfe et al. (1992), Nice et al. (1992) and Njoo and van der Does (1994) to the lack of experience of the individual therapists or their uneven level of experience.

- Eventually, Licht et al. (2007) managed to confirm good results for the reliability of the clinical examination of mTrP in a much larger population, from a total of 304 selected muscles in the trunk and buttocks. A good inter-rater reliability was achieved. Some of the Kappa values were >0.8.

- These results are only possible if both therapists have a comprehensive range of experience and the definitions are precisely determined and a standardised examination procedure has been developed.

- The very good results in the inter-rater reliability make mTrP a valuable clinical parameter for differentiating pain in the locomotor system.

- For further scientific argument, they can also be used as objective parameters for the course of progress for, e.g., checks on success and results.

13.5 TECHNICAL EXAMINATION PROCEDURES

This is where we once again emphasise the importance of investigating any possible differential diagnosis of the patient's symptoms in order to sufficiently evaluate the MPS caused by mTrPs (see Ch. 14). It is only on this solid basis that the experienced physician and therapist can, together with the patient, develop a realistic treatment plan, introduce any concomitant measures and make any statements on the prognosis of the disease.

There is currently no recognised technical investigation procedure for diagnosing mTrPs, either in laboratory chemistry or using equipment (Travell, Simons 2002). For research purposes, phenomena can be recorded using ultrasound, EMG, algometry and ESWT to show the individual properties of mTrPs. These procedures are, however, not suitable for everyday practice for determining the complexity of an MPS, nor are they required.

Currently clinical examination with targeted palpation represents the only comprehensive diagnostic basis (see Section 13.3).

13.5.1 Ultrasound

Gunnar Licht

This representation can differentiate between structural changes and movements of the muscles. With the latter, the local twitch response is of interest. This important confirmatory diagnosis criterion was recorded by Gerwin et al. using ultrasound (Gerwin et al. 1997a). However, for everyday clinical practice, the method is irrelevant as it is too costly and time consuming. The local twitch response can be triggered by experienced therapists using rapid palpation or dry needling and can almost always be palpated or even seen.

It is currently believed that structural changes, especially trophic changes in the tendons, are evidence of the long-term consequences of mTrP syndromes.

We must wait and see whether in the future higher-resolution procedures will be able to demonstrate mTrPs or trigger point zones directly.

13.5.2 Needle EMG

Gunnar Licht

Experts still do not always agree on the results of needle EMG tests. Travell and Rinzler (1952) described specific properties of mTrPs in a needle EMG, as did Hubbard and Berkoff in 1993. They described spontaneous, low-frequency pathological end-plate noise and high-frequency spike activity (Hubbard and Berkoff 1993). However, critics consider the cited needle EMG activity as normal variations in the potentials from motor unit end plates. There is still no clear scientific test in existence today. However, we can justifiably investigate the reason for the high range of variability in motor unit end-plate potentials.

13.5.3 Surface EMG

Gunnar Licht

In tests using a surface EMG we have long concentrated on the properties of a single mTrP. Some of the controversial statements have been characterised by the so-called pain-spasm cycle. We established an increased readiness to react, an increased tendency to fatigue and a delayed recovery phase for muscles affected by mTrP.

We have to thank Lucas et al. (2004) for the breakthrough in the surface EMG research which focused not on the properties of a single muscle but researched the response behaviour of different muscles during predefined movements. They showed that mTrPs crucially change the activity behaviour of the muscles during shoulder movement. A muscular imbalance occurs, which leads to ineffective performance of the movement and stress on individual muscles. After treatment of the mTrP the movement pattern is immediately harmonised (Lucas et al. 2004).

Typical function disorders, as also described in manual medicine, could in future be made visible in this manner.

13.5.4 Algometry

Gunnar Licht

Another procedure invoked for the scientific examination of mTrPs is pressure algometry. The defined load is measured in kg/cm^2 (Fisher 1986) using a feather algometer. There are also thin rubber plates which measure the pressure applied during palpation based on a piezoelectric effect. Three threshold values are measured:

- tenderness threshold,
- referred pain threshold,
- pain tolerance threshold.

The pressure needed to achieve each of the thresholds is directly read off in kg/cm^2.

The scientific method has a few weaknesses:

- the threshold limits do not tell us anything about the cause of the pain,
- the target threshold limit values can be differently interpreted based on the trigger point's location (depth and underlying structures, e.g. bones or soft tissue) and of course they vary from person to person,
- it is difficult to standardise because of the relatively complex and often underestimated demands on the therapist.

The value of these threshold measurements must be seriously questioned. Because of these problems, a standardised procedure is not really possible between and among individuals. In the opinion of the author, pressure algometry only has a certain amount of documentary value in terms of checking the progress of an mTrP, e.g. after an interventional treatment (see Fig. 13.13).

In summary, pressure algometry is an attempt to objectify the pressure used in palpation. In daily practice the finger or thumb are better, as they can both provide pressure and perceive various contact and structural qualities.

13.5.5 Laboratory tests

Hans-Joachim Schmitt, Nicolas Behrens

A laboratory screening is required:

- to investigate a differential diagnosis which can then orient the therapist to a possible suspected diagnosis,
- if there is continued pain in spite of normal diagnosis and therapeutic measures.

As part of a basic examination we recommend:

- full blood count,
- ESR,
- K^+, Ca^{2+}, creatinine, basal thyroid-stimulating hormone, possibly uric acid.

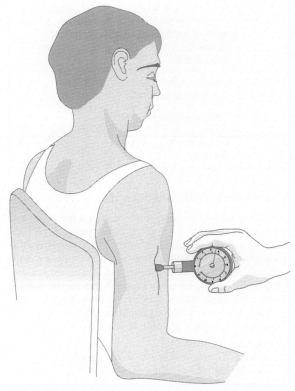

Fig. 13.13 Pressure algometer.

The following more precise tests may be required to rule out perpetuating factors, if there is a suspicion of:

- anaemia: iron serum level, ferritin, mean corpuscular volume and mean corpuscular haemoglobin, possibly differential blood count,
- vitamin deficiency: B_1, B_6, B_{12}, C, folic acid; cobalamin level,
- thyroid gland or pituitary disorders: FT3/FT4,
- diabetes: blood sugar level, glucose tolerance test,
- parasitic diseases: differential blood count/ eosinophils,
- viral diseases: possibly determination of mononuclear cells,
- Bechterew's disease (ankylosing spondylitis): HLA-B 27,
- rheumatological/autoimmune diseases (see Section 14.1.5).

13.5.6 Extracorporeal shock wave therapy

Gunnar Licht

This is not the place to go into the details of which form of ESWT, focused or radial, should be used as a diagnostic and/or therapeutic instrument. Focused ESWT can elicit individual clinical characteristics of mTrPs (Müller-Ehrenberg, personal communication 2006): the known referred pain pattern with recognition of the pain by the patient and the local twitch response. The essential diagnosis criteria, taut band and the pain of this cannot be verified.

Overall, ESWT should be considered more of a supplementary diagnostic tool and predominantly a therapeutic procedure.

13.5.7 Overview of apparatus test procedures used to rule out other disorders

Hans-Joachim Schmitt, Nicolas Behrens

Test procedures needing apparatus are only required to rule out other disorders or provide evidence of acute injuries.

CLINICAL SUSPICION OF	TEST PROCEDURE
Haematoma, bursitis, calcification	Ultrasound, X-ray, MRI
Sprain	Ultrasound, MRI
Tendon changes, (partial) tendon rupture	Ultrasound, MRI
Fracture	X-ray

Degenerative changes, segmental instabilities, erosive osteochondritis (= aseptic spondylodiscitis)	X-ray, possibly with dynamic images, MRI with contrast medium
Osteoporosis	Bone density measurement, X-ray (late stage)
Nerve lesions, compression, e.g. as a result of intervertebral disc prolapse	EMG, nerve conduction speed, possibly CT or MRI
Entrapment of a peripheral nerve	Nerve conduction speed (if serious)
Inflammatory, degenerative or timorous bone changes	X-ray, scintigraphy
Rheumatological diseases, Bechterew's disease	X-ray, CT of the iliosacral segment

13.6 MAKING A COMPREHENSIVE DIAGNOSIS WITH INSTRUCTIONS FOR TREATMENT

Nicolas Behrens

After tests have been carried out, a comprehensive structure- and function-related diagnosis should be made. We recommend the following (Senn) structure.

Each diagnosis should provide details of:

- the key findings/functional disorders including information from the history, using the rubric 'with',
- any findings which have been ruled out, under 'without',
- the underlying structural changes and conditions causing them, under 'due to'.

The advantages of this recording procedure are as follows:

- summary of the clinical picture and pathological event,
- rapid orientation when the patient attends again,
- no key findings or aspects are overlooked,
- key or supposed functional associations are worked out for therapy,
- it produces a clear treatment plan,
- this type of diagnosis is very helpful for co-therapists (physiotherapists, etc.) and is a good basis if there is a different therapist (e.g. can also be printed out and given to the patient for prescription),
- it forms the basis of an interim history and checks on findings.

This procedure is good training in clearly structured thinking and working. This diagnosis can be supplemented with notes on other important aspects such as data from the patient's life history, psychosomatic associations, ideas for approaches to treatment, etc.

13.6.1 Diagnostic documentation

Single and complex diagnoses (examples)

MPS of the hip adductors on the right

With	Partial rupture of the muscle fibres mTrP in the M. adductor magnus
Due to	Previous muscle trauma at XY

MPS of the cervical spine

With	Headaches (more pronounced on the right side of the forehead than the left) Limited rotation and rotation in flexion greater to the left than the right Active mTrP in the M. splenius capitis on the right, in the M. sternocleidomastoideus on the right, in the M. trapezius on both sides and in the Mm. levator scapulae on both sides Segmental function disorder of the upper cervical spine
Without	Relevant radiological changes Neurological symptoms
Due to	Previous whiplash injury on _____ Suspected post-traumatic stress reaction Incorrect posture in the sense of protraction of the head

Components and constituents

The following should serve the reader as a list of suggestions and a checklist. The findings and symptoms cited under 'with' suggest a list of questions and tests that is as comprehensive as possible. The excluded findings ('without') list records what has been tested without coming across any pathological findings; this will avoid any superfluous second tests. The 'due to' instructions provide an understanding of the cause and the treatment.

Possible principal diagnoses include:

- acute or chronic MPS,
- acute or chronic myofascial strain symptoms,
- acute or chronic irritation symptoms,
- segmental function disorder,

- periarthropathy (possibly in the sense of an impingement),
- contracture,
- acute or chronic lumbovertebral syndrome,
- acute or chronic radiculopathy, e.g. S1 on the left.

Essential information and findings from the history ('with')

With	Pain location and pain referral area and frequency of occurrence
	Modalities (improvement by ___, deterioration by ___)
	Type of referred pain: pain radiating from which structure? (see Section 14.2.2)
	Functional disorder and/or painful movement: restricted movement or pain caused by (attribute as far as possible)?
	Active mTrP in the . . . muscles ___ Latent mTrP with shortening of the . . . muscles ___
	Other relevant findings: segmental function disorder, segmental reflex complex, etc.
	Sensorimotor deficits

Excluded findings or disorders ('without')

Without	Neurological deficits/symptoms
	Involvement of neighbouring joints
	Relevant radiological changes

Causative somatic and mental conditions, functional associations ('due to')

Due to	Trauma
	Postural disorder (e.g. increased postural work for the 'small of the back' with weak lumbar posture)
	Chronic strain (due to work, etc.)
	Disorders of functionally associated regions (e.g. with craniomandibular dysfunction, shortening of other muscle groups)
	Mental/family stress (e.g. disturbed attitude to life, such as victim posture)
	Arthritis, deformities of the vertebral column

Practical examples

Chronic, predominantly myofascial strain symptoms of the cervical spine

With	Referred myofascial pain in the left arm (predominantly from the scalene muscles)
	Limited flexion and rotation to the left and lateral flexion to the left > right, with a muscular cause in each case
	mTrPs matching right-sided head pain symptoms in the area of the occipital part of the occipitofrontalis muscle
Due to	Incorrect posture in the sense of slight protraction of the head, interscapular 'flat back' (hypokyphosis) and shoulder protraction right > left
	Indications of an overall definitely increased muscle tone (including CMD with traces of abrasion of the teeth; patient already has a bit splint)

MFS of the trunk/pelvic girdle

With	Myositis/mTrP of the iliacus muscle > psoas on both sides, gluteus min. left and piriformis right, each correlating with known symptoms
	Trunk leans to left (right pelvis approximately 1.5 cm higher, unchanged when seated, as long as no difference in leg length) and slight torsion of the upper body to the right
Without	Indications of a relevant iliosacral joint or hip joint participation
Due to	Posture in the sense of a flexion position of the pelvis in the hip joints with slight hyperlordosis of the lumbar spine
	Indications of associations with life history; pronounced 'autonomic dystonia'
	Previous oophorectomy on the right in 1972

13.6.2 Therapeutic consequences using case studies

Patient 1

Chronic, recurring, myofascial strain symptoms of the whole vertebral column pronounced on the right and predominantly the cervical spine

With	Most likely myofascial pain referred to the forehead
	Limitation of flexion, rotation in flexion to the left (caused by left-sided upper cervical spine muscles), rotation on left/right 65°–0°–85° and lateral flexion on both sides 20° (caused by levator scapulae/trapezius desc. and paravertebral muscles) and extension to half way
	Pronounced myositis (particularly the levator scap./trap descendens and paravertebral muscles right > left)
	Involvement of the muscles of mastication (especially the temporalis) due to bruxism
	Slight shift of the vertebral column to the right and slight elevation of the pelvis on the right (sometimes because of shortening of the right flank, does not require balancing)
Without	Significant restriction of movement of the thoracic and lumbar spine
	Pain referred into the arms, neurological deficits
Due to	Pronounced increased basic tension with tendency towards a 'military posture'
	Preforaminal intervertebral disc prolapse at C6/7 on the left, which may also affect the root at C8 (findings by a third party)
	Posture in the sense of pronounced head and (shoulder) protraction and hyperlordosis of the lumbar spine, right shoulder higher than left
	Tendency towards general muscular hypertension (including bruxism); suspected life history associations

Therapy and suggestions for further treatment

After the examination, acupuncture treatment via distal points (SI 3 zone, BL 62, KI 3, stellate zone and cervical spine at C6 area on the left ear) and via mTrPs of the Mm. trapezius descendens and levator scapulae on both sides, which can achieve a definite relaxation, indicated in particular by a lowering of the left shoulder by about 3 cm. This treatment should be continued, focusing on the mTrPs in the area of the cervical and lumbar spine.

The subsequent Gua Sha ('scraping') and cupping massage can also be continued by a partner.

We very much recommend learning Jacobsen's progressive relaxation; the relevant addresses can be given to the patient.

Clarification of any life history associations is very sensible. The patient is also introduced to various possibilities for this and given addresses.

A sensible addition to treatment would be massage, e.g. in the form of reflex breathing massage or Glaser® psychotonics, and should be discussed with the patient and possibly prescribed at the next session.

Patient 2

Diagnosis 1: periarthropathia humeroscapularis on the right (impingement), predominantly myofascially caused

With	Painful arch on the right
	Isometric tension pain on elbow flexion (M. biceps brachialis) and lateral rotation of the shoulder (M. infraspinatus) as well as shoulder abduction (Mm. supraspinatus and deltoideus)
	Restricted lateral rotation on the right to 35°, on the left to 45° (more likely contracture M. subscapularis as in the sense of a capsular pattern; lateral rotation in horizontal abduction only limited at the end of the range of movement on the right)
	Slightly limited medial rotation on the right (shortening of the Mm. infraspinatus/teres minor)
	Involvement of the right acromioclavicular joint
	Disorder of the scapulohumeral rhythm on the right ('forerunning' of the right scapula during abduction and anteversion)
	Shortening/tendomyosis of the Mm. levator scapulae, M. trapezius desc., M. pectoralis major/minor (shoulder protraction, active mTrP) and M. sternocleidomastoideus
	mTrP of the Mm. supraspinatus and infraspinatus, latissimus dorsi, teres major/minor, deltoideus, subscapularis, biceps brachii
Without	Evidence of current instability
Due to	Previous shoulder dislocation on ____

Ultrasound of the shoulder: effusion in the sulcus bicipitalis consistent with biceps tendinitis; the ultrasound did not show any evidence of a Bankert lesion; rotator cuff preserved from the configuration onwards, no subdeltoid bursitis; no calcifications. The echo-poor zones in the supraspinatus were most likely a consequence of prior local trigger point treatment.

Diagnosis 2: Myofascial lumbar spine syndrome

With	Slight, left convex scoliosis of the lumbar spine
	Reduced lumbar spine presentation during flexion and restricted lateral flexion to the left greater than to the right (explained by shortening of the M. quadratus lumborum right > left)

Therapy and suggestions for further treatment

Acupuncture treatment via the distal points had already brought some improvement. Subsequent treatment of the mTrPs of the Mm. infraspinatus, latissimus dorsi, teres major/minor, supraspinatus, pectoralis minor/major and trapezius descendens on the right (dry needling) led to further improvement of mobility and pain on movement; in particular, the arch was no longer painful. The patient was shown how to extend the Mm. pectoralis major and minor. Subsequent infiltration of the right acromioclavicular joint brought still further improvement.

Physiotherapy prescription: introduction to consistent extension of the above muscles, including the paravertebral lumbar spine muscles and the M. quadratus lumborum; optimisation of shoulder joint/shoulder girdle movement; sensorimotor activation of the shoulder muscles; massage based on findings in the shoulder, neck and lumbar spine area on both sides.

If this does not lead to any permanent improvement in the symptoms, I would prescribe the use of a transcutaneous electrical nerve stimulation (TENS) device. The lumbar spine will be included in the next treatment.

Patient 3

Suspected segmental function disorders of the cervical spine (in the sense of hypomobility most likely due to degenerative changes)

With	Pain at the end of the range of movement in the area of the neck Pronounced restriction of movement (rotation left/right 10*–0°–45°, lateral flexion left/right 5°*–0°–10°, rotation in flexion left/right 5°*–0°–20°, flexion Reduced to two-thirds and externally to half
	Pronounced myoses of the paravertebral muscles, particularly the M. splenius capitis > left, M. levator scapulae and M. trapezius descendens and deep segmental muscles of the whole cervical spine
Without	Evidence of significant blocking of the occiput/C1 and C2/3 Pain referred/radiating to the extremities

Due to	Incorrect posture in the sense of slight translation of the head to the right with slightly elevated shoulders on both sides and increased kyphosis of the thoracic spine (hypomobile) and slight head and shoulder protraction right > left (shortened pectoral muscles)
	Bone-covered intervertebral disc prolapse and osteochondrosis at the level of C6/7 (current clinical relevance rather slight)
	Evidence of overall increase in muscle tension (traces of abrasion on the teeth, myoses of the muscles of mastication)
	Prior strain (see previous history)

*Severe left suboccipital pain at the end of the range of movement, rather hard feeling at the end of the range of movement.

Therapy and suggestions for further treatment

Directly after the examination, acupuncture treatment was carried out over distal points and mTrP of the M. splenius capitis on the right and the Mm. levator scapulae, trapezius pars descendens and the paravertebral segmental muscles of the upper/middle cervical spine on the left. This, in association with subsequent mobilisation in the sense of postisometric relaxation, led to a definite improvement in the range of movement and the pain at the end of the range of movement.

Targeted physiotherapy should here ideally be performed in the sense of manual therapy, e.g. using the Maitland plan.

Patient 4

Suspected slight radiculopathy most likely of the root at L5 on the right

With	Positive Lasègue sign at the end of the range of movement with simultaneous extension of the dura from proximal
	Referred myofascial pain (Mm. biceps femoris and gastrocnemius (caput medialis)/tibialis posterior)
	Slight shift of the vertebral column to the left
	Slight shortening/hardening of the paravertebral lumbar spine and the flank muscles on the right
	Slight involvement of the right sacroiliac joint (hypomobility)

Without	Evidence of segmental function disorder or restriction of movement of the lumbar spine
	Involvement of the hip joint (currently)
Due to	Previous accidental injury 1.5 years ago
	Sequestered intervertebral disc prolapse at L5/S1 on the right, affecting the root at S1 more than L5 on the right; root L5 slightly swollen (findings from elsewhere, MRI on _____)
	Pelvic obliquity on the left of 0.5 cm (recommend trying to even it out) and pronounced flat back (lower thoracic spine even slightly lordotic)
	Evidence of posterior McKenzie derangement syndrome

Therapy and suggestions for further treatment

The examination was immediately followed by treatment of the mTrP in the M. biceps femoris, M. tibialis posterior and in the M. gastrocnemius as well as supplementary treatment of the paravertebral muscles including the Mm. quadratus lumborum and piriformis. Almost the same symptoms were provoked by the trigger points during this treatment in both areas.

Physiotherapy prescription: McKenzie exercises (repetitive mobilisation of the lumbar spine into extension in the prone position supported on the arms without straining the paravertebral muscles), (introduction to) extension of the above muscles, with the ischiocrural muscles and also with flexion of the cervical spine in the supine position in the sense of extension of the dura/root mobilisation, mobilisation of the right iliosacral joint; massage based on the findings.

If long-lasting and sufficient pain improvement is not achieved by the trigger point treatment, we recommend an additional caudal block, with the possible addition of, e.g., Lipotalon on the first or second occasions.

Remarks: the patient (a mountain guide) remained completely free of symptoms after the first treatment.

Chapter | **14** |

Differential diagnosis

Nicolas Behrens, Dominik Irnich, Martin Offenbächer, Hans-Joachim Schmitt, Michael Späth, Andreas Winkelmann

The differential diagnosis of myofascial pain must be made carefully and be based on current medical knowledge. The following problems occur in practice.

- Is this primarily myofascial pain?
- Is the myofascial pain only a 'sympathetic reaction' to some other pathology?
- What part does the myofascial pain play in pain elsewhere, e.g. muscle pain with inflammatory joint disease?

In the following sections we look at the problem of myofascial pain from two different aspects.

- First, the differential diagnosis is described according to the affected structure and the cause (Section 14.1).
- Second, the clinical and practical distribution pattern of the myofascial pain is discussed; this offers a valuable basis for the consideration of a differential diagnosis (Section 14.2).

14.1 DIFFERENTIAL DIAGNOSIS ACCORDING TO AFFECTED STRUCTURE AND CAUSE

14.1.1 Muscle diseases

Michael Späth

If the cause of the pain is attributed to MPS in the course of the diagnosis and one or more mTrPs can be attributed to the local findings, the pain is usually classified initially by the patient non-specifically as muscle pain and requires consideration of a differential diagnosis, to include the whole spectrum of myopathies. This is despite only a few muscle diseases being accompanied by pain. Initially, the findings from the clinical examination are helpful in this. However, more extensive tests using different methods are usually essential.

Definition and characteristics: findings of clinical examination (key symptoms) in myopathies

Myopathies are diseases which result in structural or at least metabolically active changes to the muscles. It is necessary to differentiate between inflammatory – usually immunogenic – myositis, degenerative and metabolic disorders, typically myopathies, which are determined by molecular genetics, and toxic and endocrinal myopathies.

The clinical pattern is typically characterised by the proximal symmetrical weakness of the muscles of the extremities without sensory deficits. However, the less common distal, nuchal, bulbar or oculopharyngeal distribution types are also possible. The deep tendon reflexes are frequently not weakened until there is definite paresis. Only some of the myopathies are associated with atrophy, which is not uncommonly dependent on the severity and duration of the disease. With some muscle diseases, hypertrophy (myotonia congenita) and pseudohypertrophy (Duchenne's muscular dystrophy) are possible, as well as mixed forms (Becker's muscular dystrophy and other limb girdle dystrophies).

Most myopathies present with slightly reduced muscle tone. When considering a differential diagnosis with MPS, phenomena should be taken into account which are characterised by a change in muscle tone or involuntary muscle activity (see Table 14.1 and Table 14.2).

http://dx.doi.org/10.1016/B978-0-7020-4312-3.00014-3

Table 14.1 History and clinical findings with myalgia

Localisation	Location (anatomical), distribution (focal or generalised), referral, superficial or deep pain sensation
Pain character	Stiff muscles, cramp-like, burning
Duration and frequency	Permanent, intermittent
Worsening factors, pain provocation	Pain at rest, dependent on movement, associated with infection: environmental factors, medicines/drugs
Clinical findings and concomitant symptoms	Paresis, spasms, motion disorders, tenderness, changes in muscle tone, clinical indicators for other diseases

Other questions about history
- Start and course, dependent on time of day, temperature or food?
- Activity: increasing weakness or improved strength?
- Muscle pain at rest or during exercise?
- Loss of weight or muscle mass?
- Exhaustion?
- Muscle diseases in the family?
- Development of motor function?
- Other characteristic diseases?
- Medicines?
- Nutrition, travel?

Correlative symptoms

The individual myopathies which should be considered are summarised in Table 14.3. A correlative symptom is the sensation of muscle pain, although this can also usually be attributed to an mTrP on account of its characteristics.

Divergent symptoms

Divergent symptoms can be recognised using the symptoms described in Table 14.3. However, it should still be noted that any of the diseases mentioned can also be accompanied by an MPS without any causal association; that is, mTrPs can also be palpated.

Diagnostic and differential diagnostic procedure for myalgia

The diagnosis of myalgia is represented in Fig. 14.1 in accordance with the neuromuscular centre consensus paper commissioned by the *Deutsche Gesellschaft für Muskelkranke e.V.* (DGM, the German Society for Muscular Disease).

Table 14.2 Examination findings of 'muscle tone' and 'involuntary muscle activity'

Cramp	Temporary, involuntary, visible and painful contraction of a larger muscle area
Tetany	Syndrome of neuromuscular excitability with muscle twitches, cramps and carpopedal spasms
Fasciculation	Random, spontaneous and painless twitching of a group of muscle fibres or a motor unit, also recognisable in a movement of the overlying skin, mucous membrane or finger (with anterior horn cell damage and axonal neuropathy; benign fasciculation is possible without amounting to a disease)
Myoclonia	Short, involuntary, irregular twitching by contraction of individual or several muscles
Myokymia	Continuous wavelike movements of the superficial muscles and the overlying skin, e.g. with radiogenic neuropathy
Myotonia	Unusual muscle relaxation after voluntary activity or tapping of the muscle
Neuromyotonia	Syndrome not always clinically distinguishable from myotonia with spontaneous, continuous muscle fibre activity, associated with muscle cramps, weakness, muscle stiffness, slow relaxation and increased sweating
Contracture	Fixed restricted movement of a joint which can be caused by muscle and tendon shortening or reduced extensibility of the joint capsule
Myxoedema	Focal muscle contraction following percussion with formation of a small swelling
Rippling	Muscle contraction phenomenon with a lengthwise hollow parallel the long axis of the muscle, which moves slowly in a distal direction

14.1.2 Periarthropathies

Andreas Winkelmann

Definition

Periarthropathies can be defined as pain in the periarticular soft tissue (muscles, tendons, bursae, fascia and joint capsules) with reduced joint function capacity resulting

Table 14.3 Myalgia due to myopathy

Inflammatory myopathy	
Idiopathic inflammatory (immunogenic) myopathy	Polymyositis, einschlusskörpermyositis (mostly without myalgia), dermatomyositis (DM), interstitial myositis (concomitant myositis with inflammatory rheumatic systemic diseases)
Less common focal inflammatory myopathy	Granulomatous myopathy (e.g. with sarcoidosis), focal myositis, eosinophilic polymyositis, eosinophilic fasciitis
Pathogen-associated myositis	Bacterial (staphylococci), Coxsackie B5 virus, *Borrelia burgdorferi*, parasitosis
Degenerative myopathies	
Duchenne muscular dystrophy	Calf pain in approximately 30% of cases, predominantly in childhood
Becker muscular dystrophy	Pain more pronounced, paresis and atrophy less so
Fascioscapulohumeral muscular dystrophy	
Limb girdle dystrophy	e.g. Dysferlinopathy
Myotonia	
Myotonia congenita	Becker/Thomsen/potassium-induced, ion-channel disease
Paramyotonia congenita	Ion-channel disease
Myotonic dystrophy	
DM1 (Curschmann–Steinert)	Autosomal dominant (trinucleotide expansion); tendency to distal paresis and myotonia
DM2/proximal myotonic myopathy (PROMM)	Autosomal dominant (tetranucleotide expansion); tendency to proximal paresis with frequent myalgia, myotonia rather mild; myalgia characteristic, predominantly exercise-induced and dependent, frequently tenderness and headache
Metabolic myopathies	
Symptoms	Stiff muscles, pain dependent on exercise, muscle weakness and stiffness; possibly rhabdomyolysis and myoglobinuria with carbohydrate, fatty acid or purine metabolism disorders
McArdle's syndrome (glycogenosis type V)	Autosomal recessive (lack of muscle phosphorylase); pain can often be relieved by further muscle work ('second wind')
Tarui's disease (glycogenosis type VII)	Autosomal recessive (lack of phosphofructokinase)
Carnitine palmitoyltransferase (CPT) deficiency: CPT-I and CPT-II deficiency	Exercise dependent myalgia less pronounced than with glycogenosis; blood test using tandem mass spectrometry is cost-efficient and comprehensive
Myoadenylate deaminase deficiency (MAD deficiency)	Innervation-dependent stiffness of the skeletal muscles; enzyme histochemical evidence of the enzyme defect in the skeletal muscles; up to 75% of those affected without pain
Endocrine myopathies	
Hypothyroidism	Muscle weakness, myalgia, muscle cramps
Hypoparathyroidism	Painful tetany due to calcium and magnesium deficiency
Toxic myopathies	
Alcohol, heroin	Necrotising myopathy
Tetanus toxin, strychnine	
Drug side effects	Statins, chloroquine, colchicine, D-penicillamine, vincristine, cocaine; painful muscle cramps: clofibrate, L-dopa, salbutamol

Continued

Table 14.3 Myalgia due to myopathy—cont'd

Myalgia with rare diseases	
Stiff person syndrome	Frequent association with other autoimmune diseases
Neuromyotonia (Isaacs–Mertens syndrome)	Frequent association with other autoimmune diseases, frequently antibodies to tension-dependent potassium channels
Brody myopathy	Typically in childhood or adolescence painless muscle contractions can be provoked by muscle work and cold, but also exercise-dependent myalgia
Rippling muscle disease	Autosomal dominant and sporadic; exercise-induced myalgia and cramp-like states, frequently calf hypertrophy; percussion-induced, fast muscle contractions
Amyloid myopathy	Myalgia in isolated cases

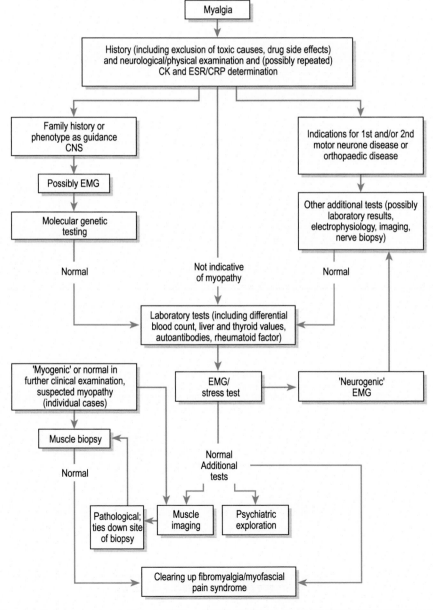

Fig. 14.1 Algorithm for diagnosing myalgia. (Berghoff et al. 2005) CK, creatinine kinase; CRP, C-reactive protein.

in reduced ability to participate in everyday life. Synonyms used for periarthropathy are the terms periarthritis (-itis = inflammation, peri = around) or periarthrosis. Periarthropathy is an umbrella term for a number of disorders and changes in the soft tissue around the joints (e.g. the shoulder, hip and less commonly the knee region).

Characteristics, findings from clinical examination (key symptoms), aetiology

With functional disorders of the joint there is usually a characteristic capsule pattern. The extent of the disorder is dependent on the soft tissue surrounding the affected joint, the perception of pain and the strategies implemented in handling the symptoms, e.g. on the postural deficit or posture correction. There is usually evidence of a taut band in individual muscle groups, and sometimes muscle contraction as well. If the joint symptoms are caused by strain on the tendons and/or muscles, the pain can be provoked by stretching and/or extending the affected muscle in the area of the joint. When testing joint mobility, the end feeling if there is limited mobility can be described as taut elastic (as with muscle contraction and MPS). Patients often report end-phase pain in this case.

With or without evidence of inflammation in the periarticular tissue, there is evidence of taut bands and mTrPs, which are usually latent.

An active mTrP should not be considered the leading cause responsible for the symptoms of periarthropathy. If this is the case, a diagnosis of MPS should be made.

Strain of one or several periarticular soft tissue structures may be cited as the cause, which can be triggered by incorrect posture, incorrect loading, trauma or ligament instability. These can cause reactive inflammation, such as bursitis or capsulitis.

Periarthropathy is most frequently observed in the shoulder area and is therefore described here as an example. As explained in detail in the following, the affected structure and/or the causing structure should also be described as precisely as possible, as well using the term periarthropathy.

If inflammation keeps occurring with periarthropathia (periarthrosis, periarthritis) humeroscapularis, calcium deposits can occur in the tissue (very often at the insertion of a tendon or along the course of the tendon, for example with supraspinatus tendon syndrome or impingement syndrome; this is also possible without calcium). This can sometimes cause a rupture of the tendon as well (e.g. supraspinatus tendon). These calcium deposits are mostly hydroxyapatite deposits (hydroxyapatite is a calcium salt compound). In an X-ray, hydroxyapatite usually looks milky and homogeneous. If the small hydroxyapatite crystals enter a synovial bursa, under certain circumstances it leads to very acute, highly inflammatory, severe shoulder pain and severely restricted movement caused by the pain, or even a completely frozen shoulder. If the joint symptoms are caused by calcium, the diagnosis of periarthropathia (periarthritis) calcarea should be selected.

Correlative and divergent symptoms

Taut bands can occur with periarthropathy and with MPS, as well as with all the diagnoses in Table 14.4. The taut band seen in MPS, and frequently also in periarthropathy, is prominent. With functional disorders of the vertebral column this is frequently referred distally into the extremities as kinetic chain tendinosis, with distally reducing taut band. Because a taut band alone does not serve to differentiate between these diagnoses, this has not specifically been cited under the findings in Table 14.4 of the correlative and divergent symptoms of MPS.

The symptoms as cited in the following table for active arthrosis can be described for periarthropathy with inflammation (bursitis).

To differentiate the arthralgia see the other sections in this chapter, especially on the topics of arthrosis and arthritis (Section 14.1.3), functional disorders of the vertebral column (Section 14.1.4), muscle diseases (Section 14.1.1), medical diseases (Section 14.1.7) and neurological diseases (Section 14.1.6).

14.1.3 Degenerative joint diseases

Hans-Joachim Schmitt, Andreas Winkelmann

Definition

Arthrosis can be described as wear and tear on the joint. As such, it is less a disease and more a natural, slowly progressive aging process. The term arthrosis covers all the degenerative diseases of the joint, which lead to increasing destruction of the joint cartilage and involve other joint structures such as bones, joint capsule membranes and surrounding muscles. There is first of all an underlying disparity between strain and resilience of the cartilaginous joint parts.

Aetiology, characteristics, findings from clinical examination (key symptoms)

There are two types of arthrosis: primary and secondary. The causes of primary arthrosis cannot be easily explained, while the causes of secondary arthritis (e.g. post-traumatic) are easier to name. They occur earlier than primary arthritis and more often affect only one joint. Signs of arthritis can

Table 14.4 Differential diagnosis of arthralgia

DIAGNOSIS	PAIN CHARACTER[1]	CLINICAL EXAMINATION (JOINT END FEELING)	mTrP[2]	LABORATORY[3]	X-RAY (FINDINGS)[4]
MPS	a) Diffuse, dull, dragging, burning, b) regional, c) pseudoradicular pain referral	Limited movement with hard elastic end feeling, end-phase pain	++ Twitch response, referred pain	–	–
Periarthropathy	a) Diffuse, dull, dragging b) regional in/around the joint, c) radicular pain referral	Limited movement with hard elastic end feeling, end-phase pain, capsule pattern	+ or ±, Not trigger of symptoms	–	Possibly calcification at tendon insertion
Arthrosis without activation	a) Diffuse, dull to stabbing, b) regional in or around the joint, mono/oligo- (large joints) or polyarticular (small joints), c) exercise-dependent	Limited movement with hard end feeling, end-phase pain, capsule pattern, some crepitation	±, Not trigger of symptoms	–	Narrowing of joint space, osteophytes
Arthrosis with activation	a) Diffuse, dull, stabbing, dragging, burning, b) regional in or around the joint, mostly monoarticular, c) exercise-dependent, pain at rest or at night	Signs of synovitis (reddening, heating, swelling or effusion), restricted movement with hard elastic end feeling, pain on movement, capsule pattern	±, Not trigger of symptoms	– (slight + possible)	Narrowing of joint space, osteophytes, joint effusion
Arthritis	a) Diffuse, dull, stabbing, burning, wearing, b) mono-, oligo- or polyarticular, c) pain at rest or at night, run-up pain, early morning wakening due to pain	Signs of synovitis (reddening, heating, swelling), restricted movement with hard elastic end feeling, pain on movement, capsule pattern	±, Not trigger of symptoms	+	Erosions, usures, demineralisation
Functional disorder vertebral column with pseudoradicular referral	a) Diffuse, dull, dragging, burning, b) regional, c) pseudoradicular pain referral	Limited movement with soft elastic (hypermobility), hard elastic (muscular strain of segmental dysfunction) or hard end feeling (degenerative vertebral column without activation), end-phase pain	±, Not trigger of symptoms	–	–

Table 14.4 Differential diagnosis of arthralgia—cont'd

DIAGNOSIS	PAIN CHARACTER[1]	CLINICAL EXAMINATION (JOINT END FEELING)	mTrP[2]	LABORATORY[3]	X-RAY (FINDINGS)[4]
Functional disorder vertebral column with radiculopathy	a) Diffuse, dull, dragging, burning, b) regional, c) radicular pain referral	Limited movement with hard elastic (with nerve extension reactive taut band) end feeling, sensory and/or motor function deficits, nerve extension tests with pain referral close to vertebral column, end-phase pain	±, Not trigger of symptoms	–	Nerve compression
Chronic widespread pain/ fibromyalgia syndrome	a) Diffuse, dull, dragging, stabbing, burning, wearing, b) multilocular/generalis, c) pseudoradicular pain referral	Little or no restriction of movement, if available with hard elastic end feeling	±, Not trigger of generalised symptoms	–	–

[1]a) Pain quality, b) pain locality, c) pain on exercise/rest
[2]mTrP: active (++), latent (+), possible (±)
[3]Laboratory: inflammatory values elevated (+); not elevated (–)
[4]X-ray (findings): normal, not relevant (–)

be found in almost everyone over the age of 65. However, younger people can also be affected, especially if their lifestyle make great demands on their joints, such as in athletes. Characteristically, joint pain dependent on strain is described as diffuse, dull, dragging, and sometimes even as stabbing, gnawing or burning.

The first clinical evidence of arthritis may be restricted movement with capsule pattern (at the beginning movement is still possible without end-phase pain). Sometimes crepitation can be felt during movement. At the end of the movement the sensation is typically hard as the joint structures touch, causing end-phase pain. When activated with recurrent synovial irritation and formation of effusion, the end sensation is usually hard and elastic when the joint structures touch at the end of the motion, and if the effusion is large the feeling is soft and elastic. If there is synovitis, pain can be caused as the motion starts and also during movement. There are normally joint problems when the arthritis is active: these include pain, restricted movement and/or signs of synovitis (reddening, heating, swelling).

The joints most frequently affected are, in descending order: knee, shoulder, hips, carpometacarpal joint of the thumb, middle and terminal phalanges of the fingers,

and vertebral joints. Factors of influence are being overweight, poor posture and endocrine factors (metabolic factors).

Correlative and divergent symptoms

Correlating to the MPS are taut bands and diffuse, dull, dragging and/or burning pain, usually regional (arthritis in the joint area), sometimes with pseudoradicular referred pain (more common with MPS). Latent or active mTrPs can also be present with arthritis. Correlating to the activated arthritis is the hard elastic end sensation at the end of joint movement.

Divergent from MPS is the capsule pattern which is typical of arthritis if there is a joint function disorder, and for non-activated arthritis it is the hard end feeling at the end of the joint movement. With arthritis, an active mTrP, if present, is not the main cause of the pain.

The signs typical of synovitis are different from those of activate arthritis: reddening, heating, swelling (effusion). A lack of mTrPs rules out MPS.

To differentiate the arthralgias see Table 14.4 and other sections, especially on the topics of periarthropathy (Section 14.1.2), arthritis (Section 14.1.3), functional disorders of the vertebral column (Section 14.1.4), muscle diseases (Section 14.1.1), medical diseases (Section 14.1.7) and neurological diseases (Section 14.1.6).

14.1.4 Functional disorders of the vertebral column

Hans-Joachim Schmitt

In many cases symptoms of the vertebral column cannot be attributed to a definite cause. The underlying cause of vertebral column pain is frequently irritation of nociceptive structures within or outside the movement segment. However, this irritation subsides in more than 95% of cases within the first 14 days, as there is a great tendency for these lesions to heal themselves. Experiencing back pain at least once a year is the rule rather than the exception in people aged over 60.

Chronic or chronically recurring back pain is a problem. These days, this is understood to be a somatic, psychological or social event where in the end a unique cause cannot be found either at the physical or the psychological level. The event is more likely to have occurred as a result of a number of factors and the factors which cause chronification are crucial:

- conviction that it can be controlled (lack of self-effectiveness),
- attitudes to disease (e.g. turning everything into a catastrophe or rigid endurance),
- workplace dissatisfaction,
- psychoemotional factors such as anxiety, depression or somatoform pain experience.

Contrary to popularly held opinion, factors such as lack of exercise, obesity, physical strain and degenerative changes are of secondary significance (Schiltenwolf, Henningsen 2007).

Nevertheless, it is essential to describe damaged structures using the findings and bring subjective symptoms into agreement with objective findings (see Section 13.5). However, this is not always possible. Making a diagnosis about the vertebral column is also dependent on training, understanding and the therapist's attitude.

> The therapist should be aware that there is as yet no generally recognised division of functional disorders and pain caused by the vertebral column. This also applies to the nomenclature that is used.

The following sections discuss the functional disorders of the vertebral column in a clinically oriented way, which is also significant for the therapeutic course of action.

Strain syndrome of the vertebral column

Definition

This is diffuse, mostly superficial pain caused by poor posture, long-term strain or too great a strain on the paravertebral soft tissue (ligaments, muscles).

Characteristics

Pain predominantly of muscular cause leads to increasing strain or after strain to swelling, diffuse dragging, sometimes gnawing/piercing, pressing local pain, which spontaneously recedes after a short period of being relieved of the load (lying down, changing position).

If the pain is predominantly caused by the ligaments, it also locally occurring, gradually increasing, dragging, burning pain, which occurs particularly after exercise at rest. It is not relieved by a relief posture alone but produces a feeling of needing to move gently.

Correlating symptoms and findings with MPS

- Dragging to burning, gradually deteriorating pain, which is made worse with increasing strain and can quickly recede with rest, although reduction of swelling may be delayed.
- Dysfunction with restricted motion at the end of the range of movement.

Divergent symptoms and findings

- Referred pain is rather seldom observed in this syndrome.
- There are local ligamental tenderpoints.

Excluding symptoms and findings

There are no symptoms or findings which definitively rule out MPS. However, if there are no trigger points with a referred pain pattern or a typical myofascial pain pattern which can be triggered by the therapist (pain which can only be reproduced by the strain situation), the diagnosis of a (musculoligamentary) strain syndrome should be made.

From clinical experience, the treatment of the paravertebral muscles is also often effective via latent TrPs, in addition to repetitive extension and posture training, etc.

Segmental functional disorder of the vertebral column

Definition

The term 'segmental functional disorder of the vertebral column' with or without pain describes limited or excessive movement in the segment, which is caused by a change in the structures of the motion segment according to Junghans and Schmorl (1951; segmental muscles, segmental facet joints, discs, ligaments, capsular structures, cancellous bone tissue).

Segmental functional disorders of the vertebral column can cause referred pain depending on the pathology. The causes can be spondylogenic, affect the intervertebral discs (derangement or prolapse with or without irritation of the root) or the facet joints or even accompany true radicular pain syndrome. There is an overlap here with the segmental muscles, an overlap which at the same time provides access for therapy via the trigger point.

> Behind many vertebral column problems which are also segmental is strain caused by excessive muscular tension, which is particularly unfavourable for the facet joints, for example, where there is concomitant hyperlordosis.

Characteristics

Spondylogenic pain – that is, pain and functional disorders caused by cancellous bone tissue – can cause segmental or polysegmental symptoms. The symptoms are spread neurotopographically and correspond not only to the myotome or the dermatome but also to the sclerotome. The pain tends to be deep-seated, dragging and oppressive and radiates far into the extremities and the strain gets worse suddenly or gradually, depending on the structure affected.

If segmental functional disorder is associated with musculoligamentary strain (see characteristics above) this frequently affects the iliolumbar ligaments at the vertebral column, or the supraspinosa and interspinosa ligaments, and less frequently the sacrospinalis and sacrotuberalis ligaments.

The term derangement describes a temporary deformity of a poorly malleable intervertebral disc, mostly after poor posture for a long time. The pain is typically on movement in the direction of the limited malleability (where the typical wedge shape can even form a bulge). The symptoms recede with repetitive small-amplitude movement in this direction, when the pain then centralises.

With facet syndrome strain of the vertebral joints with alteration of shape and/or position leads to segmental functional disorders with muscular dysfunction (taut band) or via activated inflammatory processes to irritation of the joint capsule with the stimulation of effusion. Typically, tenderness is caused on the facet or facet compression pain with ipsilateral limited rotation and extension.

On a MRI scan, erosive osteochondrosis or aseptic spondylodiscitis can be distinguished by bone marrow oedema of the vertebral body bordering the affected intervertebral disc compartment with irregular (erosive) superior or inferior end plates. When a contrast medium is administered, enrichment can be found particularly in the central intervertebral disc space, which is normally not supplied by blood vessels. The nerves have been infiltrated by the vessels and this leads to massive pain even with small movements, and moreover when strain is relieved, as in an exercise bath. The increased irritability of the segment correlates with reports from the patient that strain is suffered for days afterwards (the 'irritation condition').

Reversible functional disorders of the motion segment without structural lesion, with changed sensation at the end of the range of movement (hard elastic), stabbing pain at the end of the movement, hypertonic segmental muscles and possibly functional disorder of the segmental viscera are often also described as blockages.

Correlating symptoms and findings

Correlating symptoms are usually functional disorders with or without muscular taut bands and referred pain which does not correspond on closer examination to the supply area of a spinal nerve.

Divergent symptoms and findings

- **Musculoligamentary strain:** diffuse pain with usually static strain, functional disorder when posture is resolved.
- **Derangement:** primarily severe limitation of movement, end feeling determined by counter tension, typically tolerance of the tiniest of movements with concomitant centralisation of the pain/spread of the pain.
- **Facet syndrome:** sensation at the end of the range of movement determined by counter tension (avoidance of pain), pain typically caused in extension and rotation, stabbing, sharp pain.
- **Blockage:** reversible functional disorder of the motion segment without structural lesion. Changed sensation at the end of the range of movement (hard elastic), stabbing pain at the end of the range of movement.

Excluding symptoms and findings

- **Musculoligamentary strain:** symptoms recede at rest, no mTrP.
- **Derangement:** centralisation of the pain with small amplitude repetitive movement in the direction of the painful movement.
- **Facet syndrome:** extension–rotation pain in the lumbar spine, compression pain over the facet.
- **Blockages:** irritation zones.

Radicular syndrome of the vertebral column

Definition

Radicular symptoms arise as a result of irritation or compression of spinal nerves, for example as a result of a prolapsed disc, spinal stenosis or narrowing of the neuroforamina.

Characteristics

Radicular syndrome leads to pain projected into the periphery, which is felt as burning, stabbing, electrifying or shooting pain. The functional disorder occurs during extension or compression of the nerve structures or as a result of biochemical stimulation or through perineural and endoneural fibrosis which occurs at the chronification stage. Sensorimotor deficits may also occur. Irritation of the dura is revealed in clinical examination when the pain is felt during coughing, sneezing or straining and can even get worse in a seated position. If the symptoms have been caused by a disc lesion, they occur quickly in the causative movement with an annular cause, but there can be a delay of several days if there is a nuclear cause.

Correlating symptoms and findings

As with primary MPS, functional disorders and muscular taut bands can occur. Subtle autonomic symptoms can also occur, such as a feeling of coldness or slight neuropathic symptoms such as burning.

Divergent symptoms and findings

Divergent symptoms are stabbing, burning, electric shooting pains at rest, made worse by movement, pressure or extension of the course of the nerve. There is a response to slight cold and sensorimotor deficits.

Excluding symptoms and findings

Excluding symptoms are sensorimotor deficits attributable to the nerve supply area and positive nerve extension signs.

14.1.5 Inflammatory joint diseases

Michael Späth

Joint diseases are always manifested as arthritis. The structures associated with the joints can also be affected: they may be involved or they may be affected in isolation. If mTrPs can also be palpated during the examination, the whole spectrum of inflammatory joint diseases must be considered in terms of a differential diagnosis. Make sure that some of the systemic inflammatory rheumatic diseases are not involved at all and only the 'soft tissues' are affected.

Clinical findings (key symptoms)

Systemic inflammatory rheumatic diseases are all characterised by the release of inflammatory mediators by complex autoimmune processes which independently of any clinical picture can in the worst-case scenario destroy both joints (with all the associated morphological components) and structures close to them (tendons, tendon sheaths,

ligaments, bursae). In the case of arthritis, the pattern of attack (monoarticular, oligoarticular or polyarticular, in the last case symmetrical or asymmetrical) often helps to further the differential diagnosis (see Table 14.5).

Basically, but particularly with joint pain without swelling, symptoms of possible involvement of internal organs should be considered. Historical information on the manner in which the disease began is indispensable (e.g. possible early symptoms such as cervical syndrome or carpal tunnel syndrome with rheumatoid arthritis, gastrointestinal or urogenital infection approximately 2–4 weeks prior to the arthritis with reactive arthritis, an unusual 'sunburn' with systemic lupus erythematosus, the very sudden occurrence of myalgia of the proximal extremities with polymyalgia rheumatica). In all the examples mentioned, and in most of the other systemic inflammatory rheumatic diseases, laboratory tests and possibly also imaging tests complete the diagnosis.

Correlating symptoms

The individual inflammatory joint diseases to take into account are summarised in Table 14.6. A correlating symptom is the sensation of muscle pain, but this can usually also be attributed to one of these diseases by noting the characteristics of any mTrPs.

Divergent symptoms

Divergent symptoms can be recognised using the symptoms described in Table 14.6. However, it should still be noted that any of the diseases mentioned can also be accompanied by an MPS without any causal association (i.e. mTrPs can also be palpated).

Diagnostic and differential diagnosis characteristics

For diagnostic and differential diagnosis characteristics, see Table 14.7.

14.1.6 Neurological diseases

Michael Späth

Secondary mTrPs can be found with many neurological diseases. These can on the one hand indicate an underlying disease and, on the other, in rare cases, indicate existing muscle dysfunction as well, such as that caused by mTrPs associated with slight neurological symptoms (e.g. hyperaesthesia via mTrP, nerve-compression syndrome caused by mTrP). In any case, if neurological symptoms occur, the appropriate neurological tests can be introduced to rule out an underlying neurological disease. It can be helpful

Table 14.5 History and clinical findings for arthralgia/arthritis

History and clinical findings	
Localisation	Location (large or small joints), distribution (mono-, oligo- or polyarticular, symmetrical or asymmetrical), bordering structures affected (tendosynovitis, tendovaginitis, bursitis), myalgia (referred pain, independent muscle involvement in the sense of interstitial myositis). Tendon insertion pain with concomitant enthesopathy with seronegative spondyloarthropathy and arthritis psoriatica
Pain character	'Dragging', 'gnawing', sometimes 'stabbing' joint pain on movement, but also occurring at rest, sometimes leading to waking up at night With muscle involvement: muscle soreness, cramp-like, burning
Duration and frequency	Permanent pain, intermittent Run-up pain, frequently associated with morning stiffness >1 h Polymyalgia rheumatica: night pain with early morning wakening, improvement during the day, sometimes as far as freedom from symptoms by later afternoon
Factors which provoke pain or make it worse	Resting pain, exercise-dependent; associated with infection, environmental factors, medicines/drugs Nutrition dependent: gout (arthritis urica)
Clinical findings and concomitant symptoms	• Arthritis with swelling, reddening, overheating, restricted movement, palpable effusion • Enthesopathy with tenderness, possibly also swelling and overheating in the area of the tendon insertion • Polymyalgia rheumatica with varying paresis during the daytime; with giant cell arteritis: possibly (painful) palpable temple artery • Seronegative spondyloarthropathy: pain and restricted movement of the axial skeleton • Concomitant myositis: paresis, motion disorders, tenderness • Arthritis psoriatica: psoriasis vulgaris • Basically: all symptoms with possible organ involvement

Questions for the history
• Start and course of the disease, dependent on time of day, temperature and nutrition?
• Activity: increase in pain or deterioration of function?
• Joint pain at rest or during exercise?
• Weight loss?
• Exhaustion?
• Joint diseases in the family?
• Medicines?
• Nutrition, travel?

here to classify according to the clinical findings (key symptoms).

Clinical findings (key symptoms) with lesions of the CNS and the second motoneuron

Besides the myopathies described elsewhere (see Section 14.1.1) some diseases of both the central and peripheral nervous system can lead to increases in muscle tension (spasticity and rigor) which are manifested as pain and tension in the affected area, predominantly in the area of the extremities. The key symptoms of the central nervous innervation disorder can very often be attributed to the actual disease (see Table 14.8).

Clinical findings (key symptoms) with lesions of the peripheral nervous system

Damage to the peripheral nervous system due to various causes can be accompanied by myalgia as a non-specific symptom (see Table 14.9).

Correlating symptoms

The individual neurological diseases to take into account are summarised in Table 14.6. A correlating symptom is the sensation of muscle pain, although this can usually also be attributed to one of these diseases by noting the characteristics of a trigger point.

Table 14.6 Myalgia with inflammatory joint diseases

Chronic arthritis and seronegative spondyloarthritis	
Rheumatoid arthritis	Myalgia frequently in the prodromal stage, later occasional interstitial myositis (concomitant myositis); reduced strength caused by pain
Arthritis psoriatica	Enthesopathy
Spondylitis ankylosis	Particularly if initially sciatica-like (early morning wakening), pain also felt as myalgia (with sacroiliitis); enthesopathy
Reactive arthritis	Sciatica-like, pain also felt as myalgia (with sacroiliitis); enthesopathy
Arthritis and spondyloarthritis with inflammatory bowel disease	Sciatica-like, pain also felt as myalgia (with sacroiliitis); enthesopathy
Collagenosis and vasculitis	
Systemic lupus erythematosus	Myalgia frequently in the prodromal stage, later occasional interstitial myositis (concomitant myositis); reduced strength caused by pain
Progressive systemic sclerosis	Myalgia, occasionally interstitial myositis (concomitant myositis); reduced strength caused by pain
Sjögren's syndrome	Myalgia, occasionally interstitial myositis (concomitant myositis); reduced strength caused by pain
Mixed collagenosis	Myalgia, occasionally interstitial myositis (concomitant myositis); reduced strength caused by pain
Immunogenic myositis	See Muscle diseases
Polymyalgia rheumatica	Myalgia predominantly of the muscles of the proximal extremities, definitely pronounced at night and in the early morning, improvement during the day; paresis
Takayasu's syndrome	Myalgia possible
Panarteritis nodosa	Myalgia
Wegener's granulomatosis	Myalgia
Churg–Strauss syndrome	Myalgia possible
Cutaneous leukocytoclastic vasculitis	Myalgia possible
Behçet's syndrome	Myalgia, occasionally interstitial myositis (concomitant myositis); reduced strength caused by pain
Pathogen-associated arthritis	
Arthritis with virus infections	Myalgia
Arthritis with bacterial infections and following infection with other microorganisms	Myalgia possible
Infectious arthritis	Myalgia very rare

Table 14.7 Diagnostic anomalies with inflammatory joint diseases

Chronic arthritis and seronegative spondyloarthritis	
Rheumatoid arthritis	Symmetrical polyarthritis, predominantly metacarpophalangeal and metatarsophalangeal joints and middle joints of the hands and feet, anti-ccP antibodies
Arthritis psoriatica	Dactylitis, mono- or oligoarthritis, psoriasis vulgaris (family history!) but also possible without
Spondylitis ankylosans	Sacroiliitis, vertebral column also affected later with typical changes visible radiologically, evidence of HLA-B27 in about 95% of cases
Reactive arthritis	Previous gastrointestinal or urogenital infection, mostly monoarthritis but also oligoarthritis after 2–3 weeks' latency Evidence of HLA-B27 in about 60–70% of cases
Arthritis and spondyloarthritis with inflammatory bowel disease	Mono- or oligoarticular attack, bowel disease usually prior to the joint manifestation erythema nodosum more common in patients with arthritis than in those without arthritis
Collagenosis and vasculitis	
Systemic lupus erythematosus	Typical clinical picture with possible characteristic organ involvement (e.g. 'butterfly erythema', 'lupus nephritis') Laboratory data: anti-nuclear antibodies, anti-double-stranded-DNA antibody, but also other autoimmune antibodies possible, use of complement (C3 and C4), increase in creatinine kinase activity with concomitant myositis possible
Progressive systemic sclerosis	Various course and attack pattern (e.g. diffuse, circumscript sclerodermia, e.g. CREST syndrome), possible involvement of internal organs (particularly problematic: involvement of lungs with pulmonary hypertension), various antibody profiles, including anti-Scl-70, anti-centromere and anti-PmScl antibodies
Sjögren's syndrome	Sicca syndrome due attack of exocrine glands (e.g. parotitis); pancreas involvement also possible, definitely increased risk of lymphoproliferative disease, anti-SS-A and anti-SS-B antibodies
Mixed collagenosis	e.g. Sharp's syndrome (anti-U1-RNP antibodies) and antisynthetase syndrome, e.g. Jo-1 syndrome (anti-Jo1 antibodies) with variably good differentiation from other collagenoses, but frequently identifiable by the relevant antibody profile
Immunogenic myositis	See Muscle diseases
Collagenosis and vasculitis	
Polymyalgia rheumatica	In older patients the clinical symptoms can begin suddenly, frequently accompanied by poor general condition and B-symptoms; definitely increased humeral inflammatory parameters, 'sudden' improvement on glucocorticoids; *note*: possibly giant cell arteritis with risk of irreversible loss of sight (begin treatment promptly!)
Takayasu's syndrome	Large vessel arteritis, 'aortic arch syndrome', 'pulseless disease'
Panarteritis nodosa	B-symptoms, organ manifestations, safe diagnosis from histology
Wegener's granulomatosis	Necrotising vasculitis; organ attack with granulomatous changes in the so-called generalisation stage in 95% of cases evidence of anti-neutrophil cytoplasmic antibody

Continued

111

Table 14.7 Diagnostic anomalies with inflammatory joint diseases—cont'd

Churg–Strauss syndrome	Lung involvement, eosinophilia, granulomatous intra- and perivascular infiltrate, laboratory: leukocytosis and eosinophilia
Cutaneous leukocytoclastic vasculitis	'Hypersensitivity angiitis'; vasculitis of the small blood vessel, limited to the skin, laboratory does not provide a differential diagnosis
Behçet's syndrome	Systemic vasculitis affecting skin and mucosa, eyes and joint inflammation, genetic disposition; more common in Mediterranean and Asiatic countries
Pathogen-associated arthritis	
Arthritis with virus infections	Hepatitis B, hepatitis C, parvovirus-B-19, HIV, rubella, alphaviruses (e.g. Ross River)
Arthritis with bacterial infections and following infection with other microorganisms	Rheumatic fever, brucellosis, gonococci, syphilis, Lyme disease
Infectious arthritis	Also 'septic' arthritis: pathogens in the joint, e.g. gonococci, *Mycobacterium tuberculosis* and other mycobacteria

Table 14.8 Symptoms and classification of CNS innervation disorder

CNS DISORDER	MUSCLE INVOLVEMENT
Parkinson's disease initially	Myalgia of the shoulder and upper arm region
Thalamus lesion, e.g. bleeding	Occasionally unilateral, not easily locatable pain; malposition of distal sections possible, especially of the upper extremities
Spinal cord lesions	Myalgia projecting into the muscles, almost always accompanied by central or peripheral paresis, sensory disorders or bladder and rectal function disorders
Amyotrophic and spinal muscle atrophy	Myalgia also in the early stage (mTrPs in the sense of MPS due to posture!)
Post-poliomyelitis syndrome	Myalgia 20–40 years after poliomyelitis (possibly as a result of overtaxing paretic muscles)

Questions for the history
- Start and progress?
- Indication of cause of infection, fever, skin changes?
- Activity: increase in pain or deterioration of function?
- Myalgia at rest or during exercise?
- Muscle atrophy?
- Myalgia accompanied by further neurological symptoms?
- Exhaustion?
- Medicines?

Table 14.9 Symptoms and classification of peripheral nervous system innervation disorder

DISORDERS OF THE PERIPHERAL NERVOUS SYSTEM	MUSCLE INVOLVEMENT
Guillain–Barré syndrome (idiopathic polyneuritis)	Myalgia common and early
Acute intermittent porphyria with neuropathy	Myalgia fleeting and early
Polyneuropathy of various causes affecting both sensorimotor function and autonomic fibres	Deficiency symptoms, myalgia very rare (as stimulus phenomenon)
Intoxication of peripheral nerves	Myalgia
Bannwarth meningopolyneuritis (with borreliosis)	Multiplex mononeuritis with severe pain pronounced at night on the trunk and extremities

Divergent symptoms

Divergent symptoms can be recognised using the symptoms described in Table 14.8. However, it should still be noted that any of the diseases mentioned can also be accompanied by an MPS without any causal association (i.e. mTrPs can also be palpated).

14.1.7 Internal diseases

Michael Späth

mTrP can be found with many internal diseases and their occurrence can have various causes. There is often a segmental co-reaction, which then affects further structures as well, such as skin and connective tissue, as a motor reaction to the symptom of pain or because of specific internal diseases, such as hypothyroidism or hyperthyroidism. Sufficient treatment of the mTrP can often lead to a relief of the symptoms as well. Nevertheless, internal diseases must be ruled out if the symptoms are longstanding or immediately if the key symptoms are appropriate.

Definition and characteristics: findings of clinical examination (key symptoms) in internal diseases with myalgia

Besides the inflammatory joint diseases described elsewhere, including collagenosis (see Section 14.1.5), and also besides neurological diseases with myalgia, some internal diseases can be accompanied by muscle pain, which must be considered in case there is a different diagnosis from that of MPS (see Table 14.10).

Table 14.10 Symptoms and classification of myalgia with internal diseases

INTERNAL DISEASES	MUSCLE INVOLVEMENT
Hypothyroidism and hyperthyroidism	Myalgia (myopathy)
Inflammatory intestinal diseases	Occasionally myalgia
Hypoparathyroidism and hyperparathyroidism	Myalgia
Viral hepatitis	Myalgia
Other viral diseases (e.g. Coxsackie B, parainfluenza)	Myalgia

Questions for the history
- Start and progress, fever?
- Activity: increase in pain or deterioration of function?
- Concomitant symptoms: e.g. diarrhoea?
- Pain not felt to be attributable to the muscles?
- Weight increase?
- Weight loss?
- Exhaustion?
- Medicines?
- Nutrition, travel?

Correlating symptoms

The individual internal diseases that should be considered are summarised in Table 14.10. A correlating symptom is the sensation of muscle pain, which, however, can usually also be attributed to one of these diseases by noting the characteristics of an mTrP.

Divergent symptoms

Divergent symptoms can be recognised using the symptoms described in Table 14.10. However, it should still be noted that any of the diseases mentioned can also be accompanied by an MPS without any causal association (i.e. mTrP can also be palpated).

14.2 DIFFERENTIAL DIAGNOSIS DEPENDING ON DISTRIBUTION PATTERN

14.2.1 Locoregional and regional pain patterns

Nicolas Behrens, Dominik Irnich

mTrPs can also cause exclusively local pain and functional disorders, for example in the area of the Mm. levator scapulae or deltoideus. With local and regional pain, it is important to distinguish whether the local mTrP is actually relevant in the sense of a concomitant cause of the pain or functional disorder. With local pain and existing local mTrP pathologies in the area of the joints, the bordering (non-muscular) soft tissue and local nerves should be delimited at the same time. The history and quality of the pain often provide crucial evidence.

> The basis of the diagnosis of MPS is always the careful palpation of the locoregional mTrPs; the precise and full release of the patient's local pain justifies attempted therapy (before more far-reaching diagnostic measures are undertaken).

Demarcation of local, non-myofascial pain

Locoregional nociceptive pain can arise from various structures which must be considered in case of a differential diagnosis. These include joints with ligaments, discs, capsules, intervertebral discs, bones, inflammatory vascular structures or tumours. The quality of the pain is often not enough for decisive evidence. The process of the development of the pain is more indicative.

- If this is an acute event, inflammatory or traumatic processes or their consequences are more likely, e.g. phlebitis, inflammation of the synovial bursa. The classical signs of inflammation are clinically definitive: heat, redness, pain and tumour as well as deterioration on the application of heat.
- If joint structures, e.g. menisci, are affected, it is typical that the pain on motion is not incremental with the size of the movement but is acute when movement is tested.
- Pathologies in the area of the bone can often be recognised by direct pressure palpation with suppression of the above-lying muscles.
- Inflammatory vascular processes can also often be provoked by precise, structure-related palpation.

Delimitation of local neuropathic pain

Locally limited or regionally referred pain patterns can also be of neuropathic origin. The patient usually reports burning, shooting, electrifying pain. This should prompt a differentiated neurological examination to look for causes (nerve damage by compression, inflammation, metabolic disorders such as Type 1 diabetes, etc.). The sensory examination in these cases should include the testing of thermal and mechanical stimuli to find the sensory and pain threshold in each case. In detail these include:

- tenderness,
- pain on needle stimulation,
- sharp/blunt discrimination,
- mild mechanical stimulation (e.g. swab),
- thermal stimulation (heat, cold),
- sense of vibration (e.g. polyneuropathy),
- testing for hypoaesthesia.

Using the history, including the pain quality and the neurological examination, locally limited or locoregionally referred pain patterns of neuropathic origin can usually be definitely identified.

Overview of differential diagnoses for local and regional pain patterns

Table 14.11 shows a locally limited pain pattern and the systems to be investigated for possible differential diagnoses. If pathologies are found here that explain the findings with pain and possibly functional disorder, the relevant (specialised) therapy measures should be taken up.

If there is resistance to therapy and the findings are not conclusive, a somatoform cause of the pain or psychoemotional stress should always be considered as a differential diagnosis. In Table 14.11 commonly found empirical psychopathologies and psychological stress patterns are included for the individual areas. If the pain is resistant to therapy and there are relevant symptoms (e.g. weight loss, fever), tumours and systemic inflammatory processes must be ruled out.

If the pathology is already regional, other structures and systems have frequently already been disturbed as well (e.g. muscle function chains), or they may have been strained as they attempt to compensate. The symptoms can spread in accordance with various sometimes scientifically substantiated but sometimes also only empirically known associations over the whole body (see Table 14.12, Fig. 14.2).

> With locoregional pain note that whole muscle chains have frequently already been disturbed (including the antagonists). The pain is usually just the tip of the iceberg!

14.2.2 Referred pain

Nicolas Behrens

Pain radiating to the extremities can have various causes and be attributed to a great variety of structures. Radiated myofascial pain is one of the most common in the locomotor system. It can usually be treated easily by addressing the cause, but is often overlooked or incorrectly diagnosed ('root irritation').

As almost all referred pain has long been diagnosed as root compression or irritation, so the introduction of the distinguishing term 'pseudoradicular' was sensible. Besides segmental spondylogenic pain, however, it also includes all referred pain which is not associated with the segmental classification. We do not therefore use the term pseudoradicular, but differentiate more precisely in accordance with the underlying referral mechanism and structure (see Tables 14.2–14.4). This means that myofascial pain can be immediately recognised, the appropriate therapy applied and excessive therapeutic interventions avoided.

> The identification of radicular pain can usually be performed relatively easily by clinical examination (see below). The differentiation between segmental spondylogenic and non-segmental pain referral using the pattern of radiation is on the other hand usually more difficult (different topography, dermatome and myotome, see below).

Segmental referred pain

With segmental pain referral, a therapeutic approach as close to the cause as possible is necessary in order to distinguish between nerve root compression or irritation as a cause, i.e. radicular symptoms, and a pathology in a motion segment of the vertebral column (segmental spondylogenic pain).

With radicular referral the underlying pathology is in the area of the nerve root, while with spondylogenic referral the

Table 14.11 From the pain area to the system: pain location and possible pathological associations

PAIN LOCATION	DIFFERENTIAL DIAGNOSIS TO SYSTEMS TO BE EXAMINED
Head and facial area	• Stomatognathic system (functional unit including muscle-temporomandibular joint-ligaments) • Upper cervical spine (e.g. atlanto-occipital transition) • Paranasal sinuses • Neuropathic pain syndrome of the face area (e.g. trigeminus neuralgia) • Ear or eye disease Psychological aspect: distress as disparity between stress and recompensation
Cervical spine, shoulder neck area	• Stomatognathic system • Lymph nodes • Sternoclavicular and acromioclavicular joint, sometimes also glenohumeral joint • Segmental functional disorders of the vertebral column • Pathology referred from the lumbopelvic hip region (e.g. hyperlordosis, pelvic torsion) Psychological aspect: anxiety (in the neck), stress ('too much on my shoulders')
Thoracic spine and thorax	• Thoracic/mediastinal organs (e.g. pain derived from lungs, heart) • Rib block • Costotransversal joint, sternocostal joints ('rib block') • Segmental functional disorders of the vertebral column • Structural damage to the vertebral column (e.g. osteoporosis) Psychological aspect: anxiety ('ties up your chest') or anger
Abdomen	• Abdominal organs (e.g. pancreas, gallbladder including mesentery, possibly adhesions after operation) • Segmental functional disorders of the vertebral column • Structural damage to the vertebral column (e.g. osteoporosis) • Fascia (e.g. abdominal wall hernia) Psychological aspect: suppressed emotions such as 'rage in the belly', brooding, worries about the future
Lumbar spine and buttocks	• Lower abdominal organs (e.g. urogenital system, bowel) • Structural damage to the vertebral column (e.g. osteoporosis, erosive osteochondrosis = aseptic spondylodiscitis) • Ligaments and joints of the lumbar, pelvic and hip region (e.g. iliosacral joint, acetabulofemoral joint (hip joint)) • Fascia (e.g. inguinal hernia) Psychological aspect: often excessive supervision, anxiety, uncertainty
Extremities	• Joints including ligamentary and capsular structures • Synovial bursa • Insertion tendinopathy, periarthropathy (mTrPs of the tributary muscles are usually crucial here) • Soft tissue tumours • Bone diseases such as periostitis, osteomyelitis and tumours • Nerve irritation, nerve compression Psychological aspect: e.g. elbow and wrist: holding on and letting go

pain is referred only over the healthy nerve root. Only in the first case may a neuro-surgical intervention or local infiltration of the root be required.

With both types of segmental pain referral, the symptoms are limited to the borders of the segment. However, note that symptoms with segmental disorder are referred not only into the most well-known dermatome but also into the associated myotome and sclerotome, which are supplied by the same nerve root. These are not topographically superimposed on each other but are often far apart (see Fig. 14.3). Furthermore, the whole dermatome or myotome is not always affected. It is even more difficult if there are connections between the neighbouring spinal ganglia. If the pain referred from a segmental spondylogenic disorder radiates over two or more roots, it is almost impossible to make the diagnosis on the basis of the referred pain.

The pain topography can only provide an indication of the possibly affected roots or segments, because of the movements of dermatome and myotome. An exact attribution of the segment is only possible via the dermatome and with a needle stimulation disorder, as this is the only thing which stops directly at the dermatome border (see Fig. 14.3, 14.16). Cannulas or acupuncture needles are suitable sterile disposable tools for testing.

Segmental-radicular referred pain

Radicular pain actually caused by nerve root compression or irritation is less common in everyday practice. The pain quality is usually shooting or burning and is characterised by dysaesthesia. A simple differential diagnosis can be made here if there are definite clinical signs.

- Nerve root compression can be diagnosed by symptoms of a deficit: sensory deficits (hypoalgesia and hypoaesthesia) and paresis are characterised by appropriate reflex deficits. Note that there is often no evidence of definite findings in an EMG until 3 weeks after the start of the compression.
- Positive nerve extension tests (e.g. Lasègue for roots L4–S1) are characteristic of nerve root irritation. 'Plus symptoms' with hyperaesthesia, hyperalgesia and overreaction of the muscles, including the formation of mTrPs, are also demonstrated.

Table 14.12 Possible regional associations and pain location

POSSIBLE REGIONAL ASSOCIATION	'FUNCTIONAL CHAIN'
Above–below	• Temporomandibular joint ↔ cervical spine, lumbar, pelvic, hip region ↔ ankle ↔ arch of the foot
Back to front (segmental and functional)	• Lumbar spine pain with shortening of the M. iliopsoas or tone disorder of the abdominal muscles • Iliosacral joint: inguinal pain • Costotransversal joint: sternal pain
Left–right	• One-sided temporomandibular joint pathology with effect on the contralateral temporomandibular joint • Shoulder–cervical spine–shoulder axis, e.g. posture or protection with strain on the opposite side • Hip–pelvis–hip
Flexion side–extension side (agonist–antagonist)	• Achillodynia: M. tibialis • Weakness of the hip abductors with shortened adductors

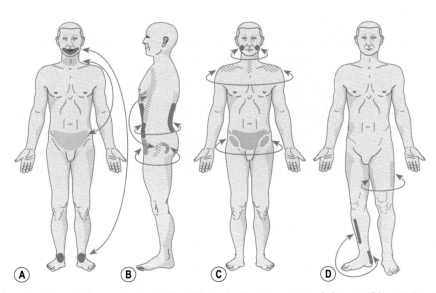

Fig. 14.2 Possible regional associations and pain location: (a) top–bottom, e.g. postural changes; (b) posterior–anterior, e.g. segmental associations; (c) left–right, e.g. consensual reactions, compensation or resistance; (d) agonist–antagonist.

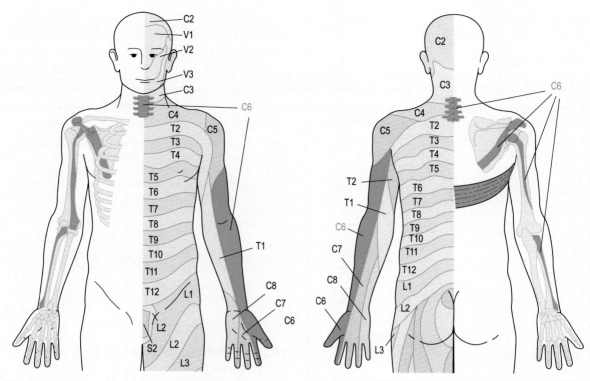

Fig. 14.3 Innervation in the area of the pain: a dermatome, myotome and sclerotome each supplied by the same spinal nerves.

> Progressive neurological changes and/or bladder or rectal disorders require immediate specialist diagnosis and treatment if necessary.

> In contrast to segmental radicular pain referral, spondylogenic referral has a stabbing, dragging or grinding pain quality (see Section 14.1.4).

Segmental spondylogenic referred pain

Spondylogenic pain is referred from the segment. The term 'motion/movement segment' originated from manual therapy (see Junghans, Schmorl 1951). It includes intervertebral discs with annulus fibrosus, ligaments, small intervertebral joints of two bordering vertebral bodies and small 'segmental' muscles. It is frequently not possible by means of clinical examination to definitely attribute the referred pain to the structure from which it is referred. Evidence from manual examination shows hypomobility (so-called blocking), and provocation of symptoms by anterior thrust of the affected vertebral body over the spiny process (posterior–anterior stress, PA stress). Local tissue swellings with tenderness (connective tissue diagnosis) provide indications.

Sometimes another differentiation of the structure is possible by using a precise reproducible blockade with LA (e.g. small vertebral joints).

Non-segmentally referred pain

The most common cause of non-segmentally referred pain is mTrPs. Other causes are listed below.

- Entrapment or irritation of peripheral nerves by various tissue structures: muscles (see Table 14.13), bony structures (e.g. brachial plexus between the clavicle and the first rib, peroneus nerve due to subluxation of the head of the fibula) and joints (e.g. following trauma).
- Joint involvement: pain can be referred distally into the extremities if there is periparthropathy both from the soft tissue coat, where the mTrP again plays a significant role, and from the actual joint.

> The deeper the structural cause, the more distal the referral.

Table 14.13 Examples of entrapment syndrome which is caused by hardening of neighbouring muscles

AFFECTED NERVE	CAUSATIVE MUSCLE
N. supraorbitalis	M. frontalis
N. occipitalis major	M. semispinalis capitis
Plexus brachialis, lower stem	Mm. scaleni
Plexus brachialis	M. pectoralis minor
N. radialis (sensitive branch)	M. triceps brachii
N. radialis, deep branch	M. supinator
N. ulnaris	M. flexor carpi ulnaris
Nn. digitales manus	M. interossei
Posterior branches of the spinal nerves	Paravertebral muscles
N. ischiadicus	M. piriformis
Deep branch of the peroneus nerve	M. peroneus longus

Arthritic pain is often stabbing and dependent on movement (movement in the joint); periarthritic pain is also dependent on movement but can also be made worse by pressure on the affected tissue (tendon insertions, synovial bursae).

With non-segmentally referred pain, somatoform pain should also be considered. Somatoform pain can be regarded as the physical expression of inner mental tension. An indication of this is pain that moves and changes in quality (e.g. alternating stabbing and burning pain) and resistance to conventional therapeutic measures (see Section 14.1.7, Table 14.14).

Important: somatoform pain is real pain and must be taken seriously, predominantly as a message of the patient's suffering.

14.2.3 Multilocular pain and fibromyalgia

Martin Offenbächer

Even though myofascial pain is usually regional, it can cause problems in investigating differential diagnoses in patients with primary MPS if this is located at more than one site, particularly if muscle function chains are affected. Manifestations of multilocular pain in the locomotor system can be:

Clinically, entrapment is characterised by a neuropathic pain quality (burning, shooting, electrifying). The neurological symptoms can range from paraesthesia to sensory deficits depending on the extent of the irritation or compression.

Table 14.14 Referred pain, differentiated according to the underlying affected structures

REFERRAL PATTERN	UNDERLYING STRUCTURE	CAUSES	PAIN CHARACTER
Segmental	Radicular (neurogenic) Spondylogenic	Nerve root compression Radiculopathy in the sense of irritation (Central) motion segment including segmental reflex complex[1]	Shooting, burning, dysaesthesia Stabbing, dragging or oppressive pain quality
Non-segmental	Myofascial Nerval	Referred pain e.g. Entrapment of peripheral nerves including thoracic-outlet syndrome (see Table 14.4)	Dull, motion-dependent Burning, shooting, electrifying
	Arthrogenic Somatoform	Arthritis Mental tension	Stabbing, motion-dependent Very variable, often demonstrative

[1]Tilscher, Eder's (1989) term for segmental reflex complex.

- MPS at more than one site,
- inflammatory diseases caused by pathogens (particularly hepatitis, borreliosis, HIV),
- inflammatory rheumatic diseases (e.g. chronic polyarthritis, seronegative spondyloarthropathies, collagenosis, myositis, vasculitis, polymyalgia rheumatica) (see Section 14.1.5),
- non-inflammatory diseases (particularly thyroid gland function disorders, neoplasia, myopathy; see Section 14.1.1),
- fibromyalgia, depression, chronic fatigue syndrome, somatoform pain disorders, irritable colon, multiple chemical sensitivity with much overlapping.

Inflammatory, rheumatic and pathogenic diseases are easily distinguished compared to primary MPS. Note that patients with these diseases can also develop secondary myofascial pain, the symptoms of which must then be treated.

> If there is musculoskeletal pain throughout the whole body, inflammatory and non-inflammatory diseases must be ruled out with clinical and laboratory findings.

On the other hand, multilocular pain causes difficulty in distinguishing differential diagnoses with fibromyalgia,

depression, chronic fatigue syndrome, somatoform pain disorders, irritable colon and multiple chemical sensitivity. These syndromes overlap and have much in common.

Many patients with the above diseases and symptoms nevertheless also demonstrate definite secondary myofascial findings, although these are sometimes also part of the clinical picture. It is therefore the diagnostician's task alone to distinguish a primary MPS. The clinical evaluation should include the whole locomotor apparatus and involve a basic medical and neurological examination.

Fibromyalgia, depression, chronic fatigue syndrome, somatoform pain disorder, irritable colon and multiple chemical sensitivity, as well as certain forms of anxiety disorder, demonstrate much in common in terms of the type of symptoms and their severity (see Table 14.15). Some of the clinical pictures are therefore classified as syndromes and no definite differential diagnoses are distinguished.

> In the end, individual treatment of the symptoms is indicated, while noting the overall context. Concomitant myofascial findings should therefore also not be regarded in isolation but should only be treated as part of a somatic and psychological overall treatment plan while identifying and solving social stress situations.

Table 14.15 Primary MPS, fibromyalgia, depression, chronic fatigue syndrome, somatoform disorders, irritable colon and multiple chemical sensitivity: commonalities in the type and extent of the symptoms

	PAIN CHARACTER	LOCATION	SWOLLEN FEELING	SLEEP DISORDER	GASTRO-INTESTINAL	MUSCLE STIFFNESS	TRIGGER
Primary MPS	Dull, pressing, dragging	Regionally restricted or classic referral pattern	No	Only with chronification	No	No	Poor posture
Fibromyalgia	Dull, pressing, dragging	Stem and/or extremities at three or more different parts of the body above and below the waist	Yes	Difficulty getting to sleep or sleeping through the night	Not to the fore	Yes	Compulsive disorder, stress and strain
Depression	Variable	Variable	Rare	Difficulty getting to sleep or sleeping through the night	Not to the fore	No, more likely muscular hypotonus	Independent mood

Continued

Table 14.15 Primary MPS, fibromyalgia, depression, chronic fatigue syndrome, somatoform disorders, irritable colon and multiple chemical sensitivity: commonalities in the type and extent of the symptoms—cont'd

	PAIN CHARACTER	LOCATION	SWOLLEN FEELING	SLEEP DISORDER	GASTRO-INTESTINAL	MUSCLE STIFFNESS	TRIGGER
Chronic fatigue syndrome	Variable	Variable	No	Difficulty getting to sleep or sleeping through the night	Not to the fore	No	Physical strain
Somatoform pain disorder	Variable	Variable	Yes	Difficulty getting to sleep or sleeping through the night	Visceral pain can be the main symptom	Frequent, if pain in the locomotor system is the main symptom	Mental stress situation
Irritable colon	Dull, variable	Frequently joints	Rare	Rare	Main symptom	Rare	Effect of food, stress
Multiple chemical sensitivity	Variable	Variable	Rare	Difficulty getting to sleep or sleeping through the night	Rare	Rare	Environmental stress

Section | 2 |

Treatment of myofascial pain

Chapter | **15** |

Principles of treatment

Dominik Irnich

15.1 DOCTOR–PATIENT RELATIONSHIP

The key influential factor for the success of treatment is a 'healing' doctor–patient relationship (Ch. 16). The patient should feel accepted and understood. It is important that the symptoms are taken seriously and regarded as real, even if the doctor finds the symptoms hard to understand. In patients with chronic myofascial pain in particular, psychosocial stress factors must also be evaluated and included early on in the consultation (see Section 13.1).

An evaluation of the strength and extent of the stress factors in accordance with the therapist's criteria must be avoided as there is no objective measuring stick for these subjective factors. The doctor–patient relationship can be permanently damaged by trivialisation or overvaluation and the success of treatment will be endangered.

At the beginning of each treatment, the patient should be asked an open question to provide an opportunity for expressing any currently important matters. The effect of the last treatment should be evaluated (e.g. for how long did the symptoms improve?) and any possible changes to the symptoms, or different symptoms, asked about. Note the key principle that focusing on positive effects and improvements supports the patient's resources and self-healing potential.

Another important aspect of treatment is motivation and maintaining exercise of the affected muscles to improve the follow-up experience (self-effectiveness).

15.2 PRACTICAL ADVICE

Before each treatment the patient should undergo another examination to locate currently active mTrPs. If relevant mTrPs are found, a series of treatments should be devised. It has proved reliable to treat the main, or the most clearly felt, mTrPs. If muscle chains are affected then proceed from central to peripheral. During palpation, note that the fingernails should be kept short, otherwise pressure on the skin is painful. To avoid guarding reactions or tickling, the non-palpating hand can be placed contralaterally and flat with light pressure.

Before treatment, night pain as a result of stiff/sore muscles should be explained to the patient, as this can occur if a muscle twitch response is obtained (post-treatment muscle soreness). Avoid letting the patient worry about the reaction; this reaction should be explained as a positive, therapeutically healing effect.

With some patients, this muscle soreness can last 1–2 days; that is, contraction of the treated muscle can feel slightly painful. This can be used for therapeutic behaviour; it is possible that mTrPs in the trapezius muscle can cause contraction, leading to pathological shoulder elevation. With sufficient mTrP treatment the shoulder is usually successfully lowered. If there is any post-treatment pain, this causes the patient to avoid contracting the trapezius muscle and lifting the shoulders. This indirectly supports the effort at treatment.

15.3 LEGAL ASPECTS

Legal considerations play an important role in the treatment of myofascial pain on several levels. The patient has a right to appropriate pain relief. On the one hand this relates to the introduction of supposedly effective treatment and on the other to not withholding from the patient any procedure generally considered to be effective. In a practical sense, this means that if the pain is severe the patient should not be deprived of an initial dose of analgesics in many cases, but effective procedures such as manual or invasive therapy should also not be withheld.

Please see the professional guidelines for the legal aspects of the treatment of myofascial pain, including any specifics of the legal aspects of pain therapy.

Any undesirable effects should also be explained to the patient before any procedures. With invasive measures, the treatment room must be equipped with the relevant emergency equipment, because e.g. the administration of LAs can lead to a life-threatening condition due to overdose or allergic reaction.

15.4 KEEPING RECORDS

For various reasons it is crucial to record the progress of the disease in detail:

- checking the success of treatment,
- departure from the natural course of the disease,

- possibilities for before and after comparisons for doctor and patient,
- formal legal reasons,
- quality assurance.

Progress can be recorded using standard pain scales (Ch. 13, Fig. 13.3) or appropriate questionnaires (Fig. 13.1). We also recommend mentioning the patient's own impression of the main symptoms or the restrictions to daily life and evaluating their severity before treatment, e.g. using a numerical rating scale (0 = no symptoms, 10 = maximum severity).

Mentioning the specific symptoms is essential for identifying changing symptoms, because the location can alter following successful therapy in patients with pain in several places and the pain can recur to the same extent and at the same intensity at other sites.

However, recording the symptoms should not be exaggerated; although it can be motivating, it can also fixate on a particular symptom. Occasionally, it is worthwhile assessing the level of satisfaction or feeling of wellbeing using a scale, in order to move from a negative view to a positive one. With chronic pain the guidelines from pain therapy agreements can be helpful (e.g. DGS questionnaire).

At the somatic level, of course, various physical function parameters can also be included (e.g. finger ground distance, etc.) as well as the findings from the manual examination. We must nevertheless be aware here that these are not usually particularly reliable and in many cases depend on motivation. The subjective findings are crucial, as are the improvement in quality of life and maintenance or restoration of the capacity to work.

Chapter | 16 |

The doctor–patient relationship in cases of chronic pain

Nicolas Behrens

The treatment of patients with chronic pain is a big challenge for which we are little prepared during our studies or in our practical (specialist) training. There are many factors to be aware of. The more chronic the symptoms the less important are the treatment prospects and the more important is a comprehensive approach, including on the level of your relationship with the patient.

This chapter provides suggestions for this approach, highlights various aspects of dealing with patients with chronic pain and offers support with a collection of treatment recommendations and tips. We also recommend the use of a range of specialist training techniques.

16.1 THE PATIENT SITUATION AND POSSIBLE OBSTACLES TO TREATMENT

- Long period of symptoms without sufficient treatment success.
- Lack of experienced pain therapists.
- Personal suffering, mental assessments and self-selected more or less helpful behaviour strategies such as endurance, victim role (with disguised recrimination or manipulation of others, the 'culprit' aspect), complaining or accusatory behaviour or dissimulation up to ignoring one's own needs, exhaustion ('I never get a break'), build-up of emotions such as anger (at the pain, etc.) and depression. These usually lead in the end to retreat: somatic (taut bands, limited mobility), mental (reduced emotionality and zest for life), social (contact with other people and range of interests are reduced) and spiritual (reduced or lost feeling of sense of life and closeness to a greater whole).
- So far no adequate explanation for the pain has been found (which can also be due to the examination:

according to the International Association for the Study of Pain, MFS and psychosomatic disorders are the most commonly overlooked causes of chronic pain), leading to the patient searching for a somatic diagnosis. In addition, other people, especially at work, cannot comprehend the disabling effect of pain ('don't talk to me about headaches – that's often used as an excuse').
- Many different previous findings and diagnoses (which sometimes also reflect the point of view and system of belief of the therapist), resulting in the patient often feeling unsure or fixated on opinions, even to the extent of an inadequate prognosis ('you'll always have symptoms with that' = 'voodoo effect').
- Anxiety, e.g. of incorrect diagnosis: cancer or other incurable disease could be hiding behind the pain.
- Worry that it is permanent and could even get worse; this is the triple rule: that one third of the pain is past experience, another third is worry that it will be the same or worse in the future and 'only' one third is current pain. If the patient can succeed in getting to the present and remaining there, the other two-thirds can be 'let go'.
- Psychological and psychosomatic diseases are often belittled in the wider population as a personal weakness. This is why the physical correlate or symptoms are imparted if necessary when visiting the doctor.
- Too little time and understanding from previous therapists as a result of a biased somatic point of view, caused also by a lack of training in psychosomatic diseases and inadequate appreciation of discussion.
- Referrals to specialists are often not done in a positive framework but to get rid of a patient who is getting on one's nerves or is too demanding (passing the patient on; the referral context of 'hot potato' or 'passing the buck').

http://dx.doi.org/10.1016/B978-0-7020-4312-3.00016-7

- Patient depressive: little motivation or capacity to change anything in one's life (use depression questionnaire).
- Conviction that others or life circumstances are to blame, and that and these cannot be changed (this is usually correct, but often stretches the patient's own point of view).
- Patient's own one-sided view of the illness as somatic, with the illness as an industrial accident. A psychosomatic treatment approach is refused; one's own part in the situation is negated, favouring the underlying attitude and behaviour pattern in the sense of a negative coping strategy.
- Experience of inadequate treatment or even devaluation by previous therapist ('just psychological' = imaginary).
- High pressure of expectation on the doctor, initially positive confirmation of the doctor ('you will be able to help me in the end', 'I set all my hopes on you').

16.2 POSSIBLE ERRORS BY THE DOCTOR OR THERAPIST

- Devaluation by previous or other therapists, accepting (inadequate) praise (warning: KKS syndrome).
- Putting pressure on yourself to achieve success.
- Allowing yourself to be pressurised by (auto) aggressive patients to undertake invasive or destructive measures.
- Seeing pain as the enemy; this one-sided pathological somatic view (technical diagnosis leaves the patient alone) leads to a risk of further chronification.
- Depriving the patient of the right to decide, not checking the patient's readiness to undergo therapy and fixating only on the symptom.
- Wanting to help the patient by 'sparing' them the experience and opportunity of the low point. This fixes the patient in a dependent role as a victim. This 'helper syndrome' by the therapist promotes chronification and leads to its own chronic overload.

16.3 SOLUTIONS

- Pick up the patient from where they are: take into account biopyschosocial diagnosis, disease pattern and the patient's expectations.
- Let the patient assess themself, noting verbal and motor reactions and social behaviour pattern. This leads to trust in your own countertransference: how do I feel about this patient?
- Have respect for a concealed sense of pain (e.g. the metaphor of the oil warning light in a car, see below)

and do not strive for a one-sided pain reduction or discontinuation.
- Handle the patient and their fate attentively, not just the pain.
- Treat the patient as an expert, and in so doing activate their own responsibility and potential.
- Remain calm, 'non-acting': accompany the patient, do not strive for success at any price.
- Have the patient keep a pain diary.
- Set out a clear concept and prognosis, and dampen unrealistic expectations: is there an available vision of a solution?
- Negotiate definite treatment instructions and agreement ('you can take a horse to water but you can't make it drink').
- Depending on qualifications and time, address life history aspects; take a systematic view. Get away from 'either body or soul' to 'both body and soul'.
- Look for the message together; try to understand, do not read your own plan into it!
- If necessary, risk a crisis (the 'initial reaction') and then resolve it together with the patient.
- Be clear about your own role and its limits, and if possible develop a coordinated treatment team.
- Use external support or supervision (e.g. pain conference or Balint group); do not become involved with the patient's support system.
- Look for solutions instead of getting lost in analysing the problem ('why?').
- The therapist needs to be positive and sensible.

> If pain has become chronic, it has lost its warning function on a purely physical level. Its final function can often be deduced in a biographical context or on a relationship level, or during physical therapy.

The body provides us with direct access to (suppressed) emotions (see Ch. 12). If this is revealed during therapy it is always a great opportunity for a leap forwards in (pain) treatment. At the same time, this makes great demands on a good therapist to act as adequately as possible. Training under supervision, for example in psychosomatics, and looking at one's own reactions to patients with difficult pain, is recommended. This can also help with the development of one's own personality and also has direct benefit for one's own life.

Pain is a crisis and as such includes both risk and opportunity. A muscle shield can be an expression of withdrawal and exercise a protective effect, but the feelings frozen in the muscles can also lead to reduced liveliness. This makes disease a warning signal of the effort to escape from oneself.

Acupuncture and mTrP therapy can be used as a comprehensive solutional approach, as they offer an opportunity for relationship medicine. However, this means that a purely mechanistic course of action has to be avoided:

- touch/treat/tackle; record/understand (e.g. palpation of CV 17); possibly find 'sore point',
- note reactions to touch or needling,
- use of known axes and attribution of function area,
- think about the whole patient; perception and reaction will be more comprehensive,
- provide training in body awareness for the patient,
- let immediate reactions (surfacing of feelings) happen and utilise them as far as possible (Ch. 12).

16.4 QUOTATIONS AND STORIES FOR UNDERSTANDING PAIN

The following are a few quotations and images for the comprehensive understanding of pain. They are also suitable for display in the waiting room.

Image of the oil warning light: if we are driving a car and the oil warning light comes on (= pain), we stop (protection for acute pain) and call a mechanic (doctor). If the mechanic cannot repair it (chronic pain) but takes the light out of the dashboard, breaks it and allows us to carry on driving (symptomatic destructive course of action) then we know that this does not make sense: we have ignored the insistent, specific message of the oil warning light. With successful, non-destructive treatment (when a change of oil level is required, via the lubrication system) the light goes out by itself.

The oil-light comparison is of course clumsy, but then in the body the symptoms can provide access to the real crux of the matter. 'There are no one-way streets in the body' (Bergsmann). This is what we use in acupuncture or trigger point therapy: the body surface addresses and influences visceral function as well as the whole psycho-neuroimmunological regulation, including the feelings.

Disease is not a defect which it is sufficient to repair. . .
Disease is nothing more than the person himself, better: the opportunity to become himself.
Conventional medicine expels the subject from medicine.

Quotations from Viktor von Weizsäcker

For Plato, pain was a spiritual experience which showed a person had lost their wholeness. Modern people no longer want to know about this spiritual aspect: with the separation of body and soul it is now sufficient to try to establish the physical causes of the pain and to eliminate them. The transformation of pain into an external threat has been particularly taken advantage of by the pharmaceutical industry, which treats the pain, and by extension the patient, as an object. Back problems are almost exclusively treated with drugs and the often underlying depressive disorders are totally unrecognised (Marcus Schiltenwolf, Professor of Orthopaedics in Heidelberg, *source*: www. FAZ.net, 8 June 2008).

On pain
Your pain is the breaking of the shell that encloses your understanding.
Even as the stone of the fruit must break, that its heart may stand in the sun, so must you know pain.
Much of your pain is self-chosen.
It is the bitter potion by which the physician within you heals your sick self.
Therefore trust the physician, and drink his remedy in silence and tranquillity:
For his hand, though heavy and hard, is guided by the tender hand of the Unseen. . .

Khalil Gibran: *The Prophet*

Disease is solely and purely corrective: it is neither vindictive nor cruel: but it is the means adopted by our own Souls to point out to us our faults: to prevent our making greater errors to hinder us from doing more harm and to bring us back to that path of Truth and Light from which we should never have strayed.

Edward Bach

You are running in circles and looking for a gap
You are running in vain – get your head around it!
Think about it –
You only have one way left –
look into yourself.

Erich Kästner

If someone is looking for health, ask him first whether he is also prepared in the future to avoid any causes of his disease – only then can you help him.

Socrates

Regarding trigger point therapy and acupuncture as 'real therapy': stop the patient running away by experiencing the needle in the 'here and now'.

The five freedoms
The freedom to see and hear what is.
Instead of seeing and hearing what should be
Or even what will be.
The freedom to say what you feel and think,
Instead of saying what you should say about it.

The freedom to feel what you feel,
Instead of feeling what you should feel.
The freedom to ask what you like,
Instead of always waiting for permission.
The freedom to take risks in your own interests
Instead of deciding
'To take the safe way out'
And 'not rocking the boat'.

Virginia Satir

It is not the world which must be changed to banish pain but your heart (open up).

Life changes when we change ourselves.

A teacher said to a pupil who was always complaining about others: 'If you really want satisfaction, try to change yourself, not others. It is easier to protect your feet with shoes than to cover the whole world with carpet (or even to demand a red carpet laid out for you).'

'The most common reason for unhappiness,' explained the teacher, 'is a decision to be unhappy. That is why, if two people are in the exactly the same situation, one feels happy and the other miserable.'

Anthony De Mello, *Eine Minute Unsinn –
Weisheitsgeschichten* (A Minute of Nonsense – Stories of
Wisdom), Herder Freiburg im Breisgau, 1993

Resistance to therapy is illustrated in a story by Nasrudin (a Sufi satirist; like an oriental Till Eulenspiegel). Nasrudin laid out a flower bed where dandelion was almost the only plant which grew. After many unsuccessful attempts to get rid of the dandelions he went to the estate gardener to get some advice. But Nasrudin had already tried all the tips that the gardener gave him. After pondering for a long time, the estate gardener finally said to Nasrudin: 'I think there is nothing left for you to do except learn to love the dandelions.'

Provide the pain, which by now should have been driven away and yet is still inseparable from the patient, with space, until it is unconditionally accepted that it cannot change and allow its nucleus/message/sense to be acknowledged and usefully integrated.

Be yourself
Find a spiritual place
For your tiredness.
Find an atmosphere
Where you can grow.
Discover that fragility is a strength
And that vulnerability creates closeness.
Build on your inner strength
(Centre, calmness, attentiveness)
Which the outer world will bear.
Determine where the centre of your life is,
And allow its value to infiltrate your life.
Let go of everything you are not.
Embrace (and be) what you are.
Look at the world with circumspection,
Love it with passion.
Grow like weeds,
Stand like a tree.
Be yourself.

From the Heiligenfeld Psychosomatic
Clinic (source unknown)

Chapter | **17** |

Selection of suitable treatments

Beat Dejung, Dominik Irnich

Selecting the procedure used for the treatment of mTrPs depends on various factors. For the therapist's part, this includes the knowledge and practicalities of each procedure and the external circumstances (place of treatment, staffing, average treatment time, etc.). We thoroughly recommend that a method of treatment with as few side effects as possible should be selected.

It is also crucial that the suggested treatment accepted by the patient. This in its turn depends on the patient's previous experiences, convictions about the illness and expectations. In the perfect case, a high level of therapeutic competence comes together with a motivated patient with reasonable expectations and a sufficient time frame.

17.1 STANDARD TREATMENTS

Beat Dejung

The diagnosis of myofascial disorders makes use of the local ischaemic situation. By stretching the diseased muscle fibres the ischaemia is made worse and the pain, which brought the patient to the doctor, is reproduced. We use a series of extension tests like this as a screening method. The ischaemic situation is also useful for actually identifying the trigger points; if the ischaemia is momentarily more strongly palpated, it can cause severe pain. This can locate the mTrPs to within a millimetre. This is indispensable for needling, an important form of treatment.

In traditional physiotherapy, attempts have been made to treat non-specific pain with stretching. Such attempts are usually useless. Stretching makes the ischaemic situation in the mTrPs, and the pain, worse. It also provokes a reflex increase in tension. Janet Travell used stretching under cold-spray application as the first actual trigger point therapy. Spraying and stretching actually inhibits the guarding spasm of the stretched muscles (Ch. 18). However, when used alone spray and stretch is only effective with fresh and not very severe pain syndromes. We have used spray and stretch regularly in the last two decades as a secondary measure after manual therapy or dry needling. Because the cold media chloroethyl and vaporised liquid nitrogen have not been covered by health insurance in Switzerland for several years, the spray-and-stretch method has disappeared from our therapeutic repertoire.

In the last few years, many have tried to influence mTrPs with postisometric relaxation, sometimes with stretching following isometric exercising of the muscles affected by the mTrP. The observed pain reduction probably has something to do with the improved perfusion of the trigger point region. This is more of a consequence of the reduction in reflex tension and not the result of dissolving the contracted sarcomere. We should probably regard the therapeutic effect of postisometric relaxation as the dropping back of a manifest MFS into latency. Severe or chronic pain syndromes cannot be treated in this way.

The most commonly used therapy for myofascial pain in the world today is probably the dry needling of trigger points with acupuncture needles (see Chs 21 and 22). This procedure was first described by Lewit (1979). It depends on finding the mTrP precisely; this can have a diameter of only a fraction of a millimetre. This normally causes a twitch in the muscle fibre with the mTrP, which many consider to be evidence that the mTrPs are actually located at the sites of the motor end plates (Travell, Simons 1983). The end plates are usually in the middle of each muscle fibre. With non-feathered muscles it is therefore possible to cause several local twitch responses, one after another, from a single puncture by searching with the acupuncture needle; we have observed more than 20 twitch responses one after the other. If a twitch response is caused,

http://dx.doi.org/10.1016/B978-0-7020-4312-3.00017-9

the patient feels an intense pain and the tension of the relevant taut band immediately drops dramatically. The mechanism of the effect of dry needling has not yet been sufficiently explained. It is possible that the contracted sarcomeres are quite simply cut by the puncture so that the ischaemic situation is removed. With chronic pain syndromes dry needling sometimes causes only hyperanalgesic pain, not a twitch response (see below for explanation). Sometimes, needling causes not just local pain but also pain referred to another region of the body (Travell, Simons 1983). The recognition of this pain by the patient lets us know for certain that we are treating the cause of an MPS.

Needling of a trigger point with concomitant infiltration with a LA is very effective (see Ch. 21). However, this injection only lasts if the local twitch response has been found. Searching the end-plate region with a thick cannula is very traumatic for the patient. If the local twitch response is not provoked by the puncture, the therapeutic pain is indeed temporarily relieved, but the actual trigger point pain returns after a few hours.

Injection therapy with botulinum toxin (see Ch. 21) is extremely effective with various trigger points. This is a precision technique that can put one or more motor end plates out of action for several months and which considerably reduces myofascial pain. However, as this method is very expensive it is not suitable as a routine treatment. Its efficacy is a strong indicator for the trigger point end-plate hypothesis which we favour.

In physiotherapy in Switzerland, predominantly manual techniques are used for the treatment of MPS. The possibility of manual treatment was mentioned by Travell and Simons (1983). The actual system of manual trigger point therapy was first described by Dejung (1988). Chapter 18 covers with it in detail (see Section 18.1).

In the last few years, orthopaedists and practitioners of sports medicine have started to treat myofascial pain with shock waves (see Ch. 20). Shock wave therapy, which has until now only been indicated for treatment of a frozen shoulder, pain in the lateral epicondyle and the calcaneal spur, has a very wide scope of application. Shock wave therapy is still very expensive, which limits its application, certainly in the field of physiotherapy. The mechanism of its effect is as yet unknown. However, users report good results on myofascial pain. As with all forms of trigger point therapy, evidence of efficacy will have to be worked on in the next few years. This will only be possible if experienced users in the periphery work closely with hospitals and health centres, the institutions that are in a position to carry out randomised studies.

17.2 OTHER (STANDARD) TREATMENTS

Besides the known procedures of infiltration, dry needling and manual mTrP therapy, a number of other methods and procedures are now being used in the treatment of mTrPs.

We have to say that there is usually still insufficient scientific evidence available for the efficacy of these procedures. However, this also means that there is no evidence either that they are not effective. After critical evaluation an assessment of those procedures can therefore be based only on empirical reports and personal experiences.

One of the procedures with the longest tradition is certainly classical needle acupuncture (see Ch. 21). As we have already seen, there are parallels between the system of acupuncture points and meridians and the system of mTrPs with corresponding patterns of referred pain (see Ch. 8). In many cases muscle tension and myofascial pain are relieved with classical Chinese acupuncture as well. Whether using the distal points of classical Chinese acupuncture, microsystem acupuncture or even Japanese acupuncture, in every case the needling procedure far from the painful site has proved reliable. If you commence acupuncture with this type of far needling, it frequently has immediate effects on the muscles. Any remaining findings can then be approached using a selection of segmental acupuncture points. This second stage has proved sensible in various systems. Local needling is not necessary until a third stage is reached. For chronic, long-term myofascial problems, a complete course of treatment of 10–12 sessions is needed.

Local mTrP treatment can also be carried out using laser acupuncture. It is important that there is a sufficiently high application of energy (see Section 22.6). The advantage of laser acupuncture is that it is non-invasive and virtually pain free. The disadvantage is that it cannot sufficiently reach trigger points located deeper in the tissue. The application of electrostimulation acupuncture is recommended if the patient complains of very intense pain; that is, acute or subacute myofascial pain (see Section 22.5).

All forms of acupuncture have in common that they do not just address one symptom but try to address the whole person in context in the inner and outer world by using additional diagnostic and therapeutic measures. This greater concept is also suitable for most relaxation techniques (see Ch. 24). Conscious movement or conscious relaxation influences not just muscle tension but also the patient's whole autonomic system. However, this can only be achieved by continuous exercising, with the active participation of the patient. The therapeutic success of the various relaxation techniques in particular depends on the patient's motivation and discipline. The therapist's task is to build up and maintain the appropriate motivation, as well as providing the patient with information. It is also crucial that the patient identifies with the relevant technique. All forms of relaxation technique are not suitable for every patient.

Some physical procedures also offer the possibility of self-treatment. TENS (see Section 20.5), the application of warmth or cupping massage are suitable for independent use. A prerequisite is that the patient is introduced carefully to the procedure. Other physical procedures are regularly applied passively. These include ultrasound, many other electrotherapy procedures and shock wave therapy (see Section 20.7).

The therapist should not in any case delay employing concomitant pharmacotherapy for patients in severe pain (see Ch. 25). A protective posture, for example, can ruin the success of one of the above procedures before a long-term effect has been achieved. Drug treatment should be individually chosen, for example according to comorbidities and effect. The principles of pain therapy apply: 'by the mouth', 'by the clock' and 'by the ladder' (see Ch. 25): the medicine should normally be administered orally, noting the timing of the effect (e.g. ibuprofen four times daily). It is rational to use combinations of different products, such as a NSAID plus mild opioid or NSAID plus muscle relaxant. The use of pharmacotherapy for a restricted period is sensible and can definitely increase the efficacy of non-medicinal procedures; by the relief of pain, the patient gains in flexibility and mobility, which is a prerequisite for overcoming myofascial pain.

For chronic myofascial pain in particular, psychosocial factors should be evaluated early on and included in the treatment plan. Taking this basic rule into account is also key to avoiding iatrogenic chronification (see Chs 13 and 16).

> Looking at the symptoms from a purely somatic point of view can be deconstructive; the patient may have chronic pain with biopsychosocial components, but the physician or the patient may consider only the application of purely somatic therapies.

Another important basic rule is to check the success of the treatment regularly but not too often. A guide would be after five to six treatments. If there is not at least some short-term success after this number of treatments, the therapy should be modified and/or altered.

Chapter | **18** |

Manual therapy and physiotherapy

Beat Dejung, Karel Lewit, Dominik Irnich, Robert Schleip

18.1 DEJUNG MANUAL TRIGGER POINT THERAPY

Beat Dejung

18.1.1 Theoretical considerations

In folk medicine it has always been known that finger pressure on a painful spot can reduce the pain. This was first described in pain medicine by Melzack in 1981. Travell and Simons demonstrated in 1983 that pressure on an mTrP can eliminate myofascial pain and attributed this effect to the removal of algogenic substances from the trigger point region and a reactive hyperaemia. In the 1950s Ida Rolf developed a slow, very firm deep massage with the aim of manually stretching the connective tissue structures. Her intention was to help her clients to improve their posture. After such treatment, patients repeatedly said that their chronic pain had been relieved permanently.

That connective tissue treatment can influence chronic musculoskeletal pain that has previously been considered completely untreatable forces us to make some theoretical considerations. In 1975 Fassbender showed that in patients with 'muscular rheumatism' the degeneration of myofibrils could often be found, even to the extent of necrosis of the contractile substance. We have to accept here that a local ischaemia causes the destruction of this muscle tissue. Ischaemic necrosis produces an inflammatory reaction, like other damaging influences on the muscle tissue. Such a reaction always follows the same typical path:

- the occurrence of hyperaemia and exudation of fluid into the tissue,

- macrophages pass through the vessel walls into the tissue and transport the tissue debris,
- stem cells differentiate into fibroblasts and angioblasts,
- fibroblasts produce collagen fibres which interlink to form scar tissue (Böcker et al. 1997).

This is how connective tissue forms in the muscles and is subject to shrinkage, as with any fresh scar tissue (van Wingerden 1995). The shrinking scar tissue evidently interferes with the shortened sarcomeres in the mTrP and hardens the contracted structures so firmly that the expected twitch response of the relevant muscle fibres during needling of the relevant mTrP becomes impossible (Fig. 18.1). We can regard this as the first stage of the chronification of MPS. The persistent nociception from the ischaemia zone of a chronic mTrP leads over time to further chronification processes in the nociceptors and the posterior horn (Mense 1997) and in certain cases also in the hypothalamus (Jeanmonod et al. 1996).

The connective tissue has now become plastic to a certain degree and, after stretching of the natural rippling, the connective tissue structures can be stretched by about 5% without tearing. If a force is allowed to work on a collagen structure slowly over a lengthy period, a reordering of the collagen fibres and the proteoglycan, and a change in the water content take place and the change in length persists (van Wingerden 1995). This mechanically improves the perfusion in the mTrP and its surroundings.

18.1.2 Connective tissue techniques

Based on these considerations, we have commenced treating chronic pain patients with connective tissue techniques. Today, we use a small treatment range of four different techniques (which can be combined or modified at will) to stretch the collagen tissue in and around the

http://dx.doi.org/10.1016/B978-0-7020-4312-3.00018-0

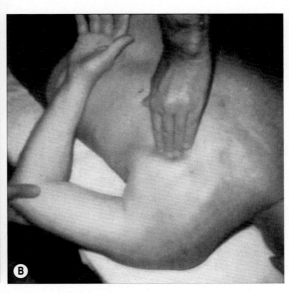

Fig. 18.1 Physiological connective tissue conditions in healthy people (a). As a result of ischaemic inflammatory processes and the formation of contracted connective tissue, the fascia in the area of the scapula can become adherent in patients with chronic pain (b).

mTrP in the area of the superficial fascia and intramuscular connective tissue structures and also between connective tissue-adherent muscles, and to restore the restricted blood flow (Dejung 1988).

Procedure

Our techniques are individually described as follows:

Technique I. The tip of the thumb presses the most sensitive site on the mTrP against a bony foundation or we compress this site between thumb and middle finger. During this, the patient actively makes repetitive movements with the muscle being treated. Pressure is maintained for 5–15 s and can be repeated one or more times after a pause. The active movement is slow and can be assisted by the therapist and does not usually cover the whole range of movement (Fig. 18.2a).

Technique II. The tip of one finger is used to make contact with the connective tissue knot which surrounds the identified mTrP. This connective tissue knot is stretched apart with a very slow, firm movement (Fig. 18.2b).

Technique III. With the nodule of a metacarpophalangeal joint or the thumb we stretch the superficial fascia of the muscle to be treated through the skin. The movement should be carried out very slowly so that a non-reversible increase in length can be made in the collagen structures. Probably, connective tissue structures which have formed inside the muscle as a result of pathological reconstruction processes can also be stretched in this way. It is important when using this technique that the muscles and their fascia are correctly stretched (Fig. 18.2c).

Technique IV. The hand is moved slowly deep between two muscles to release adhesions such as might have formed in most people in the course of their life as a consequence of muscular irritation (Fig. 18.2d).

Notes

The hand movement technique must be varied according to the local anatomical conditions. In most people, this technique can lead to a dramatic improvement in the mobility of the muscles that are treated, especially if the agonists and antagonists are stretched apart.

With any form of trigger point treatment we must remain aware that we are treating the most painful sites on the patient's body, the sites where normal palpation triggers severe pain. It is important to talk to the patient about this. The patient should be reassured that they can end any painful movements immediately at any time with the word 'Stop', if it becomes too much. The patient needs to learn to relax during painful treatment and also to learn to set their own limits. Of course, there are people who cannot accept any pain at all or for whom the allodynia due to chronification is so advanced that treatment without

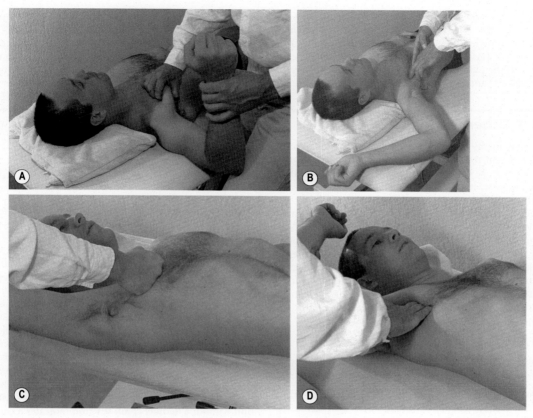

Fig. 18.2 Connective tissue techniques on the M. pectoralis major: technique I (a). Technique II (b), technique III (c) and technique IV (d): loosening fascia between the Mm. pectorales major and minor.

anaesthetic is not possible at all. However, the vast majority of patients react differently to this. Especially if they have noticed some improvement after two or three treatments, many say: 'Thank goodness I have finally found someone who has found the cause of my pain!' or 'Finally someone is being thorough with me!'

Even the therapist has to give thought to the pain. Carrying out painful treatment as a matter of routine is not for everyone. The therapist must be convinced about the method and must also be patient and not try to achieve too much at once.

After the treatment

Small impressions will be visible at the treatment site on the skin for several minutes to several hours after the treatment. Skin reddening lasts rather longer. Occasionally, small bruises can also occur, especially with elderly women. Skin injuries should be avoided. Otherwise the patient may have severe pain at the treatment site for 2 or 3 days. It is important to talk to the patient about all this.

We recommend relieving any pain that has been provoked during treatment, by using NSAIDs for a few days. This same site should not be subjected to further treatment for at least a week. There are also some absolute contraindications for trigger point therapy, such as a low score from a Quick's test and an infection in the tissue.

The patient should be advised after treatment to stretch the treated muscle daily and exercise it again as soon as this is possible without pain. A recurrence should be prevented by avoiding non-physiological exercises and postures.

Mechanism of action

We only partially understand the mechanism of action of trigger point therapy. We have already discussed above the stretching of collagen tissue and its effect on local blood flow. It cannot be ruled out that contracted fibrils in the mTrP are torn by the slowly applied force or that the contraction knots may relax because of this. Danneskiold-Samsoe et al. (1986) described evidence of such processes: during painful deep massage of muscles with active mTrPs the myoglobin level in the plasma increased to 10 times its initial value. The same massage did not have this effect on healthy muscle. After the tenth treatment on the diseased muscle (i.e. a muscle where treatment had been completed) the plasma myoglobin level was normal again (Danneskiold-Samsoe et al. 1986).

18.1.3 Other techniques

In everyday therapy we have become accustomed to combining different techniques. If the therapeutic pain is not well tolerated, we can anaesthetise the mTrP and the area of tissue to be treated with a LA. We often try to deactivate a clearly identified mTrP with precise needling. We decide that the needling is successful if we succeed in causing the local twitch response in the centre of the mTrP (see Section 22.1). For acute and subacute pain the trigger point region is then always treated manually, even if other treatment modalities are to the fore. With chronic myofascial pain, manual treatment is of greater significance as it is the only way to bring about a change leading to healing (by loosening the connective tissue structures). Nevertheless, the area must very often be pretreated with a LA.

> The experience of many therapists that the chronification of MPS may be prevented by precise trigger point treatment has still not been scientifically confirmed. Greater evidence from studies is also needed to confirm the experience that manual trigger point techniques improve pain syndromes up to a certain level of chronification and sometimes make them curable.

18.2 LEWIT TREATMENT TECHNIQUES

Karel Lewit

18.2.1 The meaning of chain patterns

From the overview of the theory in Chapter 7 you can see that the main thing with functional disorders is to establish and analyse the functional associations. These are the muscular chain patterns described in that chapter. Without exception, there are several chain reactions in each patient which come together and have an effect on each other. For example, there is a right-sided chain which extends from the M. sternocleidomastoideus to the adductors which is itself caused by the disordered interplay of the diaphragm with the M. transversus abdominis. At the same time, there is limited rotation of the trunk to the left with mTrPs in the

M. erector spinae, M. quadratus lumborum and M. psoas on the right.

A prerequisite for understanding and treating is detailed functional examination of the whole locomotor system. Otherwise it is impossible to distinguish between important and subordinate disorders. It is also not possible to target rehabilitation on the key disorder. After the examination has been completed, it is crucial first of all to recognise and analyse the chain pattern and where possible to determine the key link in the chain.

> A therapeutic procedure should therefore not be carried out before the examination is concluded.

A key link fulfils the following criteria: it must have underlying functional significance for the locomotor system, it must be associated with the intensity of the disorder and it must match patterns of the patient's medical history which expose the associations (see example below). Disorders in the area of the stabilisation system of the trunk and feet, for example, and in the area of the atlanto-occipital joint are particularly serious. Fascial 'adhesions' and scars in particular can also be key links, especially if the history shows that the patient's condition has deteriorated conspicuously after an operation. Very persistent pain at a single point without a definite chain reaction indicates a chronic mTrP with a reflex that is no longer reversible.

After treatment of the key link under suspicion, another examination is carried out to see if the chain reaction has been successfully eliminated, and whether there are any residual findings or evidence that the final result is incorrect. In this way, the therapeutic procedure also serves to help you make and determine the diagnosis.

If such an attempt is unsuccessful, it is thoroughly legitimate to address other potential key links. Occasionally it may even be sensible to choose the first procedure for diagnostic purposes. This is the case with active scars in particular. If a pathogenic scar is suspected because of numerous linked mTrPs, then you should begin here, as there is no other way of knowing its significance. However, if a relevant active scar is not treated, successful treatment is usually illusory. The following case studies serve as a illustration.

Case study 1

Patient P. A., born in 1979, had been complaining of headaches which spread into her eyes and ears since she was 18. Sometimes the pain lasted several days and it occurred about once a week. The headaches were initially accompanied by vomiting and later nausea. The headaches were independent of menstruation, although she had had menstrual symptoms since the menarche when she was 15, both in her lower abdomen and in the small of her back. The only concomitant disease she had was chronic rhinitis.

The findings on admission showed she had two flat feet and hip asymmetry on the left. There were mTrPs in the diaphragm on both sides and also in the thoracolumbar M. erector spinae and the pelvic floor. This was therefore a typical of disorder of the deep trunk stabilisers. Shallow breathing was clinically noticeable. Treatment therefore consisted of stimulating the coordination between the diaphragm and the deep abdominal muscles, at first in the supine position, then with breathing exercises sitting in front of a mirror, where the patient could exercise self-control (using her hands and eyes). Immediately after exercising, palpation of the diaphragm and back extensors was no longer painful. The patient's task was to carry out this exercise at home, at least twice a day, initially with a mirror and later without.

At the follow-up examination 2 months later the patient reported that a fortnight after treatment she had pain in the small of her back but that then the headaches and the back pain had disappeared. During examination breathing was normal and the abdominal muscles were functioning normally, although the pelvic floor (M. coccygeus) was still painful on palpation and there were still mTrPs in the adductors. However, the Vele's test was positive. With pelvic rocking exercises the mTrPs in the adductors disappeared (without local treatment of the mTrPs). The patient remained free of pain in the 2 month follow-up monitoring period.

Case study 2

Patient S. R., born in 1975, a lorry driver, had experienced of pain across the small of his back since he was 15. He had also had pain in his left shoulder for more than a year and then in his right shoulder for 6 months. Otherwise, the patient had never been ill, apart from an operation on his right knee.

The examination revealed a blockage of the left acromioclavicular joint, and mTrPs in the M. psoas and M. quadratus on the right and in the right adductors. There was also a blockage at the head of the fibula on the right with mTrPs in the M. biceps femoris and a blockage in the Lisfranc joint with mTrPs in the flexors of the sole and back of the foot. When leaning forward, automatic toe flexion was weakened.

Therapeutically, we exercised flexion of the toes when moving forward, which spontaneously released the blockage of the Lisfranc joint and the mTrPs in the foot. With repeated exercises the mTrPs on the right disappeared. On the left only mobilisation of the acromioclavicular joint was required. His homework was to continue with Vele exercises, leaning forward with swinging movements.

At the follow-up examination a month later there was just pain in the left arm, which was treated with mobilisation of the acromioclavicular joint. Treatment was not carried out until the analysis was complete.

18.2.2 Trunk stabilisation system

If the stabilisation system of the trunk is involved, our first interest is its activation, as this actually shows that most mTrPs can be made to disappear if this system is functioning again. The key is the coordinated activity of the diaphragm and the M. transversus abdominis. Clinically, its function can be seen in the tone of the lateral abdominal wall at the waist. This applies particularly when breathing in, which involves concentric contraction of the diaphragm and concomitant eccentric strain on the M. transversus abdominis. If this system is working in an uncoordinated manner, such as when continuously sitting in a bent-over position, this can lead to shallow breathing (see Fig. 18.3), which in turn leads to tension of the scaleni muscles with the upper fixators of the shoulder girdle. This causes strain on the cervical spine and by removal of the thorax from the pelvis leads to destabilisation of the lumbar spine.

The first therapeutic stage is to palpate the tone of the waist with the hands and ask the patient to exert pressure on the palpating hands with the muscles of the waist (the lateral abdominal wall). Some patients cannot do this (Fig. 18.4).

This should then be exercised by sitting upright with the lower legs hanging down while lifting the knees. This

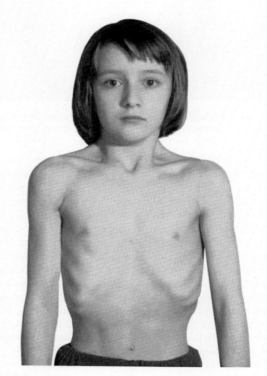

Fig. 18.3 High thoracic breathing with simultaneous 'paradoxical' breathing by pulling in the abdomen during inspiration. Note tension in the upper part of the M. trapezius, M. sternocleidomastoideus and the Mm. scaleni.

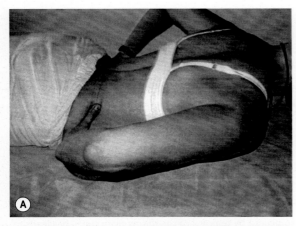

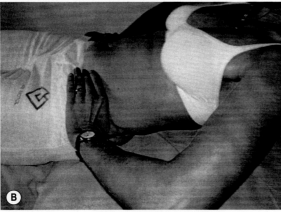

Fig. 18.4 Tension of the lateral abdominal wall when lifting the head and shoulders in the prone (a) and supine (b) positions (the patient can feel this for themselves with hands at the waist).

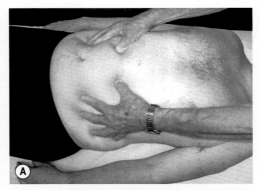

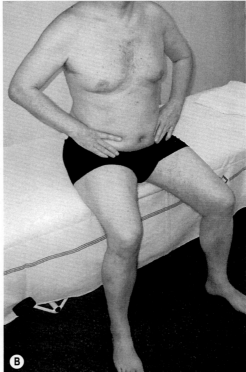

Fig. 18.5 (a) Stimulation of physiological breathing in the supine position. The therapist mobilises the thorax during expiration in a inferior direction, stimulates the lateral abdominal wall at the waist during inspiration and uses the hands to prevent lifting of the thorax during inspiration. This teaches the patient to use the deep abdominal muscles to prevent lifting the ribs during inspiration but instead to widen them. (b) Patient seated upright in front of a mirror with hands at the waist and fingertips on the side of the lower abdomen: the feet are used for support and are slightly abducted and laterally rotated. First the patient breathes out and during inspiration the lateral abdominal wall and lower abdomen tense. The patient notices in the mirror that neither the clavicle nor the ribs nor the navel are lifted. The thorax extends sideways from the waist; provide feedback with the aid of the hands and the mirror.

exercise can be carried out isometrically without the knees actually being lifted. This usually succeeds in enabling the patient to perceive the muscles of the lateral abdominal wall and even contract them in isolation by practising.

Another activation exercise is carried out in the prone or supine position: The head and shoulders are lifted while both the back extensors or Mm. recti abdomini and the lateral abdominal wall are tensed. Activation of the lateral abdominal wall relieves the lumbar spine. It is particularly important that the patient breathes out fully in the supine position so that the ribs are inferiorly mobilised, while when breathing in the thorax is cranially fixed and the patient is asked to tighten the lateral abdominal wall at the same time. This fixes the position of the thorax, which then widens but does not lift (Fig.18.5a).

If the patient succeeds in this, the next exercise is carried out in the upright seated position in front of a mirror. The patient's hands are placed on the waist. Now the patient practises breathing so that the thorax is extended by the waist but the clavicle is not lifted. Make sure, too, that the lower abdomen does not protrude and that the navel is not lifted (Fig. 18.5b).

If the patient succeeds in this, the mTrPs in the diaphragm, the scalene muscles, the pelvis and the back from the cervical to the inferior area disappear, and even disappear in the area of the lower extremities.

18.2.3 Foot stabilisation system

When dealing with the stabilisation system of the foot we are dealing predominantly with forward posture (Fig. 7.6). Correlates are mTrPs in the M. rectus abdominis, the M. biceps femoris and the feet. The first therapeutic priority is to exercise the automatic toe flexion during forward movement (Fig. 7.5). This movement can be practised with a swinging movement forwards and backwards with upright posture. If the arch of the foot is weak, the patient should concentrate on and be aware of walking on the lateral edge of the foot (even in shoes) but should not exaggerate and roll over onto the outer edge of the foot. Abduction of the big toes should be exercised, particularly if there is a tendency to hallux valgus.

The fixation of the shoulder blades plays a crucial role in functional disorders of the upper extremities. Here it is particularly important that the patient learns to voluntarily tighten the lower (ascending) part of the trapezius muscle. It is often sufficient for eliminating mTrPs and blockages of the shoulders and elbows.

The patient can also exercise on all fours, placing most of the weight on the hands pressing the thenar eminence of both hands against the mat: the shoulder blades should not stand up and should remain abducted.

Something similar also applies to the atlanto-occipital joint. Its function is to hold up the head, even under a load. Blockages of C0/1 and C1/2 with mTrPs predominantly in the M. sternocleidomastoideus and the short atlanto-occipital joint extensors can be successfully eliminated if you put quite light and fast tapping pressure on the skull in neutral upright position with a precisely centred cervical spine. The head should not sway from one side to the other nor from front to back. After practising, the patient can carry out self-treatment.

18.2.4 Neuromuscular techniques

It is often necessary to treat mTrPs and blockages over and beyond the main exercises. Neuromuscular techniques offer particular advantages as they are gentle, effective and take up little time and because they predominantly use the patient's muscles for mobilisation. This is obviously better for the patient than the muscles of even the best therapist. Furthermore, the majority of these techniques are also suitable for self-treatment.

The underlying principle of neuromuscular techniques is postisometric relaxation and reciprocal inhibition. In the simplest form, the joint (or the muscle) is tensed with minimal force. The patient then performs isometric resistance with minimal force for 5–10 s against the movement induced by the therapist. This is followed by relaxation. During relaxation the movement in the restricted direction slowly increases without the therapist actively increasing the range of movement (the therapist cannot relax the patient, that must be done by the patient themself). It is important that the therapist waits for the release (relaxation) to end, which can take 10–30 s. The rule is: the longer, the better.

Once the range of movement has been increased in this way, the exercise can be repeated in order to increase the range of movement further. This is followed by reciprocal inhibition, when the patient actively carries out the movement in the restricted direction or while the therapist provides resistance for the patient. To make sure that this does not lead to a type of duel where the patient may well be the stronger, the same effect can be achieved if the therapist repeatedly carries out the movement with minimal force against light resistance from the patient. This can be illustrated in this simplest form by restricted pronation with mTrPs in the supinator muscle (Fig. 18.6).

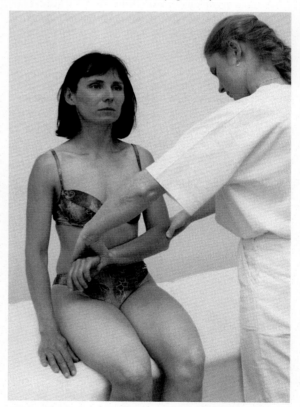

Fig. 18.6 Postisometric relaxation and reciprocal inhibition in pronation: first isometric resistance against supination, then relaxation into pronation (release). Then reciprocal inhibition by repetitive passive pronation against resistance from patient. The same technique is also used for self-treatment.

18.2.5 Breathing in and out

In most cases, postisometric relaxation is significantly more effective with the aid of other facilitation techniques. Breathing in and out and direction of sight are the first of these. In most cases, breathing in makes tension easier and breathing out makes it easier to relax.

The mobilisation of the occiput against the axis is illustrated in Fig. 18.7. The patient is in the supine position. The head rests on the palm of the therapist's hand; the therapist places their thumb and index finger on the spiny process of the atlas and presses the head with minimal pressure in a inferior direction against the atlas. The patient is then asked to look at their forehead and take a deep breath: the automatic dorsal flexion is prevented by isometric resistance. The patient is then instructed to look down at the chin. Relaxation into anteflexion occurs. Mobilisation can be repeated once this position is attained. This is a kind of double facilitation because looking upwards facilitates not only dorsal flexion but also inspiration and looking down (to the chin) helps with expiration.

Breathing in and out is particularly effective if inspiration is combined with a movement in one direction and expiration in the opposite direction. This is known as 'respiratory synkinesis'. That is also the case with the temporomandibular joint and the muscles of mastication. The muscle tension increases as you breathe out and relaxes when you breathe in, as with yawning. The patient is also asked to breathe out first and then breathe in deeply 'as if yawning' (Fig. 18.8a). Self-treatment is performed in the same manner (Fig. 18.8b).

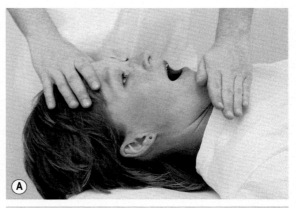

(A)

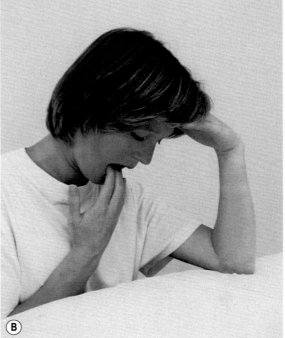

(B)

Fig. 18.8 (a) Treatment lying down. The patient opens their mouth and the therapist places one hand on the chin and instructs 'breathe out, breathe out'. Now the muscles of mastication tense during expiration. The patient is then asked to breathe in deeply while keeping the mouth open wide 'as if yawning'. This leads to relaxation of the muscles of mastication. (b) Self-treatment in the seated position: the patient holds their head above the eyes in a neutral position, places one hand on the chin, opens their mouth slightly and breathes out. Then they breathe in deeply and opens their mouth wide 'as if yawning' and repeats two to three times.

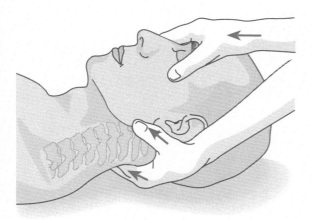

Fig. 18.7 Mobilisation of C0–C1 in anteflexion. The back of the patient's head lies in the therapist's palm, the transverse processes of the atlas are held in place by the thumb and index finger. The head is tightened in a inferior direction opposite the atlas: the patient looks to the forehead and breathes in to produce isometric tension against resistance from the therapist. Then they looks to their chin and breathing out automatically leads to relaxation (release).

We have Gaymans to thank for the particularly beneficial respiratory synkinesis. During lateral flexion of the cervical and thoracic spine in the straight segments (C0, C2, T2, etc.) resistance increases during inspiration and fades during expiration. In the segments which are not straight (C1, C3, T3, etc.), on the other hand, resistance increases against lateral flexion during expiration and fades during inspiration. Only in the cervicothoracic transition does resistance occur exclusively during inspiration with fading during expiration.

In practice, the procedure is as follows: pre-tense the cervical and thoracic spine in the lateral position. In straight segments the patient is asked to look up and breathe in slowly, hold the breath and slowly breathe out again. Towards the end of the out-breath (wait!) any resistance fades (release). Looking up facilitates breathing in and increases resistance to lateral flexion; looking down facilitates breathing out but should be avoided for the thoracic spine because the patient leans forward. In the non-straight segments, direction of sight is not used and the patient is only asked to breathe out deeply and slowly and then slowly take another deep breath. Towards the end of the inspiration any resistance fades and mobilisation begins (release) (Fig. 18.9).

It is particularly advantageous to make use of the effect of gravity. For example, the patient can extend their leg in the supine position and hold it in this position for 10–20 s, then let the leg fall and relax in this position for 20 s. This can be repeated two to three times. With the knee extended, the rectus femoris muscle is isometrically stretched; if the lower leg is hanging down it relaxes. For reciprocal inhibition the patient then strongly flexes the knee. This is self-treatment using the best physiological means and is easy to practise daily (Fig. 18.10).

18.2.6 Relaxation of the M. quadratus lumborum

In the area of the trunk as well there is the possibility of combining the effect of gravity with the breathing technique and the direction of sight. A good example is the relaxation of the M. quadratus lumborum. The patient stands with legs slightly spread apart and leans to the side. On the

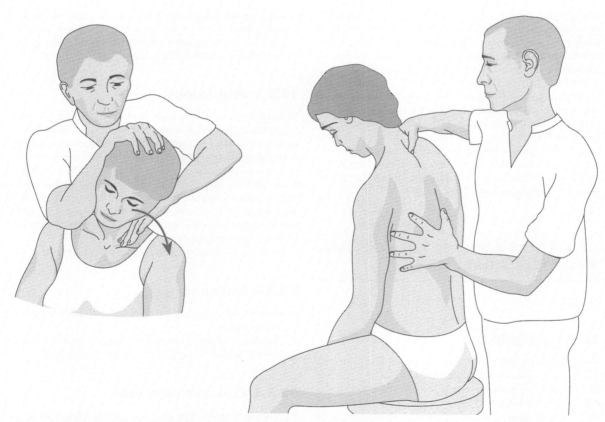

Fig. 18.9 Mobilisation into cervical (a) and thoracic (b) lateroflexion: the patient straightens up and leans the straight segments sideways, looks up and breathes in after holding their breath. They then look down and breathe out. Breathing in automatically leads to tension and breathing out to release. In the thoracic segments omit the glance downwards. In the curved segments after tension, tell the patient to 'breathe out slowly and breathe in deeply and slowly again'.

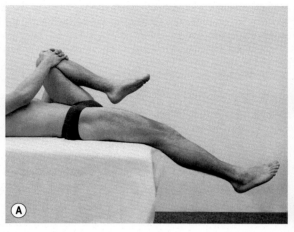 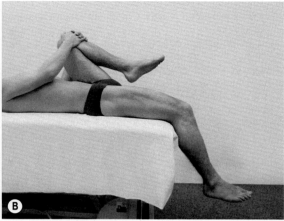

Fig. 18.10 Relaxation of the M. rectus femoris using gravity. The patient lies in the supine position and lifts the lower leg to the horizontal, holding it isometrically against gravity for 10–20 s (a). They then let it hang down relaxed for another 20 s. This is repeated two to three times. For the reciprocal inhibition the knee is strongly flexed (b).

assumption of good relaxation, optimum pre-tension can now be achieved with the aid of gravity. Then the patient looks up and breathes in slowly and deeply. With good relaxation, the patient is lifted up a small but perceivable amount by the deep breath. Now the breath is held for a moment and then the patient looks down and slowly breathes out, when the upper body leans to the side again. The manoeuvre is repeated three times. After that the patient pushes the hanging arm strongly towards the floor (reciprocal inhibition). Now the same manoeuvre is repeated. After pre-tensioning by looking upwards, inspiration is facilitated and the trunk is lifted. Looking down on the other hand facilitates expiration and gravity allows relaxation leaning sideways (Fig. 18.11).

18.3 SPRAY AND STRETCH, COOLING AND STRETCHING

Dominik Irnich

18.3.1 Definition

The spray-and-stretch technique involves cooling treatment of an mTrP with concomitant extension of the affected muscle. This treatment technique has been described in detail by Travell and Rinzler (1952). In the view of many mTrP therapists, however, the spray-and-stretch technique is only of historical significance. On the other hand, therapeutic hypoaesthesia or anaesthesia with extreme cold or ice represents a successfully applied procedure in surgery, orthopaedics, sports traumatology and sports medicine.

Very recently, Simons also told us that for environmental reasons (destruction of the ozone layer) he was against the use of a cooling spray. Nevertheless, ice massage is recommended, and this can achieve the same effect.

18.3.2 Physiology

There are only hypotheses about the mechanism of effect of cooling and simultaneous stretching. It is postulated that muscle extension is increased with simultaneous analgesia with the application of cold. The cold-pain tolerance of the skin is a limiting factor of this treatment. On the other hand, only by applying the cold for a long period does muscle temperature actually drop low enough. We must also accept that segmental reflective mechanisms and the activation or inhibition of autonomic reflexes lead to observed muscle relaxation.

There are no theories about physiological acceptance.

18.3.3 Indications

- MPS of the superficial muscles without inflammatory components.
- Treatment of acute myofascial pain, especially in the field of sports traumatology and sports medicine.

18.3.4 Contraindications

- Muscle fibre tears (partial or complete). Exception: part of a specific treatment cycle for acute muscle fibre tear in high-performance sport.
- Superficial injuries.
- Gout (uric acid crystals in the tissue).

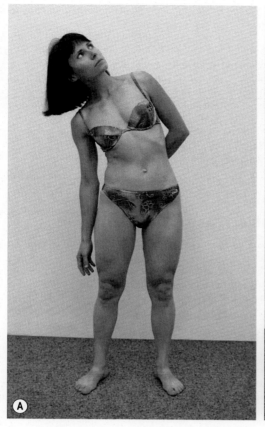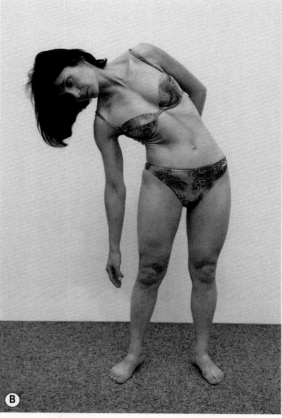

Fig. 18.11 Relaxation of the M. quadratus lumborum while standing. The patient bends to the side and then relaxes. Once relaxed, they look up and breathes in slowly and deeply (a). Deep breathing lifts the patient slightly. They then hold their breath, look down and breathe out. This leads to relaxation in lateral flexion. This is repeated two to three times. For reciprocal inhibition they press the hand hanging down towards the floor (b).

18.3.5 Undesirable effects

- Cold pain.
- Increase in reflex muscle tension.
- Freezing with formation of blisters and ulcerations if inappropriately used

See also undesirable effect from stretching (Section 19.2).

18.3.6 Practical procedure

For this technique you need a cool spray with a nozzle which can produce a fine but strong spray (e.g. no loss of pressure over 1 m). Sprays which cover a wide area are not suitable for this technique. The spray should be held 40–60 cm away from the tissue to be treated. The angle of the spray should be between 30 and 60°. As this a procedure which can cause pain or loss of sensation, it is particularly important to touch the patient first with your own hand and palpate the underlying condition of the connective tissue and the muscle.

A second possibility is cooling and stretching using ice. The ice can be frozen in a convenient form, such as in a paper cup or ice tray. If a handle such as a stick or a wooden pencil is frozen with it, handling is made easier (Fig. 18.12).

The ice is rubbed firmly over the mTrP. For longer treatment, a container that absorbs the cold should be used (e.g. metal cup, drinks can) to avoid 'water damage' (Fig. 18.13). The direct application of ice can feel unpleasant so sometimes a cooled drinks can rolled over the skin is sufficient. It is important that the patient is comfortable so that the affected muscle is in a relaxed mid-position.

> If the tension of the whole muscle is definitely increased, cold treatment should not be carried out.

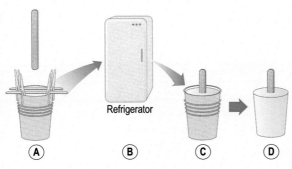

Fig. 18.12 Preparation of ice for treatment.

Treatment with jet or ice should always be carried out in one direction, as if smoothing out the mTrP. Sometimes we recommend smoothing out the mTrP in the direction of the referral zone. Usually the trigger point is parallel to the course of the muscle fibres and in the direction of the muscle insertion.

Smoothing and cooling is carried out slowly, rhythmically and dynamically. After about 20–30 s, or at the latest when definite pain from the cold is felt, the treatment should be interrupted for about 60 s. During the treatment, the muscle being treated should be passively and gently stretched. During a pause in treatment as above, continue to stretch the muscle. The stretching pressure increases during the course of the treatment if this is tolerated by the patient and not felt to be unpleasant.

After each treatment the local findings should be checked and the active motion tested.

The whole treatment may last between 15 and 20 min and should be carried out with concentration. As with all mTrP treatment techniques, make sure that the patient is still mobile after the treatment, without being overtaxed. The therapist can show the patient some simple stretching exercises (see Chs 26–34), which can then be done at home.

18.4 FASCIA TECHNIQUES FOR THE TREATMENT OF mTrPs

Robert Schleip

18.4.1 Definitions

Manual treatment modalities are designed to loosen fascial restrictions (taut bands, contractions, adhesions). The most well known of these is the Rolf method of structural integration (Rolfing), examples of which are described below.

18.4.2 Physiological basis

Ida P. Rolf, the founder of this method (and, during the Second World War, one of the first female biochemists to gain a doctorate at the respected Rockefeller Institute in New York), stressed the viscoelasticity of the fascia as one

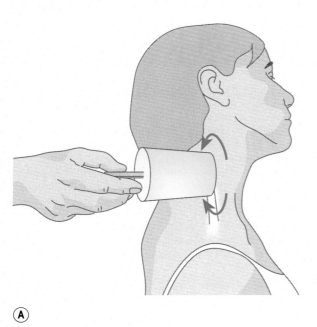

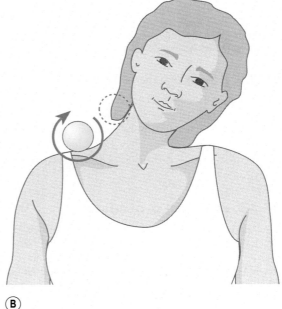

Fig. 18.13 Treatment with ice.

of the most essential physiological bases for her method, and in particular its property of reacting to strong or persistent deformation not just with temporary (elastic) but also with permanent (plastic) change of shape. She associated the tendency of colloid substances to change from a firm (gel) to a more liquid (sol) condition as a result of mechanical perturbation (thixotrophy) with the clinically observed plasticity of the fascia.

More recent ideas emphasise the abundant innervation of the fascia with mechanoreceptors as well. The stimulation of these sensory nerve endings can lead to changes in the underlying tension of the skeletal muscle (by stimulation of the Golgi receptors), to a general inhibition of the sympathicotonic activation (Ruffini receptors) and to greater hydration of the worked tissue (free nerve endings). It can also have the effect of an increase in local proprioception, particularly the reduction of a dysfunction described by Thomas Hanna (2003) as 'sensorimotor amnesia' (Golgi, Paccini, Ruffini receptors, free nerve endings).

In association with trigger points it is supposed that the hardening in the so-called taut band is relaxed by myofascial loosening (by loosening the collagen crosslinks and/or increasing the local matrix hydration) and that the stimulus threshold of the nociceptors is increased at the mTrPs by desensitisation. There is so far still only experimental confirmation of both effects, and this is not specifically in relation to trigger points. The permanent relaxing effect of myofascial manipulation on firm connective tissue has been recorded in the carpal tunnel area of human cadavers; the desensitisation of mechanosensitive nociceptors by myofascial techniques has been demonstrated on the hind legs of dogs.

Besides these specific local effects, the Rolfing therapist also assumes so far unproven acceptance that the occurrence of trigger points is favoured by so-called muscular dysbalance. This refers to the frequent chronic stiffness of certain muscle groups as described by Vladimir Janda, Ida Rolf and others (e.g. upper trapezius, levator scapulae and larger and smaller chest muscles) which are accompanied by simultaneous weakness of other muscle groups which are functionally associated (e.g. anterior neck muscles, lower shoulder blade stabilisers). The aim of the treatment is to balance these dysbalances and is usually pursued by loosening work on the hardened muscle groups. (For 'strengthening' the weakened muscle groups on the other hand there is a lack of detailed theoretical models and concrete treatment plans.)

18.4.3 Theoretical basis

Ida Rolf assumed that gravity has a pronounced lifelong influence on individual body structure and muscular dysbalance. By body structure she meant the common denominator of typical body posture. The more the body structure of a person is straightened out, the less the body must struggle with permanent muscle contraction against gravity and the less the tendency for myofascial stiffness. The use of myofascial release can tangibly reduce local hardening or adhesions, as found in everyday clinical practice, often within a few minutes. Whether these changes are permanent, however, depends – according to Ida Rolf – on whether the rest of the body returns to the old posture or whether it succeeds in bringing the whole body into a new, more economical and upright posture which then is at least as permanent as the previous stance.

According to Ida Rolf the fascial network represents the 'organ of shape'. Contractions or hindrances to smooth functioning in this bodywide network mould the body structure when standing, and in the individual gait, habitual movement during respiration and general play of movement of the joints. To release such restrictions, the therapist usually follows the premise 'Put it where it belongs and ask for movement'. The fascial layers are pushed in the direction of their physiological configuration while the client is instructed to support this grip with specific active micromovements of the region being treated. The commonly created shearing in the tissue can lead to local *wohlweh* ('good pain') sensation for the client and to temporary muscle pain after treatment. However, the therapist calculates the strength and duration of the hold very precisely in relation to the client's nervous system so that their body looks forward to each new hold with positive expectation. The training for this specific calculation and the empathy required is usually one of the most important parts of therapist training.

18.4.4 Indications

The Rolfing method is frequently also used as a non-medical measure, for example in the field of wellness. On the other hand, in the context of medical therapy this method finds increasing application for painful myofascial dysfunction associated with chronic postural deviation; this is particularly the case with hyperkyphosis, hunched shoulders, holding the head forward and leg deformities such as genu valgum/varum, pelvic tilting or hyperlordosis. For general sympathicotonic dystonia the method is frequently used for vagotonic stimulation as well, particularly through slow-motion release at the back of the head and neck, diaphragm, pelvis and abdominal area.

18.4.5 Contraindications

Absolute contraindications (red flags) are acute inflammatory musculoskeletal diseases, known aneurysm, acute phlebitis and incompletely healed wounds in the area.

Increased caution (yellow flags) applies to osteoporosis, pregnancy, cancer, arteriosclerosis, psychological diseases and long-term cortisone treatment.

18.4.6 Undesirable effects

One case is documented where an insufficiently trained therapist loosened a urethral stent by deep abdominal manipulation.

The first sessions for people with bipolar disorders should not take place during a manic phase, as this can lead to worsening of the symptoms.

Athletes may require several days to adjust to their accustomed fine level of coordination as a result of changed fascial tensions. If the type of sport that the athlete does involves a high level of coordination and precision, we therefore recommend that Rolfing sessions are not used during a competition phase but in a training phase.

18.4.7 Practical procedure (for myofascial pain)

In the Rolfing method, the therapist usually applies slow melting pressure to the hardened areas. Depending on the area and the deep layer of interest, this is performed with the fingertips, knuckles, back of the hand or the elbow. The first contact (landing) of the hand doing the work is very gentle in every case. The second hand then usually rests on another associated part of the body.

Using 'kinaesthetic empathy' the therapist forms an inner relationship with the working area; e.g. with the perception of this area in the therapist's own body and the prior expectation of having a beneficial effect not just on the client's body but also on one's own. The client may be asked to look at this area in their mind. Not until both the client and the therapist are giving their full attention to the working area does the working hand begin to increase pressure and push the skin and the subcutaneous tissue against the underlying deep fascia. It is almost always a shearing movement (which stimulates the Ruffini receptors in particular) so that the treated fascial structures are stretched rather than compressed.

In some movements, the therapist's hand or elbow may slide several centimetres during the movement. Once the limit of the skin's mobility has been reached, there can still be skin-on-skin movement, making use of the slight film of moisture usually created locally after several seconds of slow pressure. Only in rare cases, such as with very hairy skin, is the additional use of skin cream required (but not oil, otherwise the intended slow stretching effect on the deeper tissue layers is lost).

The direction of the working hand – or the direction of the sliding movement – is decided so that the collagen fibres in the treated layer are subjected to unaccustomed stretching. This can be longitudinal to the dominant direction of the fibres in the area, or it may be perpendicular. If the working area is close to the skeletal insertion of the same fibres, the sliding movement is always directed away from the insertion.

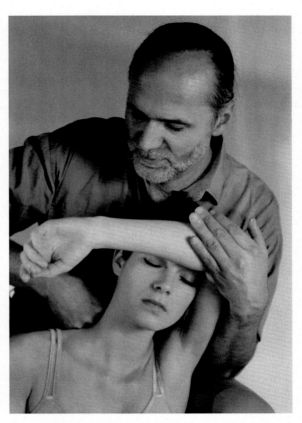

Fig. 18.14 Example of a myofascial loosening grip of the upper trapezius muscle during a Rolfing session. The therapist uses slowly increasing manual pressure in a slightly inferior direction while the patient is told to place their forehead against their elbow (Schleip 2002).

In all other cases, however, there are usually several different direction options for effecting stretching of the fibres. It is then often proprioceptive considerations that decide which direction is most likely to be relieving for the client's nervous system. In the area of the upper trapezius muscle (Fig. 18.14), for example, this is usually not in a superior but a inferior direction.

The sliding movement may last for up to 2 min and the mechanical pressure from the working hand may sometimes increase considerably (often by more than 100 N, comparable to 10 kg). The precise direction of stretching and strength of pressure depend on the optimum release effect on the hardened tissue and often require great local empathy to determine. The typical 'release' feeling is then usually experienced by both the therapist and the client as a slow, soft melting of the formerly hardened fibre bundle structures. To refine the therapist's perception, it can be useful to imagine large numbers of the tiniest organisms in the treatment area (Fig. 18.15). As soon as one of these therapist simultaneously moves the elbow and head rather more to the left. The principle of 'less is more' applies to these active support movements by the client. The slower and finer these movement are, the greater their efficacy. This principle is supported by appropriate coaching and numerous encouraging verbal reminders from the therapist.

The majority of treatment movements are carried out with the client lying on an upholstered bench. At the end of a treatment session in particular, however (this typically lasts 50–75 min in Rolfing), the movements often take place with the client in a seated or other active position. In the movement shown in Fig. 18.14 the client is asked to lean the upper body forward (as if trying to fall asleep in a moving bus) so that the upper back extensors particularly are extended and relaxed. The therapist's left hand supports the weight of the upper body and at the same time can feel to what extent the client is ready to let their head fall forward at any moment.

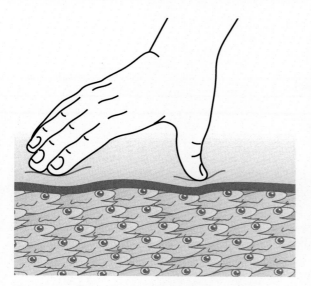

Fig. 18.15 A frequently used trick for increasing tactile awareness: the therapist imagines the tissue is inhabited by a number of tiny organisms. As soon as one of the organisms releases itself from the surrounding areas, the therapist slows the movement and directs it to this site and the neighbouring areas (Schleip 2002).

organisms releases itself from the surrounding areas, the therapist slows the movement and directs it to this site and the neighbouring areas.

During the procedure the client often supports this with active internal micromovements. In some – albeit rare – cases these are fine tensioning of the treated muscle fibres (to stimulate the fascial Golgi receptors). Usually, though, they are movements which open the treated area and support the therapist's direction of stretching. In Fig. 18.14, for example, they are slight snuggling movements of the client's forehead against the skin of the elbow or the slow downward movement of the right shoulder while the

18.4.8 Clinical studies

There are a good dozen uncontrolled clinical studies on the Rolfing method, and so far two published studies with randomised control groups. In the first, in 10 Rolfing studies a positive effect was shown on a general anxiety state which was still definitely noticeable 5 weeks after the last treatment (Weinberg, Hunt 1979). The second study recorded that a single Rolfing treatment on the pelvis led to a significant improvement in vagal tone and horizontalisation of the pelvis (less pelvis tilting) (Cottingham et al. 1988). The vagal tone was an indicator of the health of the autonomic nervous system. Studies without control groups showed improved balance regulation, more economical muscle activation in everyday movements, a pain-relieving effect on patients with chronic pain, a functional improvement in children with mild cerebral palsy and patients with chronic tiredness said they felt better. Admittedly, all these studies were clinical trials with relatively small trial groups ($n < 35$). An overview of these and other published Rolfing studies can be found at www.rolfing.org.

Chapter 19

Treatment plan for myofascial trigger point therapy

Roland Gautschi

Trigger point therapy as a treatment technique: as a treatment technique, trigger point therapy aims to deactivate active mTrPs. Various techniques have been developed for this: manual (Chs 18 and 19), physical (Ch. 20) and invasive (Chs 21 and 22) techniques.
Trigger point therapy as a treatment plan: for the long-term treatment of myofascial pain, trigger point therapy is necessary as a treatment technique; if it is the only approach, however, it is often insufficient. Experience shows that, especially if symptoms have become chronic, it is necessary to include other factors in the trigger point treatment plan for lasting elimination of myofascial problems:

- first, it is necessary to treat the reactive changes in the connective tissue simultaneously with the trigger point itself,
- second, it is necessary to recognise the causative and supportive factors and integrate them into the mTrP treatment plan.

Based on Dejung trigger point manual therapy (Section 18.1) the Interest Group for Myofascial Trigger Point Therapy (IMTT) has developed a treatment plan for mTrPs which has proved reliable in everyday therapy. There is now a six-stage treatment programme (the Swiss approach): four manual techniques (Section 19.1) are supplemented by detensioning/stretching measures (Section 19.2) and functional strengthening of the muscle (Section 19.3). To improve everyday poor posture, patients are also made aware of the ergonomic aspects (Section 19.3).

In a comprehensive sense the treatment plan is open to integrating other therapeutic measures such as joint- and nerve-specific techniques, strategies for stress management and nutritional aspects, among others.

19.1 MANUAL TECHNIQUES AND DRY NEEDLING

In the trigger point therapy treatment plan, deactivation of the trigger point (manual techniques, dry needling) and the release of connective tissue adhesions (manual techniques) have a key place.

19.1.1 Manual techniques

The manual procedures for the treatment of mTrPs give equal weight to both the mechanical and reflex influence on the mTrP and the treatment of reactively changed connective tissue structures. These techniques have been summarised in the section on Dejung manual trigger point therapy (Section 18.1) and in Table 19.1.

19.1.2 Dry needling

Manual techniques and dry needling (Section 22.1) can be combined and can mutually strengthen the effect. The treatment of mTrPs using acupuncture needles makes it possible to deactivate the diseased muscle fibre sections precisely to within millimetres. This provides long-term support for the effect of manual techniques I and II. Particularly in body regions where the mTrPs of the muscle to be treated are covered by other muscle layers, dry needling provides the chance of working precisely and specifically deep in the muscle, for example:

- treatment of the M. glutaeus minimus through the Mm. glutaeus medius and maximus (Sections 32.12),

http://dx.doi.org/10.1016/B978-0-7020-4312-3.00019-2

Table 19.1 Treatment plan for trigger point therapy: manual treatment techniques and their local effects (Gautschi 2008)

Technique I	Ischaemic compression of the mTrP	• Pressing out the 'inflammatory soup' and the local oedema • Reactive hyperaemia following ischaemia → Increase in metabolism • Reflective detensioning of the taut band belonging to the mTrP

Technique II	Manual stretching of the mTrP region	• Pressing out the 'inflammatory soup' and the local oedema
		• Reactive hyperaemia following ischaemia
		   → Increase in metabolism
		• Reflective detensioning of the taut band belonging to the mTrP
		• Destruction of the local rigor complex
		• Stretching reactive connective tissue adhesions (pathological crosslinks) and contractures
		   → Improvement in intramuscular supply and suppleness

Technique III	Fascia stretching technique
	Manual stretching of the superficial and intramuscular fascia
		• Loosening reactive connective tissue adhesions (pathological crosslinks) and contractures
		   → Improvement in intramuscular mobility and supply
		   → Better muscle extension
		• Stimulation of fascial mechanoreceptors
		   → Reflective detensioning of the taut band belonging to the mTrP
		   → Lowering of sympathetic nerve activity, lowering of basic global tension

Technique IV	Fascia separation technique Manual loosening of intermuscular fascia adhesions	• Loosening of adhesions between fascia of neighbouring muscles → Improvement in intermuscular mobility
Technique V	Stretching – detensioning (stretching by therapist, autostretching) (see Section 19.2)	• Detensioning → Improvement in stretchability of the muscle
Technique VI	Functional training – ergonomics (see Section 19.3)	• Physiological weight-bearing and exercise support the regeneration process and make the muscles more resilient • Ergonomy reduces incorrect strain on the muscles

- treatment of the deep paravertebral muscles (multifidii and rotator muscles) of the M. erector trunci through the superficial back muscles (Section 32.1),
- treatment of the M. supraspinatus through the M. trapezius (Section 28.2).

Techniques

Various dry needling techniques are applied (Section 22.1), as follows.

- With 'deep dry needling' the needle penetrates the mTrP directly. This mechanically destroys the trigger point region. Typically, there is a brief twitch of the muscle fibres where the mTrP lies (local twitch response). This deep form of needling is described as 'intramuscular stimulation' (or IMS).
- By contrast, during 'superficial dry needling' the needle is just placed superficially, 1–2 mm below the skin, in the area over the mTrP. This form of dry needling is

described as 'superficial afference stimulation' (or SAS), and is intended to detension the deep-seated mTrP in a reflex reaction.

It is important to remember that with dry needling the connective tissue components of a myofascial problem – which is frequently a peripheral chronification factor with long-term symptoms – have not been sufficiently treated. For chronic pain, manual connective tissue techniques (techniques II–IV) are of great significance and are essential.

Treatment intensity

The manual techniques and dry needling methods described here are often painful. They demand a good relationship between the therapist and the patient. The patient must be informed about the sense and purpose of the pain during the therapy. The patient must understand that the pain caused by the therapy serves to release the contraction knots and the connective tissue and that this is the most direct way to achieve the therapeutic objective. Before manual therapy you must agree upon a mutually understood signal so that painful treatment can be interrupted at any time, such as when they say 'Stop!' The therapist should keep strictly to the agreement: the patient determines how strong the painful therapeutic intervention is and how long it lasts.

Highly irritated tissue should be treated with low pressure and for short periods of time in an individual session and mildly irritated tissue can be treated for longer and more intensively. The treated tissue is often reddened after treatment and sensitive to pressure for 2–3 days. Patients should be advised of these possible side effects beforehand. Any severe pain can be dulled with NSAIDs for a few days. If, after treatment, the pain is worse for more than 2 days or if there is a bruise as a result of weak connective tissue or too much pressure then the intensity of the treatment should be reduced (less pressure, longer pauses between treatments).

> The irritability of the tissue should define the intensity of the treatment.

Building up treatment

The sequence of manual techniques I–IV and dry needling should be adapted to the actual situation. With certain muscles, always begin with manual technique IV based on the anatomical conditions. For example, to treat the subscapularis muscle directly with techniques I and II, the articular space between the M. serratus anterior and M. subscapularis must first be released using the fascia separation technique (technique IV). Not until these two muscles have been separated from each other is the way open for the therapist's fingers to treat the trigger point in the M. subscapularis directly. With fresh, acute problems, the use of techniques I and II or dry needling directly 'on the spot' are likely to be successful.

For patients with chronic pain or high tissue irritability, it is appropriate to begin slowly and extensively with technique III. This prepares the tissue and also allows the therapist to touch the client more firmly without causing pain. Gentle stretching of the muscle to which technique III is applied makes it easier to palpate the taut bands, which are the key structures for identifying a trigger point. The active trigger point can then be thoroughly treated using techniques I and II. Technique IV is used to release the fascial

adhesions of neighbouring muscles, which is especially relevant for antagonistic muscle groups. Substantial and lasting improvement in motion restrictions can be achieved by this measure. The sequence of manual therapy is often concluded with technique III. At the right level, most clients find it pleasant and beneficial. By stimulating the fascial mechanoreceptors it helps to lower sympathetic activity (Schleip 2003).

Duration of treatment: for acute symptoms two to four treatments are often enough to provide lasting relief from a myofascial problem. A definite improvement should be expected for chronic pain conditions after a few trial treatments. If there is no improvement after three to five treatments, the indication and treatment strategy should be checked.

Summary

The aim of trigger point therapy is to provide a permanent cure for myofascially caused pain and functional disorders. This requires:

* finding the relevant active trigger point,
* deactivating the relevant trigger point using manual techniques and/or dry needling,
* providing thorough manual treatment of the connective tissue changes which occur as a reaction, especially with chronic symptoms,
* recognising the factors which cause the problem to persist and including them in the treatment process.

19.2 EXTENSION AND RELAXATION/ STRETCHING AND DETENSIONING

In practice it has proved reliable to stretch the affected muscles after manual treatment (techniques I–IV) or dry needling of the mTrP. Stretching is integrated in the treatment plan for trigger point therapy as technique V.

19.2.1 Effects of stretching

In this chapter 'stretching' (or extension) describes the process by which the origin and insertion of a muscle are distanced from each other. When the therapist carries out an extension manoeuvre, a soft elastic stop is tangible at the end of the range of movement. The patient personally perceives how extension is increased. 'Stretching' in this context is a term from everyday language and describes the subjective feeling that something is being 'stretched'. If the patient says during extension or after stretching that it now feels 'less tense' or 'is stretching better' and the 'movement is going further', it is not conclusive in the scientific sense that the mechanical extension of a morphological structure has been carried out. The changed feeling of extension and the measurable gain in movement can be caused by various factors (Lindel 2006, Zahnd 2005):

- biomechanically structure-specific components have a traction effect on:
  - muscles (titin (connectin) filaments transfer traction within the extended muscle from Z-line to Z-line as molecular, highly elastic springs),
  - connective tissue (pathological crosslinks, contractions, unorganised alignment of collagen) with its intramuscular and extramuscular parts;
- reflex components lead to detensioning (neuromuscular inhibition): afferences of muscle spindles and Golgi receptors influence the tension in the muscles;
- psychological components (becoming accustomed to extension, changed pain acceptance, etc.).

We are not yet in a position to distinguish precisely in clinical practice to what extent structural factors were mechanically influenced by improved mobility or a less unpleasant end feeling, to what extent reflex processes led to detensioning of the muscle or to what extent a greater tolerance of stretching in the individual plays a part. We basically suppose that reflex processes dominate if there is a sudden, pronounced change. The mechanical treatment of structural muscle and/or connective tissue parts will show slower results in smaller steps, as direct mechanical influence on structurally contracted muscles requires long-lasting and repeated force. This should have the effect of increasing the sarcomeres, which are connected in series (Freiwald et al. 1999). However, the intention is to release contractions and pathological crosslinks in the intramuscular connective tissue. Long-term extension stimulates the fibroblasts to release collagenase which should reduce pathological crosslinks (van den Berg 2001). Experimental tests *in vitro* have shown that extension lasting about 3 min causes the release of collagenase (Carano, Siciliani 1996).

19.2.2 Biomechanical, structure-specific components

mTrPs lead to the formation of taut bands. In the area of the trigger point the myosin and actin filament complex remains in a contracted position (Fig. 19.1; rigor complex, in the central area: 'contraction knots'). The sarcomeres of the neighbouring muscle fibre sections compensate by lengthening. Overall, the affected muscle fibres are shortened. Compared to the surrounding muscle tissue, these shortened bands of muscle are palpable as taut bands.

The taut bands can be responsible for a whole series of negative effects, independently of pain caused directly by mTrPs and/or functional disorders; motion restrictions are very often the result of muscle shortening (Table 19.2).

To release the taut bands and eliminate the resulting negative consequences, extension techniques are frequently recommended and used in physiotherapy. If a muscle is

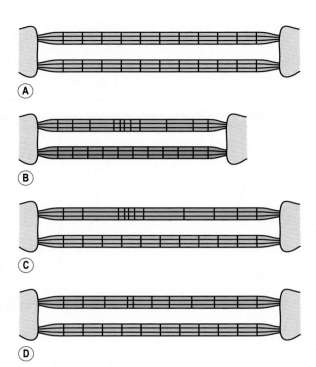

Fig. 19.1 Effect of stretching on healthy muscle fibres or muscle fibres contracted as a result of trigger points (taut bands). (a) Muscle fibres in healthy muscle: sarcomeres all the same length. (b) Muscle fibres with mTrP (top): shortening of the length of the sarcomeres in the trigger point zone is accompanied by compensatory lengthening of the bordering sarcomeres (taut band), this shortening of the muscle fibres. Normal muscle fibres adapt to the shortening (bottom). (c) Stretching without prior mTrP therapy (top): the muscle fibres with trigger points remain contracted in the trigger point zone. In the area of the rigor complex, myosin and actin filaments cannot be released from each other; the bordering and already lengthened and weakened sarcomeres are additionally traumatised and the previously intact sections of the muscle fibres may also be damaged as a result of too strong traction forces. Normal muscle fibres return to their original length (bottom). (d) Stretching after successful trigger point therapy (top): the mTrP zone is weakened by manual therapy or destroyed by the dry needling: gentle extension supports the reorganisation processes in the area of the former knotted contraction. Bordering muscle fibre sections are not additionally traumatised. Normal muscle fibres return to their original length (bottom).

extended, the taut band is the first to be under traction. The mechanical stretching will predominantly overextend the muscle fibre sections directly bordering the trigger point zone, which are already lengthened as a reaction and therefore weakened (Fig. 19.1). At these places in the muscle, which are the determining cause of the shortening of the muscle fibres – the mTrP – extension cannot have a releasing effect if the contraction knots have already been there for a long time and have become fixed structures.

Table 19.2 Effects of muscular taut bands

CONSEQUENCES OF MUSCULAR TAUT BANDS	EFFECT
Shortening of the muscles	Restricted movements, motor function disorder
Disorder of intramuscular coordination	Motor function disorder
Disorder of intermuscular coordination	Motor function disorder
Increased pressure on the intramuscular blood vessels (venous and arterial)	• Strangulation of the blood vessels • Local perfusion disorder and thus damage to the tissue metabolism
Increase in pressure on the extramuscular blood vessels (especially the leg veins) and lymph vessels	Increased formation of oedema (e.g. along the bundles of vessels and nerves through the soleus muscle)
Increase in pressure on the nerve pathways if these run through muscle or between muscular taut bands and bone structures	• Entrapment with metabolic blockage of nerve tissue conduction • Nerve dysfunction (dysaesthesia, metabolic disorder)
Taut bands reduce the full contraction and release capacity of the muscle and thus reduce the effect on the muscles as a muscle pump (peripheral heart)	Increases oedema

- If the stretching is too strong, the neighbouring sarcomeres can be damaged in unfortunate cases (Fig. 19.1c), predominantly by traumatisation of the membranes in the area of the Z-lines (van den Berg 2001).
- If the stretching is not too strong, the relevant muscle fibres will be detensioned for a short while and with long-term extension there may follow a length adaptation of the muscle fibres by new formation of additional sarcomeres (Freiwald et al. 1999, van den Berg 2001).

This, admittedly temporarily, reduces the traction on the trigger point zone and may also temporarily eliminate the symptoms, but the cause has not been treated.

> Treating the cause of contracted muscle resulting from taut bands consists of deactivating the sections of muscle fibre incapable of decontraction (the mTrP) using manual techniques or dry needling and releasing the connective tissue changes that have occurred as a reaction (pathological crosslinks, contractions).

This creates the prerequisite for the muscle tissue to reorganise itself in the previously pathologically changed muscle section. During the reconstruction phase, gentle, appropriate, pain-free or low-pain extension is helpful. This tells the muscle to what length the muscle tissue should regenerate (Fig. 19.1d).

19.2.3 Reflex components

Reflex detensioning of the muscle fibres by extension exercises relieves the mechanical traction on the mTrP. As long as the contraction knots are not fixed structures, spontaneous recovery of the trigger point is favoured. However, the rigor complex of structurally manifest contraction knots and reactive connective tissue changes cannot be released as a reflex.

19.2.4 Non-specific effects of stretching

A patient who regularly carries out repeated extension exercises throughout the day does not just benefit from the specific effects of the stretching (improvement in range of movement, increase in stretch tolerance of the muscle, signal effect to the muscle tissue regenerating after manual trigger point therapy, etc.). A number of other factors are positively influenced at the same time:

- reduction in poor muscle posture thanks to interruption of one-sided posture and/or monotonous movements,
- effects on other non-muscular structures (non-specific nerve mobilisation, pressure changes on blood vessels, etc.),
- development of body sensations,
- psychological effects (feeling of wellbeing, calmness, collectedness).

These non-specific effects of extension are often desirable and welcome in the management of chronic pain.

153

Summary

Treating the cause of the taut bands – and also the contracted muscles – consists of deactivating the trigger point causing the taut bands and releasing the connective tissue changes which have occurred as a reaction (pathological crosslinks, contractions).

- Deactivating the mTrP (manual techniques I and II, dry needling).
- Releasing connective tissue adhesions and contractions (techniques II, III and IV).
- Extending the affected muscles (technique V).

19.2.5 Forms of extension

Extension can be carried out in different ways (Table 19.3). The type of extension used is decided on a case-by-case basis.

- As manual trigger point therapy and dry needling are hands-on techniques, the patient should be instructed in a form of self-extension (self-stretching) whenever possible. With self-stretching, the patient can make an active contribution to the treatment in the form of a home programme. Self-stretching can be carried out statically or dynamically in the form of slow, rhythmical see-saw movements.
- Static extension emphasises the mechanical effects on the tissue properties of muscles and connective tissue (Fig. 19.2a and b).
- Dynamic extension uses predominantly the reflex components for detensioning the muscles (Fig. 19.2c).
- If the relevant trigger points are distributed in various muscles (often in muscle chains such as trigger points in the M. quadratus lumborum, M. tensor fasciae latae, Mm. gluteus medius and minimus), global extension is helpful (Fig. 19.3).
- Global extension is also applied if predominantly the non-specific effects of extension are desired (e.g. interruption of one-sided posture and monotonous movements; see above).
- If only one muscle is affected by trigger points, selective extension of the affected structure is recommended (Fig. 19.4).

If the patient carries out an extension exercise as part of a home programme it is worth being pragmatic: as a trial treatment after successful treatment of the mTrPs we recommend instructing the patient in an extension exercise for the muscle affected by mTrPs as a home programme. In the next therapy session, you can evaluate whether the exercise has become part of the daily routine, and the patient's experience with it. The extension positions should be adapted to the patient's everyday situation (Fig. 19.5) and not be unpleasant. This lowers the resistance threshold and increases the probability that the client will do the exercises every day. If static extension is unpleasant, dynamic extension should be tried, and vice versa.

> With the aid of extension the patient can learn (if instructed appropriately) to be more aware of themselves and to listen to what their body is telling them. If extension remains unpleasant in spite of modifications after several therapy sessions then the extension exercises should be stopped.

Table 19.3 Forms of extension

How stretching is performed	
Static stretching	The stretch is held for a short time (5–15 s) or for a longer time (> 60 s)
Dynamic stretching (ballistic stretching, intermittent stretching)	Rhythmical, slow intermittent movements are carried out at the end of the range of movement
Neuromuscular stretching techniques	Stretching after prior contraction of the affected muscle (use of postisometric relaxation) extension of the muscle while the antagonistic muscles are active (use of reciprocal inhibition)
What is stretched	
Selective stretching	Stretching of a specific muscle has specific effects (see Fig. 19.3)
Global stretching	When stretching whole muscle chains non-specific effects are more important (see Fig. 19.4)
Who does the stretching	
Stretching by therapist	The therapist stretches the muscle
Self-stretching	The patient stretches the muscle themself (self-stretching), following a programme at home (see Fig. 19.5)

Fig. 19.2 Stretching curves. (a) Lengthwise strain curve of connective tissue: in the matrix strain area a collagen structure can be lengthened without increasing the strain. If the structure is also lengthened, the collagen fibres are significantly strained. Distortion of the collagen fibres occurs in the creep area. If further strain is added, this leads to traumatisation (van den Berg 2001). (b) Static stretching: increasing the length of a muscle tendon complex if constant traction (i.e. without movement) is applied repeatedly to the end of the range of movement (Taylor 1990, in van den Berg 2001). (c) Dynamic stretching: changing the tension (detensioning) a muscle tendon complex with constant stretching at the end of the range of movement using repeated slow, rhythmical movements (Taylor 1990, in van den Berg 2001).

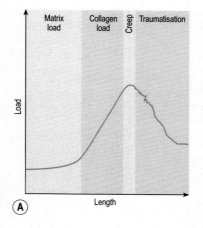

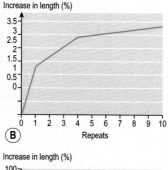

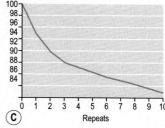

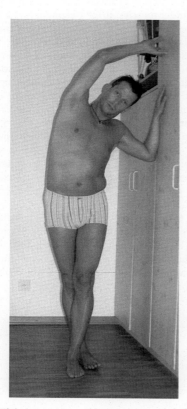

Fig. 19.3 Global stretching of the M. quadratus lumborum, together with the M. tensor fasciae latae and the M. latissimus dorsi.

Summary

With respect to trigger point therapy, gradually increased stretching of the muscles which demonstrate trigger points is sensible for the following reasons:

- it has been tried and tested in practice,
- after prior trigger point treatment (manual and dry needling), a gradual increase in extension is valuable in the regeneration phase as an information signal,
- if stretching is regularly carried out throughout the day the non-specific effects of extension should not be underestimated.

The topic of 'extension' should always be examined and treated in association and under continuous awareness of the mTrPs and the associated taut bands. The primary aim of extension is the release of taut bands and not an undifferentiated or forced lengthening of the muscle. To achieve this aim we use the biomechanical and reflex effects of the manual techniques of trigger point therapy and dry needling, and local treatment of the causes of contracted muscle fibre zones (contraction knots with muscular and connective tissue components) followed by a subsequent gradual build-up of stretching.

19.3 FUNCTIONAL TRAINING AND ERGONOMICS

One of the most common causes of mTrPs is acute or chronic overload of the muscles. Overload can be defined as an imbalance between strain and the ability to withstand

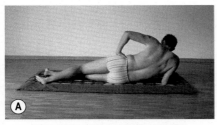

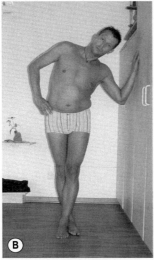

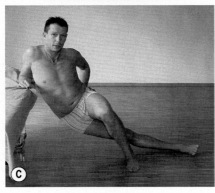

Fig. 19.4 Selective stretching using the M. quadratus lumborum as an example (with different starting points, a–c).

load. Predisposing factors (e.g. poor condition of the muscles), causative factors (e.g. trying to prevent a fall, repetitive movements at work, overload in sports, accidents) and maintaining factors (e.g. sitting or standing for long periods at work, one-sided training in sport, chronic stress) work together. The balance between strain and ability to withstand load can be distorted (Fig. 19.6):

- because the strain is too great, i.e. non-physiological,
- because the ability to withstand stress is reduced,
- because strain is increased at the same time as ability to withstand load is reduced.

Functional training (technique VI) increases the ability to withstand stress: well-trained muscles are less likely to be overloaded. Ergonomic measures and functional training in the sense of practising activities of daily living (ADLs) help to reduce poor posture.

Taking ergonomic aspects and the functional training of the muscles into account are therefore sensible key components of any myofascial treatment. They have been integrated into the treatment plan for trigger point therapy as technique VI and are crucial in determining the long-term success of the trigger point therapy.

Physiological strain and motion:

- promotes perfusion and metabolism in the muscle,
- supports the regeneration process,
- preserves and improves tissue mobility,
- increases the muscle's ability to withstand strain.

mTrPs lead to motor function disorder (Travell, Simons 2004, Dejung 2006). Using the shoulders as an example, Lucas et al. (2004) showed that mTrPs induce a significant change in the timing of the muscle activation pattern of all the shoulder muscles. mTrP treatment had a normalising effect on the muscle activation pattern of the muscles involved (Lucas et al. 2004, Gautschi 2007).

From research into low-back pain we know that the capacity to activate the local stabilisers at the correct time (Mm. multifidi, M. transversus abdominis) significantly reduces the rate of recurrence (Hodges, Richardson 1996). The economical or correctly timed activation of both the local stabilisers (Hodges, Richardson 1996) and the globally stabilising and dynamic muscle systems (Zahnd 2005) are a prerequisite for the locomotor system to reach its full functioning capacity. As this timing can be irritated by mTrPs, effective coordination and reconstructive training is only possible in association with deactivation of mTrP.

Because trigger points can be the cause of disorders of function, the relevant kinetic chain should be consistently examined for the presence of mTrPs before any active muscle rehabilitation. If mTrPs are present they should be adequately treated before active training. This is a prerequisite for effective functional training.

> Effective coordination and reconstructive training are only possible in association with deactivation of mTrPs.

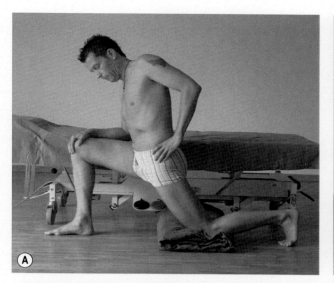
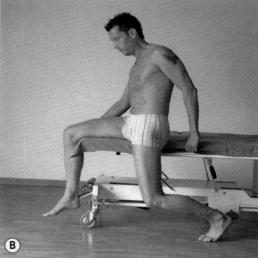
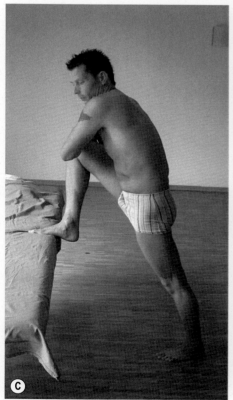
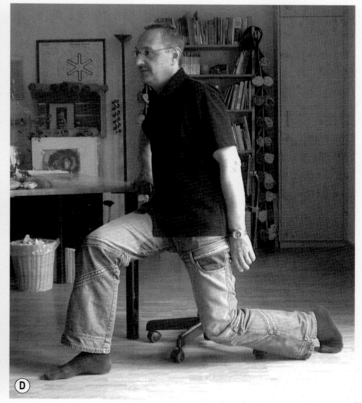

Fig. 19.5 Situative stretching using the iliopsoas muscle as an example (with different starting points): stretching the iliopsoas for athletes and other individuals (a); after implantation of a full implant (b); for lorry drivers (c); in the office (d).

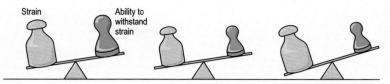

Fig. 19.6 Strain: the mismatch between load and load-bearing capacity.

Summary

The treatment of myofascial pain can in many cases only be permanently successful if at the same time the necessary attention is given to the influences which chronically overload the muscle as well as to the local treatment of mTrP. Otherwise, recurrences inevitable. Predisposing and perpetuating factors must be recognised and included in the treatment strategy in the form of ergonomics and functional training of the muscles.

Chapter | **20** |

Physical procedures

Hans-Joachim Schmitt, Raymund Pothmann, Winfried Banzer, Markus Hübscher, Markus Maier, Martin Kosub

20.1 ULTRASOUND THERAPY

Hans-Joachim Schmitt

Basic principles: the ultrasound waves used in ultrasound therapy represent mechanical oscillation of a frequency of 800 kHz–1 MHz. The waves are transferred to the body from the sound head using a suitable conductive medium (mineral oil, water or gel). The ultrasound spreads through the body as a mechanical longitudinal wave; the diameter of the sound bundle changes insignificantly. The sound is absorbed by the tissue and transformed into heat (ultrasound diathermy). To avoid the interference of sound waves in the tissue in front of the sound head with the consequence of increasing intensity, the sound head must be kept moving during treatment by the therapist in continuous circular movements. The sound is absorbed to varying extents by the tissue (the heating in the tissue layers also varies). There is a small amount of absorption and heat development in the fatty tissue, a moderate amount in the muscles and organs and a high amount in the bones. The depth of penetration is reduced corresponding to the range of absorption. This is about 7 cm. A type of vibration massage can be considered by using additional sound pressure from pulsed sound (50 Hz).
Indications: superficial subacute to chronic muscular ligamentary tissue changes, reflex tension in the muscle, the formation of scar tissue.
Contraindications: areas with abnormal sensitivity, fresh bleeding, fresh thrombosis, parenchymatous organs (heart, spinal cord following laminectomy), malignant tumours.
Dosage: treatment of MPS is carried out if the trigger point is superficial with a dose of 0.8–1.2 W/cm^2 with a treatment duration of 10 min. With pulsed ultrasound, dosages of up to 2 W/cm^2 can be used.

20.2 HOT AND COLD THERAPY

Hans-Joachim Schmitt

20.2.1 Heat therapy

Basic principles: tissue warming can be carried out directly using a hot pack by means of convection or conduction, or as heat radiation from a source of radiation (infrared); it can also be carried out directly by means of energy absorption, with heat formation taking place in the tissue, as for example with ultrasound therapy (see the section above).

The procedures used for heat therapy are:

- moist heat applications (see Fig. 23.3), wraps, hay sacks (see Fig. 23.2), hot rolls,
- packs (peat mud, paraffin, volcanic mud, silt),
- partial and full baths (possibly with additives),
- showers, drenches,
- hot air bath (sauna, steam bath, hot air bath),
- infrared radiation,
- ultrasound.

Effects:

- local/systemic arterial and venous widening of the blood vessels,
- reduction in peripheral vessel resistance, lowered blood pressure,
- increase in vasomotion, increase in lymph formation and lymph flow,
- consensual reaction in regions of the body not immediately influenced,
- increase in tissue clearance,
- improvement in metabolism as a result of influx of oxygen and nutrients,

http://dx.doi.org/10.1016/B978-0-7020-4312-3.00020-9

- improvement in immunological situation by the supply of antibodies and white cells,
- anti-inflammatory effect,
- relief of pain,
- detensioning of skeletal muscles; improved stretchability of tissues,
- reduction in viscosity of body fluids,
- the subsequent cooling of segmental visceral organs due to warming of the surface,
- psychological relaxation and sedation.

Indications: subacute and chronic conditions, inflammatory and degenerative joint and vertebral column diseases, subacute soft tissue rheumatic changes, functional perfusion disorders, chronic paranasal sinus problems, relief of pain and gastrointestinal and urogenital symptoms; post-traumatic or postoperative subacute conditions of the locomotor apparatus.

Contraindications: acute inflammatory processes, severe arterial perfusion disorders, oedema, infections, dermatitis, sensory deficits, bleeding.

Procedure: for the treatment of MPS, we recommend the application of moist hot packs locally over the trigger point area (such as a damp cloth with a hot water bottle, a hay sack or a hot roll (a rolled towel with hot water poured onto it and then the individual layers are wrapped up and rolled onto the skin in rocking movements). A sauna is also a well-tested method of detensioning the skeletal muscles. This is good for preventing the activation of latent trigger points by avoiding a hypoxic tissue situation in the mTrPs.

Duration of treatment: treatment with local applications is 20 min for a hot air cabin, and a maximum of 15 min for a sauna. These procedures are particularly suitable for patients in the treatment-free intervals during specific treatment by the doctor or therapist.

20.2.2 Cold therapy

Basic principles: there is a difference between the techniques of cold therapy and cryotherapy:

- cold therapy is carried out within the range of 0–35 °C and uses cold compresses, cold towels, drenches, wraps, cushions, covers and additives such as alcohol or quark cheese;
- cryotherapy uses temperatures below 0 °C to remove heat and also uses ice in various conditions (crushed, like an ice block (see Section 18.3), spray, ice chips and others).

Effects:

- influence on muscle tone: increased with short-term use, reflex lowering of muscle tone when applied for longer than 5 min,
- analgesia,
- better perfusion in the arterial system and promotion of venous flow,
- reduction in swelling,

- activation of cutivisceral reflexes,
- spasmolysis.

Indications:

- pulled muscles or tendons, bruises,
- arthritis pain,
- strains,
- mTrPs.

Contraindications:

- sensitivity to cold,
- vascular occlusion,
- lack of resistance,
- neuropathy.

Procedure and duration of treatment: the duration of cold therapy is the crucial factor that depends on the constitution and current condition of the patient. It is therefore important to check the effects on the individual, particularly before using a series of treatments. To lower muscle tension, a treatment time of 1–10 min (cryotherapy) is needed up to a maximum of 20 min (cold therapy). Make sure the treatment is not used too often – a maximum of twice a day – and that the patient is not chilled. Short-term rubbing with ice or an ice massage are suitable for mTrPs, possibly with concomitant extension, or cold treatment for 10–20 min using a cold towel or wrap with the addition of alcohol or chilled quark cheese (see Section 23.3.5).

20.3 ELECTROTHERAPY

Hans-Joachim Schmitt

20.3.1 Low-frequency electrical stimulation (Bernard diadynamic electricity)

Basic principles: low-frequency electrical stimulation provides uni- or bidirectional electrical impulses alternating periodically between two impulse frequencies of 50 or 100 Hz, as a combination of direct current and alternating current (diadynamic). Polarity is adjusted via the electrodes. The cathode is the stronger analgesic electrode. The analgesic effect is caused by the stimulation of A-delta and C fibres. With unidirectional currents, if the electrode is not far enough from the skin there is the risk of burning the skin by electrolysis when using viscose swabs. With diadynamic currents there are four different types of current relating to the direct current part or the periodic sequence.

- mf (monophase fix), 50 Hz, smallest direct current components, most effective stimulation with the greatest analgesic effect, for acute injuries;
- cp (courtes periodes), alternating impulses of 50 and 100 Hz, effective on subacute soft tissue pain, promotes absorption;

- lp (longues periodes), impulses of 50 and 100 Hz alternating with double 100 Hz periods and amplitude swelling, chronic soft tissue symptoms, detensioning;
- df (diphase fix), always 100 Hz, usually direct current, chronically painful soft tissue changes (less muscular cause), analgesic, soothing.

Indications: connective tissue changes in the locomotor apparatus, acute, subacute and becoming chronic, persistent pain and trigger points, mesenchymal and muscular structures of the locomotor apparatus with dysfunction pain.

Contraindications: muscle inflammation, application of electrode over skin lesions, sensory deficits with the risk of burning, implanted electronic devices, inflammatory vessel changes, severe heart failure, severe cardiac rhythm disorders.

Procedure: for the treatment of MPS note that when applying the electrodes stimulation can be greater if different (small-surface-area) cathodes are used over the trigger point area, with a large-surface-area anode on the opposite side of the body. Alternating cp and lp currents are very suitable for use during treatment.

Duration of treatment: treatment lasts 12–15 min.

20.3.2 Middle-frequency therapy

Basic principles: this first-line treatment for muscle or muscle fibres uses a frequency of between 1 and 100 kHz. This leads to activation, physiological stimulation or contraction in the muscle. It represents a volume effect and is apolar (in contrast to low frequency). When applying the electrodes, the same activity applies to both. Large-surface-area rubber electrodes should be used and should be placed at least 1 cm apart. Because of the use of alternating current, these electrodes can be placed directly on the skin without the risk of electrolytic damage and middle-frequency therapy can be combined with low-frequency therapy in the so-called Wymoton method. In this procedure 250 kHz, from the low-frequency range, is combined with 11 kHz from the middle-frequency range and so has the effect of combining an analgesic treatment with a muscle activation treatment.

Indications: lack of muscle sensation, muscle weakness, voluntary innervation weakness and reflex muscle tension. The active cooperation of the patient (with instructions from a physiotherapist) is required to optimise voluntary muscle function so that the muscle can be used effortlessly.

Contraindications: metal implants in the through-flow area, implanted electronic devices, application of electrodes to skin lesions and inflammatory vascular diseases are relative contraindications. The treatment of infants is absolutely contraindicated.

Procedure: painful muscle and tendon diseases such as active muscular mTrPs can be treated, where possible with the above Wymoton method of combination of using middle and low frequencies. Middle frequency is suitable for the treatment of the affected muscles where there is latent myofascial pain to improve control, perception and, finally, relaxation.

20.3.3 Trancutaneous electrical nerve stimulation (TENS)

Also see Section 20.5.

Indications: tendomyopathy, arthralgia, neuralgia, headache, dystrophy, visceral pain, perfusion disorders.

Contraindications: implanted electronic devices, application of the electrodes to skin lesions, severe heart failure, severe cardiac rhythm disorders, anxiety about the treatment procedure.

Procedure: for the treatment of MPS, the adhesive electrodes should be placed immediately in the area of pain. The cathode should lie directly over the trigger point area and the anode in the proximal segment. Low frequency should be selected and the intensity individually adjusted to the tolerance of the patient.

Duration of treatment: treatment should last 20–30 min as a sufficient analgesic effect is not noticeable until then.

20.4 CUPPING (BAGUANFA)

Hans-Joachim Schmitt

Basic principles: there are two types of cupping: dry cupping and cupping with blood letting. The decision as to which method is used depends on the assessment of the tissue according to its emptiness or fullness (i.e. perfusion). Sources are sought in the connective tissue or muscles in the connective tissue zones (segmentally oriented to the head zones) described by Dicke et al. (1982; Fig. 13.8). Finding these connective tissue zones can also be done using a dermographism assessment (fingernail test) in the skin region. If it is empty, a white dermographism forms, if full the dermographism is red. The method of cupping treatment is derived from this. Dry cupping is used for emptiness, blood letting for fullness.

Indications: for MPS with local ischaemia in the contraction knot, dry cupping is an additional possibility for treatment of mTrP regions. This particularly applies to persistent myofascial pain involved with medical diseases.

Procedure: the simplest method of treatment uses a suction bell. Traditionally, the vacuum is created in the cup by using fire (note that there is a danger of burning the patient). The hyperaemia that is created helps to reduce tissue tension as the haematoma fades. This improves the stretchability of the tissue (manual mTrP treatment).

20.5 TRANSCUTANEOUS ELECTRICAL NERVE STIMULATION (TENS)

Raymund Pothmann

20.5.1 History

Even the Egyptians made use of the electricity in fish to relieve the pain of gout. In the 19th century electrical current was used to provide short-term analgesia (Colwell 1922). It was not until the pain research of the 1960s, however, and in particular the publication of the gate control theory by Melzack and Wall (1965), that the prerequisites for the neurophysiological understanding of stimulation analgesia were created. TENS (or TNS) was introduced into Germany in the mid-1970s and has found a place in almost all pain therapy institutions.

20.5.2 Definition

TENS means the application of electrical impulses which work through the skin to affect the nerves to avoid or relieve pain.

20.5.3 Neurophysiology

Muscular pain occurs in the body periphery as a result of mechanical, inflammatory or chemical damage or central nervous decompensation of pain control. After an initially very fast impulse via myelinised A-delta or A-beta fibres the pain, which has become chronic, spreads slowly via the non-myelinised, thin C fibres.

In animal experiments, electrical nerve stimulation led to a significant reduction in pain impulses through heat stimulation of the skin (Zimmermann, Handwerker 1984). In the clinical setting this produces an approach that uses vibration or transcutaneous electrical stimulation of the trigger point via the myelinised nerve fibres to modulate the pain.

From our understanding of the gate control theory (Melzack, Wall 1965) central descending pain inhibition is generally accepted today to be more important than segmentally distributed pain inhibition. Serotonin-like descending tracts have an indirect inhibiting effect on the spinal level of entry via the periaqueductal grey matter and the release of endorphins there. However, this control mechanism is restricted predominantly to low-frequency (1.5 Hz) electrostimulation and can be controlled by placebo through the administration of naloxone (Eriksson, Sjölund 1979, Zimmermann, Handwerker 1984).

20.5.4 Method

Technical prerequisites

- Mini-stimulator.
- Electrode cable.
- Rubber surface electrodes of about 10 cm² in size.
- Electrode gel and plaster for fixing or self-adhesive electrodes.

Stimulation parameters for 'conventional' TENS

- Biphasic right-angle impulses.
- Impulse duration of 0.1–0.5 ms.
- Current strength of between 1 and 50 mA, continuously adjustable.
- Frequency range of 1–100 Hz.
- Burst stimulation (1–3 Hz).

The burst stimulation is associated with the release of endorphins similar to the effects caused by (manual) needle stimulation. It is therefore also referred to as 'acupuncture-like' TENS. A combined high frequency of 70–100 Hz makes it possible to apply better-tolerated higher currents which can reach deeper muscle nerves, which are more difficult to stimulate (Eriksson, Sjölund 1979).

TENS stimulation is carried out below the pain threshold: this is achieved by means of the lower longitudinal resistance of the stimulated myelinised nerve fibres.

Treatment prerequisites

- Suitable indications.
- Sufficient referral to hospital or practice.
- Sufficiently successful treatment during admission.

Means of treatment at home

- Use once to three times per day, more often as required.
- Stimulation of 30–45 min or longer.
- Electrode plates can be left in place for several hours.
- We recommend a break during the night for the skin to recover.

Applying the electrodes

Applying the electrodes depends on:

- location of the pain,
- extent of pain in the segment,
- the nerve affected,
- active trigger points,
- position of sympathetic ganglia (Jenckner 1980, Eriksson, Sjölund 1979),
- crosswise (e.g. for joints).

An electrode plate is usually fixed over the painful site and felt to be active (with the biphasic mode usually only a 'relative cathode' is used). With nerve injuries and direct nerve stimulation the 'cathode' is placed distally.

Electrode differentiation does not play any part in paravertebral arrangement and the same applies to bifrontal stimulation. The electrodes must be individually arranged and changed if insufficiently intensive; painless stimulation is not sensed over areas that are not well innervated. With biphasic stimulation electrode differentiation still plays only a subordinate role.

Equipment

There are a large number of TENS devices on the market. The main differences are in design, handiness, rental service and price (Fig. 20.1). A modern TENS device should include as a minimum:

- a constant current circuit to avoid current spikes as a result of moving the electrodes,
- two channels,
- a biphasic impulse generator,
- high-frequency 'conventional' burst stimulation,
- low-frequency ('similar to acupuncture') burst stimulation,
- an 'anti-habituation programme' with alternating frequencies and intensities for long-term stimulation.

20.5.5 Indications

The indications for TENS as part of trigger point stimulation are divided into a few main categories.

Main indications

- Pain in the locomotor apparatus.
- Nerve pain, also supported by the sympathetic.

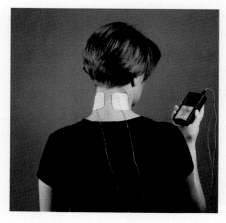

Fig. 20.1 A TENS device being used.

Individual clinical indications

- Joint pain, especially in the sense of referred pain.
- Shoulder–arm syndrome.
- Epicondylitis.
- Tunnel syndrome.
- Cervical syndrome.
- Tension headaches, migraine.
- Lumbago.
- Phantom/stump pain.
- Trigeminal neuralgia.

Pain in the locomotor apparatus with typical tender and trigger phenomena is the most important. Back and neck pain predominate, but peri-articular muscle pain with epicondylitis or gonarthrosis are also important. In childhood clinical conditions such as torticollis, cervical spine syndrome following whiplash trauma or chrondropathia patellae are also significant.

Nerve pain in the form of neuralgia of the trigeminal nerve is eminently suitable for TENS, and indeed in the form of contralateral or cervical stimulation. The ipsilateral trigger point must be avoided during this treatment.

With stump pain it is usually sufficient to affix two electrodes in the area of the individual mTrP of the end of the stump (e.g. medial and lateral). In keeping with the 'stump beat' a slow frequency of 2–4 Hz is selected here (Gessler 1996).

Another indication is traumatic lesions of the peripheral nerves, tunnel syndrome in the initial stage, or to bridge the gap until surgical treatment with regular electrophysiological checks, and polyneuropathic pain especially in the distal area of the lower extremities (Jenckner 1980, Eriksson, Sjölund 1979).

Tension headaches and cervical spine syndrome – also after whiplash injury – currently appear to be one of the most important indications for TENS in adults and children. There are underlying mTrPs in three-quarters of cases. In children treatment usually leads to complete remission within a few months (about one-fifth of cases). The use of slow stimulation frequencies (2 Hz) and suboccipital application are obligatory.

Measured against the technical, financial and time costs, TENS is a reserve method for acute therapy and prophylaxis of migraine (Appenzeller 1978, Goepel et al. 1985). The efficacy of TENS for migraine is less than for acupuncture, and significantly less effective than musculoskeletal TENS indications. The poor migraine response is probably attributable to the longer duration of the disease or its vascular character; patients with 'pure' migraine are also rarely found with trigger points (Larbig 1982).

20.5.6 Contraindications

Relative contraindications are:

- large metal implants,
- psychogenic pain (usually multifocal),

- visceral pain and cardiac rhythm disorders,
- age-related contraindications are pain in infants and young children.

An absolute contraindication is the presence of a pacemaker in the immediate vicinity (Eriksson 1975). This does not apply when the location of the TENS device has been checked by electrocardiogram (ECG) with varying frequencies and intensities.

20.5.7 TENS application in practice

The loan or prescription of a TENS device may be paid for by health insurance, or provided free of charge. We recommend checks every 4–6 weeks. Modern devices even allow control of the times of application in a memory chip.

Stimulation time, duration and strength of pain during treatment should be recorded by the patient in a pain diary. The patient should be motivated to try out the best electrode position.

20.5.8 Clinical results

TENS is generally used for symptomatic treatment if used for chronic pain (Loeser et al. 1975, Eriksson, Sjölund 1979, Jenckner 1980). On average, a clinically satisfactory response can be estimated in about 50–60% of the cited indications during the first 3 months. Then the original effect recedes slightly over the course of a year (Eriksson, Sjölund 1979). Overall, 40–50% of patients continue to use TENS long term.

The results for children and juveniles are better; treatment for longer than 3 months is usually the exception. This can be attributed to the better prognosis with a shorter course of the disease or a lower level of chronification. The most important indications are tension headaches with known trigger points in the trapezius muscle (Pothmann 2003).

20.6 LASER THERAPY

Winfried Banzer, Markus Hübscher

20.6.1 Definition

Laser therapy is the therapeutic application of laser light in medicine. Musculoskeletal and myofascial symptoms are the main indications.

20.6.2 Physical and technical principles

There have been detailed reports since the development of the first laser in 1960. The acronym laser stands for light amplification by stimulated emission of radiation. The term makes it clear that the generation of laser radiation is based on a physical phenomenon, so-called stimulated emission. If energy from outside is added to an atom, this moves from the ground state to a higher energy level. Accordingly, this comparably energy-rich state of the atom is described as excited. The excited atoms return after a very short time, typically a few picoseconds or microseconds, to their initial stable state, releasing the previously taken up energy in the form of photons, without external influence (spontaneous emission) (Cotton 2004). If such a photon now collides with another excited atom whose energy corresponds exactly to the energy of the photon, this is also reduced to its ground state and emits another photon with the same wavelength, phase and vector (direction of spread) as the induced photon. This process is described as stimulated emission.

A laser system consists basically of three components: a laser medium (laser-active material or gain medium), an energy source (pump source) and a resonator (Fig. 20.2).

By adding energy via a pump (e.g. electrical, optical or chemical energy) the atoms of the laser-active material are energetically excited. The aim is to induce population inversion, i.e. to put more atoms in the excited state than in the ground state. The process of stimulated emission leads to an exponential increase in photon density. As the process takes place in a space surrounded by reflective surfaces, the resonator, the photons are continuously reflected back and forth between these surfaces so that the emission of photons keeps on increasing. One of the mirrors is partially transparent and allows the exit of laser radiation (Philipp, Berlien 2003).

Collimated (parallel) laser light can be created in the visible, infrared and ultra-infrared spectrum and spreads in phases in spatial and time coherent optical waves of one wavelength (monochromasia). The combination of these three properties (collimation, coherence, monochromasia) is the crucial difference between lasers and normal light sources (Philipp, Berlien 2003, Cotton 2004, Simunovic 2000).

Depending on the laser medium used, the following laser types are distinguished:

- body-fixed laser: e.g. ruby, neodymium-yttrium aluminium garnet (Nd-YAG),

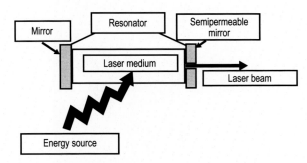

Fig. 20.2 Diagram of a laser. *(Modified from Cotton 2004)*

- gas laser: e.g. helium–neon (HeNe), argon, carbon dioxide,
- diode laser: e.g. gallium–arsenide (GaAs), gallium–aluminium–arsenide (GaAlAs),
- dye laser: e.g. rhodamine G6.

For musculoskeletal and myofascial symptoms low energy, athermic devices (soft lasers) are available for low-level laser therapy (LLLT). Soft lasers are divided into red light (helium–neon; ≤ 10 mW) and infrared (diode) lasers (5–150 mW, sometimes higher performance). The most commonly used lasers are:

- helium–neon, wavelength 632.8 nm, red light,
- gallium–arsenide, wavelength 840 nm, infrared light,
- gallium–aluminium-arsenide, wavelength 820 nm, infrared light.

Lasers are also distinguished by their mode of operation. Laser radiation is emitted continuously (continuous wave, cw) or in the form of short individual impulses (pulsed, p) (Fig. 20.3).

The depth of penetration of laser radiation is not precise. Besides the wavelength of the laser light it depends on the individual optical properties of the tissue (e.g. thickness of the epidermis, pigmentation), blood volume and vessel architecture. The penetration depths given in the literature range from about 0.5 cm for red laser light to about 1 cm or more for radiation in the infrared range (Hawkins et al. 2005).

Laser parameters

The relevant parameters include:

- wavelength in nanometres (nm),
- laser performance in milliwatts (mW),
- treatment duration in seconds (s),
- dose in joules (J),

- radiation surface in square centimetres (cm^2),
- density (mW/cm^2).

The dose is calculated from the laser performance and the duration of radiation:

Dose (J) = laser performance (W)
$\times$ treatment time (s) (see dosage recommendations)

Light and tissue interactions

Based on the underlying optical laws, the interaction of laser and tissue (Fig. 20.4) takes place as:

- reflection,
- transmission,
- scattering,
- absorption.

A therapeutically relevant tissue effect occurs only with the absorption of photon energy, whereby the extent of the effect depends on the wavelength used and the performance or energy density determined (Almeida-Lopes et al. 2001, Khadra et al. 2005, Azevedo et al. 2006).

20.6.3 Physiological principles

Although the therapeutic mechanism of effect underlying soft laser treatment has so far been only partially explained, non-thermal, photochemical processes at the cellular level have been postulated (Knappe et al. 2004). The applied laser energy can be absorbed by endogenous photosensitisers such as porphyrin, mitochondrial cytochrome, flavoprotein and NADPH oxidase (Lubart et al. 2005, 2006). The activated photosensitisers form reactive oxygen species (ROS), which have an essential function in cell proliferation and cell regulation besides their pathophysiological effects (Burdon 1995, Finkel 2000, Lubart et al. 2005). In this connection, *in vitro* studies by Passarella et al. (1988)

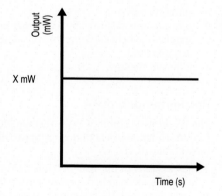

Continuous wave output

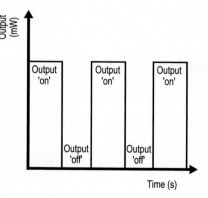

Pulsed output

Fig. 20.3 Forms of laser radiation.
(Modified from Baseter 1994)

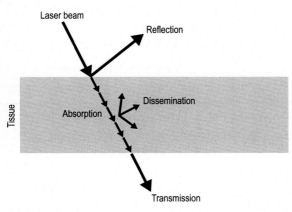

Fig. 20.4 Interaction between laser and tissue. *(Modified from Niemz 2003)*

and animal experiments *in vivo* by Mochizuki-Oda et al. (2002) showed laser-induced activation of enzyme complexes of the electron transport chain with consecutive increases in mitochondrial ATP production. Other *in vivo* studies demonstrated biostimulative effects of soft lasers on the proliferation of human fibroblasts (Azevedo et al. 2006, Pal et al. 2007) and animal osteoblasts (Garavello-Freitas et al. 2003, Stein et al. 2005). There has also been evidence of inflammation-inhibiting effects in the sense of reduced concentrations of inflammatory markers (prostaglandin E_2 (PGE_2), TNF, IL-1, cyclooxygenase 2 (COX-2); Bjordal et al. 2006).

Microvascular and neurophysiological mechanisms, as part of laser-inducible therapy effects, are also under discussion. Studies by Flitney and Megson (2003), Karlsson et al. (1984) and Maegawa et al. (2000) indicated that NO/cyclic GMP produced relaxation of smooth vessel muscle cells with consecutively increased microcirculation. Neurophysiological experiments by Tsuchiya et al. (1993) and Kasai et al. (1996) demonstrated reduced impulse transmission of peripheral sensory nerves.

20.6.4 Indications

The main indications in the area of the locomotor system are:

- MPS,
- fibromyalgia,
- gonarthrosis,
- rheumatoid arthritis,
- syndesmosis injury,
- peroneal tendon injury,
- pull/tear of the fibulocalcaneal ligament,
- tendon sheath inflammation of the toe extensors,
- pull/tear of the anterior fibulotalar ligament,
- subtalar sprain and instability,
- sprain injury (talocalcaneal joint),

- plantar fasciitis,
- achillodynia,
- epicondylitis.

20.6.5 Contraindications

The contraindications include:

- photosensitivity (e.g. light dermatosis),
- sunburn,
- direct radiation into the eyes,
- irradiation of the fetus,
- radiation of a neoplasm.

20.6.6 Practical procedure (for myofascial pain)

The following treatment principles should be considered when using LLLT for mTrPs:

- explanation to the patient,
- placing the patient in a relaxed position,
- exact location of mTrPs using palpation,
- pretreatment of skin:
  - thorough skin cleansing (oil removal) with alcohol,
  - possibly hair removal (reflex reduction),
- selection of device/radiation dose based on established recommendations (see dose recommendations, below),
- focus of spot radiation,
- laser-beam application over mTrPs in direct contact with the skin and vertically to the radiation surface (reflex reduction, optimisation of energy density),
- note the accident-prevention regulations 'Laser radiation' BGV B2 (see laser safety notes, below).

Laser application can be carried out as:

- monotherapy,
- a complementary therapy with other procedures (e.g. manual medicine, osteopathy, physical medicine, acupuncture),
- adjuvant therapy.

Recommended dose

The World Association of Laser Therapy (2005) published recommendations on LLLT dosing for two different types of laser (Table 20.1):

- laser class 3 or 3b, 780–820 nm GaAlAs laser, continuous or pulsed, performance >0.5 W,
- laser class 3 or 3b, 904 nm GaAlAs laser, maximum pulse performance >1 W.

For treatment of mTrPs dose recommendations can be derived from current randomised controlled studies. The 632.8 nm HeNe Laser (Ilbuldu et al. 2004) and 904 nm

Table 20.1 Dosage recommendations for laser class 3 and 3b, 780–820 nm GaAlAs lasers (output >0.5 W) and 904 nm GaAs lasers (output >1 W), continuous or pulsed, output >0.5 W

	POINTS OR CM²	JOULES 780–820 NM	JOULES 904 NM
Tendinopathies			
Carpal tunnel syndrome	2–3	12 (min. 6 J/point)	4 (min. 2 J/point)
Epicondylitis humeri lateralis	1–2	4 (max. 100 mW/cm²)	1 (max. 100 mW/cm²)
M. biceps humeri capitis longus	1–2	8	2
M. supraspinatus	2–3	10 (min. 5 J/point)	3 (min. 2 J/point)
M. infraspinatus	2–3	10 (min. 5 J/point)	3 (min. 2 J/point)
Trochanter major	2–3	6	2
Patellar tendon	2–3	3	2
Iliotibial tract	2–3	8 (max. 100 mW/cm²)	2 (max. 100 mW/cm²)
Achilles tendon	2–3	12 (max. 100 mW/cm²)	2 (max. 100 mW/cm²)
Plantar fasciitis	2–3	3 (min. 6 J/point)	3 (min. 2 J/point)
Arthritis			
Finger PIP or MCP joints	1–2	62	2
Wrist	2–3	10	3
Humeroradial joint	1–2	4	2
Elbow	2–3	10	3
Glenohumeral joint	2–3	15 (min. 6 J/point)	6 (min. 2 J/point)
Acromioclavicular joint	1–2	4	2
temporomandibular joint	1–2	6	2
Cervical spine	2–3	15 (min. 6 J/point)	6 (min. 2 J/point)
Lumbar spine	2–3	40 (min. 84 J/point)	10 (min. 4 J/point)
Hips	2–3	40 (min. 8 J/point)	10 (min. 4 J/point)
Anteromedial knee	2–4	20 (min. 5 J/point)	6 (min. 2 J/point)
Ankle	2–4	15	6

max., maximum; min., minimum; MCP, metacarpophalangeal; PIP, proximal interphalangeal.

GaAs laser (pulsed) have proved particularly therapeutically effective. The relevant dose is 1.5–5 J/mTrP.

We recommend either a daily treatment for a period of 2 weeks or every other day for a period of 3–4 weeks. Treatment should begin with the stated dose and reduced by 30% as symptoms improve (World Association for Laser Therapy 2005).

Laser safety

In medicine high-energy lasers (surgical laser; class 4) should be distinguished from low-energy lasers (low power laser, or LPL; class 3). Taking into account their damage potential, the following types of laser are distinguished according to their danger classifications (Philipp, Berlien 2003).

- Class 1: generally accessible lasers are not dangerous to skin or eyes but are unsuitable for therapeutic purposes (e.g. as used in a CD player).
- Class 2: these laser beams are only emitted in the visible spectrum. They are not dangerous to eyes because of the lid protection reflex and the very short duration of radiation associated with them. These include HeNe laser pointers.
- Classes 3a and 3b: class 3a lasers represent a danger to the eyes if the diameter of the beam is narrowed by optical instruments (e.g. an endoscope) and shone directly into the eyes. They are not dangerous to the skin. The beams from class 3b lasers are dangerous if shone directly into the eyes.
- Class 4: both direct and reflected beams are dangerous to the eyes and skin. These include surgical lasers (argon, Nd-YAG, carbon dioxide). There is a risk of explosion or fire.

Devices used in LLLT are usually class 3b lasers. These can damage the eyes if inappropriately handled and should therefore be used in a manner compliant with the accident prevention instructions 'Laser radiation' BGV B2. These require:

- appointment of a laser protection officer,
- enclosing and marking the laser area during operation,
- wearing suitable laser protection goggles,
- instructing the people staying in the laser area.

20.6.7 Scientific data, studies

Against the background of current research it is not possible to make a conclusive assessment of the efficacy of LLLT, taking account of the association of dose with effectiveness. Interpretation of the information is particularly problematic as there are great differences between the laser parameters used (wavelength, dose, treatment frequency); this is made even more difficult as there are often methodical weaknesses in the available studies. Nevertheless, some studies show specific and clinically relevant effects in the treatment of musculoskeletal and myofascial pain. It is worth noting the following:

- myofascial shoulder and neck pain (Gur et al. 2004, Hakgüder et al. 2003, Ilbuldu et al. 2004, Ceylan et al. 2004),
- fibromyalgia (Gür et al. 2002a, 2002b),
- dysfunctions of the temporomandibular joint in connection with myofascial pain (Fiká·ová et al. 2007),
- arthrosis of the knee joint (Bjordal et al. 2007),
- spontaneous osteonecrosis of the knee joint (Banzer et al. 2008),
- rheumatoid arthritis (Brosseau et al. 2000),
- achillodynia (Bjordal et al. 2006).

20.7 SHOCK WAVE THERAPY

Markus Maier, Martin Kosub

20.7.1 Definition and physiological principles

Extracorporeal shock waves are individual acoustic waves of extremely short duration. They release their energy on the border layers of tissue of different acoustic density. The usual physical unit used today is energy flow density (EFD), given in mJ/mm^2 (Gerdesmeyer et al. 2002).

Clinically, extracorporeal shock waves have been used for more than 20 years for shattering symptomatic organ stones. Shock waves have also been used since the 1990s in the treatment of diseases of the supportive and locomotor apparatus. Today, studies are available that explain the mechanism of effect of extracorporeal shock waves in individual indications (Maier et al. 2003, Hausdorf et al. 2004) (Fig. 20.5, Fig. 20.6).

The application of extracorporeal shock waves for pain therapy is based on the symptoms and is also described as trigger shock wave therapy (Maier 2003). The applied EFD is directed to the region to be treated: near air-filled hollow spaces such as the lungs or the bowel, the EFD used should be as low as possible, but away from these organs, such as on the extremities, it is possible to use a higher EFD.

The use of radial shock wave technology in particular is now well established in trigger point treatment and represents the current treatment standard.

20.7.2 Indications

The standard indications for traditional shock wave therapy on the supportive and locomotor apparatus are:

- tendinosis calcarea of the shoulder,
- fracture healing disorders,
- plantar fasciitis,
- epicondylitis radialis humeri.

Trigger shock wave therapy is particularly indicated for:

- all chronic MFSs with trigger points in body areas which allow low-energy shock wave treatment,
- concomitant myofascial disorders (e.g. lateral epicondylitis) in combination with traditional shock wave indications,
- post-traumatic muscle lesions in the subacute stage.

20.7.3 Contraindications

As there so far have not been sufficient studies on the effects and side effects of low-energy shock waves in muscle treatment, it is important to adhere to a low-risk application.

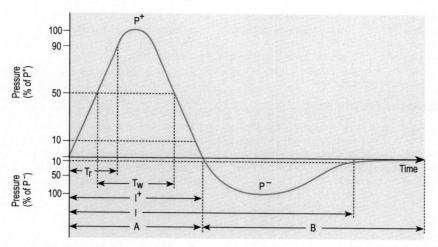

Fig. 20.5 Graphic representation of a standardised shock wave. The shock wave pressure is expressed as a function of time (from Gerdesmeyer et al. 2002): first part of the shock wave with positive pressure (a), second part of the shock wave with negative pressure (b). Abbreviations: P$^+$, positive peak pressure; P$^-$, negative peak pressure; T$_r$, rise time; T$_w$, pulse width; I$^+$, standard time interval to calculation of the so-called 'positive energy' of the shock wave; I, standard time interval to the calculation of the so-called 'total energy' of the shock wave.

Fig. 20.6 Diagram of a radial shock wave source. *(From Gerdesmeyer et al. 2002)*

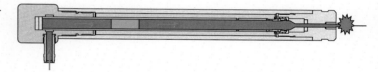

The known contraindications for traditional shock wave therapy must therefore be strictly considered. Applications with high EFD in the area of the chest or lungs, use on nerve structures or vessels and in patients with clotting disorders or who are undergoing anticoagulant therapy must be avoided, even if there are as yet no known serious complications.

20.7.4 Practical course of action

The following treatment recommendations are based on the authors' many years of experience with radial shock wave technology.

- Before treatment, make sure that all the muscle areas to be treated are covered with a sufficient quantity of contact medium as most treatment covers a large surface. Insufficient contact can lead to subcutaneous bleeding as a result of the cavitation effect. Apart from the usual ultrasound gels, oils (such as castor oil) can also be used as contact medium. This makes it easier to slide the applicator over the skin.
- For superficial mTrPs, an applicator of at least 10–15 mm diameter should be chosen. A narrow treatment head (5 mm) is only recommended for interdigital application (e.g. Mm. interossei). A trigger point applicator should be used for deeper-seated mTrPs.
- Pressure during treatment also depends on the depth of the mTrP.
- The optimum treatment frequency for shock waves is 10–15 Hz.
- There are two supplementary techniques for muscle treatment:
  - the first local technique serves to release the mTrP under the assumption that this releases the contracted shortened actin–myosin filaments of the sarcomere,
  - a second stroking technique is intended to reduce hypertension in the affected muscle. A possible cause of the detensioning effect of this technique is stimulation of the muscle spindles or Golgi tendon organs.
- The mTrP should first be treated with 400–600 impulses. This requires precise location of the applicator. A check is made using repeated palpation and biofeedback while the patient is asked about the pain maximum during the application. The energy of the treatment is based on the position of the muscle and the depth of the trigger point.

After local therapy, treatment should be carried out length-wise along the muscle fibres over the area of the muscle. This is described as smoothing. This treats the whole tensed fibre bundle and possibly concomitant insertion trigger points. Depending on the size and diameter of the muscle 1000–2000 impulses are applied for this.

20.7.5 Follow-up treatment

After carrying out shock wave therapy, follow-up treatment of the affected muscle is worthwhile. Measures for further reduction of tension or muscle-extension techniques have proved particularly effective for this. The following treatment techniques are recommended:

- spray and stretch (Section 18.3),
- postisometric relaxation,
- reciprocal inhibition,
- muscle energy techniques.

If necessary, another tension-lowering effect can be achieved by stimulating the mechanoreceptors of the skin. Stretching the skin over a muscle contributes to the reflex inhibition of the muscle lying under the stretched skin by activity of the antagonists. Such reflex therapy can be carried out by using elastic acrylic-coated tapes. Known as kinesiotape, this is used predominantly in sports medicine and can be ideally combined with trigger shock wave therapy and worn for several days after treatment.

Chapter | **21** |

Trigger point infiltration

Hans-Joachim Schmitt, Dominik Irnich

The infiltration of trigger points is one of the most significant and highly efficient techniques in the treatment of myofascial pain and restricted function. Optimum success is assured by using a precise procedure, suitable materials (thin needles, only as long as necessary) and appropriate medication in as low concentrations as possible. The more chronic the mTrP, the more restrained the infiltration techniques should be, so that the chronic complex problems are not made worse when the attitude of many patients is limited to the somatic (iatrogenic chronification). A different attitude is indispensable for optimum application of this technique. There is an obvious difference between treating a young athlete with mTrPs and a patient with chronic back pain.

21.1 INDICATIONS AND CONTRAINDICATIONS

21.1.1 Indications

There is an indication for infiltration of a trigger point if:

- manual trigger point therapy or stretching has had an inadequate effect,
- manual trigger point therapy or stretching cannot be adequately carried out because of severe pain,
- acute severe pain and functional problems are to the fore,
- there are additional diagnoses for which manual therapy is unsuitable or may be contraindicated (hypermobility, calcinosis, etc.),
- the post-treatment soreness that occasionally occurs with dry needling is undesirable.

21.1.2 Contraindications

- Anticoagulant therapy.
- Taking acetylsalicyclic acid in the last 3 days.
- Anxiety.
- Known drug intolerance.

The number of injection treatments depends on:

- the selection of trigger points which determine the symptoms (5–10 points possible in one session),
- the precision of the injection,
- concomitant/instructed stretching of the affected muscles by the patient or therapist.

We recommend at least 3 days between invasive treatments, or better still 7–8 days, and exercise can be intensified during this time.

21.2 INJECTANTS

The choice of injectant depends on a phased plan, whereby local anaesthetic (LA) is the first choice. When choosing the substance, first assess the duration of effect and the myotoxicity (i.e. the potential cause damage to the skeletal muscle tissue, leading to myonecrosis). A rule of thumb is that the shorter the duration of effect and the lower the concentration, the lesser the myotoxicity and cell infiltration into the tissue.

> Avoid the addition of adrenaline (epinephrine) because of the occurrence of muscle necrosis.

http://dx.doi.org/10.1016/B978-0-7020-4312-3.00021-0

The injection of bacteriostatic (alcohol) or physiological saline is very effective compared to LA.

For trigger points at a muscle insertion (with inflammatory components) we recommend the admixture of a crystalline corticoid, but only to a maximum of three times. Infiltration is performed around the tendon.

If non-invasive (manual trigger point therapy) and invasive methods of dry needling and injection as well as combinations of them do not lead to the desired result, the injection of botulinum toxin A is indicated for severe distress in exceptional cases.

21.2.1 Local anaesthetics

Basic principles

LAs work by binding to the tension-dependent sodium channels in the nerve membranes. The LAs interact in their ionised form with the amino acids phenylalanine and tyrosine, which leads to a blockade of sodium inflow. At high concentrations other ion channels are also blocked. The blockade of sodium permeability leads to both depolarisation and the spread of the excitation wave being suppressed. This interrupts the conduction of pain signals.

The following factors affect the length of time the LA remains at the site of application and the effect:

- the pH value determines the level of lipid solubility: the further from the physiological pH value of 7.4, the less effective is the LA (e.g. inflammation),
- local perfusion,
- enzymatic hydrolysis with ester-type LAs.

In the bloodstream ester-type LAs such as procaine and tetracaine are split by plasma cholinesterase. The split products are ineffective as LAs and are non-toxic in their resulting concentrations. Breakdown in the liver is of secondary significance.

Amide-type LAs such as lidocaine are mainly oxidatively dealkylated or hydroxylated and enzymatically hydrolysed by carboxyesterase, located in the endoplasmic reticulum. Amide-type LAs are more slowly metabolised (half-life of between 1.5 and 3.5 h) compared to ester-type LAs (e.g. procaine has a half-life of 0.5–1 h) in the plasma and tissue (Table 21.1).

LAs can also be classified by their duration of effect:

- short duration: procaine 30–60 min,
- average duration: lidocaine, mepivacaine, prilocaine 60–120 min,
- long duration: ropivacaine and bupivacaine up to 400 min.

Substances

Because of its proven low myotoxicity we recommend lidocaine 0.2–0.5%, mepivacaine 0.2–0.5%, prilocaine 0.2–0.5% and bupivacaine 0.125% or less (a higher dosage is potentially myotoxic). Because of their low lipophilia of the esters procaine and tetracaine have the lowest level of myotoxicity, although esters are estimated to have a higher allergic potential. Low concentrations of LA are usually sufficient to obtain the desired effect. A high dilution also avoids affecting motor fibres.

If this is the first diagnostic injection (i.e. to find out whether the mTrP is actually causing the pathology) for reasons of practicality a short-acting LA should be used (e.g. procaine, lidocaine, prilocaine). The advantages are the fast onset of effect (allowing rapid review) and the shorter duration of effect (meaning safe management in the outpatient setting).

If these are therapeutic injections, short- and long-acting LAs can be combined. This ensures a rapid onset of effect which lasts a long time, with longer desensitisation.

Side effects

Myotoxicity: LAs are indeed the substance of choice for local infiltration; however, they can also be myotoxic. Initially, intracellular membrane systems are affected with subsequent formation of oedema in myocytes. As a consequence this can lead to areas of necrosis, although without sequelae because of regeneration. Basically, all LAs can have myotoxic effects, although the myotoxic potential of the individual LA varies. In animal trials, procaine leads to only minimal structural changes, while the worst damage has been observed with bupivacaine (in high concentrations). Pathophysiologically, myotoxicity is based on a pathologically increased intracellular free calcium (Ca^{2+}) concentration in monocytes. Many LAs induce Ca^{2+} release, depending on concentration, from the sarcoplasmic reticulum and at the same time prevent Ca^{2+} reuptake. This effect depends on lipophilia and stereoisomeric configuration. The clinical significance of myotoxicity induced by LAs is controversial, as toxic muscle damage is extremely rarely reported after infiltration of mTrPs. Ca^{2+} deposits can best be avoided with procaine.

> LAs can also cause various undesirable reactions and effects. The systemic toxic effects and the very rare allergic reactions play a particular role because of their potentially threatening nature.

Systemically toxic side effects: these occur as a result of overdose or inadvertent intravasal injection. They occur primarily as disorders in the CNS or the heart. Cerebral disorders are usually found initially and cardiovascular disorders so not usually occur until the plasma concentrations are higher (Fig. 21.1).

Table 21.1 Clinical application of LAs (with or without adrenaline). The maximum dosages are only recommendations as different maximum dosages are given in different countries. The duration of effect depends on the blockade technique and the quantity of LA injected (Larsen 2006)

SUBSTANCE	CONCENTRATION (%)	VOLUME (ML)	ONSET OF EFFECT (MIN)	DURATION OF EFFECT (MIN)	MAXIMUM INDIVIDUAL DOSE (MG)
Amide-type LAs					
Lidocaine	0.5–1	–	–	–	200 without adrenaline, 500 with adrenaline
	1–1.5	30–50	10–20	120–240	–
	1–2	15–30	5–15	30–90	–
	5, hyperbaric	1–2	5	30–90	–
Prilocaine	0.5–1	–	–	30–90 without adrenaline, 120–360 with adrenaline	400 without adrenaline, 600 with adrenaline
	1–2	30–50	10–20	180–300	–
	2	15–30	5–15	150–600	–
Mepivacaine	0.5–1	–	–	45–90 without adrenaline, 120–360 with adrenaline	300 without adrenaline, 500 with adrenaline
	1–2	30–50	10–20	180–300	–
	1.5–2	15–30	5–15	60–180	–
	4, hyperbaric	1–2	5	–	–
Bupivacaine	0.25–0.5	–	–	120–240 without adrenaline, 180–420 with adrenaline	175 without adrenaline, 225 with adrenaline
	0.25–0.5	30–50	15–30	360–720	–
	0.25–0.75	15–30	10–20	180–300	–
	0.5	2–4	10	75–250	–
Levo-bupivacaine	0.25–0.5	1–60	1–5	–	175 without adrenaline 225 with adrenaline
	0.25–0.5	30–50	–	–	
	0.25–0.75	10–30	8–20	–	–
	0.5	2–4	10	75–250	–
Etidocaine	0.5–1	30–50	10–20	360–720	400 with adrenaline
	1	15–30	5–15	180–300	–
Ropivacaine	0.2–0.5	1–100	1–5	120–360	300
	0.5–1	15–30	15–30	360–720	–
	0.2–1	15–30	10–20	180–360	–
Ester-type LAs					
Procaine	0.5–2%	10–20	10–15	30–60	–

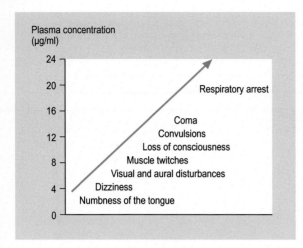

Plasma concentration (μg/ml)

Respiratory arrest

Coma
Convulsions
Loss of consciousness
Muscle twitches
Visual and aural disturbances
Dizziness
Numbness of the tongue

Fig. 21.1 Signs of brain toxicity.
(From Larsen 2006)

Neurotoxicity: in animal experiments high concentrations of LA can damage nerve tissue. However, this is not to be expected as long as the usual clinical concentrations are used. Individual reports are available of long-term damage as a result of intraneural injection.
Allergies: allergies occur extremely rarely. These are more commonly described for LAs from the ester group. With amide-like LAs, allergies to the added stabilisers have been described (e.g. *para*-hydroxybenzoic acid methyl ester). Allergic reactions can occur as allergic dermatitis, asthma attacks or anaphylactic shock.
Vasovagal reactions: these can occur with any method of sampling blood or injection and must be distinguished from allergic reactions. As prophylaxis patients should be treated lying down.

Dosage

A quantity of about 0.2–0.5 ml should be used for infiltrating each mTrP so that even if 10–15 mTrPs are injected there is no danger of exceeding the approved overall dose.

21.2.2 Physiological saline solution

This is used for treatment in some studies. The effect is to some extent comparable to a LA but this has not been reflected in all studies. It is probably based on the alcoholic, bacteriostatic mixtures used and the mechanical lesion at the mTrP caused by the traumatising injection needle or the infiltrated volume (dry needling). An injection with physiological saline should always be considered if the patient is known to be intolerant or has an allergy to LAs.

21.2.3 Corticosteroids

Corticosteroids cause inhibition of the release of arachidonic acid and a reduced formation both of thromboxanes and prostaglandins (inflammatory mediators), as well as normalisation of the increased capillary permeability in the inflamed tissue (oedema reduction). This also leads to reduction of fibroblast proliferation and collagen deposits ('scarring') as well as reduced leucocyte infiltration (inflammatory pain).

An immediate injection in the mTrP is not recommended (danger of rupture); the infiltration of the insertion site with a combination of LA and steroid can be balanced for a short time (maximum of three injections) with inflammatory participation.

We tend to recommend crystalline solutions with a mild systemic effect and longer duration of effect, and which are applied in a comparatively low concentration (e.g. 10 mg triamcinolone/ml). An injection directly into a tendon itself should be avoided!

21.2.4 Botulinum toxin A

Basic principles

Published applications of botulinum toxin A (or BTX-A) include spasticity, dystonia, achalasia, tremor (essential), piriformis muscle syndrome and myofascial pain (US Food and Drug Administration). However, according to the current literature there is insufficient evidence that the injection of botulinum toxin A into mTrPs is effective.

Substances

Botulinum toxin is produced by *Clostridium botulinum*, an anaerobic Gram-positive bacterium. It blocks ACh release at the cholinergic neuromuscular synapse. This block is irreversible and is the cause of a long-term effect lasting about 2–3 months. Re-innervation of the target tissue does not occur until new axons are produced from the peripheral nerves. This process has been observed, according to the literature, up to 40 times so far.

Indications

Individual indications are spasticity, dystonia and tremor. In the treatment of mTrPs it is only indicated in the rarest of cases and after all other treatment measures have been exhausted.

Side effects

There is no organ toxicity apart from in the target muscle. Possible side effects are:

• weakness of the target muscle with a reduction of physiological function and the resulting biomechanical consequences,

- a temporary functional disorder in the neighbouring muscle and glandular tissue,
- a systemic feeling of weakness (although because of the low dose this is rather rare), shortness of breath, difficulties swallowing and accommodation disorders,
- occasionally flu-like symptoms (systemic side effect or immunological reaction).

Dosage

The effective strength is measured as a biological unit in mouse units (MU). One MU corresponds to the LD_{50} of botulinum toxin for a mouse population. An immediate comparison of the effective strength of the products on the market is not available because of the different bioassays of the individual companies producing the toxin. The known highest dose in one session is 800 MU.

21.3 TECHNIQUE

- Disinfect the area.
- Palpate the taut band in the muscle: find the mTrP or trigger point region based on the local pain maximum.
- The point or region is isolated by holding it between thumb and index finger (Fig. 21.2a) or using the Y-grip between the index finger and the middle finger, holding it in place by pressing against the underlying tissue (Fig. 21.2b).
- Apply the above grip with pre-tension (extension) of the muscles being sought (this is recommended for deeper-seated muscle layers, e.g. gluteal).
- During the exploratory injection, the support of the hand guiding the cannula provides security.
- The syringe is usually steadied on the webbing between the second and third fingers with support from the fifth finger or the hypothenar eminence. Pressure on the plunger is exercised by the thumb (Fig. 21.3a).
- The syringe can be held for vertical insertion like a dart between the thumb and digits III–V and the therapist supports himself on the hypothenar eminence or the pisiform bone. Pressure on the plunger is from the index finger (Fig. 21.3b).
- Further protection over the thoracic region is provided by a flat almost tangential angle of insertion and at a right angle to the course of the ribs, using the Venetian-blind-like effect of the ribs and support from the hand (Fig. 21.4).

An attempt at aspiration is usually made before injection to rule out intravasal positioning of the cannula. With deep injection close to large vessels, aspiration should be performed in two planes (= double aspiration with turning of the needle tip through 90°).

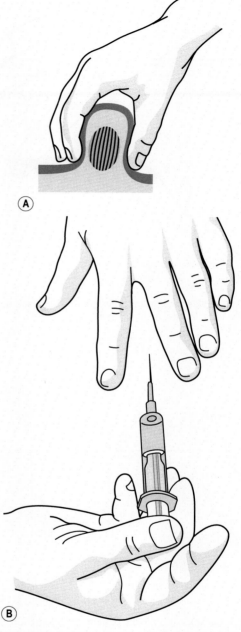

Fig. 21.2 Fixation of the point or region with a pinch grip between thumb and index finger (a) or the Y-grip between the index finger and the middle finger and with a fixing pressure against the underlying tissue (b).

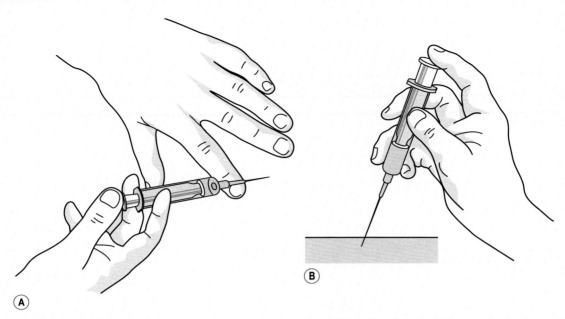

Fig. 21.3 Holding the syringe between the thumb and the third and fourth fingers (a) and between the little finger, the thumb, and the third, fourth and fifth fingers (b).

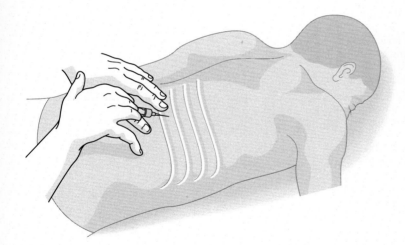

Fig. 21.4 Further protection over the thoracic region is provided by a flat almost tangential angle of insertion, using a Venetian-blind-like effect of the ribs and by support from the hand.

After prior explanation to the patient and instruction about the twitch reaction that is to be expected, disinfection is followed by insertion of the injection needle (guage 21, 25 or 27). It is quickly pushed through the skin then slowly pushed forward in the direction of the mTrP. A fan-shaped forward movement procedure with the injection needle may be required in the fixed area in order to find the mTrP (Fig. 21.5).

The correct position of the needle in the mTrP is controlled by the visible or tangible twitch response (or also

EMG-controlled). The volume to be injected at the mTrP is about 0.2 ml.

It is possible to inject both at the mTrP and at the insertion (possibly infiltrating by using a simplified technique with rather more volume). A disadvantage of infiltration is the lesser effect and the lack of control over the needle position in the T-point.

This probe technique with twitches is an mTrP injection technique that is more painful than usual for patients, it has to be performed with confident verbal

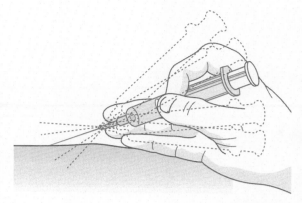

Supporting
the hand

Fig. 21.5 Superficial probing with the injection needle.

reassurance and breathing instructions (expiration). It is usual for patients to cry out, yawn or laugh. Occasionally, tears are observed as an expression of pain or in memory of pain previously suffered. Seeing this should prompt the therapist to respond and if necessary include it in the discussion of the treatment plan with the patient (psychosomatic).

An absolute prerequisite for injection is knowledge of the precise regional anatomical conditions and knowledge of possible risks. It is imperative to explain about possible complications (infection, bleeding, pneumothorax, haematoma, blood vessel or nerve lesion, allergic reaction, cardiovascular toxicity, sensory deficits), including their documentation.

Chapter | 22 |

Acupuncture and related procedures

Dominik Irnich, David Euler, Jochen Gleditsch, Winfried Banzer, Jürgen Bachmann

22.1 DRY NEEDLING (TRIGGER POINT ACUPUNTURE)

Dominik Irnich

22.1.1 Definitions

Dry needling is a functional anatomical locoregional needling technique for the treatment of myofascial symptoms. The aim of needling is to find the exact site of an mTrP and to cause a local muscle twitch reaction (Travell, Simons 2002). There are various forms of this technique:

- direct dry needling of the mTrP,
- dry needling of the affected muscle fascia,
- superficial dry needling.

22.1.2 Physiological principles

Touching a mTrP leads to stimulation of the muscle end-plate zone and subsequently to a local muscle twitch reaction and subsequent relaxation of the muscle. The physiological principle of this mechanism has still not been conclusively explained. Although part of the effect of mTrP needling with the mechanical destruction of the mTrP has been explained, this concept seems too mechanistic. It is better to accept that the severe contraction of an already shortened muscle fibre bundle leads to microtrauma. This could in its turn be the cause of the dispersion of the contracted myofilaments.

The subsequent stretching recommended in practice allows the contracted muscle fibre bundle to be brought back to its original initial length. It is even conceivable that the cell destruction caused by the needling leads to a change in the biochemical milieu, which explains the subsequent

muscle pain and also leads to increased perfusion with the re-establishment of neurotransmitter homeostasis in the surrounding area. One of the key neurotransmitters could be ATP, which is released inside the cell during cell destruction by the needle.

22.1.3 Principles of treatment

Dry needling is a highly effective form of therapy for many mTrPs. The use of dry needling requires intuition and experience. First experiences with needling should be gained with superficial mTrPs, for example in the area of the wrist extensors. With needling in the area of the thoracic aperture and the deep trunk muscles, special techniques must be applied in order to avoid complications such as pneumothorax and nerve injuries.

The aim of dry needling is to trigger the local muscle twitch reaction. Through manual contact the therapist should try to note this reaction and regard it as a sign of needling efficacy (Fig. 22.1).

Depending on the individual pain sensation, the patient may find this muscle twitch reaction surprising and unpleasant but also as 'beneficial pain'. It is a brief, twitching pain like a short fasciculation, which may be converted into muscle soreness or a feeling of heaviness after treatment (post-treatment soreness). This sensation can occur immediately after treatment is finished but can also develop in the first 24 h after treatment. It lasts a maximum of 48 h.

If the patient feels this pain, the affected muscles should be kept relaxed. This can also be regarded as therapeutically beneficial. If the mTrP is the result of incorrect posture or strain (e.g. raised shoulders), the patient should avoid this posture while the post-treatment sensation lasts and this will lead to improved posture. This 'follow-up pain' is basically a positive, therapeutically meaningful phenomenon.

http://dx.doi.org/10.1016/B978-0-7020-4312-3.00022-2

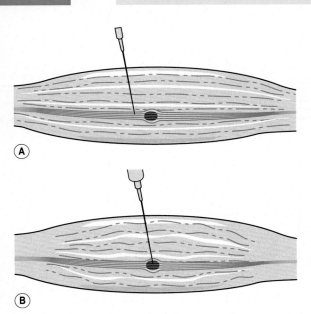

(A)

(B)

Fig. 22.1 Causing a local muscle twitch reaction (a and b).

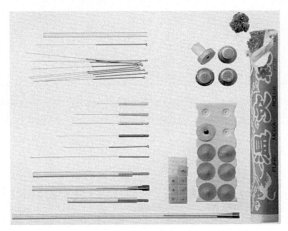

Fig. 22.2 Choice of acupuncture needles (with guide tubes). Moxibustion rolls are shown on the right.

The muscles are a sensitive organ and increased muscle tension can be the expression from a psychosomatic point of view of mental conflict or insufficiently processed emotions or the expression of a physical, spiritual or emotional strain. The muscle becomes a defence shield against the environment (muscle shield). In these cases proceed cautiously and sensitively during needling. Acupuncture can also be used to improve body awareness.

22.1.4 Your explanation to the patient

The method of treatment, including the effects to be expected during and after treatment, must be explained to the patient beforehand (the muscle twitch response, follow-up soreness, etc.). A patient who understands the reason for the needling and is motivated to get better will usually not find the pain caused by the needling unpleasant. Experience teaches us that this pain is felt to be 'good' as in the end someone has 'found the spot'.

22.1.5 Technique

Acupuncture needles have proved reliable for conducting needling because they slide in so easily compared to an injection needle. The rounded edge of the acupuncture needle tends to displace the tissue to be penetrated and leads to less bruising compared to the 'cutting' action of the injection needle.

The choice of needle should be made according to the principle of being 'as thin as possible and as long as necessary'. The needle lengths on the market are usually sufficient. Only with obese patients and for some very deep lying muscles (such as the Mm. interspinales) are lengths of more than 80 mm required, in which case spinal needles can be used (Fig. 22.2).

The use of very thin (or fine) needles has proved highly appropriate for pain-sensitive patients. However, it takes some practice to insert the needles quickly so that they do not bend when you try to penetrate the skin. Insertion must be vertical and be carried out with a firm, concerted movement. To make insertion easier, guide tubes are available (Fig. 22.2). The pressure of the guide tube on the skin also serves to activate mechanosensitive low-threshold/swelling afferences, which may inhibit the noxious input to the level of the spinal cord caused during insertion and the central transfer of the pain and any possible guarding reactions. This effect can also be achieved by exercising finger pressure directly next to the insertion site (Fig. 22.3c). We recommend placing the whole hand flat; this not only inhibits pain but also allows the therapist to perceive the autonomic status of the patient, the patient's reaction to the needling and the local muscle twitch response in the superficial muscles. If you notice a 'mental' withdrawal of the patient from the treatment situation or a definite guarding reaction, it may be necessary to interrupt the treatment to prevent a traumatic experience.

22.1.6 Types of dry needling

Direct dry needling

Direct dry needling aims to probe the mTrP and cause the local twitch response. This is the most traumatic form of dry needling. Throughout the needling process, the therapist

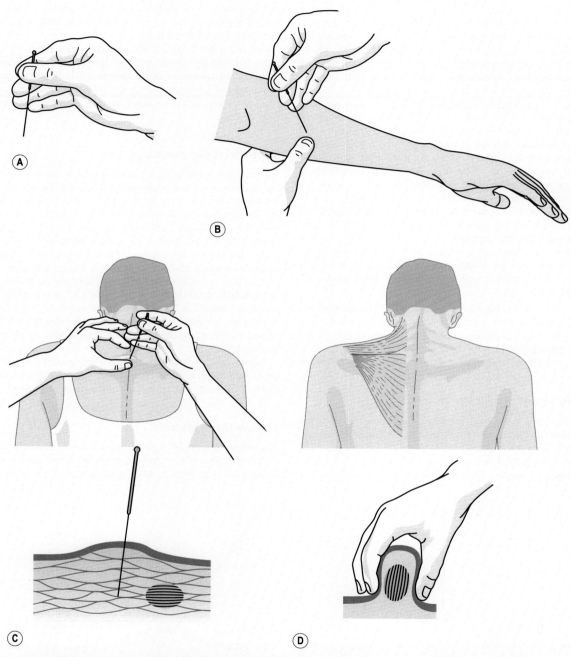

Fig. 22.3 Techniques for holding the needle and insertion: hold the needle with three fingers (a), tighten soft tissue (b), insert with thumb pressure (c), grasp the muscle (d).

should concentrate on the tip of the needle to perceive the consistency of each tissue (connective tissue, fascia, muscle). The first quick and painless insertion is made through the cutis to the subcutis. Now the therapist deliberately reduces the speed of the needling to penetrate the muscle and find the mTrP. Great sensitivity is required for this. With practice, when the tip of the needle encounters the mTrP, an increasingly rubber-like consistency is felt. Now smaller, low-level movements of the needle's tip are enough to cause the twitch response. If the therapist has definitely reached the mTrP and does not succeed in causing the twitch, the needle is withdrawn up to maximum of 1 cm and probed again. If this still does not cause a twitch response, further intramuscular manipulation does not usually bring success. Nevertheless, a definite improvement can be seen after treatment.

If the location of the mTrP cannot be found as the needle is pushed forward, the needle is withdrawn as far as the subcutis and the direction of insertion changed slightly so that the needle can slowly be pushed forward again (Fig. 22.1). If several changes of direction fail to find the mTrP, the working hypothesis and technique must be reconsidered. Causes can be:

- the palpated hardening is not an mTrP (lymph nodes?),
- the mTrP is in a different layer or another muscle,
- the patient's change of position between diagnosis and therapy lead to the mTrP having changed location,
- insufficient material is used, e.g. the needle is too short.

Dry needling via the muscle fascia

A local twitch response can often be achieved by irritation of the outer fascia of the affected muscle. Insertion through the cutis is made quickly as far as the connective tissue. In contrast to direct dry needling, the needle is now moved along the outer muscle fascia above the mTrP. Rapid needle movements are now used to cause high-frequency stimulation of the fascia (Fig. 22.4). In many cases this causes a local muscle twitch reaction.

This technique is gentler and less complicated for the patient. It is suitable predominantly for superficial muscles such as the trapezius or the levator scapulae. There is also less danger of a pneumothorax. On the other hand, the local twitch response is not caused as often as it is with direct dry needling.

Superficial dry needling

Superficial dry needling is a particular form of dry needling. The acupuncture needles are only pushed superficially into the tissue over the mTrP by about 5–10 mm. The needles are then left in this position for about 30 s (Fig. 22.5). Now the needles are removed again and the tenderpoint is palpated and assessed at the same time to see whether any relaxation has taken place. If not, the needles are put in position again and left for about 2–3 min. The aim is not to cause a local muscle twitch reaction but an indirect relaxation of the mTrP (neuronal cause?). If there is still no reaction, proceed as for the techniques above or leave the needles in place for 20–30 min with occasional stimulation (rotation, lifting and lowering) as for traditional acupuncture treatment.

Superficial dry needling is particularly suitable for patients with a high readiness to react who often suffer a strong reaction to a minor stimulus (check the patient's history).

Follow-up treatment

After releasing an mTrP we recommend further treatment of the muscle. This can be carried out using various extension techniques (see Section 19.2, extension and relaxation/

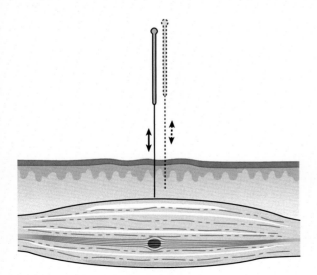

Fig. 22.4 Dry needling via the muscle fascia.

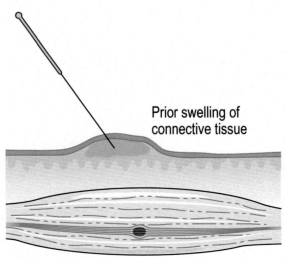

Prior swelling of connective tissue

Fig. 22.5 Superficial dry needling.

stretching and detensioning) or superficial smoothing of the slightly extended muscle in the direction of the fibres. With chronic myofascial symptoms it is necessary to combine dry needling with manual therapy, physiotherapy, physical therapy, natural remedies and/or psychological or medical treatment. During additional behavioural therapy and physical exercises the patient can be prompted to distance themselves from the pain and be motivated to exercise on their own. With chronic disease, the aim should be to encourage the patient as far as possible to take on the responsibility of managing the pain and its effects. The choice of effective therapeutic approach is very specific to the individual.

Dry needling and acupuncture

Techniques similar to dry needling have already been described in traditional Chinese acupuncture texts. It is only with recent research that the associations with function and anatomy have become known (see Ch. 8). It is advantageous to have knowledge and practical experience of traditional acupuncture for dry needling. An experienced acupuncturist has usually mastered quick, pain-free needle penetration and can distinguish different structures in the tissue with the needle. In view of the high correlation of traditional acupuncture points and mTrPs (see Ch. 8) the finding of mTrPs is routine.

The effect of mTrP acupuncture can be optimised by additional needling in accordance with the criteria of traditional Chinese acupuncture and needling of microsystem points (e.g. points on the ear). In this case, the distal points, chosen according to meridian theory, should be treated first. This can relieve local pain during the following trigger point needling. This effect can also be achieved by prior needling of microsystem points. Under favourable conditions far-point needling alone can lead to the disappearance of the mTrP and make local treatment superfluous.

For anxious patients or those with very strong local sensitivity, relief can be achieved initially through contralateral needling.

Short course of treatment

History

- Differentiate the pain according to:
  - quality: usually dull and oppressive.
  - intensity: from mild to the most severe pain, measurement using the visual analogue scale,
  - modulating factors: e.g. increase in stress (extension or contraction of affected muscles).
- Careful questioning about painful movements or limited function.

Examination

- Instruction to the patient to report any pain provocation during the mobility examination.

- Detailed functional anatomical or manual therapy examination to identify the affected muscles.
- Careful palpation of the painful or movement-restricted muscles to locate active mTrPs:
  - initially crosswise palpation to locate the taut band,
  - if a taut band has been located, palpation along the taut band until and mTrP can be identified,
  - examination for pain on pressure, extension and contraction,
  - compression of the trigger point for 10 s to cause referred pain symptoms.

Implementation

- Explain to the patient and allow time to think about it if necessary.
- Make sure the treatment atmosphere is relaxed, place the patient and muscles in a relaxed position (so that patient, therapist and muscles are all relaxed!).
- Before local treatment, needle the distal points, as local treatment is then less painful.
- Choose sterile acupuncture needles with a length corresponding to the depth of the mTrP; with long and very thin needles, a guide tube is helpful.
- Locate the mTrP in the tissue (enclose the mTrP with a pinch grip between thumb and index finger or with two fingers).
- Quick insertion as for traditional needling.
- Probing the mTrP and causing a local twitch response when it meets the mTrP exactly, warning: muscle twitches can be painful and lead to muscle pain which lasts for several hours, so it should be used intermittently and be adjusted to the patient's reaction.
- Discontinue if there is any burning pain.
- Remove the needles after sufficient stimulation or leave in place for 30 min as for acupuncture. As the muscle can continue to work, especially after a local twitch response has been caused, intramuscular needles should be withdrawn as far as the subcutaneous tissue.
- Checking the findings and treat any residual findings if necessary.
- After treatment stretch the relevant muscles, e.g. with postisometric relaxation (tense, relax, stretch).

Indications and contraindications

Indications

Dry needling is suitable for the treatment of most mTrPs. It is the treatment of choice for:

- patients with acute MPS and the wish for immediate treatment at the first appointment,
- athletes wishing for fast recovery,
- therapy resistance to manual medicine and physiotherapy.

Dry needling is one part of a treatment plan for chronic myofascial symptoms caused or maintained by mTrP, such as:

- temporomandibular pain syndrome,
- lateral and medial epicondylitis,
- periarthropathy (shoulder, hips),
- tendinosis,
- insertion tendinopathy,
- arthritis,
- degenerative cervical, thoracic or lumbar spine syndrome,
- spinal syndrome with segmental functional disorder,
- visceral pain syndrome.

A good success rate has also been achieved with pain diseases where the muscles have taken on a trigger function:

- migraine,
- tension headaches.

> For chronic pain with biopsychosocial components there is the risk of iatrogenic chronification caused by simple, monocausal models of explanation and invasive monotherapy. For these patients, the application of dry needling should be only part of a comprehensive, multimodal, interdisciplinary, individual treatment plan.

Contraindications

- Manifest blood clotting disorder.
- Epilepsy.

Undesirable effects

Injuries to the internal organs cannot be regarded as an undesirable effect but only as an error on the part of the therapist as a result of lack of knowledge or experience. Other undesirable effects include:

- the undesirable effects that apply to traditional acupuncture, including pneumothorax,
- subsequent muscle pain.

Scientific data, studies

Specific evidence of efficacy for trigger point acupuncture in accordance with the criteria of evidence-based medicine is not available. The methodological problem is the absence of a proper placebo control. Various clinically controlled trials show evidence for the efficacy of dry needling for myofascial pain. These include:

- myofascial pain (Lewit 1979),
- cervical spine syndrome (Irnich et al. 2001, 2002),

- myofascial shoulder pain (Ceccherelli et al. 2001),
- lumbar myofascial pain (Ceccherelli et al. 2002),
- in a controlled study on migraine prophylaxis, trigger point therapy was as effective as metoprolol (Hesse et al. 1994),
- in a systematic overview no difference could be found between the injection of substances and direct needling for myofascial pain (Cummings, White 2001),
- in a meta-analysis in 2008 there was a positive tendency in the direction of dry needling (Tough et al. 2008).

22.2 TRADITIONAL ACUPUNCTURE

Dominik Irnich

22.2.1 Definitions

Acupuncture is the most well known therapy in traditional Chinese medicine (TCM). It uses the insertion of metal needles at precisely established points on the skin for diagnostic and/or therapeutic purposes with functional, reversible diseases or disorders; these points may be spontaneously painful or tender (de la Fuye's definition).

Moxibustion is an important component of acupuncture and is indicated for so-called empty or cold syndromes (frequently due to chronic diseases, sensitivity to cold or exhaustion). Heat is produced over the acupuncture point by burning *Artemisia vulgaris* (moxa, mugwort) using moxa cigars, moxa cylinders (which can be fixed to the handle of the placed needle) or moxa containers.

The traditional acupuncture point is defined by a more or less exact anatomical location. It is the site of the transfer of a stimulus. Each acupuncture point has local effects and specific effects are attributed to certain points after transfer along the meridian to functions of the whole organ or one of its areas.

Ah-shi points are the pressure-sensitive points in the painful region which do not lie at traditional locations but may be part of a point plan because of their sensitivity. Ah-shi points correspond to cutaneous, ligamentary, myofascial or bony trigger points or tenderpoints.

A meridian (or channel) comprises a mainly vertical series of acupuncture points to which similar effects are attributed.

Corresponding to traditional Chinese thinking, Qi describes the fundamental substance of the universe. In relation to humans, the term Qi describes the essential substance of the human body and the resulting functions which sustain life. According to TCM, the harmonious circulation of Qi in the meridians, tissues and organs means health.

De Qi feeling describes the subjective feelings caused when an acupuncture point is touched or activated. It comprises various sensations which are described as a dull, dragging feeling, heaviness, heat or numbness or slight pain mainly along the relevant meridian (PSC, propagated sensation along the channels).

22.2.2 Physiological principles

Evidence has been shown for the analgesic effects of acupuncture (overview in Irnich, Beyer 2002, Pomeranz 1999). The short-term effects of acupuncture analgesia are produced by the activation of endogenous opioid antinociception and descending pain-inhibition systems. Some acupuncture analgesia can be explained by spinal segmental and heterosegmental inhibition mechanisms. Activation of supraspinal diffuse pain inhibition (diffuse noxious inhibitory control, or DNIC) through acupuncture has to be presumed.

Various endorphins, serotonin, noradrenaline (norepinephrine), CGRP, corticoptropin (adrenocorticotrophic hormone, ACTH) and oestrogens have been described among others as neurotransmitters and hormones that participate in the acupuncture effect. Potential long-term effects cannot be sufficiently explained with the available results, but there is evidence of spinal and neuromodulatory effects and the participation of the limbic system.

The effect of acupuncture on myofascial pain is probably based on the cited spinal, reflex and systemic inhibition mechanisms. Added to this is the local effect of the needle when it meets the mTrP (see Section 22.1).

22.2.3 Theoretical principles of acupuncture

The theoretical principles of traditional Chinese acupuncture are based on ancient Chinese philosophical thinking and have gone through changes over time in the area of tension between Confucianism and Taoism and are also dependent on scientific knowledge, socioeconomic demands and political and religious movements (Unschuld 2003, Ots 2002). An essential characteristic is the descriptive, phenomenological procedure without any causal or analytical relationship construct.

22.2.4 Yin and Yang counterpart system

The Yin and Yang counterpart system is a historical dialectical system for the interpretation of natural phenomena.

- Yin and Yang represent opposites (e.g. day and night, water and fire, motion and rest).
- Yin and Yang are dependent on each other and mutually influence each other.
- The nurturing substance of the body is attributed to Yin and the functional activity to Yang.

- Disease can basically be interpreted as a predominance of Yin or Yang: with chronic empty and cold diseases Yin predominates, while acute, full and hot diseases correspond to Yang.
- In relation to the body, Yang is outside and above, while Yin is inside and below.
- Meridians and organs are attributed either to Yin or to Yang.

22.2.5 Theory of Qi, blood and body fluids

- Qi, blood and body fluids are fundamental substances which sustain the function of the organism and are distributed throughout the whole organism.
- Qi corresponds to Yang, blood corresponds to Yin.
- Qi sustains the functions of the organs, meridians, tissues and fluids and has warming, moving, controlling, guarding, sustaining, nurturing and activating functions.
- Qi is divided into innate Qi (Yuan Qi, roots in the kidneys), breathing Qi (Zong Qi, stored in the lungs), nurturing Qi (Yingqi, produced in the stomach and spleen) and guarding Qi (Wei Qi, body surface).
- The meridians and organs possess some specific Qi.
- Blood is formed as red fluid in the spleen and stomach from the essence of food, and is circulated in the vessels.
- Blood is moved by the heart and controlled by the spleen (e.g. held in the vessels); the liver stores the blood and controls the blood volume.
- Blood nourishes and moistens tissue and organs, is responsible for the movements of the extremities and the eyes and for mental function.
- All other fluids, such as saliva, tears and gastric juices, count as body fluids (Jingye). They are divided into clear (Jing) and cloudy (Ye) fluids and are functionally associated with Qi and blood.
- Localised stabbing pain and pathological tissue collections (e.g. haematoma, tumour) are described as blood stagnation.
- Diffuse, referred and colic-like pain is described as Qi stagnation.
- Vomiting or coughing is described as rebellious Qi.

22.2.6 Theory of the Zang-Fu organs

In TCM, certain physiological functions are attributed to the organs and these are extended around functions or jurisdictions (Table 22.1) in accordance with the theory of the five phases of transformation (circles of function). Twelve main organs are described which correspond with the 12 main meridians and these are divided into six Zang organs (hollow organs, Yang) and six Fu organs (storage organs, Yin). Pathologies of the individual organs are

185

Table 22.1 Overview of the functions of the organs according to TCM with common syndromes, analogies to diagnoses and the interpreted relationship to psychological and emotional factors

ORGAN	TCM FUNCTION	CHOICE OF COMMON SYNDROMES ACCORDING TO TCM	EXAMPLES OF SYMPTOMS AND DISEASES	INTERPRETATION BASED ON BASIC PROPERTIES AND FUNCTIONS OF HUMANS
Lungs, Yin	Takes up breath Qi, distributes Qi, controls breathing, responsible for mucous membranes, skin and hair	Lungs Qi weakness, invasion of wind, moisture, mucus	Bronchitis, bronchial asthma, skin diseases, weak defence mechanism	Capacity to grieve, let go, interact with environment, rhythm of life Intuitio from Jung Sanguine person from Hippocrates Spirituality from Paracelsus
Large intestine, Yang	Transport function, excretion	Cold or heat in large intestine	Constipation, diarrhoea	
Stomach, Yang	Moves Qi down Storage and separation function	Yin deficiency symptoms	Vomiting, heartburn	
Spleen, Yin	Transport, implementation Keeps the blood in the vessels Rules thinking Nourishment of muscles, fat and connective tissue	Spleen Qi weakness Spleen Yang emptiness Spleen Yin emptiness	Meteorism, connective tissue weakness, perfusion disorders, loss of appetite, digestive disorders, dysmenorrhoea	Interaction, acceptance Digestion, integration Connection, encounter Future, overcoming limits Rationality from Jung Melancholic person of Hippocrates Ens veneni of Paracelsus
Pericardium, Yin	Protection of heart from external damaging influences		Circulatory dysregulation, tight chest, nausea, vomiting	
Three-warmer, Yang	Guarding against external damaging influences, water balance	Mucosa moisture in the middle warmer	Imbalance between thorax, abdomen and retroperitoneum	
Gallbladder, Yang	Storage and excretion of bile Function of the tendons	Gallbladder Qi deficiency Moisture heat in the gallbladder	Digestive disorders, musculoligamentary symptoms	
Liver, Yin	Regulated and distributes the Qi stores the blood	Liver Qi stagnation increase in liver Yang liver blood emptiness conflict with spleen	Irritability, hypertension digestive disorders, dysmenorrhoea visual disorders	Emotionality, courage, mobility, self-assertion, sense of proportion, perseverance, motivation, id personality, the present time, emotions from Jung, choleric person of Hippocrates, Ens astrale of Paracelsus
Heart, Yin	Seat of Shen (mind) controls the blood vessels	Heart Qi weakness, Heart Yin weakness, heart blood emptiness	Palpations, functional heart symptoms, hectic pace, nervousness, unrest, concentration disorders	Speech, communication, joy, rest, exudation, being one, love, spirit, conjunction according to Jung, Ens die according to Paracelsus

Table 22.1 Overview of the functions of the organs according to TCM with common syndromes, analogies to diagnoses and the interpreted relationship to psychological and emotional factors—cont'd

ORGAN	TCM FUNCTION	CHOICE OF COMMON SYNDROMES ACCORDING TO TCM	EXAMPLES OF SYMPTOMS AND DISEASES	INTERPRETATION BASED ON BASIC PROPERTIES AND FUNCTIONS OF HUMANS
Small intestine, Yang	Fluid excretion	Qi stagnation in the small intestine, heat in the small intestine	Digestive disorders	
Bladder, Yang	Takes up fluid and excretes it	Moisture, heat in the bladder	Bladder symptoms	
Kidneys, Yin	Seat of congenital Qi (root of life), seat of willpower, controls sexual function, development and aging, water regulation	Kidney Qi weakness, kidney Yin weakness, kidney Yang weakness	Urogenital symptoms, disorders of sexual function, anxiety, back pain	Security, reliability, sense of purpose, stability, sexuality, intent according to Jung, phlegmatic person according to Hippocrates, Ens naturale according to Paracelsus

described as a syndrome in TCM (= internal diseases). Circles of function are attributed to the organs. A circle of function comprises, in relation to nature (the macrosmos), the elements, points of the compass, seasons, development stage, environmental factors (e.g. wind) and taste. In relation to the human organism (the microcosmos) the attributions comprise sensory organs, tissues, psychoemotional factors and, as a Western interpretation (Wancura 2009, Gleditsch 2005), psychosomatic aspects.

22.2.7 System of meridians

The meridian system (Jing luo) consists essentially of 12 main meridians and eight extraordinary meridians (or special meridians, miracle meridians, extraordinary vessels). The 12 main meridians are listed below, with descriptions of their course in the neutral position (see Fig. 22.6).
- Three Yin meridians of the hand: course from the thorax to the fingertips (medial side):
  - lung meridian (LU): 11 points, anteromedial course (radial side),
  - pericardial meridian (PC): nine points, centromedial course,
  - heart meridian (HT): nine points, posteromedial course (ulnar side).
- Three Yang meridians of the hand: course from the fingertips to the head (lateral side):
  - large intestine meridian (LI): 20 points, anterolateral course (radial side),
  - triple heater meridian (TH): 23 points, lateromedial course,
  - small intestine meridian (SI): 21 points, posterolateral course (ulnar side).

- Three Yang meridians of the foot: course from the head to the tips of the toes:
  - stomach meridian (ST): 45 points, anterolateral course,
  - gallbladder meridian (GB): 44 points, lateromedial course,
  - bladder meridian (BL): 67 points, posterolateral course.
- Three Yin meridians of the foot: course from the tips of the toes to the thorax:
  - spleen meridian (SP): 21 points, anteromedial course,
  - liver meridian (LR): 14 points, centromedial course,
  - kidney meridian (KI): 27 points, posteromedial course.

Joined meridians (Yin–Yang association) with complementary/augmenting function:
- hand: LU–LI, PC–TH, HT–SI,
- foot: SP–ST, GB–LR, BL–KI.

Corresponding meridians (Yang–Yang axes):
- LI– ST (Yang Ming, anterior),
- TH–GB (Shao Yang, lateral),
- SI–BL (Tai Yang, posterior).

Circulations/rotations (Yin and Yang joined meridians of the hand and foot): a circulation consists of four meridians which belong together energetically and anatomically and run in each case in the rhythm Yin → Yang → Yang → Yin:

1. or anterior circulation: LU → LI → ST → SP,
2. or posterior circulation: HT → SI → BL → KI,
3. or lateral circulation: PC → TH → GB → LR.

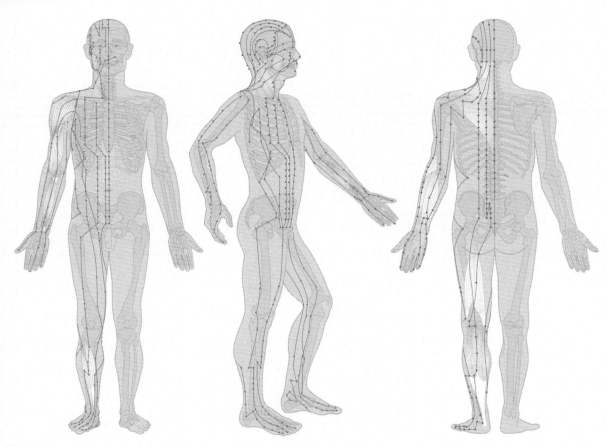

Fig. 22.6 The meridian system in Chinese medicine.

Extraordinary meridians: only two of the extraordinary meridians have their own points:

- anterior midline meridian = conception vessel (CV), 26 points, course anterior from the anus to the lower lip above the anterior midline of the body,
- posterior midline meridian = governing vessel (GV), 28 points, course from posterior of the anus along the whole vertebral column over the head to the upper lip.

These two meridians are the only unpaired meridians. The six remaining extraordinary meridians consist of a combination of points from various main meridians. They have a subordinate function.

22.2.8 Acupuncture points

- Each acupuncture point has local effects and can therefore be used for local treatment.
- Some meridian points have an especially strong effect along the meridian and are used as distal points.
- Some acupuncture points have a particular effect on individual symptoms and are selected appropriately.

- Some points have superordinate functions (control or system points).
- Many of the predilection sites for mTrPs correspond to the traditional acupuncture points.
- Tenderpoints which do not correspond to traditional acupuncture points are described as Ah-shi points. The needling of these points is an important component of local acupuncture.

Location of the acupuncture points is performed using characteristic anatomical landmarks. LIstances are given using the cun unit of measurement. This is an individual measurement based on the patient's finger width (most likely at the extremities), or it can be a proportional measurement as a defined distance on the body divided into equal parts (most likely at the trunk) (see Fig. 22.7):

- 1 cun = width of the patient's thumb,
- 3 cun = width of four fingers (digits II–V) at the level of the interphalangeal joint,
- 5 cun = distance of the upper margin of the symphysis to the navel,
- 8 cun = distance between the nipples,

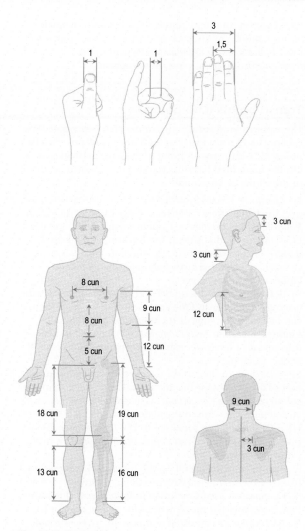

Fig. 22.7 Cun measurement.

- 8 cun = distance from the xiphoid to the navel,
- 12 cun = crook of the elbow to the crook of the wrist,
- 16 cun = middle of the patella to the lateral malleolus (highest measurement),
- 19 cun = greater trochanter to middle of patella.

Eight influential points (master points)

The points have special effects on certain structures and functions. They are used in accordance with their area of influence.

LR 13 *Location*: At the lower margin of the free end of the 11th rib *Chinese connection*: Zang organs *Indication*: Upper abdominal pain.

CV 12 *Location*: In the middle between the navel and the xiphoid *Chinese connection*: Fu organs *Indication*: Abdominal pain.

CV 17 *Location*: Midline of the sternum at the level of the fourth intercostal space between the nipples (in men) *Chinese connection*: Qi *Indication*: Thoracic pain, tight feeling, affective increase in pain.

BL 17 *Location*: 1.5 cun lateral spinous process of T7, approx. level of the angulus inf. scapulae *Chinese connection*: Blood *Indication*: Upper abdominal pain.

GB 34 *Location*: With bent knee in the hollow in front of and below the head of the fibula *Chinese connection*: Tendons *Indication*: Pain in the locomotor system.

LU 9 *Location*: In the transverse wrist crease, radial to the radial artery *Chinese connection*: Vessels *Indication*: Perfusion disorders, hypotension or hypertension.

BL 11 *Location*: 1.5 cun lateral spinous process of T1 *Chinese connection*: Bones *Indication*: Bone pain, degenerative diseases.

GB 39 *Location*: 3 cun above the lateral malleolus, at the anterior margin of the fibula *Chinese connection*: Bone marrow *Indication* Cervical spine pain, abdominal pain.

Switch points (synonym: cardinal, confluence or key point)

These points influence the region of the meridian switched on. They are effective distal points. Combination Yin–Yang linked switch points are a reliable combination e.g. SI 3–BL 62.

PC 6 *Location*: 2 cun proximal to the middle of the palmar wrist crease between the tendons of the Mm. flexor carpi radialis and palmaris longus *Coupled meridian*: Yinwei mai *Area of influence*: Thorax, heart.

SP 4 *Location*: In the hollow over the transition from the base of the shaft of the first metatarsal bone at the change of colour of the skin *Coupled meridian*: Chong mai *Area of influence*: Lower abdomen, uterus.

SI 3 *Location*: With the fist closed on the ulnar side on the back of the hand in the hollow behind the end of the top fold of the palm *Coupled meridian*: GV (Du mai) *Area of influence*: vertebral column.

BL 62 *Location*: Under the tip of the lateral malleolus *Coupled meridian*: Yangqiao mai *Area of influence*: Lateral vertebral column, head, eyes.

TH 5 *Location*: 2 cun proximally to the middle of the dorsal wrist crease, opposite PC 6 *Coupled meridian*: Yangwei mai *Area of influence*: Lateral side.

GB 41 *Location*: In the proximal angle between metatarsal bones IV and V *Coupled meridian*: Dai mai *Area of influence*: Lumbar region, dorsal–ventral connection.

LU 7 *Location*: 1.5 cun proximal to the transverse wrist crease, over the radial artery *Coupled meridian*: CV (Ren mai) *Area of influence*: General condition and autonomic nervous system.

KI 6 *Location*: Under the tip of the medial malleolus *Coupled meridian*: Yinqiao mai *Area of influence*: Lower abdomen, legs, eyes.

Source points (Yuan points)

These points have a particular effect on the associated organ. The combination with the relevant Shu point is well-proven. Source points lie in the area of the wrist or the ankle.

LU 9 *Location*: In the transverse wrist crease, radial to the radial artery *Chinese connection*: Lungs *Indication/area of influence*: Respiratory symptoms, wrist.

LI 4 *Location*: On the back of the hand at the highest point of the muscle bulge between metacarpals I and II *Chinese connection*: Large intestine *Indication/area of influence*: Pain, particularly headaches, dyshidrosis, influence on the function of the intestines and the uterus.

ST 42 *Location*: At the highest point of the instep (A. dorsalis pedis) *Chinese connection*: Stomach *Indication/area of influence*: Gastric pain, meteorism, foot.

SP 3 *Location*: Just proximal to the proximal phalanx of the big toe, on the tendon of the M. abductor hallucis *Chinese connection*: Spleen *Indication/area of influence*: Symptoms of dysentery and gastritis, poor digestion.

HT 7 *Location*: Ulnar wrist fold, radial side of the pisiformis bone *Chinese connection*: Heart *Indication/area of influence*: Heart function symptoms, regulates the autonomic nervous system, mild anti-anxiety agent.

SI 4 *Location*: Ulnar side of hand, transition between red and white flesh, at the base of the fifth metacarpal/articular space to the hamate bone *Chinese connection*: Small intestine *Indication/area of influence*: Wrist.

BL 64 *Location*: Lateral margin of foot, behind the tuberosity of the fifth metatarsal at the colour change of the skin *Chinese connection*: Bladder *Indication/area of influence*: Lumbago, eyes.

KI 3 *Location*: Between the strongest protrusion of the medial malleolus and the Achilles tendon *Chinese connection*: Kidneys *Indication/area of influence*: Lumbar spine symptoms, knee, ear.

PC 7 *Location*: In the middle of the palmar wrist crease between the tendons of the Mm. flexor carpi radialis and palmaris longus *Chinese connection*: Pericardium *Indication/area of influence*: Heart symptoms, psychosomatic disorders.

TH 4 *Location*: Groove lateral to the tendon of the M. extensor digit. long. at the level of the wrist crease *Chinese connection*: Triple heater *Indication/area of influence*: Shoulders, back, wrist.

GB 40 *Location*: At the intersection of the horizontal through the tip and the vertical at the front, through the biggest circumference of the lateral malleolus, over the calcaneocuboid joint *Chinese connection*: Gallbladder *Indication/area of influence*: Eyes, upper abdomen, ankle.

LR 3 *Location*: In the proximal angle between metatarsal bones I and II, on the back of the foot *Chinese connection*: Liver *Indication/area of influence*: Hypertension, dysmenorrhoea, pain, especially headache.

Transit points (Luo points)

These points produce a connection with the associated meridian. The 12 main meridians, CV and GV all possess a Luo point. M21 is the transit point of the large network vessels. On the main meridians the transit points mostly lie distal to the elbow or knee joint.

LU 7 *Location*: 1.5 cun proximal to the transverse wrist crease, over the radial artery *Connection*: Large intestine meridian *Indication/area of influence*: Cough, wrist, cervical spine.

LI 6 *Location*: Radial side of the forearm, at the lateral margin of the radius, 3 cun proximal to the wrist crease *Connection*: Lung meridian *Indication/area of influence*: Upper extremity, ear, eye.

ST 40 *Location*: Mid-distant between the highest point of the external malleolus and the articulation of the knee joint, 2 cun lateral to the edge of the tibia *Connection*: Small intestine meridian *Indication/area of influence*: Limited movement of the lower extremities, paresis as a result of stroke, facial paresis.

SP 4 *Location*: In the groove over the transition from the base of the shaft of the first metatarsal bone at the change of colour of the skin *Connection*: Stomach meridian *Indication/ area of influence*: Pain in the abdomen.

HT 5 *Location*: 1 cun proximal to HT 7 *Connection*: Small intestine meridian *Indication/area of influence*: Pain in the forearm and wrist.

SI 7 *Location*: Dorsolateral on the forearm, 5 cun proximal from SI 5; on an intended connection line between SI 5 and SI 8 *Connection*: Heart meridian *Indication/area of influence*: Pain and restricted movement of the upper extremities.

BL 58 *Location*: 1 cun distal and later BL 57 *Connection*: Kidney meridian *Indication/area of influence*: Limited movement, paresis of the legs.

KI 4 *Location*: At the upper margin of the calcaneus, 0.5 finger widths behind the medial malleolus *Connection*: Bladder meridian *Indication/area of influence*: Heel pain, lumbar spine symptoms.

PC 6 *Location*: 2 cun proximal to the middle of the palmar wrist crease between the tendons of the Mm. flexor carpi radialis and palmaris longus *Connection*: Triple heater meridian *Indication/area of influence*: Pain in the area of the forearm, chest pain, stomach pain.

TH 5 *Location*: 2 cun proximally to the middle of the dorsal wrist crease, opposite PC 6 *Connection*: Pericardium meridian *Indication/area of influence*: Pain/limited movement/sensory deficits of the upper extremities/shoulder/neck.

GB 37 *Location*: 5 cun above the lateral malleolus *Connection*: Liver meridian *Indication/area of influence*: Pain, limited movement, knee paresis, lower extremity.

LR 5 *Location*: At the medial edge of the tibia 5 cun above the medial malleolus *Connection*: Gallbladder meridian *Indication/area of influence*: Pain in the leg, pain in the lower abdomen.

GV 1 *Location*: Between the coccyx and the anus *Connection*: Governing vessel *Indication/area of influence*: Lumbar spine pain, headaches with feeling of heaviness.

CV 15 *Location*: 1 cun below the xiphoid *Connection*: Conception vessel *Indication/area of influence*: Heart and chest pain, stomach pain.

SP 21 *Location*: Medioaxillary line, sixth intercostal space *Connection*: Large vessel network *Indication/area of influence*: Pain in the thorax, generally with pain or weakness of the joints, wandering pain.

Shu and Mu points (warning and back transport points)

- **Indications:** visceral pain, segmental function disorder of the vertebral column, organ dysfunction as in TCM.
- **Principle:** segmental inhibition, activation of the cutivisceral reflex.
- Simultaneous needling of neighbouring segments strengthens the effect.

Depending on the preferred school of acupuncture, additional toning and sedation points, si cleft point, ancient Shu points, etc., may be used.

Other important acupuncture points in pain therapy

Besides the points already mentioned, there are other important acupuncture points which can be selected for their function, flow area (route of meridian) and tenderness.

Points on the large intestine meridian

LI 14 *Location*: On the lateral side of the upper arm, just over and in front of the insertion of the M. deltoideus *Function*: Local *Indication/area of influence*: Pain, paresis in the arm/shoulder, neck.

LI 15 *Location*: If the arm is lifted sideways in the anterior area of the two grooves below the acromioclavicular joint between the anterior and middle third of the M. deltoideus (in the posterior groove lies TH 14) *Function*: Local *Indication/area of influence*: Pain, limited motion, paresis in the shoulders and arms.

WARNING POINT (MU POINT)	BACK TRANSPORT POINT (SHU POINT)	CHINESE ORGAN CONNECTION	SEGMENT	INDICATION/AREA OF INFLUENCE
LU 1	BL 13	Lungs	DFS T3	Cough, cervicothoracic transition, shoulders
CV 17	BL 14	Pericardium	DFS T4	Tight feeling
CV 14	BL 15	Heart	DFS T5	Tight feeling
LR 14	BL 18	Liver	DFS T9	Pain/feeling of fullness, intercostal neuralgia
GB 24	BL 19	Gallbladder	DFS T10	Pain in the upper abdomen
LR 13	BL 20	Spleen	DFS T11	Pain in thorax, intercostal neuralgia
CV 12	BL 21	Stomach	DFS T12	Pain and epigastric heaviness
CV 5	BL 22	Triple heater	DFS L1	Abdominal pain
GB 25	BL 23	Kidneys	DFS L2	Intercostal neuralgia
ST 25	BL 25	Large intestine	DFS L4	Pain and feeling of tension in the abdomen
CV 4	BL 27	Small intestine	For. sacr. 1	Lower abdominal pain
CV 3	BL 28	Bladder	For. sacr. 2	Lower abdominal pain

Points on the stomach meridian

ST 5 *Location*: On the anterior margin of the insertion of the masseter to the mandible – blow out the cheeks – over the palpation site of the facial artery *Function*: Local *Indication/area of influence*: Cheek pain, facial paresis, trigeminal neuralgia.

ST 6 *Location*: 1 cun in front of or above the mandibular angle *Function*: Local *Indication/area of influence*: temporomandibular joint arthritis, neck pain, paresis in the area of the face.

ST 7 *Location*: Below the middle of the zygomatic arch *Function*: Drives out wind, relieves pain *Indication/area of influence*: Restricted movement of the mandible, facial paresis, trigeminal neuralgia.

ST 8 *Location*: In the angle of the forehead and temple, 3 cun above and 1 cun behind the orbital/zygomatic bone angle *Function*: Drives out wind, relieves pain *Indication/area of influence*: Forehead and one-sided headache.

ST 44 *Location*: Interdigital crease between the second and third toe close to the proximal phalanx of the second toe *Function*: Drives out wind, relieves pain *Indication/area of influence*: Pain in the foot, head and abdomen.

Points on the spleen meridian

SP 6 *Location*: 3 cun above the highest point of the medial malleolus on the posterior margin of the tibia *Function*: Crossing point of the 3 Yin meridians *Indication/area of influence*: Limited movement, sensory deficits, pain, paresis of the lower extremities.

SP 9 *Location*: With the knee bent in a hollow under the medial tibial condyle at the same level as GB 34 *Function*: Meer-he point *Indication/area of influence*: Pain/swelling in knee, pain/feeling of tension in the abdomen.

Points on the heart meridian

HT 3 *Location*: With maximum flexion of the arm between the end of the crook of the elbow and the ulnar epicondyle *Function*: Meer-he point *Indication/area of influence*: Pain and limited movement of the elbow joint.

HT 5 *Location*: 1 cun proximal to HT 7 *Function*: Transit point (Luo point) to SI 4.

Points on the small intestine meridian

SI 6 *Location*: In a hollow just proximal and radial to the ulnar styloid process *Function*: Xi cleft point *Indication/area of influence*: Symptoms in the area of the forearm, shoulder and neck pain.

SI 9 *Location*: 1 cun above the end of the axillary fold with the arm hanging down *Function*: Important local point for shoulder symptoms *Indication/area of influence*: Pain, limited motion in the shoulder blade region and upper extremity.

SI 10 *Location*: Lower margin of the spina scapulae, vertically above SI 9 *Function*: Crossing point of the Yang wei mai and Yang qiao mai *Indication/area of influence*: Pain, weakness, limited movement of the shoulders and arms.

SI 11 *Location*: Middle of the infraspinata fossa at the level of the spinous process of T5 *Function*: Local *Indication/area of influence*: Pain in the shoulder blade, in the lateral and posterior arm and elbow

SI 12 *Location*: If arm is lifted sideways, in a hollow in the middle of the suprascapular fossa *Function*: Local *Indication/area of influence*: Pain in the shoulder blade region, sensory deficits, pain in the arms.

SI 13 *Location*: In the middle part of the supraspinata fossa where the spina scapulae bends; in the middle between SI 10 (lower border of the scapula, vertically above the axillary fold) and the spinous process of T2 *Function*: Drives out wind, relaxes tendons and muscles, relieves pain *Indication/area of influence*: Pain, stiffness, limited movement of shoulders and neck.

SI 14 *Location*: In the upper scapular region; 3 cun lateral to the lower border of the spinous process of T1 *Function*: mTrPs in the M. levator scapulae *Indication/area of influence*: Pain in the back, shoulder, limited movement, pain in the neck.

SI 18 *Location*: At the anterior border of the insertion of the masseter at the maxilla; teeth biting together or mouth open wide *Function*: Local, especially for wind diseases in the area of the head *Indication/area of influence*: Facial paresis, facial spasms, trigeminal neuralgia.

Points on the bladder meridian

BL 2 *Location*: Intersection of the medial end of the eyebrow/eyelid – supraorbital foramen *Function*: Local *Indication/area of influence*: Frontal headaches, migraine, facial paresis, trigeminal neuralgia.

BL 10 *Location*: Insertion of the trapezius at the external occipital protuberance *Function*: Local *Indication/area of influence*: Neck stiffness and pain, cervical and lumbar spine symptoms, headaches.

BL 13 *Location*: 1.5 cun lateral to the spinous process of T3 *Function*: Back transport point (Shu point) lungs *Indication/area of influence*: Bronchitis, cough, sleeplessness, exhaustion.

BL 14 *Location*: 1.5 cun lateral to the spinous process of T4 *Function*: Back transport point (Shu point) pericardium *Indication/area of influence*: Tight feeling.

BL 15 *Location*: 1.5 cun lateral to the spinous process of T5 *Function*: Back transport point (Shu point) heart *Indication/*

area of influence: Pain in the area of the thoracic spine, thorax, lateral costal arch.

BL 16 *Location*: 1.5 cun lateral to the spinous process of T6 *Function*: Back transport point (Shu point) Du mai *Indication/area of influence*: Thoracic spine or thoracic pain.

BL 18 *Location*: 2 cun lateral to the spinous process of T9 *Function*: Back transport point (Shu point) liver *Indication/area of influence*: Pain in back, lateral rib region.

BL 19 *Location*: 1.5 cun lateral to the spinous process of T10 *Function*: Back transport point (Shu point) gallbladder *Indication/area of influence*: Pain in the thoracic spine, thorax, lateral costal arch.

BL 20 *Location*: 1.5 cun lateral to the spinous process of T11 *Function*: Back transport point (Shu point) spleen *Indication/area of influence*: Pain/feeling of tension in the thoracic and lumbar spine and abdomen.

BL 21 *Location*: 1.5 cun lateral to the spinous process of T12 *Function*: Back transport point (Shu point) stomach *Indication/area of influence*: Pain in the thoracic spine, lumbar spine, epigastrium.

BL 22 *Location*: 1.5 cun lateral to the spinous process of L1 *Function*: Back transport point (Shu point) triple heater *Indication/area of influence*: Lumbar spine symptoms, feeling of tension in the abdomen.

BL 23 *Location*: 1.5 cun lateral to the spinous process of L2, i.e. lateral to SI 4 *Function*: Back transport point (Shu point) kidneys *Indication/area of influence*: Chronic knee symptoms.

BL 24 *Location*: 1.5 cun lateral to the spinous process of L3 *Function*: Back transport point (Shu point) Ren 6 *Indication/area of influence*: Lumbar spine symptoms.

BL 25 *Location*: 1.5 cun lateral to the spinous process of L4 *Function*: Back transport point (Shu point) large intestine *Indication/area of influence*: Pain and restricted movement in the lumbar spine, hips, lower extremities.

BL 26 *Location*: 1.5 cun lateral to the spinous process of L5 *Function*: Back transport point (Shu point) Ren 4 *Indication/area of influence*: Lumbar spine symptoms, diseases of the sciatic nerve.

BL 27 *Location*: 1.5 cun lateral to the posterior midline next to the first sacral foramen *Function*: Back transport point (Shu point) small intestine *Indication/area of influence*: Symptoms in the lumbar spine/iliosacral joint, pain in the lower abdomen.

BL 28 *Location*: 1.5 cun lateral to the posterior midline next to the second sacral foramen *Function*: Back transport point (Shu point) bladder *Indication/area of influence*: Symptoms in the lumbar spine, sacral region.

BL 30 *Location*: 1.5 cun lateral to the posterior midline next to the fourth sacral foramen *Function*: Back transport point (Shu point) perineum *Indication/area of influence*: Symptoms, cold sensations in the lumbosacral area or hip region.

BL 31 *Location*: In the first sacral foramen *Function*: Strengthens the kidneys and the lumbar area *Indication/area of influence*: Lumbar spine symptoms, pain, limited movement of the knee.

BL 32 *Location*: In the second sacral foramen at the same level as BL 28 (back transport point bladder) *Function*: Supports the lower back *Indication/area of influence*: Pain in the lumbar or sacral region.

Bl 33 *Location*: In the third sacral foramen *Function*: Supports the lower back *Indication/area of influence*: Pain in the lumbar or sacral region.

BL 34 *Location*: In the fourth sacral foramen *Function*: Supports the lower back *Indication/area of influence*: Pain in the lumbar or sacral region.

BL 36 *Location*: In the middle of the gluteal fold *Function*: Supports the lower back *Indication/area of influence*: Lumbosacral or gluteal pain, pain and sensory deficits of the lower extremities.

BL 39 *Location*: Lateral (Yang) of the Wei zhong point at the medial side of the biceps tendon *Function*: Lower Meer-xiahe point *Indication/area of influence*: Knee and lumbar spine symptoms.

BL 40 *Location*: In the middle of the knee joint transverse crease between the tendons of the semitendinosus and biceps *Function*: Meer-he point, master point for back and lumbar region *Indication/area of influence*: Limited movement, sensory deficits, pain, paresis of the lower extremities.

BL 41 *Location*: 3 cun lateral to the posterior midline at the level of the spinous process of T2, lateral to BL 12, at the medial scapular border *Function*: Crossing point with small intestine meridian *Indication/area of influence*: Pain or restricted movement/sensory deficits of shoulder, thoracic spine, neck, elbow, arms.

BL 42 *Location*: 3 cun lateral to the posterior midline at the level of the spinous process of T3, lateral to BL 13 (back transport point LU), at the medial scapular border *Function*: Regulates Lu-qi *Indication/area of influence*: Pain in the thoracic spine and shoulder, neck stiffness.

BL 43 *Location*: 3 cun lateral to the posterior midline at the level of the spinous process of T4, lateral to BL 14 (back transport point PC), at the medial scapular border *Function*: Important point for deficiency syndromes *Indication/area of influence*: Thoracic spine symptoms.

BL 44 *Location*: 3 cun lateral to the posterior midline at the level of the spinous process of T5, lateral to BL 15 (back transport point HT), at the medial scapular border *Function*: Regulates Qi *Indication/area of influence*: Thoracic spine symptoms.

BL 45 *Location*: 3 cun lateral to the posterior midline at the level of the spinous process of T6 (SI 10), lateral to BL 16 (back transport point SI), at the medial scapular border *Function*: Ends pain *Indication/area of influence*: Thoracic spine or shoulder symptoms.

BL 46 *Location*: 3 cun lateral to the posterior midline at the level of the spinous process of T7, about the level of the inferior scapular angle, lateral to BL (back transport point diaphragm) *Function*: Makes the meridians open *Indication/area of influence*: Thoracic spine symptoms.

BL 47 *Location*: 3 cun lateral to the posterior midline at the level of the spinous process of T9, lateral to BL 18 (back transport point LR) *Function*: Promotes harmonic Qi flow *Indication/area of influence*: Symptoms in the thorax, thoracic spine, lumbar spine, at the lateral costal arch.

BL 48 *Location*: 3 cun lateral to the posterior midline at the level of the spinous process of T10, lateral to BL 19 (back transport point GB) *Indication/area of influence*: Symptoms in the thorax, thoracic spine, lumbar spine, at the lateral costal arch.

BL 49 *Location*: 3 cun lateral to the posterior midline at the level of the spinous process of T11, lateral to BL 20 (back transport point SP) *Indication/area of influence*: Pain in the thoracic/lumbar spine.

BL 50 *Location*: 3 cun lateral to the posterior midline at the level of the spinous process of T12, lateral to BL 21 (back transport point ST) *Function*: Removes stagnation *Indication/area of influence*: Pain in the thoracic spine, lumbar spine.

BL 51 *Location*: 3 cun lateral to the posterior midline at the level of the spinous process of L1, lateral to BL 22 (back transport point TH) *Function*: Disperses nutritional stagnation *Indication/area of influence*: Feeling of tension in the abdomen.

BL 52 *Location*: 3 cun lateral to the posterior midline at the level of the spinous process of L2, lateral to BL 23 (back transport point KI) *Function*: Strengthens lower back *Indication/area of influence*: Lumbar spine and knee symptoms.

BL 53 *Location*: 3 cun lateral to the posterior midline at the level of the spinous process of S2, lateral to BL 28 (back transport point BL) *Function*: Strengthens lower back *Indication/area of influence*: Pain in the lumbar spine or lumbosacral region.

BL 54 *Location*: 3 cun lateral to the posterior midline at the level of the spinous process of S4, lateral to BL 30 and BL 34 *Function*: Strengthens lower back *Indication/area of influence*: Symptoms in the lumbar spine or sacral area.

BL 57 *Location*: In the angle between the two gastrocnemius muscles; standing on the toes; middle between BL 40 and BL 60 *Function*: Strengthens lower back *Indication/area of influence*: Limited movement of the lower extremities.

BL 60 *Location*: Middle between the Achilles tendon and the highest point of the lateral malleolus *Function*: Jing river point *Indication/area of influence*: Neck stiffness, pain in the shoulders, back, arms, weakness and paresis of the lower extremities.

Points on the kidney meridian

KI 3 *Location*: Between the strongest protrusion of the medial malleolus and the Achilles tendon *Function*: Source point (Yuan point) kidneys *Indication/area of influence*: Lumbar spine symptoms, knee, ear.

KI 7 *Location*: At the anterior border of the Achilles tendon behind the M. flexor digit. long, 2 cun above the greater prominence of the medial malleolus = 2 cun above KI 3 *Function*: Jing river point *Indication/area of influence*: Limited movement of the lower extremities, lumbar spine symptoms.

KI 16 *Location*: 0.5 cun lateral to the median, at the level of the navel, i.e. next to Ren 8 *Function*: Crossing point with the Chong Mai *Indication/area of influence*: Pain and feeling of tension in the abdomen.

KI 27 *Location*: At the lower border of the sternoclavicular joint *Function*: Thoracic pain, cough *Indication/area of influence*: Relaxes the thorax.

Points on the triple heater meridian

TH 3 *Location*: Between the fourth and fifth metacarpals on the back of the hand in the groove proximal to the metacarpophalangeal joint with balled fist *Function*: Bach-shu point *Indication/area of influence*: Pain or limited movement in the forearm, hand, headaches.

TH 8 *Location*: 4 cun proximal to the middle of the posterior wrist crease *Function*: Crossing point of the three Yang meridians *Indication/area of influence*: Pain or sensory deficits in the arms, shoulders, neck, pain in the thorax.

TH 14 *Location*: With arm lifted in the hollow behind and under the acromion, between the middle and posterior part of the deltoideus muscle (in front LI 15) *Function*: Local *Indication/area of influence*: Shoulder symptoms, pain, limited movement of the arm.

TH 15 *Location*: At the superior scapular angle, middle between GB 21 (highest point of the shoulder, middle between acromion and spinous process of C7) and SI 13 (in the medial part of the supraspinata fossa, at the bend of the spina scapulae!) *Function*: Crossing point with Yang Wei mai *Indication/area of influence*: Shoulder or neck pain or stiffness, cervical spine syndrome.

TH 17 *Location*: At the anterior border of the mastoid *Function*: Crossing point with gallbladder meridian *Indication/area of influence*: Facial paresis, trigeminal neuralgia.

TH 19 *Location*: 1 cun above the middle of the mastoid process (TH 18) *Function*: Eliminates wind *Indication/area of influence*: Headaches, tinnitus.

TH 21 *Location*: At the level of the Incisura supratragica, with the mouth open, in the groove above the mandibular condyle *Function*: Local *Indication/area of influence*: Pain in the temporomandibular joint, maxillofacial diseases.
TH 23 *Location*: In a hollow at the lateral end of the eyebrow *Function*: Local *Indication/area of influence*: Headaches, facial paresis.

Points on the gallbladder meridian

GB 1 *Location*: 0.5 cun lateral from the outer angle of the eye *Function*: Drives out wind *Indication/area of influence*: Headaches, facial paresis.
GB 2 *Location*: With mouth open in the groove in front of the incisura intertragica, behind the ascending branch of the mandible *Function*: Local *Indication/area of influence*: temporomandibular joint pain, maxillofacial diseases, migraine.
GB 8 *Location*: 1.5 cun above the tip of the external ear *Function*: Relieves pain *Indication/area of influence*: One-sided headache, migraine.
GB 14 *Location*: 1 cun above the middle of the eyebrow, mediopupillary line *Function*: Drives out wind *Indication/area of influence*: Frontal headache, facial paresis.
GB 20 *Location*: Behind the mastoid between the trapezius and the sternocleidomastoideus muscle at the lower occipital border *Function*: Drives away inner and outer wind *Indication/area of influence*: Neck and pain at the back of the head, trigeminal neuralgia, facial paresis.
GB 21 *Location*: At the highest point of the shoulder, midway between the acromion and spinous process of C7 *Function*: Local shoulder point *Indication/area of influence*: Neck stiffness, pain and functional disorder of the shoulder, restricted movement of the upper extremities.
GB 26 *Location*: In the anterior axillary line, in front of the highest point of the iliac crest at the level of the navel *Function*: Crossing point of the Dai mai *Indication/area of influence*: Pain in the lumbar or thoracic region, intercostal neuralgia.
GB 27 *Location*: 3 cun below the level of the navel (at the level of Ren 4), in front of the superior anterior iliac spine *Function*: Crossing point of the Dai mai *Indication/area of influence*: Lumbar spine and hip symptoms.
GB 28 *Location*: 0.5 cun below the superior anterior iliac spine *Function*: Regulates the Dai mai *Indication/area of influence*: Lumbar spine and hip symptoms.
GB 30 *Location*: On the connecting line between the greater trochanter and the sacral hiatus, at the transition from the lower to the middle third *Function*: Drives out wind *Indication/area of influence*: Pain in the lumbar region, hips, sensory deficits, pain of the lower extremities.

GB 31 *Location*: Laterally on the thigh, where the middle finger points on the outer trouser seam when the arm hangs down loosely *Function*: Local *Indication/area of influence*: Restricted movement, pain, sensory deficits of the leg.

Points on the liver meridian

LR 8 *Location*: With bent knee in the groove in front of the end of the medial knee joint fold *Function*: Meer-he point *Indication/area of influence*: Knee symptoms, pain in the abdomen, lumbosacral region.

Points on the governing vessel

GV 3 *Location*: Under spinous process of L4; affects the superior opposite pole as a result of influence on the lower section of the vertebral column *Indication/area of influence*: Pain in the coccyx, weakness and numbness of the lower extremities.
GV 4 *Location*: Below spinous process of L2, laterally to BL 23 and BL 47 *Indication/area of influence*: Lumbar spine symptoms with feeling of cold and weakness, back stiffness, sciatica.
GV 5 *Location*: Below spinous process of L1, lateral to BL 22 *Function*: Strengthens Qi in lumbar spine *Indication/area of influence*: Lumbar spine stiffness.
GV 14 *Location*: Below spinous process of C7 *Function*: Sea of Qi point *Indication/area of influence*: Neck stiffness, back muscle tension.
GV 16 *Location*: 1 cun above the occipital hairline, in the groove below the external occipital protuberance *Function*: Lets out wind *Indication/area of influence*: Headaches, neck stiffness.
GV 20 *Location*: On the connection line of the two auricular apices *Function*: Sea of Qi point *Indication/area of influence*: Headaches, heavy feeling in head.
GV 24 *Location*: Median, 0.5 cun inside the hairline on the forehead *Function*: Eliminates wind *Indication/area of influence*: Headaches.

Points on the conception vessel

CV 6 *Location*: 1,5 cun below the navel *Function*: Strengthens Yang *Indication/area of influence*: Lower abdominal pain, severe paraumbilical pain.
CV 22 *Location*: Middle of the jugular *Function*: Crossing point of the Yin wei mai *Indication/area of influence*: Cough, hoarseness.
CV 24 *Location*: In the middle of the mentolabial furrow *Function*: Disperses wind *Indication/area of influence*: Anaesthesia point for tooth extraction, facial paresis, trigeminal neuralgia.

Extra points

Abbreviations: Ex-HN, extra point head and neck; Ex-AH, extra point arm and hand; Ex-B, extra point back; Ex-LF, extra point leg and foot.

Ex-HN 1 *Location*: Four points each 1 cun anterior, posterior, medial and lateral from GV 20 *Function*: Calms spirit *Indication/area of influence*: Headaches, dizziness.

Ex-HN 3 *Location*: In the middle between the eyebrows *Function*: Disperses wind *Indication/area of influence*: Headaches.

Ex-HN 4 *Location*: Middle of the eyebrows, vertically above the pupils if looking straight ahead *Function*: Relieves pain and tension *Indication/area of influence*: Eye pain.

Ex-HN 5 *Location*: Palpable hollow 1 cun posterior to the midpoint between the lateral end of the eyebrow and the lateral canthus *Function*: Disperses wind *Indication/area of influence*: Frontal headaches, migraine, facial paresis, trigeminal neuralgia.

Ex-AH 7 *Location*: Two points on the back of the hand between the second and third and fourth and fifth metacarpal bones, 1 cun distal to the dorsal wrist crease *Function*: Harmonisation of Qi and blood flow *Indication/area of influence*: Lumbago, sciatica.

Ex-AH 8 *Location*: On the back of the hand between the second and third metacarpal bones, 0.5 cun proximal to the metacarpophalangeal joint *Function*: Harmonisation of Qi and blood flow *Indication/area of influence*: Neck and shoulder pain, cervical syndrome.

Ex-AH 9 *Location*: Four points on the back of the hand at the transition from light to darker skin, in the middle of the webbing (digits II–V) *Indication/area of influence*: Arthrosis and arthritis in the fingers.

Ex-B 2 *Location*: 17 pairs of points which each lie 0.5 cun lateral to the lower borders of the spinous process, on both sides of the vertebral column in the area of the small vertebral joints; 12 thoracic points lie between T1 and T12, five lumbar points between L1 and L5 *Indication/area of influence*: Intercostal neuralgia.

Ex-B 6 *Location*: 3 cun lateral to the lower border of the spinous process of L4 or on the lateral branch of the bladder meridian at the same level as BL 25 *Function*: Activates blood circulation *Indication/area of influence*: Lumbago.

Ex-LF 1 *Location*: Pair of points lying 2 cun above the patella and each 1.5 cun lateral and medial to ST 34 *Function*: Make meridians open, stop pain *Indication/area of influence*: Pain in the hip and knee joint.

Ex-LF 2 *Location*: With slightly flexed knee, in the middle of the upper border of the patella *Indication/area of influence*: Knee and leg pain.

Ex-LF 5 *Location*: With flexed knee in two hollows medial and lateral to the patellar ligament below the patella; the lateral eye of the knee corresponds to ST 35 *Indication/area of influence*: Diseases of the knee joint.

Ex-LF 10 *Location*: Four points on the back of the foot in the middle of the webbing *Function*: Disperses wind, relieves pain *Indication/area of influence*: Arthrosis and arthritis of the toes.

22.2.9 Disease theory, symptoms and pain

Diseases or symptoms can become apparent in the meridians (rather superficially; e.g. headaches, locomotor system) or affect the organs (meaning internal disease). This is how TCM distinguishes between external and internal diseases. An internal organ dysfunction can be the basis for an external meridian disorder. Inner disorders are frequently distinguished according to complex Zang-Fu theory (Chinese organ theory). Fig. 22.8 shows the process of diagnosis in TCM.

There are also simple general causes of disease such as trauma, overexertion, stress, poor diet and an unhealthy lifestyle. In certain cases, a distinction can also be made between external factors (cold, wind, moisture, heat, dryness, summer heat) and internal factors (fear, anxiety, brooding, sadness, annoyance, joy, worry).

Depending on the symptoms and findings, there can also be a disorder of the blood, Qi or essences. There are also many other points of view and traditions within TCM which are also differently evaluated depending on differences in time and geography.

Diagnosis

Four diagnostic methods

- **Inspection:** constitution, posture, skin colour, mucous membranes, tongue, sensory organs.
- **Auscultation and odour:** speech, respiration, odours.
- **Listening:** history of illness, symptoms, lifestyle.
- **Palpation/examination:** pulse, area of pain, meridians, acupuncture points, functional examination muscles, joints, vertebral column, neurology.

Eight diagnostic principles

The eight diagnostic principles are Yin and Yang, interior and exterior, emptiness and fullness, and cold and heat.

Yin–Yang:
- superordinate criterion,
- fullness, heat and exterior are attributed to Yang,
- emptiness, cold and interior are attributed to Yin.

Interior–exterior: internal diseases:
- differentiation from Zang-Fu theory or theory of Qi and blood,
- external diseases: distinction based on meridian theory.

Emptiness–fullness: crucial for stimulation (intensity):
- empty signs can be: long course of disease, deep-seated pain, paleness, sensitivity to cold, autonomic and/or psychoemotional exhaustion, and hypotension; these require less needling, little stimulation (filling stimulation) and moxibustion,

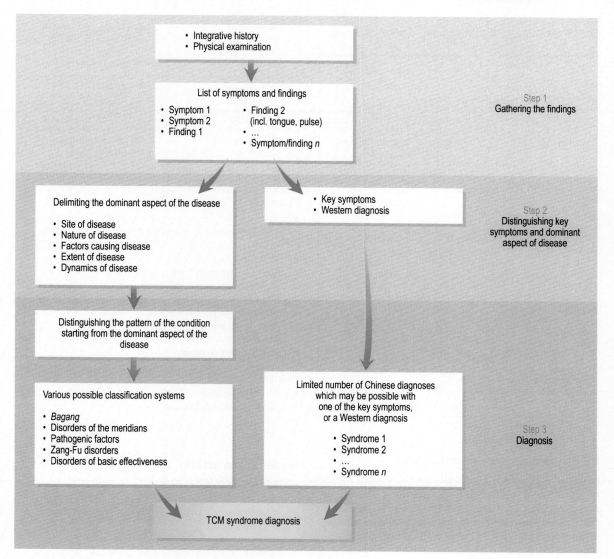

Fig. 22.8 The process of syndrome diagnosis from TCM.
(From Bäcker, Hammes 2004)

- full signs can be: acute symptoms, reddening, severe pain and hypertension; these require more needling, stronger stimulation (diverting stimulation techniques), cupping and micro bloodletting;

Cold–heat: crucial for the type of stimulation: moxa, cupping, micro bloodletting:

- heat symptoms may be: reddening, fever, thirst, constipation and deep yellow urine,

- cold symptoms can be: pallor, sensitivity to cold, lack of thirst, clear urine, pale tongue and slow pulse,
- caused by exogenic cold or Yang weakness.

Classifying pain qualities in TCM

Myofascial pain can be classified in many cases using the Chinese picture of 'Qi stagnation'. If there is local pain without referral, from the point of view of TCM the term 'blood stagnation' can apply. Depending on the cause, the relevant acupuncture points are then used, as shown here.

PAIN QUALITY	EVIDENCE OF	ACUPUNCTURE POINTS
Referred, changing, distending, diffuse pain	Qi stagnation	LR 3, ST 36, LI 4
Distending pain with headache	Heat/fire	ST 44, LR 2, micro bloodletting at Tai yang
Sharp, stabbing, localised pain	Blood stagnation: micro bloodletting	LI 4, SP 10, probing, micro bloodletting
Pain with feeling of heaviness	Moisture is blocking Qi and blood	SP 9, ST 40
Pounding, pulsing pain (e.g. migraine)	Liver disorder	LR 2, LR 3, GB 34, TH5
Burning pain	Pathogenic fire/ heat, Yin weakness	GV 14, LI 11, TH5
Astringent, dull cold pain	Pathogenic cold, Yang-qi weakness	CV 6 (moxa), KI 3, heat application

Indications and contraindications

For acute and chronic myofascial pain and limited motion with myofascial involvement, acupuncture has a predominantly analgesic and muscle-relaxing effect. Depending on the location and the severity of the myofascial symptoms, various forms of acupuncture can be used (microsystem acupuncture, meridian and functional anatomically based selection of points, dry needling).

Other important indications are listed here.

- Mild to moderately severe acute pain (use with severe or very acute pain, only by experienced therapists with the additional aid of special stimulation techniques)
- Analgesia for smaller diagnostic and therapeutic procedures (e.g. for patients with analgesic/anaesthetic intolerance): endoscopy, puncture
- Tension headaches, migraine
- Facial pain
- Temporomandibular syndrome
- Periarthropathies
- Tendinopathies
- Cervical spine syndrome
- Epicondylopathy
- Overload syndrome
- Impingement syndrome with muscular involvement
- Post-thoracotomy syndrome
- Segmental function disorder of the vertebral column
- Functional visceral pain syndrome
- Lumbago and sciatica with musculoligamentary involvement
- Post-traumatic pain
- Piriformis syndrome
- Coxarthrosis
- Gonarthrosis, chondropathia patellae, muscular imbalance of the M. quadriceps femoris

---

Some specific circumstances require close indication and many years of experience:

- acupuncture during pregnancy (back pain, carpal tunnel syndrome, analgesia during birth, child in incorrect position),
- tumour pain,
- neuropathic pain (better response to electrostimulation acupuncture, ESA),
- fibromyalgia,
- somatoform pain disorder.

Negative indications:
- irreversible conditions,
- spinal canal stenosis,
- cluster headaches.

Contraindications:
- clinically manifest clotting disorder for deep needling,
- life-threatening diseases,
- epilepsy,
- psychosis.

Undesirable effects

- haematoma,
- prolonged local pain,
- hypotensive circulatory reaction (needle collapse),
- increase in pain,
- nerve lesion,
- causing an epileptic attack in epileptics,
- infection (especially dangerous with long-term needles),
- pneumothorax (the most common serious adverse event).

Large studies have shown that acupuncture is a safe procedure with few side effects.

Course of action

Prerequisites
- Patient agreement and short explanation (form-free documentation).
- Certain diagnosis before acupuncture.
- No delay with diagnosis and therapy of acute diseases.
- Practical application requires sufficient theoretical and practical training.

- For patients suffering from chronic pain, only use acupuncture as part of a multimodal treatment plan.
- For pain in the locomotor system, combination with physiotherapy and physical medicine.
- No delay if invasive measures are indicated for impingement syndrome.
- Acupuncture should be used in cooperation with the patient as active/activating therapy for chronic pain syndrome:
  - which points/techniques are felt to be effective?
  - self-treatment of effective points/acupressure/ partner massage.
  - increase in body perception by control of the de Qi feeling.

Number of needles and duration of treatment

- On average, between 4 and 24 needles are used.
- Treatment lasts between 20 and 45 min.
- Treatments are usually carried out once or twice a week or up to twice a day if symptoms are acute.

Positioning the patient

- Treatment is usually on a bed or couch because of the risk of collapse.
- Use cushions or a knee roll, etc. for optimum positioning of the patient with the muscles relaxed.

Carrying out the needling

An important criterion for choosing the points in question is to use palpation to detect any increased sensitivity to pressure.

- Needle insertion: hold the needle with the first three fingers and place the other hand, thumb or second and third fingers next to the acupuncture point, pressing gently and lightly supporting the needling hand (ulnar border of the hand, little finger); insert the needle quickly to the subcutaneous level and probe deeper with light right–left rotational movements (depending on the tissue and the point) and cause the de Qi needle sensation (see Fig. 22.9).
- Only use sterile disposable needles.
- On the face and in tissue with little subcutaneous fatty tissue or muscles and for microsystems, only use short, thin needles (10–15 mm long, 0.10–0.20 mm diameter; often written as 0.10–0.20 × 10–15), needle tangentially if necessary and/or form skin folds (see Fig. 22.9).
- Needle tangentially at the thorax (note: pneumothorax).
- Needles should be as long as necessary (usually 30 mm, with deep needling, e.g. lumbar, pelvic and hip region up to 80 mm).
- Begin with distal points (distal meridian points, microsystem points, general analgesic points such as LI 4, ST 36, LR 3).

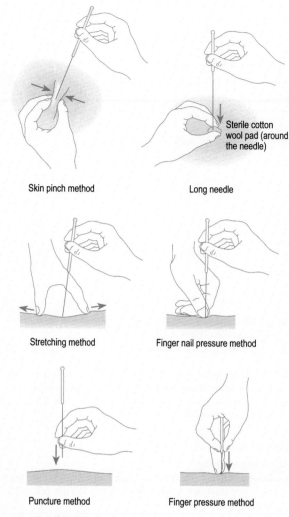

Fig. 22.9 Insertion methods. *(From Focks, Hillenbrand 2006)*

- The intensity of the local treatment depends on the patient's reaction.
- Remove any needles causing pain or correct the position.
- Individually determine the number and choice of points (see Fig. 22.10):
  - depending on effect delivered,
  - depending on the location of the pain,
  - depending on the tenderness of the points on palpation,
  - depending on the patient's condition,
  - depending on the local findings,
  - depending on the symptoms which are currently to the fore.

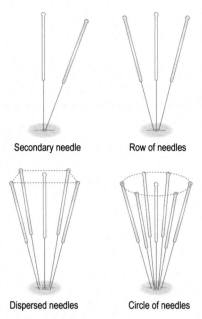

Fig. 22.10 Number of needles used.
(From Focks, Hillenbrand 2003)

- The intensity of the needle stimulation is based on the patient's condition according to the fullness/emptiness rules (see Eight diagnostic principles, Section 22.2.9, above; see also Fig. 22.11).

Special techniques

Micro bloodletting
- Lesion with the intended letting of blood after needling with acupuncture needle, three-edged needle (Chin.) or cannula.
- Indicated for severe pain at certain points (e.g. BL 40, Tai yang).

Cupping (see Section 20.4)
- Drawing-out procedure performed with glass cups.
- Low pressure is created by means of a rubber valve or heat.
- Indicated for pain in the locomotor system (e.g. on mTrPs) or as a segmental treatment for visceral pain.
- Cupping massage over the paravertebral muscles (bladder meridian) and as massage by a partner.

Clinical studies

Several hundred randomised controlled clinical research projects have been carried out on the use of acupuncture for a very wide range of topics. It is therefore one of the best researched procedures in pain therapy. For the indications of postoperative toothache and nausea and vomiting

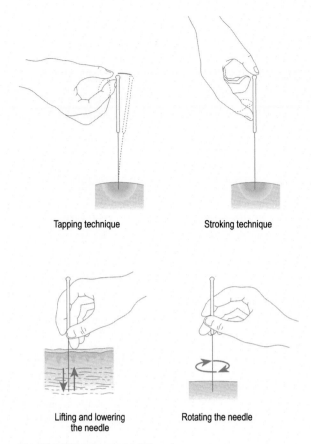

Fig. 22.11 Needle manipulation.

(postoperative and chemotherapy-induced) it is evidence based (Level 1). For some other indications such as migraine, tension headaches, lumbar spine pain, temporomandibular dysfunction, fibromyalgia, pain from knee joint arthritis and epicondylopathy there is a predominance of positive study results. In spite of this large number of studies, views on the efficacy of acupuncture are inconclusive, mostly due to study design (therapist blinding is not possible; no real, generally recognised placebo control procedures; many different forms of the application of acupuncture), so comparison of study results can only be limited.

The biggest studies so far have been carried out by health insurance companies on the indications of headaches, back pain and gonarthrosis (ART, GERAC). However, they still could not definitely explain the efficacy of the technique. This led to statements by opinion formers and in some of the lay press that 'acupuncture is a placebo', which is not fair from a scientific point of view. However, various authors offered different interpretations (Bäcker et al.;

Deutsche Ärztegesellschaft für Akupunktur (the German Society of Acupuncture Doctors)):

- verum acupuncture basically showed clinically relevant effects in all the indications investigated,
- the therapeutic efficacy corresponds to that of standard therapies. For gonarthrosis and chronic back pain, acupuncture showed greater therapeutic success than conventional standard therapy,
- in some studies verum acupuncture proved superior to minimal acupuncture,
- for migraine the therapeutic effect was comparable to pharmacological therapy (beta-blockers),

Acupuncture can be classified as a safe procedure where severe undesirable events occur extremely rarely (Melchart et al. 2004).

There are few randomised controlled studies available on the efficacy of acupuncture specifically for myofascial pain:

- with temporomandibular syndrome, which is frequently associated with a myofascial disorder, it can be assumed that acupuncture provides good pain relief (Rosted 2001),
- for patients with chronic myofascial cervical spine symptoms, a single acupuncture treatment showed an immediate effect of relief of pain and improvement in mobility (Irnich et al. 2002),
- there is also definite evidence that patients with chronic cervical spine symptoms in particular benefit from a course of acupuncture treatment if the main cause of the symptoms is a MPS (Birch, Jamison 1998, Irnich et al. 2001).

A clinically relevant effect from acupuncture for myofascial pain has been observed in most cases but the specificity of the acupuncture points and concepts has not yet been sufficiently demonstrated (Cummings, White, 2001).

22.3 KIIKO MATSUMOTO ACUPUNCTURE

David Euler

22.3.1 Introduction

Development of the method

In her acupuncture method, Kiiko Matsumoto combines the approaches of many leading Japanese acupuncturists with her own clinical experience and ideas. She worked closely with Dr Manaka (whose approach also drew from many sources) and the teachers Nagano and Kawai. After long and intense clinical work, and study and interpretation of Chinese classicists, Kiiko has brought together various approaches to form a coherent, very effective and unique method.

In a large number of diagnostic and therapeutic measures in this acupuncture method there are references to various acupuncturists as well as to traditional Chinese acupuncture. In general the actual acupuncture is very much based on the use of immediately palpable changes in the patient's body but is closely associated with the methods used in Nan Ching, Su Wen, Ling Shu, etc.

In the method described here, many ideas from these classical works, written in an unclear way that is difficult to understand, have been practically implemented and combined with modern Western medicine. David Euler's careful work has created a coherent combination between traditional Chinese acupuncture and the theories of Western medicine. This combination makes the method extraordinarily learnable but still allows the user to comfortably grasp Eastern and Western terminology.

The main characteristic of this method of acupuncture is the very close relationship between the various medical theories and the human body. Such a relationship is achieved by palpation and verification of acupuncture points as further explained later in this introduction. In general the acupuncture points are chosen according to their positive effect on the body, which is verified by palpation, feeling the pulse or measuring other changes in the body. Many reflex zones relate to various possible pathological changes.

The expression 'reflex zones' or 'reflex' is occasionally used to describe areas of the body which react to the acupuncture point stimulation and are of diagnostic value. For example, the areas between KI 15 and ST 27 on the left side are regarded as reflex zones for blood stagnation in the abdomen (*Oketsu*). Pain on pressure of the *Oketsu* sign subsides with correct needling of LR 4 and LU 5 (reflex reaction).

> The treatment points that successfully reduce tenderness are used both for diagnosis and for treatment.

Basic treatment

Basic treatment that targets the cause of the disease forms the basis for almost all acupuncture procedures in this method, without taking into account specific symptoms. The underlying diagnosis and therapy are based on palpable findings, clinical symptoms and history. The treatment is adapted to the problems presented, which have led to a specific clinical symptom or which block the natural healing mechanisms of the body. The positive effect of local or specific treatment approaches that treat the main symptoms does not often last for long without basic treatment.

If the basic treatment is not carried out at first, the treatment of a specific problem can make this worse or the treatment does not work at all. This frequently occurs with patients with a stomach Qi deficiency, adrenal deficiency and/or blood stagnation in the abdomen.

Other basic problems such as structural imbalance, scar tissue, hormonal disorders or disorders of the autonomic nervous system can also display a profound effect on the body.

> From the experiences of many well-known practitioners, from our own clinical experience and from reading traditional Chinese works and from Nagano's teaching it clear that treating the patient's symptoms alone does not lead to 'healing' or to permanent relief.

Underlying disorders which have produced a specific disease or prevent the body from recovering must first be treated or integrated into the treatment plan.

This approach is not new and is taught and practised in many schools. There are many ways of describing these underlying disorders. You can use for example, the five elements theory, the Zang-Fu theory, the eight principles, the extraordinary meridians or root and branch.

In the following text we refer mainly to 11 main categories of disharmony at which basic treatment is aimed:

- blood stagnation in the Hara (Oketsu), the head and the vertebral artery,[1]
- abnormal immune system,
- stomach Qi deficiency,
- birth trauma, shock and trauma or 'navel disorder',
- systemic detoxication,
- disorders of the autonomic nervous system,
- blood pressure disorders and cardiac disease,
- hormonal disorders,
- disorders caused by scar tissue,
- structural imbalance,
- vessel compression (in the neck, the vertebral artery and the thigh).

Each of the above disorders develops specific reflexes. As soon as one of these disharmonies is present, these reflexes are activated, as are specific symptoms; the therapist looks for these in order to diagnose and treat the underlying weaknesses. If these disorders are treated first or therapy of these disorders is added to a specific treatment, the body is supported in its recovery, leading to more thorough, complete healing.

In many cases, only very few specific points are required after treatment of the underlying disorders to help patients to full recovery of health. These 11 underlying disorders are interrelated and are mutually influential; each can cause or influence almost all patient symptoms.

Example: a patient complains of continuous sprained ankles. According to his history chart he suffered frequently from streptococcal angina as a child. There are immune reflexes in the Hara and the neck. Therapy should therefore include acupuncture points directed at the immune system. As it is mostly one leg that is affected, which can lead to damage to the ligaments of the other leg, measures against the structural imbalance are carried out on the patient. After treatment of the painful reflex zones of the body and significantly lower tenderness, measures can be carried out directly on the ankle.

This treatment can include distal points, which reduce tenderness on the ankle. Direct treatment is possible with silver diode chains, triple cords and Pachi-Pachi igniter (using Master Kawai's method) or sometimes with moxibustion and needling at the ankle (a prerequisite is that the ankle must no longer be painful). After successful basic treatment and distal needling, the ankle is often less painful so direct treatment is not always necessary.

22.3.2 Technique

In the acupuncture methods introduced here relatively thin needles are used to stimulate the points. The acupuncture points where there are no deep muscles are usually treated with 30 or 40 mm needles of 0.16–0.18 mm diameter.

Point location and selection

In general, acupuncture points are selected and needled if they demonstrate a clinical effect (by cross checking, see below). The needling angle and the individual location of the points are crucial for the success of the treatment and can deviate from the traditional location description of the point and may be different from one patient to another. Both the exact location of an acupuncture point and the angle of needling are adjusted in accordance with the changes in the affected region (symptomatic or reflex zones). Some of the points used for these acupuncture methods are of diagnostic value and are not necessarily needled; in these cases, treatment strategies should be used which reduce tenderness at these points.

Besides the very precise needling techniques, certain measures require the use of special instruments or aids. Most of these aids are very simple and inexpensive. They may include the following: superclean moxa, tiger warmer, various magnets, Manaka hammer and dowel, Shiunko cream, ion pumping cord, Pachi-Pachi igniter, triple bypass cord, diode ring, silver diode chains and Ito magnet stimulator.

---

[1]The treatment of the vertebral and basilar arteries should also be considered from a morphological point of view.

The acupuncture points are chosen according to their capacity to relieve tenderness at the reflex zones or in affected symptomatic regions. After determining the exact insertion angle and the precise location, needling is carried out to relieve tenderness and/or improve the symptoms in the affected region.

Palpation

Palpation is the main clinical approach. Most of the information received from this method has been developed by blind practitioners. The focus of the professional training of blind practitioners in Japan is in the teaching of palpation techniques for diagnosis and therapy. Because of the lack of visual control, blind students have to rely on pulse diagnosis, meridian palpation and abdominal diagnosis. This part of the clinical training makes them extremely sensitive to tactile information from the patient's body. The tendency to rely strongly on palpation findings is widespread in Japanese acupuncture.

Sensations felt by palpation are often difficult to describe adequately; this is why adjectives such as 'rubbery', 'delicate', 'hard', 'jelly-like', etc. are used in the text to aid communication of the different sensations during palpation. To understand these techniques you have to gather your own experiences of palpation.

It is possible to diagnose areas of unusual sensations, pain and tension from palpation. Particularly important are the abdomen (Hara diagnosis), neck, vertebral column, scars, the area of the main symptoms and specific acupuncture points over the whole body.

The patient usually reports a main symptom or pain for which there is a point at another body site that is associated with it. Pressure on the corresponding point should quickly and directly cause the principal pain to subside (partially or completely).

The point that relieves the principal pain is determined by the pattern of the patient's disease and the causative factors. If the patient does not feel any pain associated with the symptoms, there are still specific areas that are characteristically sensitive to palpation and are associated with the symptoms. These areas are known as reflex zones or reflection zones. To instigate healing, it is important to eliminate the tenderness of a reflex zone. If an acupuncture point is found which directly relieves the pain associated with the main symptoms, that indicates the correct disease pattern. This concept was described very early on in *Ling Shu*:

> ... *If you want to determine an acupuncture point precisely, you should press firmly on one site after another. At the right point the patient will feel a relief of pain (or at least a lessening of the pain).*

Huang Ti Nei Ching, *Ling Shu*, Chapter 51
(Treatise on back Shu points)

Cross-checking

The location of significant treatment points for the relief of pain and disease is achieved by intense learning of body palpation and so-called cross-checking. This is a procedure for proving whether pressure on an acupuncture point causes a reflex reaction at another point or another area of the body.

- First, the main area of the disorder to be relieved of pain or tension must be determined with the aid of the case history, the Hara diagnosis and the palpation of other reflex zones of the body.
- A point is then selected which most probably exercises a positive effect on the main area of disorder.
- This point is massaged or pressed,[2] for about 10–20 s and then held, and the main area sought again to determine the extent of the change.
- If it has led to a significant reduction in pain or tension, it is worth treating the point further, as it will probably relieve the main area even more.

When acupuncture points and treatment strategies are described in the course of the text, these are usually main treatment points and complementary treatment points. The main treatment points are almost always points which have relieved or significantly reduced tenderness at another body site (a reflex area or a painful area of symptoms). For treatment to be successful, it is very important that the main treatment points are used correctly. This means that the exact location and exact angle of stimulation must be found so that the best possible relief of tenderness can be achieved at the reflex area or the place of the pain. In many cases, the main treatment point will not be exactly at the traditional location as described in books on point location, but in neighbouring areas.

For the inexperienced, the exact finding of the angle and location is often a lengthy process. After each needling or moxibustion, the relevant areas should be examined again to ascertain whether the treatment is effective.

Example: Examination of a patient showed tenderness at TH 16, which can be an expression of weakness or disorder of the immune system. The relief point was found to be a 'rubbery', painful area at 'Nagano's immune point' (area at LI 10) and was vertically pressed for 20 s. Afterwards, TH 16 was palpated again (the distal point on the arm was pressed meanwhile). The patient reported that the pain was still there but not as severe as before.

A second possible treatment point close to the first was selected. Pressure on this point was not as painful for the patient but the therapist thought he felt a knot under the skin. This time the patient reported that the tenderness at TH 16 had disappeared.

---

[2]With each breath, Qi and blood move 5 cun; therefore, if a treatment point is relatively distant from the reflex zone which needs to be relieved, allow the Qi enough time to reach the reflex zone.

The point on the arm was needled in accordance with the palpation findings in the exact location and at the exact angle. The needle was inserted until the therapist could feel the knot. Further needle manipulation was not required (to achieve a de Qi feeling, this technique is not required). As mentioned above, the relief of the tenderness at the reflection zone is the desired response of the body.

Practical course of action

The constitutional basic treatment is combined with a specific treatment where not too many needles should be used at once. The treatment is divided into three 15 or 20 min phases of needling: the first 15 or 20 min are directed at the basic and organ pattern treatment points on the anterior side of the body. The second part of the treatment usually targets specific symptoms such as headaches, depression, breast cysts, elevated liver enzymes, pain in the small of the back, etc.

The selected points or point combinations should relieve the tenderness at the reflex zones or reduce the specific (symptomatic) pain and restricted movement.

> Needling should not be carried out in a painful reflex zone or a painful region, although distal points in these areas can be used to reduce tenderness.

Sometimes a selected acupuncture point is very painful on palpation. In this case the pain at the acupuncture point should first be reduced by distal treatment before directly needling the point.

Example: When specifically treating the adrenal glands it was ascertained that KI 6 and KI 27 relieves the pain at the navel (reflex zones of the adrenal glands). However, KI 27 was very painful on compression for this patient. A solution was produced by using HT 7 (ipsilateral to the painful KI 27) to relieve the pain at KI 27. After the needling of HT 7 had achieved the desired effect, KI 6 and KI 27 could successfully be used to relieve the pain in the area of the navel.

The last 15 or 20 min of the acupuncture treatment are usually directed at points on the posterior side of the patient. The patient lies on the abdomen or side (in the lateral decubitus the patient usually has to turn from one side to the other). The treatment points on the back usually comprise both basic points and symptom- or disease-related treatment points.

Example: The treatment of BL 35 on the left side to relieve pain in the area around BL 17 on the right (basic treatment of liver stagnation), points on the sacroiliac joint (structural imbalance), Huato at TH 10 (sugar point) and dragon technique at SI 11 (specific heart treatment).

A small 'freshening up' treatment is added (usually this additional treatment lasts no longer than 10 min), particularly if the patient is still showing serious symptoms (in spite of successful basic treatment with reduction of pain at the relevant reflex zone). Additional treatments can include:

- Yin–Yang stimulation by Pachi-Pachi,
- direct Hukaya moxibustion on LU 10 (to relieve pain in the small of the back at the M. quadratus lumborum),
- setting the patient's ankles in the correct anatomical position, etc.

These short additional treatments are based on the symptoms and are very effective after successful basic treatment. At the end of the treatment, magnets, pressure objects or intradermal needles are used in the area of the most effective points to prolong the effect of the treatment.

Treatment for myofascial pain

The generally muscle-relaxing points are used for the treatment of myofascial pain:

- SP 3 on both sides,
- ST 22 on the right ('sphincter of Oddi point'),
- Huato Jiaji in each relevant area of the back.

The precise location of these points should be found and needled at the corrected angle to reduce pain and tension in the affected muscles. If the area around SP 3 is very sensitive on palpation, distal points should be needled beforehand. Instead of SP 3, SP 5 and SP 9 (metal and water) can also be used.

The general muscle relaxing points can be used for all symptoms in the area of the muscles and are therefore only mentioned here. Specific point recommendations for symptoms of specific muscles are mentioned in each relevant chapter (see Chs 26–34).

22.4 MICROSYSTEM ACUPUNCTURE

Jochen Gleditsch, with the collaboration of Dominik Irnich

22.4.1 Definition

Microsystem acupuncture is a reflex-therapy-based form of acupuncture on small body areas (microacupuncture system, MAPS) not based on traditional Chinese principles (Gleditsch 2007). The most well-known types are ear acupuncture, Chinese scalp acupuncture, Yamamoto new scalp acupuncture (YNSA), oral acupuncture and Korean hand acupuncture.

According to Gleditsch's definition (Gleditsch 2005), microsystems are the cartographic visualisation of functions of the whole organism on one of its body parts. The complete cartographies can be found on the external ear and the soles of the feet (foot reflex zones).

22.4.2 Physiological principles

The physiological principles of microsystem acupuncture are largely unexplained. The activation of endogenous pain-inhibition systems (mediated by opioids, diffuse noxious inhibitory control, descending pain inhibition) as a mechanism of effect is accepted in analogy to body acupuncture but there is only anecdotal evidence so far for MAPSs.

Ear acupuncture has been the best researched: one study found almost 70% agreement between the specificity of the ear points and the clinical diagnoses. There is as yet no confirmation of these results. Via the multiple nervous innervation of the ear are connections to the trigeminus nuclei, the sympathetic nervous system and the spinal nerves, which may all be stimulation-control structures.

22.4.3 Scientific principles

There is a series of clinical studies available on ear acupuncture, which suggests efficacy for various indications. More recent studies in particular have shown that ear acupuncture can be particularly effective as a postoperative analgesic. The use of ear acupuncture for various addictions also has a scientific basis as part of an overall treatment plan. There are no specific studies available on MPS.

22.4.4 Characteristics of microsystems

Reactive occurrence: switch-off phenomenon

The points of meridian acupuncture are always present and detectable because of their amalgamation in the energy cycle of all meridians. The microsystem points occur according to an 'on/off principle' (i.e. after the underlying organ disorder has subsided they are inactive again) or 'switched off'. Simultaneously, the analogue stimulation points of the rest of the microsystems, which react at the same time, are also deactivated and 'silent', without having to be treated 'on site'. This 'switch-off' phenomenon indicates that treatment carried out on MAPSs has an all-embracing regulation impulse.

Diagnosis–palpation–detection

For point therapy and diagnosis via microsystems it is advantageous if the therapist is familiar with two or more MAPSs. This allows comparative testing to show which of the point systems is the strongest. The success of therapy is longest lasting if particularly active points are selected (see Fig. 22.12).

Point testing is preferably carried out using palpation or even better fine detecting with a detection instrument (electrical device or fine ball probe). Gleditsch's Very Point technique is a particularly effective method. The active points are felt during testing and distinguished from the surroundings by their changed reactivity.

Point location using the Gleditsch Very Point technique involves gentle tangential tapping of acupuncture points/areas with the acupuncture needle. The patient can usually report a particularly sensitive point (Very Point) which is immediately needled (see Fig. 13.10).

Advantage: exact location of the most sensitive points in the microsystem with specific point density (ear, scalp); quick, because the needle is used for both diagnosis and therapy; practice is required.

The more definitely a specific point – a 'maximum point' – is registered, the more suitable it is as a treatment site. Needle stimulation is particularly suitable as a regulation impulse – applied as precisely as possible to the point – but pressure massage (acupressure) or laser irradiation are also suitable. The systemic networks lead to distant effects, which spread far beyond the local response.

Rapid onset of effect

The effect of microsystem acupuncture generally occurs faster than that of traditional body acupuncture. This applies particularly to the treatment of disorders of the locomotor system and especially for myofascial symptoms. For chronic diseases in particular it is necessary to include TCM in order to access the deep-seated, mostly psychosomatic associations as well. Microsystem therapy is sensible at the entry level as the rapid effect also motivates the patient for further treatment measures.

Geometric point classification

Microsystems demonstrate geometric point classification:

- as means of spreading along a beam or belt as for ear geometry,
- as double location on the anterior or posterior side (outer ear),
- as double location at the medial or lateral side of a tissue (e.g. lips),
- as horizontal-linear point spread into the segments (so-called belts).

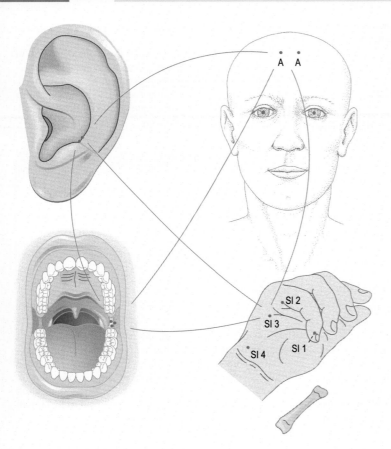

Fig. 22.12 Analogue points and areas for the cervical spine in various microsystems: treatment is preferably commenced at the most definitely reactive points (see Fig. 13.10).

Autoregulative functional mechanisms

The functional and the autoregulative mechanisms form the basis for an understanding of both TCM and modern Western microsystems. A mutual cause and effect relationship applies to organ function. The interactions of various organs and body areas can be interpreted as systemic networking.

According to scientific theory, functions can be both linear and causal as well as non-linear and acausal (Essler). Their interrelation serves the purpose of the whole in the combination of several factors. Endogenous regulation is aimed at the maintenance or restoration of homeostasis according to L. von Bertalanffy's 1940 definition of equifinality. A regulative therapy such as acupuncture or microsystem therapy is, in this sense, an ordering therapy, as defined by Bachmann, the founder of acupuncture in Germany.

Cybernetic interpretation

Expressed in terms of cybernetics, MAPSs are homeostats. They offer an exchange of information between the the environment and the inside of the human organism to ensure inner stability. Each functional disorder of an organ is reflected immediately in all microsystems, depending on the type of resonance phenomenon.

Fractal theory is an approach for explaining the microsystem phenomenon. Self-similarity has been recognised as a basic principle of self-organisation in nature. In the sense of fractalisation the body creates a number of reflections of itself, which are manifested on specific areas of the body surface. The biological purpose of these many self-reproductions can best be interpreted informatively and cybernetically as multiple insurance. Information or strengthening information is capable of reducing the extent of disordered multiplicity.

Summary

- Each point has a specific correlation with a certain organ function or a certain system of association (meridian, circle of function).
- The points occur as a reaction in the sense of an on/off principle and in this manner 'register' a specific function disorder in each case.
- The stimulated points can be used for both diagnosis and therapy and are also suitable for follow-up checks.
- Finding the exact microsystem point is crucial for the success of treatment. The effect of MAPS therapy usually occurs faster than with body acupuncture, especially for diseases of the locomotor system.
- The individual microsystems and their points interact with each other.
- The level of stimulation of analogue points on different MAPSs is however often variable. This makes it easier to decide on the therapeutic course of action.
- The various MAPSs are networked with each other so that the preferred therapy for a microsystem and its points can switch to the analogous points of other MAPSs if successful.
- The switching off phenomenon is also evidence that the target organ has been addressed and the organism is open to regulatory measures.
- The microsystem points can spread linearly and are duplicated on the anterior and posterior sides between the medial and lateral sides of MAPS areas.
- The most likely explanation for the multifaceted phenomena of MAPS is the systemic connections and informative resonance reactions.
- The mechanisms of effect and contraindications of microsystem therapy are the same as for body acupuncture. MAPS therapy is definitely superior for the treatment of numbness and neurological deficits and as additive acupuncture as part of the treatment of addiction.

22.4.5 The ear microsystem

Individual ear points were known and used as part of traditional Chinese acupuncture, without a system being developed from it. The discovery and systematic breakdown of ear somatotopy was the work of Dr P. Nogier from Lyons, France, the founder of Western auriculotherapy. Ear point stimulation was probably practised in Persia and Egypt 2000–3000 years ago. The first descriptions in Europe originate from the 17th and 18th centuries.

Orientation, innervation and representation on the outer ear

Finding the points for auriculotherapy and diagnosis requires some practice in orientation because of the extremely individual shape of the outer ear. The first orientation is the image of the homunculus in the outer ear (the embryo standing on its head). According to this, the head organs are inferiorly represented and the extremities superiorly (see Fig. 22.13a).

It seems not insignificant that for ear somatotopy the outer ear is innervated by three different nerves (see Fig. 22.13b):

- the concha is innervated by the auricular branch of the vagus nerve,
- the majority of the ear is supplied by part of the third trigeminus branch,
- the earlobe together with part of the border of the helix is supplied by the great auricular nerve from the cervical plexus.

The distinction by Nogier (1983) into entodermal, mesodermal and ectodermal areas of representation with relevant areas of life and key points is revealing, although these are largely covered with the three main innervation areas.

INNERVATION	PROJECTION ZONE	AREA OF LIFE	OMEGA POINTS (SEE FIG. 22.16)
Vagus innervated concha	Entodermal zone	Metabolic area: internal organs Superior concha with digestive tract and urogenital tract Inferior concha with respiratory tract	Omega 1 point
Trigeminus innervated part	Mesodermal zone	Motor function area: locomotor system	Omega 2 point
Area supplied by the cervical plexus	Ectodermal zone	Projection of head and CNS as superordinate control	Omega point

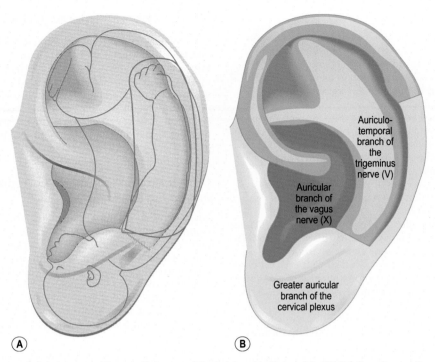

Fig. 22.13 Diagram of the outer ear: (a) symbolic image of the 'embryo' in the auricle; (b) the three innervation zones.

Representation of internal organs: enterodermal zone

Nogier assumed the points were associated with the relevant organs and named them after those organs (see Fig. 22.14). In contrast, the Chinese school of ear acupuncture sets out areas using numerals. Within these projection areas – depending on the clinical picture or affected organ region – stimulation points can occur at various locations. Even though the knowledge of the individual schools does not cover everything, each of them provides important additional knowledge.

Representation of the locomotor system: mesodermal zone

On the arch of the anthelix the points display the whole vertebral column (see Fig. 22.15a). For myofascial symptoms the area lateral to the projecting ridge of the anthelix is significant: the area of the paravertebral muscles and tendons (see Fig. 22.15b). For pain therapy the sympathicus border band with its ganglia (Fig. 22.15b) is of significance. The upper extremities are represented on the scapha – between the antihelix and the helix: the shoulder, elbow, arm and hand run in a line from bottom to top. The lower extremity is represented in the area of the triangular fossa. The inordinately large image of the fingers and toes occurs in the superior projection area of the locomotor system (see Fig. 22.15c).

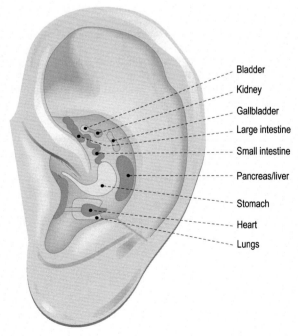

Fig. 22.14 Representation of the internal organs in the concha diagram from Nogier (1983).

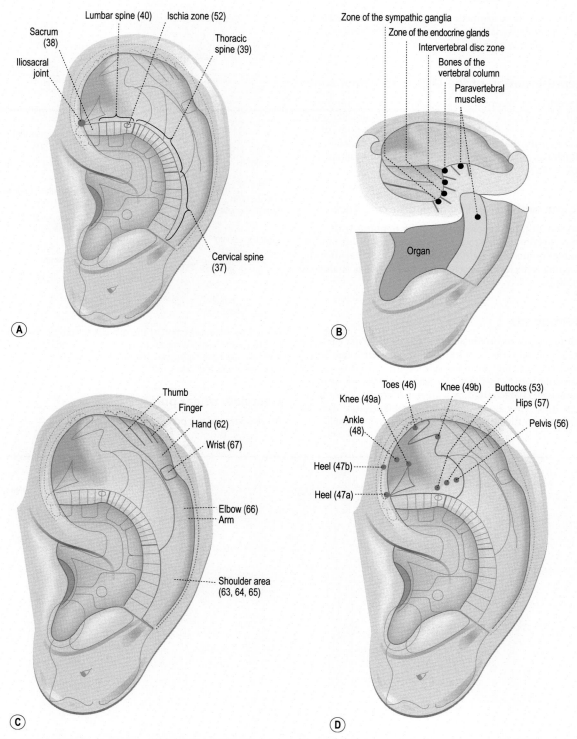

Fig. 22.15 Representation of the locomotor system on the ear: (a) vertebral column and (b) transverse section to demonstrate the location of the individual segment areas, (c) upper extremity, (d) lower extremity.

Here there is no distinction according to the affected structures. For myofascial disorders stimulation within the whole projection zone of the relevant extremity can occur.

Representation of the CNS: ectodermal zone

The ectodermal zone hides the projection of the central organs such as the nervous system, the brain stem and the spinal cord. That is why there is a representation point of, for example, the thalamus, on the medial side of the antitragus which has proved particularly reliable in pain therapy (see Fig. 22.16).

Points with a specific direction of effect

Ear somatotopy demonstrates a series of points with a specific direction of effect via the organ-related points; for example, points with pain-relieving, defence-strengthening, swelling-reducing and even psychotropic effects analogous to drugs.

Retropoints

For many points on the anterior side of the outer ear there are points with the identical indication at analogue 'insertion' sites on the posterior side of the ear. This applies particularly to points of the locomotor system whose retropoints are characterised by a greater effect on motor function (see Fig. 22.17). The retropoints should not be forgotten in the treatment of myofascial symptoms!

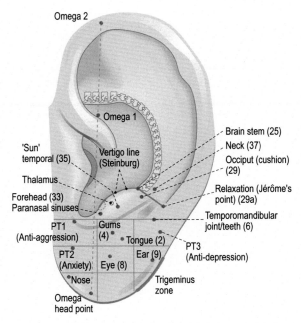

Fig. 22.16 Representation of the nervous system on the outer ear: head and sensory organs in the antitragus and lobulus area and balance zone from von Steinburg (hidden points represented as a circle).

Overview of ear points

An overview of ear points is given in Fig. 22.18.

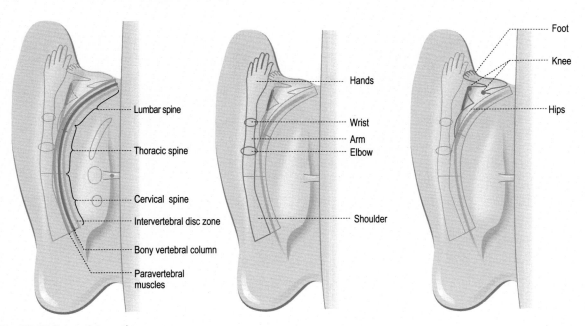

Fig. 22.17 Retropoints on the ear.

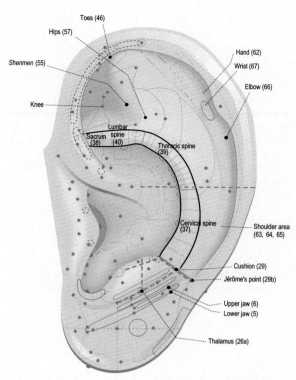

Fig. 22.18 All ear points suggested for the treatment of mTrPs in the various muscle areas (see Chs 26–34).

22.4.6 Reflex zones on the scalp: Chinese scalp acupuncture

Specific scalp acupuncture has been passed down in China and is frequently used; it is especially suitable for neurological diseases. Sensorimotor deficits and Parkinson's symptoms can be influenced from certain point lines and zones on the surface of the scalp.

The reaction lines in each case occur contralaterally to the deficit, corresponding to the known crossing of the pyramidal tracts. Additional therapeutic impulses can be activated by homolaterally situated reaction points, the efficacy of which is explained via the autonomic tracts. Four parallel treatment lines on the anterior scalp run from the median in the direction of the temples: the lines for sensation, motor function, antitremor and vasoaction. There are specific treatment regions in the area of the occiput on both sides: the speech zone, the balance and vertigo zones (supra- and retroauricular) and a vision zone not far from point GB 20.

Naturally, the motor function zone is of special significance in the treatment of myofascial symptoms. The arrangement of the treatment areas and points is associated with the 'homunculus' of the cerebral cortex.

The projection lines should be located as precisely as possible before treatment. As orientation you start from

the motor function line. This represents the linear association between a point on the top of the scalp (one finger width dorsal from GV 20) and a point in the area of the temples (one finger width in front of the tragus). The sensory and Parkinson lines each run at a distance of 1.5 cm occipital or frontal from the motor function line.

22.4.7 Yamamoto new scalp acupuncture (YNSA)

In the 1970s the Japanese physician Toshikatsu Yamamoto developed a new form of scalp acupuncture, YNSA (Yamamoto 1997). He had distinguished a series of point systems on the scalp each with 12 correspondence points to the meridian system. Yamamoto had started from Japanese abdominal wall diagnosis (see Fig. 22.19): treatment on the recently found scalp points immediately relaxed the specific abdominal wall zones. The simultaneous therapeutic effect related to each of the meridians determined by the topography of the abdominal wall point. This led Yamamoto to trace the somatotopic fields in the area of the scalp.

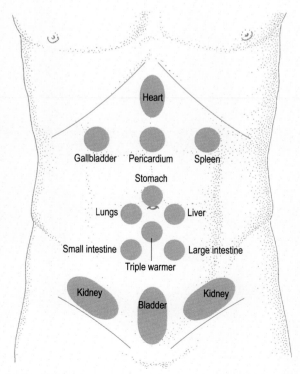

Fig. 22.19 The abdominal wall zones as a representation of the internal organs for Japanese abdominal wall diagnosis.

The points

Ypsilon (Y) points

The MAPS on the scalp related to the meridians are known as Ypsilon (Y) points (see Fig. 22.20). In accordance with the initially decoded temple somatotopy in the area of the temporalis muscle, Yamamoto found an occipital reflective Y field with identical correspondences. Yamamoto also discovered another 12-point meridian somatotopic arrangement on the neck, in the area of the sternocleido-mastoideus muscle and on the anterior cervical triangle. He used the latter for diagnosis, which made the time-consuming palpation of the abdominal wall superfluous. The meridian-related Y microsystem on the temples is the most commonly used system.

Basic points

Yamamoto found another treatment area at the border to the cranium viscerale, specifically on the forehead hairline. He called this the base zone or base points. This is a unique microsystem related to the organs. Base zones A–E are

distinguished as well as specific points for all sensory functions and 'brain points' (see Fig. 22.21). In addition to the base points are reflections in the same arrangement on the occiput.

Of particular relevance for therapy are the base zones, A, B and C, located on the frontal hairline for the treatment of head, cervical spine, neck, shoulder and hand. Zone A, a finger width from the median on both sides, represents the cervical spine and C1 is set superiorly and C7 inferiorly within the zone. Below (towards the nose) zone A are points on both sides for the sensory functions of the eyes, nose and mouth; above zone A are cerebrum and cerebellum points ('brain points'). Directly over the base zones B and C – the latter for shoulder, elbow and arm – are additional points H and I for the lumbar spine, specifically for the treatment of sciatica.

Other points for the locomotor apparatus are point D on the temple hairline for the lumbar spine, E above the eyebrows for the thoracic spine, F dorsally at the mastoid for sciatica and zone G around the lower margin of the mastoid for the knee. Five points in a row immediately in front

Fig. 22.20 Ypsilon points.

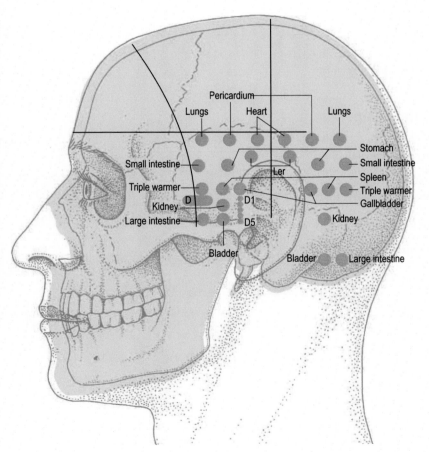

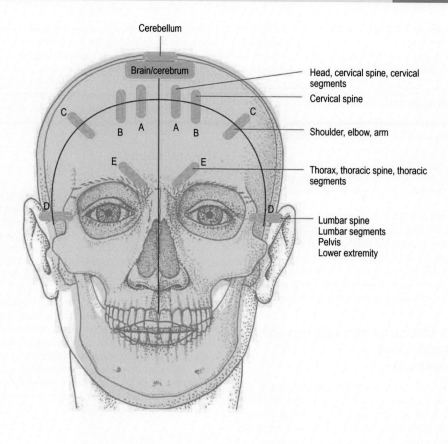

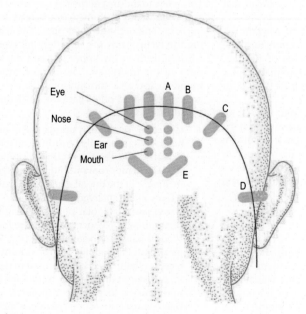

Fig. 22.21 Base points.

of the facial insertion of the outer ear represent the lumbar spine area for segments L1–L5 (points D1–D5). Apart from the base points in the area of the forehead the relevant reflective occipital points can also be considered for therapy.

Indications and practical advice

Yamamoto has been using his scalp acupuncture for 30 years for many acupuncture indications, but with particular success in the various forms of paralysis and sensorimotor deficit (with treatment repeated daily if possible). Needling on the skull usually stimulates the periosteum, which is not without significance for these types of indication.

The significance of YNSA when treating myofascial pain and functional disorders is in the treatment of acute symptoms. Besides the immediate relief of pain and improvement in function, local treatment can also be made easier and less painful. The stimulation points or areas to be treated are located according to their extreme sensitivity (detection by palpation or using the Very Point technique).

22.4.8 The terminal measurement points system: Voll's electroacupuncture

The points situated at the two nailfold angles of fingers and toes are particularly suitable for technical diagnosis procedures. The specificity of these so-called terminal or angle points is that on both sides 12 of these points are either start or end points for a main acupuncture meridian and demonstrate a particular interrelation with the organ that gives its name to the relevant meridian.

The specialisation required for precise work using the relevant technique described places electroacupuncture and other related methods in a specialised area of practice. The diagnostic possibilities of this procedure mainly play a role in the testing and restoration of fault fields and for detoxification (e.g. using nosode therapy).

Knowledge is generally empirically acquired. There is insufficient quality evidence available in the literature on the effect of these techniques on mTrPs. Attempts at disturbed-field therapy appear justified for chronic, treatment-resistant symptoms, and experiences in individual cases show definite improvements as a result of disturbed-field elimination.

22.4.9 Oral somatotopy

The discovery of specific oral mucous membrane points and their systematic recording as a microsystem in the 1970s go back to our own (J.G.'s) observations, which have been confirmed by numerous therapists in the meantime. The points on the mucous membranes of the mouth correlate with the 12 acupuncture meridians and produce a full picture of the functions of the organism. The distal effects which can be caused by the oral points occur in accordance with a set of rules and are reproducible, which is the crucial criterion for a somatotopy or a microsystem.

Several topographically different oral point systems have been produced: the biggest system is in the points in the vestibulum, and the most impressive therapeutic effects have been with the retromolar points.

The oral points

Vestibular points

The vestibular points are in the atrium of the mouth immediately next to the teeth. There is one point per tooth, although there can be two for the wisdom teeth (see Fig. 22.22). In the area of the lips the mucosal points are opposite the crowns of the teeth (i.e. distant from the fold where the dentist injects anaesthetic). In the premolar and molar area the points are increasingly closer to the tooth or the alveolar margin.

Indications: there are some very specific indications relating to the circle-of-function correlations. The points in front of the lower canine teeth, attributed to the liver–gallbladder system, have proved particularly helpful in the treatment of hip and knee symptoms. Treatment is carried out for acute symptoms ipsilaterally to the picture of symptoms. Bilateral therapy is preferred for chronic clinical pictures. This also applies to the retromolar points discussed below.

Retromolar points

This refers to the area of the jaw described as the retromolar area and extends from the wisdom teeth as far as the swelling at the end of the alveolar ridge. The alveolar ridge holding the teeth forms the maxillary tuberosity distal to the wisdom teeth in the upper jaw and the retromolar trigonum in the lower jaw. The main retromolar points are found in the area surrounding this so-called retromolar area which would offer space for the fictitious ninth tooth.

Indications:

- Upper jaw retromolar points: the main indications are headaches, especially tension headaches, migraine, dizziness and shoulder–arm–elbow symptoms. For CMD or temporomandibular joint symptoms, treatment in the buccal distal upper jaw retromolar area relaxes the M. pterygoideus lateralis.
- Lower jaw retromolar points: indications are predominantly associated with the locomotor system: cervical pain, lumbago, sciatica (Fig. 22.22) and particularly the atlanto-occipital joint and the neck receptor field. Injections are used in the retromolar area – i.e. distal to the wisdom teeth – for lumbago/sciatica in the buccal area, and for iliosacral symptoms in the lingual area. The M. pterygoideus medialis can be relaxed as a reflex response with CMD by a distal

Fig. 22.22 Points for oral acupuncture.

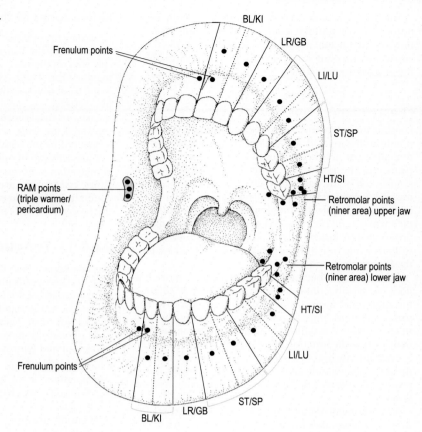

- Frenulum points
- BL/KI
- LR/GB
- LI/LU
- ST/SP
- HT/SI
- Retromolar points (niner area) upper jaw
- RAM points (triple warmer/pericardium)
- Retromolar points (niner area) lower jaw
- HT/SI
- LI/LU
- Frenulum points
- ST/SP
- LR/GB
- BL/KI

lingual injection in the retromolar area in the lower jaw.

- Retromolar point priority: stimulation by the vestibular points can often be 'switched off' by treatment in the retromolar area, but not vice versa. The retromolar points evidently have priority over the vestibular points.

Ramus ascendens mandibulae (RAM) points

Another group of points is to be found at the anterior margin of the ascending mandible. These ramus ascendens mandibulae (RAM) points correspond to the meridian pair triple warmer/pericardium, which is not represented in the vestibular system. They have proved particularly suitable in migraine therapy, vertigo and endocrine disorders.

Frenulum points

The two midline meridians GV and CV each lead to the oral cavity and end at the upper or lower lip ligaments. There are thus meridian connections between the anal and genital 'pole' with the oral cavity as the upper 'pole'. From the

upper frenulum, disorders of the mucous membranes of the anal area (haemorrhoids, anal fissures, etc.) can be influenced and from the lower frenulum genital function disorders. However, functional disorders of the spine, along which runs the GV meridian, can respond to treatment of the upper frenulum point. Correspondingly, treatment of the lower frenulum point can have a regulatory effect on the anterior median and its dominant Yin components.

Extraoral points

Extraoral points are found predominantly in the area of the lips, in an analogous location to the inner mucosal point (location by needling). They demonstrate the same indications as the intraoral points and can strengthen these in their effect. The extraoral points lie close to the lips, each half a finger width above or below the lip seam, and their position is best found by the use of a Very Point needle stroked along the horizontal tangent. The extraoral point in front of the lower canine tooth is especially effective in the treatment of hip and knee symptoms.

The detection of the extraoral points is made by gentle non-traumatising stroking of the cheek area with the finest flexible acupuncture needle. Each stimulation point traced emerges with a pinpoint of blood and/or a definite reddening of its surrounding area.

Practising oral acupuncture

Locating the oral points is not possible because of the moisture from the mucous membranes. The diagnosis and de-limitation of irritated point areas is there made by palpation. This is easier to do in the area of the vestibular points than in the retromolar area, as with the Very Point method. Palpation begins on the right or left, and the sides are compared while the thumb moves along the outside of the lip seam and the palpating pad of the index or middle finger on the inside. Any wounds on the oral mucosa should be ruled out by inspection beforehand (ulcers, prosthesis pressure sites, etc.).

Point therapy is best performed using injection of a low-dose LA, possibly diluted with sodium chloride solution; the addition of a vasostringent must be avoided. Homeopathic solutions, organic products, etc. can also be used. In areas where it is difficult to see, the palpating finger remains where the irritation point is found and the injection is made directly next to the finger tip marking the spot. The mouth is then gently closed to relax the muscles during treatment in the retromolar area after the injection has been given.

After treatment, the area should be palpated to check that the tenderness or induration of the point has been released.

22.4.10 Reflex zones and points on the outer and inner nose

Outer-nose point system

Nasal acupuncture also draws on the wealth of experience of traditional acupuncture; it is not very widespread and not as effective as, for example, ear and scalp acupuncture. The point lines defined on the external nose form a somatotopic point system.

The reaction points on the external nose are characterised by three marking lines:
- motor function line: at the lateral border of the nose and the nostril as a projection of the locomotor apparatus (motor function line),
- Yin line: a chain of points over the midline of the nose associated with the internal organs (lungs, heart, liver, kidneys, spleen),
- Yang line: in the middle between the motor function line and the Yin line as a representation of the so-called hollow organs of the digestive system and the urogenital tract (gallbladder, stomach, small intestine, large intestine, bladder).

Reflex zones of the inner nose

Excited by the new publications by Head and Mackenzie in around 1890 the Berlin physician W. Fliess explored specific sites on the nasal mucosa and their interrelation with the organism. Using cocaine or by cauterising certain sites in the nasal conchae, he caused specific, that is predictable, distal effects. It was natural to attribute these reflex sites in the nose to Head's segmental system; this is also how Fliess explained the wide range of symptoms which could be influenced by the nasal mucosa.

Today, instead of using cocaine or cauterisation, therapy is preferably performed using massage of the nose reflex zones; essential oils are used for this and are applied using cotton buds. In lectures, N. Krack described and developed the procedure of vibration massage.

22.4.11 Tongue somatotopy

We have known since time immemorial that the conditions and functions inside the body are somatotopically reflected on the surface of the tongue. Although no therapy is performed here, the significance of the tongue for diagnosis should not be underestimated. In TCM tongue diagnosis also assesses the moisture or dryness of the tongue and the colour and type of coating.

Changes to the tongue mucosa: the criteria are the coating, discoloration, drying and any fissures or indentations.
- Acute diseases: changes to the overall appearance of the tongue.
- Chronic diseases: changes limited to specific areas can indicate a specific organ.
- In the interpretation of these markings, the experiences of Eastern and Western medicine largely agree.

Innervation of the tongue: significance of changes which become visible on the surface.
- Apex and corpus are treated by the lingal nerve (connection to the parasympathetic nervous system via the tympanic cords and the submandibular ganglion).
- The glossopharyngeus nerve, which sensitises the posterior part of the tongue, is connected to the vagus, facial and sympathicus nerves via the ganglion geniculi.
- The most posterior part of the tongue is supplied by the vagus nerve.
- Here, as with the outer ear, there is a great diversity of innervation.

Tongue discoloration: assessing the tongue's colour allows derivation of diagnostic indications.
- Greyish black coating: indicates disorders in the kidney–bladder system.
- White coating: indicates a gastroduodenal syndrome.
- Yellowish coating: points to the liver and gallbladder system.
- Brown coating: indicates enteric symptoms.

- Garland-shaped impressions at the edge of the tongue with a slightly bloated, spongy body of the tongue: evidence of a functional weakness in the spleen and pancreas system.

22.4.12 Iris somatotopy

In view of the numerous somatotopic microsystems that are represented in the area of the various sensory organs, it would be logical to assume that the eye also demonstrates a somatotopy. Iris diagnosis is still denied any scientific validity; however, a serious, open-minded, scientific examination has not yet been carried out.

22.4.13 Microsystems on the hands

There are both reflex zones and several microsystems on the hands. A non-systematic transfer of points of so-called Chinese hand acupuncture is also known. The number of microsystems on the hand by far exceeds the wealth of experience on the foot. If you consider the very intense innervation of the hand and the oversized representation on the homunculus on the fields of the cerebral cortex, the special case of the hand is obvious.

Chinese hand acupuncture

In TCM there are some very effective individual points where needling or pressure massage can lead to immediate relief of symptoms. This applies to 'point 1' of Chinese hand acupuncture for the indications lumbago and sciatica. It consists of two adjacent points which lie in the metacarpal spaces between the second and third and fourth and fifth metacarpals. The palpating finger is pressed into the metacarpal space until it finds the optimum stimulation sites for treatment.

Hand point 12, between the proximal phalanges of the second and third finger, is ideal for treating throat and neck symptoms. Other points of Chinese hand acupuncture are covered by the extra systems discovered on the metacarpals and are arranged there.

Handline II: embryo containing the information of the whole organism (ECIWO)

A microsystem on the second metacarpal has been used for more than three centuries. It was first described by Zhang Yingqin, who was originally a biologist. Zhang's thesis concerned the line-shaped point system on the second metacarpal which in his view also applied to other MAPSs: he explained the microsystems as being of embryonic origin and of very early differentiation of the cell complexes in various parts of the body or specific organs. However, according to Zhang, the omnipotent valencies remain in these structures and so the latent information for the development of the whole organism is maintained in these

partial systems throughout life. This explanation is the basis of the description chosen by him for the MAPS on the second metacarpal: ECIWO. He assumed self-similarity, known from the plant and animal worlds. According to Zhang, morphological similarity is a principal phenomenon of nature, which lends additional informative and potentially regenerative power to each partial area of the organism.

Orientation: the somatotope on the second metacarpal represents a reflection of the upright human. The head and the head organs are represented in the area of the proximal phalanx, the lower body and lower extremities in the area of handline II near the wrist. Pressure palpation along the second metacarpal often produces surprisingly sensitive points. Five regions can easily be delimited along this line. Even if treatment is not on handline II, the initial palpation findings can supplement the diagnosis and later serve to check the treatment.

Indications: the numerous publications and reports of experiences (over 600 so far) mean that ECIWO treatment can also be effective in all types of indication relating to functional disorders. However, the sensitive points of handline II are mostly very effective for head and face pain, especially for trigeminus neuralgia.

Needling is performed by radial insertion close to the metacarpal bone to cause some periosteal stimulation.

Handline V

Particularly effective points can also be found in the area of the fifth metacarpal with immediate and distal effects of the same type, as displayed in the MAPS. The hand points described lie on the small intestine meridian or close by its course (see Fig. 22.23). However, they are connected to

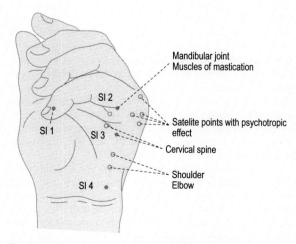

Fig. 22.23 Points in the area of the fifth metacarpal or in the area of the small intestine meridian (handline V).

the switch-off phenomenon that applies between the rest of the MAPSs and the point sequence is analogous to the arrangement of the representative body areas.

Orientation: part of the small intestine meridian runs over the hand as handline V and careful detection can be used to identify other indications. These affect the head, temporomandibular joint, cervical spine and shoulder.

- Point area SI 2 at the distal fold on the proximal phalanx: pain and function disorders in the stomatognathic system; temporomandibular joint, muscles of mastication, e.g. trismus (lockjaw).
- Point area SI 3 at the proximal swelling of the proximal fold at the proximal phalanx: pain and motor disorders especially in the throat and neck region and the cervical spine. Point SI 3 (GV switch point) is known to influence the vertebral column, especially the line of spinous processes.
- V-shaped area between the two folds at the proximal phalanx: strengthening of the point effect of SI 2 and SI 3 as well as a psychotropic effect.
- Point area between SI 3 and SI 4, one finger width proximal from SI 3: shoulder point; further proximally it lies next to the points for the thoracic spine and elbow.

In contrast to handline II, digital palpation is not sufficient here: it requires detection with a fine instrument or a Very Point needle.

Korean hand acupuncture

The idea that the hand reflects a picture of the whole person may stem from the vivid image that the fingers represent the extremities.

Su-Jok

The Su-Jok method is a version of Korean hand acupuncture, which is widespread, not just in Korea but also in Russia: literally: 'hand and foot'. In Su-Jok, the thumb is interpreted as a representation of the head and neck, the outer fingers (index and little fingers) as the upper extremities and the middle and ring fingers as the lower extremities. At the proximal phalanges are the projection areas of the shoulders and hips; at the middle phalanges are the areas of the elbows and knees. The terminal phalanges represent the wrists and ankles. The visceral organs are represented on the palm of the hand and are distributed similarly to the hand reflex zones.

An instrument with a fine rounded tip is suitable for point detection; each of the stimulation points reacts very strongly to that type of fine detection and is often favourably influenced just by the pressure of the instrument. Needling of the palmar points is performed using a very fine, short needle which is applied with the aid of an applicator device. Nevertheless, these methods are usually felt to be very unpleasant by the patient; by using the applicator, it is also not as easy to insert the needle as precisely as with the Very Point technique.

Koryo hand therapy

This form of Korean hand acupuncture sees the basis of its system in the dorsal and palmar median of the hand which continues into the middle finger. Dorsal and palmar medians correspond here to the midline meridians GV and CV and the tip of the middle finger represents the top of the scalp with a point analogue to GV 20; the meeting of the two meridians in the analogue image of the hand consequently lies on the pad of the middle finger.

However, all 12 main meridians have their representation on the fingers and hand with a large number of points, the Yang meridians on the back and the Yin meridians on the palm.

Fingers I and V here represent the lower extremities, and fingers II and IV the upper extremities. The projection of the large joints to the proximal, middle and terminal phalanges of the fingers is analogue to Su-Jok, but differently distributed on the phalanges, with the exception of the index finger.

The same point detection and insertion techniques apply as for Su-Jok.

22.4.14 A microsystem of the lower extremities: new selective pain and organ therapy

Based on his experiences with neural therapy, especially in pain therapy, Rudolf Siener discovered some very effective therapy points on the lower extremities. His first experiences were related to the distal points in the area of the medial and lateral malleolus, which were suitable for the treatment of hip and knee symptoms (see Fig. 22.24). The points described by Siener (1996) are not identical to traditional acupuncture points in the ankle region, such as B 60, B 62, N 3 and N 6.

Siener later discovered specific points on the knee with distal effects on the head organs. He was also able to produce an overall picture representing the face in points on the patella and the organs of the side of the head (tonsils, paranasal sinuses, ears) on the sides of the knee, both lateral and medial. The cervical spine was projected onto the median of the back of the knee and the middle of the cervical spine in the poplitea. The posterior midlines of the lower leg represented the individual levels of the thoracic spine and the heel medians the lumbar spine and the sacrum. The most pressure-sensitive points were to be found in the area of the heel in cases of lumbago, sciatica and especially intervertebral disc symptoms. They are to be found and treated close to the dorsal heel median.

After working out the organ representation on the lower leg, Siener continued to develop his method, originally called new point pain therapy, which is *Neue Punktuelle*

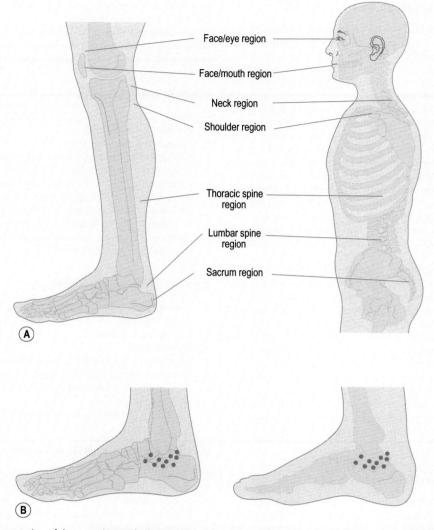

Fig. 22.24 Representation of the organism at the lower extremities. (a) Overview of the equivalent zones on the lower leg/foot from Siener; (b) special point areas on the medial and lateral malleolus for the treatment of hip and knee symptoms.

Schmerz in German, or NPS, adding an O for 'organ therapy' (NPS-O).

Siener also discovered specific pain therapy points on the upper extremities as well, again in peripheral application of the kinetic muscle chains. These points are preferably located on the hand. Siener found a correspondence point for the elbow in particular on the ring finger along the course of the triple warmer meridian. This point on the middle phalanx of the finger proved a particularly effective treatment point for a variety of elbow pains.

Siener performed the therapy with LA injections but the Siener points can be treated equally effectively using acupuncture.

22.5 ELECTROSTIMULATION ACUPUNCTURE

Dominik Irnich

22.5.1 Definition

Electrostimulation acupuncture (ESA) is the electrical stimulation of needles in acupuncture points to strengthen the needling effect.

22.5.2 Physiological principles

The physiological effect of ESA has been the object of numerous studies and experiments (e.g. Irnich, Beyer 2002). These basically demonstrated a similar mechanism of effect to needle acupuncture, particularly in the area of acupuncture analgesia. The distribution of various neurotransmitters and hormones has been shown several times following ESA (beta-endorphins, encephalin, dynorphin, orphanin Q, serotonin, noradrenaline, corticoptropin, oestrogen, gestagen, cytokine, CGRP and many more). These neurotransmitters and endogenous messenger materials display their efficacy at various sites on the organism: in the brain (periaqueductal grey matter, hypophysis–hypothalamus axis, limbic system and others), in the spinal cord and locally at the insertion site. This leads to systemic pain inhibition (e.g. endorphins in the blood), descending pain inhibition (serotonin, noradrenaline), segmental inhibition (encephalin, dynorphin) and local reactions (CGRP).

As most test results stem from animal studies (Han 2003, 2004), the detailed interplay of various antinociceptive systems in the production of acupuncture-induced analgesia in humans has not been conclusively explained. However, there are very good indications that low-frequency stimulation (2–15 Hz) leads to strong distribution of endorphins while high-frequency stimulation (80–200 Hz) is more likely to activate descending pain inhibition. The combination of both frequencies either alternately or one after the other has proved very effective in pain therapy.

Investigations on the specific efficacy of ESA for myofascial pain have not yet been carried out. A muscle-relaxing effect as described for needle acupuncture is also to be accepted for ESA.

22.5.3 Scientific principles

The clinical efficacy of ESA has been examined for some indications. Positive studies exist (e.g. Stör, Irnich 2009) for postoperative (dental) pain, fibromyalgia syndrome, hot flushes during menopause, rehabilitation after stroke and neuropathic pain. There are no high-quality studies on ESA for myofascial pain.

22.5.4 Theoretical basis

From the viewpoint of Chinese medicine this type of stimulation is a reducing technique. There have been occasional reports that low-frequency stimulation (2–15 Hz) has a somewhat filling effect (previously: tightening) and high-frequency stimulation (80–200 Hz) has a diverting effect (previously: sedative), but this cannot be proved and does not match the author's experience.

Basically any acupuncture point that can be needled according to the therapist's plan can also be electrically stimulated. In particular, if great fullness is present, such

as is frequently seen with moderately severe to severe pain, ESA has proved very effective.

With neuropathic pain, we recommend choosing points which have an influence on the relevant nerve structure, for example PC 6 and LU 5 for carpal tunnel syndrome.

22.5.5 Indications

- Severe pain.
- Nausea and vomiting.
- Stump and phantom pain.
- Analgesia for diagnostic and therapeutic procedures.
- Peripheral vascular perfusion disorders.
- Adjuvant therapy in functional neurological rehabilitation following cerebral and spinal ischaemia and incomplete nerve lesions (treatment should only be attempted by sufficiently experienced therapists and there must be some residual function present).
- Pain therapy during childbirth.

22.5.6 Contraindications

- Fear of electricity.
- Metal implants.
- Cardiac pacemaker.
- Defibrillators.
- Local skin or tissue defects, local collection of moisture.
- Manifest clotting disorder (relative contraindication depending on extent; cases should be individually considered).
- Pregnancy (relative contraindication)

22.5.7 Undesirable effects

- Pain.
- Too much stress for anxious patients.
- Needle collapse.
- Microtrauma to the muscles following muscle stimulation mode.
- Muscle contraction (leads to extension).

22.5.8 Practical course of action

A knowledge of electrotherapeutic and anatomical principles is required for using this method. ESA is basically part of a traditional acupuncture session with the difference that some of the points selected for treatment are electrically stimulated as well, depending on the available equipment. The points envisaged for ESA can be both local and distal points. Of the distal points, points with a very strong systemic effect are frequently chosen, such as LR 3, ST 36, SP 6, GB 34, TH 5, PC 6 and LI 4. The electrical stimulation of local points can be very effective but can also be unpleasant. It is therefore particularly important to take note of the patient's reactions!

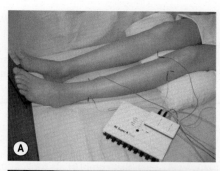

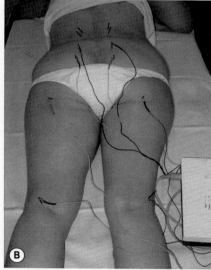

Fig. 22.25 Electroacupuncture. Treatment of knee pain with muscular dysbalance with mTrPs in the Mm. vastus lateralis and medialis (a). Treatment of mTrPs of the dorsal muscle function chains (b).

As there are two electrodes for electrical stimulation (cathode and anode), two points are stimulated at the same time. These should not be too far away from each other (same side of the body, same extremity, etc.). The electrode poles are of secondary importance as alternating current is used. This also means that burns or marks should not be treated (see Fig. 22.25).

In particular for the treatment of disorders in the area of the peripheral nerves it is worthwhile noting the neurophysiological criteria; that is, needling at the margins of sensory disorders (hyperaesthesia, dysaesthesia, anaesthesia, allodynia) or immediately at the affected nerve (e.g. GB 34 and GB 39 for peripheral fibularis function limitation, PC 6 and LU 5 for carpal tunnel syndrome).

The following therefore applies to ESA:

- apply neurophysiological criteria when selecting the point and the stimulation parameters (e.g. points over nerves),

- be aware of the variability of individual electricity tolerance,
- it is possible that neuropathic pain can worsen temporarily,
- carry out a specimen test beforehand to use for diagnostic and therapeutic procedures,
- points should be individually chosen,
- needle insertion can cause release of the Qi (making the insertion or placing the needle vertically or tangentially),
- connect the stimulation electrodes,
- the needle and electrodes may need to be fixed in place (adhesive tape),
- adjust electrical stimulation according to individual sensitivity (muscle twitches or paraesthesia/referred sensation) ('can definitely feel it, but no pain'),
- low-frequency stimulation (2–15 Hz) leads to muscle contractions with activation of endorphin distribution, whereas high-frequency stimulation (80–200 Hz) leads to paraesthesia (pins and needles) with activation of descending pain inhibition,
- adjust stimulation intensity regularly (no abrupt changes),
- duration: at least 20 min (note the acupuncture rules),
- remove needles,
- if muscle contractions occur in low-frequency mode we recommend stretching and/or extending the muscle to avoid muscle pain.

22.5.9 Use of ESA for myofascial pain

ESA can often be used very effectively on acute severe myofascial pain for general analgesia. The choice of point depends on the acupuncture criteria. Points such as LI 4, LR 3, ST 36, Gb 41, GB 34, TH 3, TH 5 and PC 6 have proved to have a particularly strong analgesic effect.

The direct intramuscular treatment of trigger points using needles in the mTrPs can be very effective in individual cases but not all patients can tolerate this extreme stimulation. A less-intensive treatment is to place the needle outside the muscle in the connective tissue above the mTrP. This treatment is indicated in the 'fullness syndromes' of TCM if the symptoms are accompanied by myofascial findings.

22.6 LASER ACUPUNCTURE

Winfried Banzer, Markus Hübscher

22.6.1 Definition

In laser acupuncture traditional acupuncture points and mTrPs are stimulated with low-energy lasers. There are practical and methodical advantages to this procedure compared to needle acupuncture: application is free of pain, there is no risk of infection, application is simple and not time-consuming, the stimulation technique and the parameters can be standardised and a physiologically inert placebo control can be carried out. An up-to-date overview of this procedure can be found in Whittaker (2004).

22.6.2 Equipment

The following equipment is used for laser acupuncture:

- rod lasers and laser pens,
- laser 'needles':
  - semiconductor laser diodes,
  - 35–80 mW power,
  - emission wavelengths of 685 nm (red) to 885 nm (infrared),
  - continuous wave mode.

In the traditional method of laser acupuncture, individual points are stimulated one after the other with a laser device, which because of its outer shape may be described as a rod laser or laser pen. In contrast, there is a comparatively new method of laser needle acupuncture where light-wave conductors, so-called laser needles, are applied with their distal light-exit surface in direct contact with the skin (without penetration). Depending on the type of equipment, between eight and 12 acupuncture points can be stimulated simultaneously (Litscher, Schikora 2005, Weber 2005).

The selection of suitable equipment in specific treatment situations is made according to the depth of the point to be stimulated. The selection criterion is the wavelength-dependent penetration depth of the laser. For body acupuncture, lasers are recommended that emit radiation in the red or infrared range, whereas green lasers are particularly appropriate for ear acupuncture because of their shallow depth of penetration.

Please refer to Section 20.6 on laser therapy for the physical and technical principles of lasers, dose recommendations and safety aspects.

22.6.3 Physiological principles

With regard to the underlying mechanism of effect for laser acupuncture, the question remains open as to what extent the same neurobiological systems are activated by laser stimulation and needle acupuncture. It is better to assume that laser acupuncture demonstrates mechanisms on at least two different physiological levels of effect:

- on the one hand, photophysical and photochemical effects may be expected which depend on the described light and tissue interaction (see Section 20.6 on laser therapy and physiological principles),
- on the other hand, there is the hypothesis of the local and systemic effects of acupuncture which still appear dubious because of the different physical properties of

the two methods and require more precise scientific investigation (Whittaker 2004).

There are currently only few studies of this type available for microvascular, endorphinergic and cerebral mechanisms. Banzer et al. (2006) found specific effects for laser acupuncture on the peripheral cutaneous and subcutaneous microcirculation. In a pilot study Whittaker (2006) succeeded in finding evidence for an opioid-produced analgesic effect in an animal model. Some of the first functional MRI (fMRI)-based analyses in humans showed comparable cerebral activity patterns to those described for needle acupuncture (Litscher et al. 2004, Siedentopf et al. 2002, 2005).

22.6.4 Indications

The main indications in the area of the locomotor system are:

- MPS,
- fibromyalgia,
- gonarthrosis,
- chronic back pain (cervical spine, thoracic spine, lumbar spine),
- shoulder and neck pain,
- patellofemoral pain syndrome,
- achillodynia,
- epicondylitis.

22.6.5 Contraindications

The contraindications include:

- photosensitivity (e.g. light dermatosis),
- sunburn,
- direct radiation into the eyes,
- irradiation of the fetus,
- radiation of a neoplasm.

22.6.6 Practical procedure (for myofascial pain)

In the treatment of myofascial pain using laser acupuncture, in addition to the point treatment of mTrPs (see Section 20.6), traditional acupuncture points are also stimulated in accordance with the criteria of TCM and microsystem points (e.g. ear points) (see Sections 22.2 and 22.4). The practical procedure is based on the principles of low-level laser therapy (see Section 20.6):

- explanation to the patient,
- positioning of the patient in a relaxed position,
- exact location of mTrPs using palpation,
- exact location of acupuncture points,
- pretreatment of skin:
  - thorough skin cleansing (oil removal) with alcohol,
  - possibly hair removal (reflection reduction),
- choice device according to depth of penetration,

- laser beam application over mTrPs and acupuncture points in direct contact with the skin, positioning vertically to the radiation surface (allowing reduced reflection and optimisation of energy density).

Laser application can be carried out as

- monotherapy,
- complementary to other procedures (e.g. manual medicine, osteopathy, physical medicine, acupuncture),
- adjuvant therapy.

22.6.7 Clinical studies

Systematic evaluation of the evidence for the efficacy of laser acupuncture for selected orthopaedic clinical pictures was the aim of an overview by Schüller and Neugebauer (2008). Overall, the investigations present inconsistent results and deliver a low level of evidence, which is also caused by the limitations of the methods used. Nevertheless, the likeliest positive results are in the treatment of myofascial pain in the shoulders, neck and back areas if traditional acupuncture points are treated in combination with mTrPs. It is also worth mentioning that in studies that found insignificant results only HTNe lasers were used, which have comparatively shallow penetration (see Section 20.6). On the other hand, there have been positive results in the use of gallium–arsenide (GaAs) and infrared diode lasers with deeper penetration.

22.7 PREUSSER GELOPUNCTURE

Jochen Gleditsch

22.7.1 Definition

Preusser gelopuncture is the treatment of points known as geloses (i.e. superficial knots which occur in the connective tissue) using acupuncture needles or injection. This method of treatment is not seen as mTrP therapy but as an early treatment for a frequently segmental regulation disorder which can later be expressed in the formation of mTrPs as well.

22.7.2 Historical background

The significance of colloid was first researched and described by W. Ostwald in his work *Die Welt der vernachlässigten Dimensionen* (*The World of Neglected Dimensions*) (1915). He wrote:

All life processes are reflected in a colloid system.

H. Schade published several works on his observations and experiences with 'geloses' between 1919 and 1926. He noticed that these were not 'myogeloses' but palpable changes in the colloids of the controlling mesenchymal connective tissue. The significance and conceptualisation of this point of view have largely been pushed into the background in modern medicine.

We have Pischinger (1980) to thank for extending our understanding of the function of connective tissue as a 'cell milieu system' or as a 'basic regulatory system', in which the connective tissue structures form a functional unit with the finest blood and lymph capillaries and the fine network of autonomic nerve fibres to the same extent. This predominantly theoretical hypothesis finds a great deal of scientific confirmation in some areas today if we look at the latest information on the significance of the fascia and other connective tissue structures (see Ch. 9).

Preusser saw the subcutaneous superficial formation of gelose as an expression of an early regulation disorder. Head (1898) and MacKenzie (1909) describe how regulatory disorders go through three phases:

- primarily as an autonomic reaction with fine autonomic signs in the cutis; these include colloid changes,
- second they lead to functional symptoms including taut bands, trigger points and similar,
- the third phase, which cannot be repaired, is tissue destruction.

22.7.3 Practical course of action

Compared to mTrPs, geloses cannot be found by palpation without specific experience and additional measures. Preusser's optimum solution for this was to coat the skin with oil before palpation. Gentle or smoothing palpation is then carried out so that fine geloses can be found and locally delineated.

Gelopuncture is then carried out by inserting an acupuncture needle or by superficial LA injection directly into the centre of the gelose. If the gelose is precisely encountered, it feels as if it is 'broken apart' by the tip of the needle. Occasionally you can hear a fine noise like the bursting of a blister. This experience is also found in acupuncture: as part of YNSA skull acupuncture in particular, the therapist frequently experiences this fine 'pop', which here too is explained as a release of a connective tissue thickening. If the connective tissue gelose is found exactly it is not just the knot which is released; the surrounding tissue is also loosened.

Treatment of geloses is particularly sensible and effective as part of segment therapy. The fine gelotic changes in the skin can be used as diagnostic evidence of a functional disorder of the visceral organ to which the particular dermatome is attributed. mTrPs on the other hand far less often signify any diagnostic evidence for the irritation of a visceral organ. Head indicated that from certain points in the segment, which then usually also demonstrate fine changes, the treatment of visceral disorders is possible whereby the selection of treatment points ('maximum points' according to Head) is crucial.

Gelopuncture can represent an optimum measure that is supplementary to trigger point therapy. After switching off the trigger point – whether via distal points as with acupuncture or by dry needling – you can check each area using oil and palpation to see whether the skin is now soft and smooth and there are no more geloses hiding in it. Otherwise, the geloses can be switched off with a few superficial injections or needling to optimise the therapeutic effect. If a large number of geloses remain in the area, the 'prior damage' remains trapped in the segment and can soon lead to a recurrence.

22.8 TUINA

Jürgen Bachmann

22.8.1 Definition and principles

The most commonly used Chinese terms for Chinese manual therapy are *Tuina* and *Anmo*. These words are made up from individual labels for manual techniques. In the basic meaning, *tui* stands for pushing, *na* for pulling and taking, *an* for pressure and *mo* for rubbing. The compound words Tuina and Anmo describe Chinese manual therapy, and the terms are frequently used in different ways regionally.

Specifically in the Chinese tradition of forms of manual therapy, as opposed to those forms found in other cultures, the actions also target specific points in the human body, the same as the acupuncture points, to affect the physiological and pathophysiological processes. In this way it is close to acupuncture procedures but also to the treatment techniques aimed at deactivating mTrPs, as these are also of pathophysiological significance in some places and have the potential for therapeutic intervention.

Chinese manual therapy has grown into a unique medical treatment system within Chinese medicine. There are various schools and family traditions of manual therapy. The manual techniques in each of these individual schools and traditions are not the same, although they all basically strive to achieve successful treatment without injury to physical integrity and usually without the use of pharmaceuticals in a simple manner using the body's own natural endogenous regulation and reflexes. The therapist's hands are used to transfer energy with various movements and to create a mechanical effect.

22.8.2 Methods/application

Tuina, acupuncture and TCM

Chinese manual therapy and acupuncture share the principle that the therapeutic method used is an influence on the internal processes of the body through the external structures, the skin and even the myofascial soft tissue. Even the key theorems of Chinese medicine, such as teaching the meridians, teaching Qi and blood or teaching Zang-Fu (internal organs), are a common component of their theoretical structure. The methods of acupuncture and manual therapy demonstrate essential internal differences in the relationship between therapist and patient, besides the abovementioned phenomenological difference.

> Manual therapy is characterised by a greater closeness, a lack of mediating agent, the needle, between the two subjects and a constant presence of the subjects over the period of treatment. Manual therapy does not allow for concomitant treatment of several patients.

Areas of application for Chinese manual therapy

Chinese manual therapy comprises, like any manual therapy, a wide spectrum of application, which makes it part of the list of the most common different forms.

Health maintenance massage (*bao jian an mo*): one of the oldest forms of massage, which strengthens the life force and which should build up the body (*yang sheng jian shen*). It uses exercises (*dao yin*), acupuncture points (*xue wei*) as the object of gentle pats, massage (Tuina), breathing in and out as well as automassage of the head, thorax, abdomen and lumbar area.

Massage of the internal organs (*zang-fu an mo*): this massage relates especially to chronic and internal diseases.

Meridian massage (*jing luo an mo*): the basis of this massage is the theorem of meridians and vessel networks. The acupuncture needle is replaced by the therapist's finger, which carries out the manipulation at specific acupuncture points. It is related to the concept of acupuncture and is therefore especially suitable for combined therapy. These underlying individual techniques are:

- *an*: pressing very hard on a point,
- *dian*: pressing on acupuncture points with a finger,
- *qia*: pressing between two fingers or with a fingertip,
- *rou*: circular massage.

Qigong massage (*qigong an mo*): Anmo, Daoyin and Qigong are combined here as a complex system in which the somatic effects on the patient are achieved by mental induction.

Traumatological Tuina (*zhenggu*): this includes the manual reposition of injured tissue, zhenggu, the soft tissue and bones, which has developed in traumatological and trauma surgery treatment as a unique system of traditional Chinese orthopaedics with various manipulations.

Childhood Tuina, childhood Anmo: this form is a unique specialism within paediatrics in Chinese medicine in which

Tuina again represents a particular specialist method. Priority actions in the area of the hand and back are used, which demonstrate an especially good effect on small children.

Sports massage (*yun dong an mo*): this form of massage is part of the tradition of Chinese martial arts. It is used before and after sporting activity or for the treatment of sports injuries.

Relaxation massage (*fang song an mo*): in former times this was carried out as a treatment for privileged patients and also in the world of martial arts. For example, the technique *na yun fang shui,* a gentle massage in the area of both lower carotids, is applied with the aim of promoting sleep and achieving general relaxation.

Chinese manual therapy in the treatment of myofascial disorders

The function of Chinese manual therapy in the treatment of mTrPs extends basically over four levels.

- First are the direct effects on the damaged muscle. This includes not only direct trigger point deactivation but also the additional necessary muscle stretching, levelling out of stimulation and local pain guarding (nocifension) in accordance with the concept of trigger treatment.
- At the level of the functional unit the relevant joint – arthromotor unit – is treated.
- At the level of functional arthromotoric chains the therapist can treat various functionally associated units, e.g. the static muscles of posture.
- The level of central nervous function associations finally distinguishes between the activation of segmental and central nocifension.

22.8.3 Treatment principles

For the implementation of treatment principles according to the current state of understanding of Tuina an immanent procedure according to the theories of Chinese medicine is enough to be a leading treatment. Apart from a primary diagnosis according to Western standards and the appropriate exclusion of other diagnoses, a Western diagnosis with the treatment principles of Tuina is not yet forthcoming. Indeed, its translation to the concepts of Western treatment for myofascial disorders is still nascent. The following initially demonstrates the treatment principles of Chinese medicine in their various facets. Nevertheless, a hypothetical classification and attribution of the therapeutic function of the individual techniques are carried out here for the first time from a Western viewpoint and on the basis of the pathophysiological mechanisms of painful myofascial disorders. The sequence of this attribution is carried out according to the value which the pathophysiological mechanisms have according to the current state of theory formation.

Theorems of TCM

Meridians (jingluo)

Theorem: the body is full of meridians which allow the Qi to circulate. This must flow freely so that the physiological functions can be maintained. However, if this flow is blocked functional disorders occur, particularly pain. Injury can prevent the free flow of Qi, as can scarring along the flow of the meridians.

Guiding principles:

- *bu tong ze tong*: literally: non-openness causes pain.
- *tong ze bu tong*: literally: openness causes non-pain.

Qi and blood (Qi-Xue)

Theorem: all physiological functions are based on the presence and supply of Qi and Xue. Qi represents breath, steam, function, life force and vital energy, translations with increasing Western cultural association. Xue is blood in its basic meaning and represents the structural, material aspect of the duo Qi-Xue, where Qi represents the functional. This corresponds to the dialectic natural philosophy under the terms Yin and Yang. The flow of the structure blood/Xue is associated with sufficient function of Qi; if there is an injury and an outflow of blood/Xue and stasis, several stages of solidification set in:

- *zhong*: swelling,
- *yu*: bleeding,
- *ji*: hardening,
- *jie*: nodules.

Guiding principles:

- *tiaohe qi-xue*: Qi and blood adapt,
- *xiaoji pojie*: drive out hardening, destroy nodules,
- *huoxue huayu*: move blood, change bleeding.

Tendinomuscular meridians (jingluo)

Theorem: the body contains meridians at the level of the tendons and muscles. These are revealed by the feeling of referred pain along muscles and therapeutically the palpable structures of Jin/muscle and tendon tissue.

Guiding principles:

- *shusong jingluo*: loosen meridians,
- *jiechu nianlian*: loosen adhesions,
- *songcouli*: loosen tissue structure.

Six pathogenic factors (liu xie)

Theorem: diseases arise as a result of the penetration of pathogenic, predominantly climactic factors such as cold, heat, wet or wind. The resistance of orthostatic endogenous guarding resists this penetration. Excessive exposure or a weakness in the body's defence system and penetration of such so-called oblique (Xie) factors into the body leads to disorders of the channels, e.g. the flow of Qi and blood. The model of pathogenic factors can be formulated in relation to the various layers of the body thus including the theorem of the main meridians, and especially the theorem of the tendinomuscular meridians, and leads with the latter to disorders on the myofascial level.

Guiding principles:

- *wenjing sanhan*: meridian warming, cold dispersing,
- *qufeng sanhan*: drive out wind, disperse cold.

Five change phases (Wuxing) and the circle of function (Zang-Fu)

Theorem: natural processes allow all the five elements to be captured in one model under five phases of change in static formulation. This attributes the various categories of natural phenomena to one of the generic terms of fire, earth, metal, water and wood. An emblematic arrangement of this type is known in the West from humoral theory and the four traditional elements.

Yin–Yang

Theorem: this is a superordinate theorem of dialectic natural philosophy in Taoist tradition. The dual term Yin–Yang represents the unity of opposites and their coming together and wrestling with the conditions of balance in natural processes. At the same time, the duo functions as a superordinate emblem of any opposites. Note that this is a relative qualitative arrangement of Yin and Yang and not an absolute attribute. Qualitative attribution to Yin or Yang can only be carried out according to category or from the viewpoint of the opposite.

Effects on the locomotor system

The hand movements of Anmo and Tuina should be directed at the local point noting the nutritional energy, the defence energy for the production of good flow of Qi and blood. This includes various basic effects to approach the underlying pathology and pain. The five main underlying conceptional formulations of Chinese medicine, their rough translation and a clinical example may explain this, as follows.

Shu jin huo luo jie chu luan tong (relax muscles, activate meridians, relieve cramp and pain)

The hard, cramp-like, tense taut bands in the area of the extensors in cases of tennis elbow are a clinical example of the area of application of this theorem. Treatment addresses not just the release but also the realignment of the 'muddled' directions of the tendons in order to drive away the pain and make the meridians open.

Huo xue hua yu xiao zhong zhi tong (move blood and change stasis, reduce swelling, soothe pain)

This describes the clinical situation which may be present, for example with post-traumatic swelling in the area of the ankle in a footballer. The aim of the massage treatment is to promote circulation and removal of the swelling by stretching and careful movement, release blood stasis (Xueyu), increase perfusion and fight the pain.

Li shun jin luo zheng fu cuo feng (order muscles and course of tendons, reduce dislocation)

Ordering the tendons and meridians in this case means rearranging 'false seams'; that is, according to traditional ideas, dislocated or at least restricted suture lines or joints.

Shun tong jing luo xuan tong qi-xue (making meridians and vessel network open, stimulating the flow of Qi and blood)

This assumes the pathogenetic idea that Qi and blood cannot move unhindered through large areas until the openness of large areas of meridians and vessel networks is restored to ensure the unhindered flow of Qi and blood.

Wen jing san han qu feng ding tong (warm meridians, disperse cold, drive out wind, settle pain)

This relates predominantly to the pathogenetic factors of cold and wind, which are tackled by warming of the meridians, driving out cold and wind as a treatment principle. Clinically relevant pictures are usually characterised by an aversion to the relevant pathogenetic factors.

Effects on Zang-Fu

Manual therapy is applied here under the premise of 'A thousand (all) things always move within the framework of the five phases of change, the treatment of disease always moves within the framework of the five organs (*wan wu bu li wu xing, zhi bing bu li wu zang*)'. The cited procedures are based in their explanation and indication on the theory of Zang-Fu and the resulting differential diagnosis (Bianzheng).

Examples of terms from Zang-Fu-Anmo:

- *shu gan li qi*: deaden liver, order Qi,
- *qing fei kuan xiong*: relieve lungs and widen thorax,
- *qing wei jian pi*: relieve stomach, build up spleen,
- *qiang xin huo xue*: strengthen heart, move blood,
- *an shen ding zhi*: calm soul, strengthen spirit.

Effects on meridians

Besides the concept of particular stimulated points, the meridians and their course in the body stem and extremities become noticeable. Analogous to the direction of insertion of an acupuncture needle, the direction of the treating hand dictates the calming or stimulating effect of manual therapy:

- *xun jing luo*: moving the massage hand along the meridians,

- *xun ze bu*: smoothing along the meridians as a method of stimulation,
- *ni ze xie*: stroking against the flow of the meridian as a method of calming.

Simple techniques

There are several dozen basic techniques, depending on the school of thought. The main basic techniques are listed below.

A hypothetical classification and attribution of the therapeutic functions of the individual techniques is presented here for the first time from a Western viewpoint and on the basis of the pathophysiological mechanisms of painful myofascial disorders. The order of each of the following arrangements characterises the status attributed to the pathological mechanisms according to this view.

An: pressing

Implementation: pressing on a site whereby the palm, the finger or the elbow can be used. No movement takes place (see Fig. 22.26a, b, d).
Function from the point of view of Chinese medicine:
- *tongjing huoxue*: make the meridian open, move blood,
- *sanfeng zhitong*: disperse wind, stop pain.
Function in the treatment of mTrPs:
- direct trigger point deactivation,
- muscular extension,
- levelling of stimulation and local nocifension,
- activation of segmental nocifension,
- activation of central nocifension.

Mo: rubbing

Implementation: placing the hands on a region and rubbing, superficially or deeply, gentle circular movements or in one direction. Pressure, speed and duration are always adjusted to the constitution and condition of the patient and the course of the treatment, frequently as an introductory or final activity. The development of a feeling of warmth on the skin or in the deeper tissue layers is desirable. Different variations and other actions have been developed from this (see Fig. 22.26c).
From the point of view of Chinese medicine:
- *shengre sanhan*: creating warmth, dispersing cold,
- *jiechu jingluan*: releasing cramp,
- *xiaoji zhitong*: taking away the peak, stopping the pain.
Function in the treatment of mTrPs:
- levelling of stimulation and local nocifension,

- muscular extension,
- activation of segmental nocifension,
- activation of central nocifension.

Cuo: reverse rubbing

Implementation: placing the hands around an extremity with reverse rubbing (see Fig. 22.26e).
From the point of view of Chinese medicine:
- *shusong jingluo*: loosen the meridian,
- *tiaohe qi-xue*: adapt Qi and blood.
Function in the treatment of mTrPs:
- levelling of stimulation and local nocifension,
- activation of segmental nocifension,
- activation of central nocifension,
- treatment of a functional arthromotoric unit,
- muscular extension,
- treatment of a functional arthromotor chain.

Rou: circling

Implementation: placing the hands or fingers in a constant position on the surface; deep circular movements adjusting pressure speed and duration; most common activity (see Fig. 22.26f and g).
From the point of view of Chinese medicine:
- *wenjing sanhan*: meridian warming, cold dispersing,
- *huoxue huayu*: move blood, change stasis,
- *xiaozhong zhitong*: reduce swelling, stop pain.
Function in the treatment of mTrPs:
- direct trigger point deactivation,
- muscular extension,
- levelling of stimulation and local nocifension,
- activation of segmental nocifension,
- activation of central nocifension.

Na: squeezing

Implementation: squeezing between thumb and the other fingers, lifting and pressing. Adapt pressure and duration (see Fig. 22.26h).
From the point of view of Chinese medicine:
- *tongjing huoluo*: make the meridian open, move collaterals,
- *jiejing zhitong*: release cramp, stop pain,
- *sanhan qutong*: disperse pain, drive away pain.
Function in the treatment of mTrPs:
- muscular extension,
- direct trigger point deactivation,
- levelling of stimulation and local nocifension,
- activation of central nocifension,
- activation of segmental nocifension.

Dianxue: pressing on the acupuncture point

Implementation: pressing on the acupuncture points with the fingertips, the elbow or similar, as a localised adapted

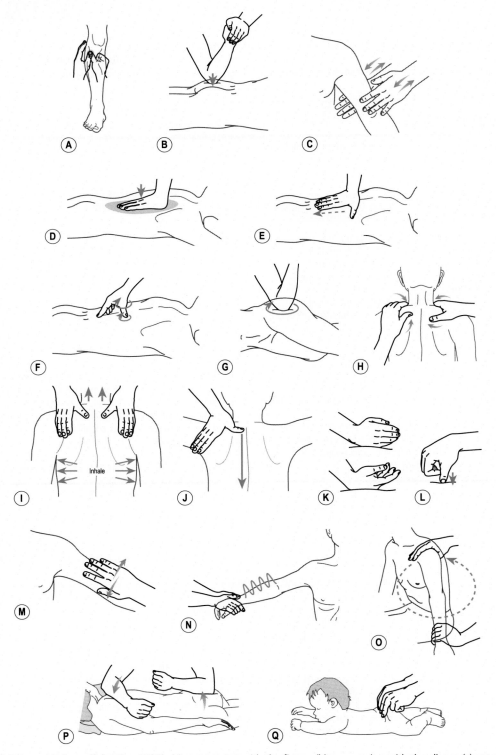

Fig. 22.26 Tuina techniques (from Han 2005): (a) *an*, pressing with the finger; (b) *an*, pressing with the elbow; (c) *mo*, rubbing; (d) *an,* pressing with the palm; (e) *cuo,* reverse rubbing; (f) *rou,* circling with the finger; (g) *rou,* circling with the elbow; (h) *na,* squeezing; (i) *dianxue,* pressing on the acupuncture point; (j) *tui,* pushing (from Han 2005); (k) *gun,* rolling; (l) *san,* spreading, (m) *yao,* turning; (n) *dou,* shaking; (o) *qia,* deep pressure; (p) *ban,* manipulation; (q) Tuina for children.

form of stimulation; a replacement for needle stimulation (see Fig. 22.26i).

From the point of view of Chinese medicine:
- *tong jingluo*: making meridians and collaterals open,
- *xiaoji pojie*: taking away the peak, destroying nodules,
- *xiaozhong zhitong*: reduce swelling, stop pain.

Function in the treatment of mTrPs:
- direct trigger point deactivation,
- activation of central nocifension,
- activation of segmental nocifension,
- levelling of stimulation and local nocifension,
- muscular extension.

Tui: pushing

Implementation: pushing the tissue in one direction, straight, transverse or diagonal to the end of the extremity or the muscle bands on the back using the finger, thumb, thenar or palm; used especially in the area of the back (see Fig. 22.26j).

From the point of view of Chinese medicine:
- *tongjing huoluo*: make the meridian open, move collaterals,
- *huoxue jiejing*: move blood, release cramp.

Function in the treatment of mTrPs:
- levelling of stimulation and local nocifension,
- activation of segmental nocifension,
- muscular extension,
- treatment of a functional arthromotor chain,
- treatment of a functional arthromotor unit,
- activation of central nocifension.

Gun: rolling

Implementation: placing the back of the hand on a region and rolling over the ulnar part with a supination movement holding back the hand with pronation (see Fig. 22.26k).

From the point of view of Chinese medicine:
- *tongjing huoluo*: make the meridian open, move collaterals,
- *xingqi huoxue*: promote Qi, move blood,
- *huanjie tengtong*: dissolve pain,
- *tongli guanjie*: get joints working again,

Function in the treatment of mTrPs:
- levelling of stimulation and local nocifension,
- muscular extension,
- direct trigger point deactivation,
- activation of segmental nocifension,
- treatment of a functional arthromotoric unit,
- treatment of a functional arthromotoric chain,
- activation of central nocifension,

San: dispersing

Implementation: place the root of the hand and move forward over a region with a rapid ulnoradial movement of the hands (see Fig. 22.26l).

From the point of view of Chinese medicine:
- *shujin huoxue*: arrange tendons, move blood,
- *sanyu xiaozhong*: disperse stasis, reduce swelling,
- *jiejing zhitong*: release cramp, stop pain.

Function in the treatment of mTrPs:
- levelling of stimulation and local nocifension,
- activation of segmental nocifension,
- activation of central nocifension,
- muscular extension,
- treatment of a functional arthromotor chain,
- treatment of a functional arthromotor unit.

Yao: turning

Implementation: turning an extremity around the axis of the joint to be treated, e.g. the shoulder, where the movement is passive; the treated joints include wrist, shoulder, hip, knee and ankle (see Fig. 22.26m).

From the point of view of Chinese medicine:
- *shujin huoxue*: arrange tendons, move blood,
- *jiechu nianlian*: loosen adhesions,
- *huali guanjie*: mobilise joints.

Function in the treatment of mTrPs:
- treatment of a functional arthromotor unit,
- treatment of a functional arthromotor chain,
- muscular extension,
- activation of segmental nocifension.

Dou: shaking

Implementation: grasp the end of the extremity away from the body with two hands and use a shaking movement of the extremity while adjusting the speed so that the movement continues centrally (see Fig. 22.26n).

From the point of view of Chinese medicine:
- *shutong jingluo*: arranging meridians and collaterals and making them open,
- *huali guanjie*: mobilise joints.

Function in the treatment of mTrPs:
- treatment of a functional arthromotor chain,
- treatment of a functional arthromotor unit,
- activation of segmental nocifension,
- activation of central nocifension,
- levelling of stimulation and local nocifension,
- muscular extension.

Qia: deep pressure

Implementation: deep pressure from the thumbnail or index fingernail in a region, possibly with smoothing, deep, in one direction, often periosteal (see Fig. 22.26o).

From the point of view of Chinese medicine:
- *kaiqiao xingshen*: opening body orifices, clearing the spirit,
- *tongjing huoxue*: make the meridian open, move blood,
- *xiaozhong quyu*: disperse stasis, reduce swelling,
- *sanfeng quhan*: drive out wind, disperse cold.

Function in the treatment of mTrPs:

- activation of segmental nocifension,
- activation of central nocifension,
- treatment of a functional arthromotor unit,
- direct trigger point deactivation,
- treatment of a functional arthromotor chain.

Ban: manipulation

Implementation: joint mobilisation with fast impulses beyond the end of the physiological range of movement, analogous to chirotherapeutic manipulation (see Fig. 22.26p).

From the point of view of Chinese medicine: *fuwei cuowei*: reposition poor posture.

Function in the treatment of mTrPs:

- treatment of a functional arthromotor unit,
- muscular extension,
- treatment of a functional arthromotoric chain,
- activation of central nocifension,
- activation of segmental nocifension.

Complex techniques

As an example, we now describe treatment sequences on the cervical spine and in the knee region.

Cervical spine

Stages 1–3 of the treatment comprise *rou* and *na*, followed by *duan* and finally *qian*.

- *rou*: Treat in the above manner with two fingers on the paravertebral muscles while supporting the head so that the patient does not actively tension the muscles that support the head. If both sides are included it is known as *na*.
- In a second step the head is supported with the two ring fingers below the mandible and the thumb in the occipital area, then on the patient's shoulder and superior traction with concomitant acupressure stimulation by *Feng chi* (GB 20). The head is moved gently forwards and backwards to create an additional loosening effect. This is followed by lateral flexion in slight rotation. The movement swings do not exceed 10°.
- The third movement also consists of traction via the mandible, although here the head is placed in the crook of the therapist's elbow and at the same time the index finger and thumb carry out acupuncture-point stimulation and traction simultaneously on the dorsal side at *Feng chi* (GB 20) in the sense of *na* or *duan*. This can also be combined with lateral flexion and particularly rotation movements, the latter also with transition to a rotation manipulation.

Knee region (xi guan jie san yao liang qu fa)

The treatment plan is called 'three turns and two bends of the knee joint'. If there are retropatellar symptoms a preparatory technique is used first (*gua*): deep friction of the parapatellar capsule structures. The preparatory relaxing procedure is followed by individual turning movements (*yao*) and flexion movement (*qu*).

- First *yao*: with the hip flexed at 90°, knee flexion and *rou* in the area of the parapatellar structures; turn the lower leg in a cone shape and in the other direction.
- First *qu*: flexion is reduced and resistance is produced with the arm close to the body under the knee joint with the first gentle traction to relax the structure; then increase flexion so that the arm close to the therapist's body acts as a hypomochlion in the popliteal area.
- Second *yao*: with the leg extended and the hips slightly spread apart and flexed, apply slight traction via the ankle which is clasped between the therapist's legs. After prior traction then make a circular movement of the knee joint under gentle additional flexion and simultaneous pressure (*an*) or pressure on the acupuncture point (*dian*) in the area of the front of the knee or the trigger point in the parapatellar structures.
- Second *qu*: the affected ankle is placed on the opposite knee joint with 90° knee flexion and lateral rotation of the hips, like a figure 4. At the same time the medial knee joint space or the medial structures are treated using *rou* by the therapist's hand.
- Third *yao*: now in a seated position with the knees hanging down in 90° flexion and 90° hip flexion, a circular movement of the lower leg is carried out while holding the back of the foot and behind the Achilles tendon, under traction in a inferior direction.
- The treatment is completed with rapid movements over the surface for relaxation (*san pai da*).

22.8.4 Indications and contraindications

Indications

Locomotor system

The range of indications for Chinese manual therapy on the locomotor system is very wide. To the fore are functional disorders and pain, at the level of both the joints and supportive tissue, and especially that of muscular and nervous control. Structural lesions are not an indication per se but those functional disorders associated with injuries, the consequences of injuries or degeneration can also be influenced by Tuina.

Specific indications:

- myofascial disorders and trigger point syndrome,
- sprains and contusions on the four extremities and in various sections of the vertebral column,
- any 'subluxation' or functional blocking of the small vertebral joints,
- symptoms following injury or surgery such as restricted movement of the extremities, atrophy, adhesions,

- chronic pain symptoms, e.g. in the area of the shoulder, elbow, vertebral column and knee, which are described as chronic injuries (*lao sun xing bing*),
- degenerative changes which are associated with limited function of the four extremities

Internal medicine and gynaecology

Under the premise of an effect on the flow of Qi and blood, manual techniques can also be sensible in the context of internal medicine and gynaecology. Manual therapy of the acupuncture points can be particularly effective when applied to the affected circle of function, on the relevant meridian and also the Mu and Shu points of the circle of function. Symptomatic points also occur in accordance with the usual rules of acupuncture. Manual techniques can also be used in the area of the upper, lower or middle warmer, or regional treatment on the trunk.

Specific indications are:

- cold-like diseases,
- headaches,
- dizziness,
- disorders of the sensory organs and the head such as tinnitus, earache, short-sightedness, tears, sore throat, vocal disorders, nosebleeds,
- cramp,
- thoracic pain,
- abdominal pain,
- stroke,
- hypertension,
- gastrointestinal disorders such as vomiting, diarrhoea, constipation,
- urological disorders,
- menstrual disorders,
- disorders associated with pregnancy and childbirth.

Paediatric medicine

Paediatrics became a separate specialism early on in the development of TCM (see Section 22.8.2). The application of Tuina in children is a special case because the child is not fully developed. Specific body regions apply as treatment areas because the meridians and acupuncture points are also not yet mature. The strength of stimulation is usually calculated to be small and is adapted to the constitution of the small patient, apart from the areas of the palms and the soles of the feet. The range of diseases comprises primarily uncomplicated functional disorders, frequently based on an external disease with filling (*shi*) as a result of penetration of pathogenic factors.

Specific indications:

- fever,
- cough,
- vomiting,
- abdominal pain,
- digestive disorders,
- constipation,

- cramp,
- enuresis,
- sleep disorders.
- muscular torticollis,
- foot deformities,
- dental symptoms.

Contraindications

The contraindications to Chinese manual therapy are reported as follows:

- early-stage broken bones,
- limited blood clotting and bleeding,
- reddened swelling, i.e. acute inflammation and also swelling of unknown cause,
- skin diseases associated with skin injuries or defects, pus formation or contagious skin diseases,
- malignant tumours, osteomyelitis, osteotuberculosis and severe skeletal system diseases such as severe osteoporosis,
- limited cardiovascular function,
- psychiatric disorders,
- pregnancy with known tendency for spontaneous abortion,
- pronounced weak condition.

Side effects

- Tiredness,
- Feeling of warmth.
- Muscle stiffness and pain.
- Worsening symptoms.
- Autonomic reactions: change in micturition, change in bowel movements, change in menstruation.
- Skin irritation.

Practical aspects

Professional prerequisites

From a professional point of view it should be mentioned that the therapeutic techniques of acupuncture such as Tuina are so extensive that in the Chinese context unique paramedical professions (acupuncturists and manual therapists), with a usual training period of 3 years, have become established. Similar to the situation in Western countries, this methodologically defined professionalisation allows for an individualised and extensive treatment plan such as through a traditional Chinese orthopaedist to appropriately qualified colleagues, acupuncturists or Tuina therapists.

Medical prerequisites

For the application of Tuina as a complementary procedure in the context of modern medicine an orthodox diagnostic investigation must be carried out. This serves first of all to find a diagnosis and as a matter of priority to recognise promptly the necessary diagnostic and therapeutic steps of modern medicine and not subject them to delay. The above key contraindications must also be ruled out. Even if the orthodox medical diagnosis does not provide any information beyond the umbrella term of 'functional disorder', the indication and especially the arrangement of treatment principles is based on a thorough diagnosis in the area of TCM.

Space prerequisites

Space prerequisites for Tuina treatment:

- surroundings at a comfortable temperature, as treatment in this context is usually on a partially clothed patient,
- peaceful treatment atmosphere so that even longer treatment sequences can be carried out in a relaxed state,
- sufficient space to allow the therapist access to the treatment couch from all sides,

- treatment should be possible in a seated position,
- the treatment couch should be height-adjustable,
- the treatment couch should have a nose hole to enable a rotation-free prone position for the cervical spine,
- the treatment couch should be as adjustable as possible so that positioning can be adapted, e.g. in extension and release positions.

Training prerequisites

The Tuina therapist must pass a clinical course covering the indications and contraindications, know the legal prerequisites of manual therapy and besides the manual techniques and skills also create the basis for his or her own physical fitness, stamina, strength and coordination. Tuina therapy is strenuous, and this applies to beginners as well. Besides the above educational content, there should also be exercises for physical training in these aspects included in the educational programme. Tuina textbooks frequently include sections showing exercises for the therapist. These exercises are often based on traditional martial arts.

Chapter 23

Complementary and alternative therapies and naturopathic treatments

Dominik Irnich

Complementary and alternative methods (CAM) are widespread in clinical practice. Because of different definitions, there are no precise data for Germany on the level of self-medication and treatment outside the official supply sectors. In Europe 40–74% of the population is treated with CAM (Fisher, Ward 1994). Depending on the specialism required in the training, up to 80% of doctors are interested in complementary procedures and basically approve their application (Haltenhof et al. 1995).

23.1 DEFINITIONS

The term complementary and alternative methods includes various areas of non-conventional procedures which have so far not found a way into current expert opinion and are not represented in guidelines. Some 100–150 methods have been classified as complementary or alternative procedures (see Table 23.1).

A number of other labels have been used as an umbrella term for these methods, such as alternative medicine, paramedicine, holistic medicine, naturopathic treatments, empirical medicine and regulation medicine. However, these terms are frequently associated with a subjective evaluation or are uncritically applied to all procedures like the actually defined term 'naturopathic treatments'. The neutral term CAM is therefore used in the following, as it corresponds to current international usage (Zollmann, Vickers 1999b).

23.1.1 Complementary and alternative medicine

According to the definition by the Cochrane Collaboration, complementary and alternative medicine refers to 'a wide spectrum of potential healing methods, which embraces the healing system, modalities and practices including the underlying theories and assumptions which lie outside the prevailing health policy system of a specific society or culture at a given time. CAM includes practices and ideas which are used according to the definition of the user to prevent disease, to treat, to promote health and to improve wellbeing. The borders within CAM and the dominant system are not sharply defined or static.'

23.1.2 Traditional (Western) naturopathic treatments

To distinguish them by content and medical history, traditional (Western) naturopathic treatments consist of the five pillars of hydrotherapy and thermotherapy, phytotherapy, breathing and exercise therapy, nutritional therapy and ordering therapy (see Fig. 23.1). They are based on the Hippocratic medicine of antiquity, which is itself based on naturopathic factors and summarised by the Kneipp system. A considerable number of the methods have found a place in physical medicine, balneology, conservative orthopaedics, pharmacology, psychology, psychotherapy and even in conventional pain therapy.

23.1.3 Traditional Chinese medicine

Traditional Chinese medicine (TCM) can be compared to traditional Western naturopathic treatments, which also have a long tradition and continuity of application and also have certain parallels to the content of naturopathic treatments. Because of their special significance, the various procedures of TCM (acupuncture, Tuina and Qigong) are represented in other chapters (see Sections 22.2, 22.8 and 24.3).

http://dx.doi.org/10.1016/B978-0-7020-4312-3.00023-4

Table 23.1 Selection of complementary and alternative methods (in alphabetical order)

Acupressure	Environmental medicine	Regulation thermography
Acupuncture	Enzyme therapy	Reiki
Alexander technique	Eutonia	Ozone and oxygen therapy
Anthroposophic medicine	Feldenkrais therapy	Schüssler biochemistry
Aroma therapy	Felke therapy	Shiatsu
Art therapy	Fasting	Spagyric medicine
Astrology	Homeopathy	Speleotherapy
Autogenic training (AT)	Homotoxicology	Spiritual healing
Autohaemotherapy	Hydrotherapy	Symbiosis control
Ayurvedic medicine	Hyperthermia	Tai chi
Bach flower remedies	Hypnosis	Therapeutic touch
Balneotherapy	Jacobsen progressive muscle relaxation (PMR)	Thermotherapy
Bioresonance therapy	Kinesiology	Thymus therapy
Breathing therapy	Kirlian photography	Tuina
Chiropraxis	Magnetic field therapy	Visualisation
Climate therapy	Manual medicine	Voll's electroacupuncture
Colon hydrotherapy	Massage	Yoga
Colour therapy	Meditation	
Cytoplasmic therapy	Neural therapy	
Electrotherapy	Nosode treatment	
Elimination therapy with:	Nutritional therapy (>200 diets)	
• baunscheidt procedure	*Ordnungstherapie* (regulative therapy/ordering therapy)	
• blood letting	Organotherapy	
• cantharide plaster	Orthomolecular therapy	
• cupping	Osteopathy	
• fontanelle	Phytotherapy	
• leech therapy	Qigong	
• purging	Reflexology	

23.2 PRINCIPLES

The theoretical principles of CAM are manifold. Most procedures are based on the stimulation–reaction principle. For traditional naturopathic procedures in particular, there is a rule that weak stimulation promotes, strong stimulation inhibits and the strongest stimulation inhibits life activity (Arndt, Schulz 1953). The intensity of the stimulation depends on the individual condition and the patient's type of constitution.

CAM includes various diagnostic procedures and methods. The basis is the detailed history, where special

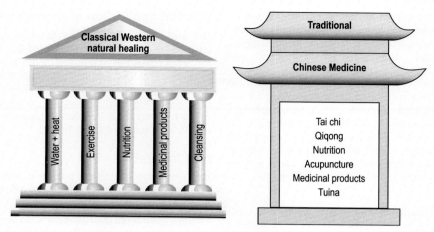

Fig. 23.1 Western and Chinese temples. (From the course script of the German Society of Acupuncture Physicians)

value is placed on the way the patient feels and their sensitivity, and the physical examination focusing on functionally disturbed, segmental reflective and constitutional aspects. Some of the newer CAM therapies make use of apparative measuring techniques and laboratory tests for their diagnosis. The separation of reliable and non-reliable methods based on validation studies in this area seems urgently required. There is a steady transfer to conventional techniques.

The aim of intervention is usually to activate the patient's powers of self-healing and stimulate the body to regulate itself. The adaptation processes stimulated must be regarded as a central biological mechanism. The specificity of the stimulus is not always in evidence but is also not always accepted in a theoretical context.

A scientific evaluation of the hypothesis formulated must be critically but openly undertaken for each individual procedure. Individual case descriptions, views of experts and explanations using only analogical conclusions do not represent scientific evidence of efficacy. Because of general interest increased research efforts in this area should be demanded. However, a prerequisite for this is its promotion by the relevant institutions and cost units, as there is ever-dwindling financial support for research in this field.

23.3 TREATMENT PROCEDURES

Because of the great number of CAM, an individual evaluation of all the methods for myofascial pain cannot be carried out. Some of the procedures are part of complete healing systems with their own view of health and disease. It is necessary to look at the relevant basic works for information on their theoretical principles and philosophical, socioeconomic and historical backgrounds.

The evaluation of the procedures has been carried out essentially using the available scientific studies on their efficacy for myofascial pain. Overall, there is a definite lack in most fields of high-quality scientific studies. However, it should be noted that an appropriate placebo-controlled study in accordance with drug trials cannot be carried out or not sufficiently carried out for many of the alternative procedures or in physiotherapeutic or other 'hands-on' procedures because of the lack of a proper placebo control.

The following selection of complementary and alternative procedures is based on subjective, empirical experience, but it also tries to include scientific aspects and relates to the efficacy for myofascial pain. The five pillars of traditional naturopathic treatments are first described; then there are the procedures which have been classed as naturopathic treatments by various authors. The procedures of TCM are discussed only briefly, as individual procedures are described in their own chapters because of their special significance.

23.3.1 Hydrotherapy and thermotherapy

The application of water in various combined conditions and hot and cold applications are components of traditional naturopathic procedures and a significant strand of Kneipp therapy. They have a broad spectrum of effect on the muscles. Besides local tissue effects on perfusion, metabolism, lymph circulation, muscle tension and use of oxygen, positive effects have been described on the neuroautonomic system (Brenke, Polonius 2002).

The duration and strength of the stimulus are adapted to the current patient condition and the patient's constitutional prerequisites. Because of the many levels of application possibilities, stimulation is very varied and individual.

In practice, hydrotherapy and thermotherapy can be favourably combined with many procedures used in the treatment of myofascial pain. Many of the techniques can also be used by the patient after appropriate instruction.

Randomised, controlled studies on hydrotherapy and thermotherapy for chronic pain are not available in sufficient quality, however, so the following instructions are based on empirical evidence or studies on different indications.

Practical application of hydrotherapy

The application of hydrotherapy can be divided into two approaches to the treatment of mTrPs.

Local treatment: mTrPs can be directly treated with a moderately strong stream of lukewarm water. The pressure of the stream of water can be varied, depending on the position of the mTrP: the deeper the mTrP, the stronger the stream. As a guideline, the stream of water should cause a 'dent' of 1–2 cm during treatment. There should be a pause after 30–45 s to allow the whole muscle to stretch for about 60 s. This process can be repeated up to 10 times. This technique also includes underwater massage using jets. Make sure that the water temperature remains close to that of body temperature.

Systemic relaxation: this is the traditional neuroautonomic mood-changing technique of traditional Kneipp treatment. It includes applying water jets to specific parts of the body such as the lower leg, leg or back, and whole body jets. The techniques described in the relevant books lead to neuroautonomic mood changes and can contribute to normalisation of muscle tension.

Note the following principles of hydrotherapy:

- note the condition of the cardiovascular system (medical investigation),
- psychoemotional stress situations and concomitant psychiatric diseases can be a contraindication,
- the first treatment should be a test run,
- begin treatment with gentle stimuli (cold, warmth; warning: ice, heat),
- increase the intensity of the stimulation in stages,
- do not apply cold or ice if patients are feeling cold,
- the patient should not eat immediately before treatment,
- acute symptoms tend to respond to cold treatment, chronic symptoms to warmth,
- do not use warmth or heat for inflammatory back pain,
- direction of jets, washes and rubs: away from the heart after close to the heart, peripheral after central, down after up, lateral after medial,
- gentle mobilisation or bed rest after treatment.

Practical application of thermotherapy

The well-known rule applies in most cases: for acute traumatic injury of the muscle, cold should be applied, for longer existing symptoms warmth has frequently proved helpful. The choice of procedure therefore depends on the acuity and cause of the mTrPs. The information from the patient, however, is crucial as to when and to what extent heat or cold is beneficial. This information should usually be discovered in the history.

Heat therapy

Heat therapy as a physical procedure is described in Ch. 20. Real applications are described here, which have proved reliable for myofascial pain.

Peloids: peloids include the application of peat from a peat bog or therapeutic earths. The application of packs which are just warm and not too hot has proved useful in the treatment of mTrPs. These are applied to the affected sites and left to work for about 15–20 min. To keep the heat in, the packs are covered with a cloth or towel.

Hay bag (see Fig. 23.2): hay bags are available from pharmacists or health shops. They are heated over steam and are then applied to the affected site for about 10 min (keeping in the warmth, see above). Exercise caution with patients who have allergic diseases. Requirements: hay bag, a towel in the middle, an outer towel, steam with a sieve insert or a wide saucepan with a drainer.

Mustard pack (see Fig. 23.3): the mustard develops a strong local heat reaction. Be careful with sensitive patients that the mustard does not come into contact with the skin. It is possible to get black mustard powder (semen sinapis powder) directly and mix it with hot water, or to pulverise mustard grains in a mortar with the addition of hot water. The mass is spread thinly between two thin gauze compresses or between layers of a rather thicker compress and placed in position. The application is wrapped with a cotton towel. The compresses should stay in place for about 5 min until there is a definite reddening of the skin, without the patient feeling any pain. The skin can then be rubbed with oil.

Cold therapy

The application of ice or strong cold is only recommended for mTrP for the spray and stretch procedure (see Section 18.3). Some patients report an improvement from cold application, for example by applying a terry towel cooled by holding under cold water to the affected muscle (see Section 21.2).

23.3.2 Phytotherapy

The medicinal use of monosubstances from plants is one of the key principles of modern medicinal pain therapy. These include morphine, capsaicin, salicylic acid and

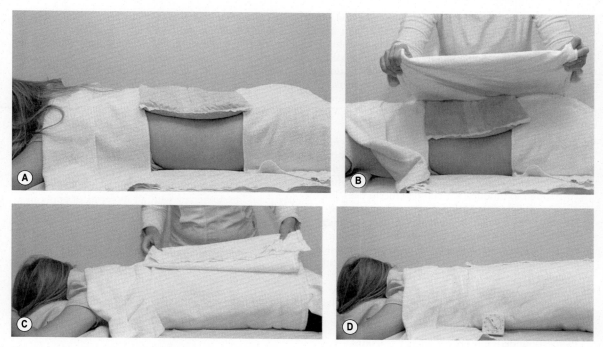

Fig. 23.2 Heat therapy using a hay bag.

Fig. 23.3 Heat therapy using a mustard powder pack.

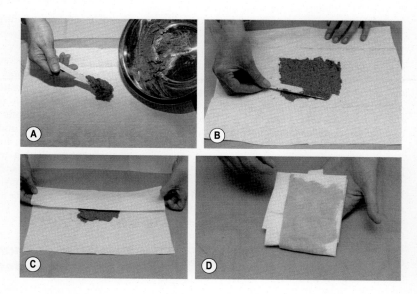

tetrahydrocannabinol. Phytotherapy is the use of mixtures of ingredients from plants, plant parts and their preparations. Phytotherapeutic products are available in a variety of forms: tablets, extracts, tinctures, oils, juices, teas or distillates. The World Health Organization (WHO), the European Union (EU), the European Scientific Cooperative on Phytotherapy (ESCOP) and the Committee of the Federal Institute for Drugs and Medicinal Products are busy with a scientific evaluation of phytotherapeutic products.

No phytotherapeutic products have been specifically trialled for myofascial pain. Nevertheless, there are positive study results for back pain for willow bark (*Salicis cortex*), the South African devil's claw root (*Harpagophyti radix*) and a compound product made of aspen (*Populus*), ash bark (*Fraxinus* sp.) and golden rod (*Solidago*) (Phytodolor®). However their analgesic potency lies in the lower to middle range. For chronic myofascial pain, an attempt at treatment can be justified if the patient requests 'plant' products.

Practical course of action: for back pain the following phytotherapeutic products can be recommended as adjuvant pain therapy based on the available evidence.

- Willow bark (*S. cortex*): anti-inflammatory, analgesic, liquid or solid administrative form, average daily dose corresponding to 60–120 mg total salicin; interactions and undesirable effects can theoretically occur which correspond to products containing salicylic acid, but clinical studies indicate that these products are better tolerated; a frequent ingredient of compound products.
- South African devil's claw root (*H. radix*): analgesic effects especially for degenerative back pain, evidence of inhibition of leukotriene synthesis, predominantly in tablet form, daily dose 1000–1400 mg.
- Bromelain (pineapple extract): anti-inflammatory, analgesic, predominantly available in tablet form, daily dose 500–1000 mg; contraindications: clotting disorder (do not give before operations), allergic diathesis; undesirable effects: allergic reactions, bloating, meteorism, nausea, interactions with antibiotics.
- There is evidence of the analgesic and anti-inflammatory effects of the compound product Phytodolor® (Ernst 1999).

The external application of phytotherapeutic products such as camphor, arnica, eucalyptus, spruce and pine needles, cayenne pepper and similar as ointments, creams, essential oils, extracts or solutions has a local hyperaemic or cooling astringent effect, depending on the composition. Good analgesic effects have also been achieved on occasion. They can lead to local allergic reactions in rare cases.

23.3.3 Breathing therapy

Breathing therapy includes a wide field of various techniques. Physiotherapeutic breathing therapy is predominantly for treating diseases of the organs of respiration. On the other hand, there are psychological and physiological forms of breathing therapy have been developed in the context of naturopathic treatments from the point of view of relaxation, body perception and meditation which have also found a place in psychosomatic medicine.

One of the most well-known forms of breathing therapy is the 'breath experience' method from I. Middendorf. This is an active exercise procedure, which tries to make the patient healthy. Eutonia describes a mentally and physically balanced state of suspense. The therapist instructs specific exercises, which the patient does on their own. This is not a perfectly external exercise but an holistic awareness of self and of conscious breathing. The aim of the therapy is to enable the patient to actively control the pain. Consistent practice of the exercises is considered a prerequisite for the success of the therapy.

There is much evidence of the physiological effects of breathing therapy, although there are no specific studies on myofascial pain (Middendorf 1995).

23.3.4 Motion/exercise therapy

Exercise therapy in the sense of naturopathic treatments includes exercises for whole-body fitness with moderate but regular stamina training and the creation of an everyday plan. Physiotherapy with all its forms of application and techniques and training of body posture are other components.

Many of these procedures have found a use in conventional treatment but they are still used in various forms in the naturopathic context. Basically any form of exercise therapy can be helpful for patients with chronic myofascial pain to overcome the pain and increases physical fitness. The procedures relevant to myofascial pain are given in Ch. 24 under relaxation techniques or as exercises specifically for the individual muscles (see Chs 26–34).

23.3.5 Dietary treatment

The influence of nutrition on the course of chronic diseases has long been known and has been shown to be especially relevant for cardiovascular and metabolic diseases. As part of losing weight because of obesity and back pain or as part of health education and as an addition to behavioural therapy, dietary treatment can be a valuable part of a multimodal treatment plan. It includes general knowledge about nutrition and physiology, the psychosocial significance of food, individual nutritional advice and the creation of a plan for everyday eating. We advise against short-term dieting and monodiets because of the lack of long-term effects and rebound weight gain. For the treatment of chronic myofascial pain a balanced and healthy diet can contribute to general wellbeing and indirectly to overcoming pain.

23.3.6 *Ordnungstherapie* (regulative therapy/ordering therapy)

We can regard *ordnungstherapie* as an holistic general term for a healthy lifestyle. The naturopathic treatment rules and advice about ordering therapy go back to Hippocrates (*diaita*), Kneipp (*Ordnungstherapie als 5. Säule der NHV*, or ordering therapy as the fifth pillar of natural healing) and Bircher-Benner (*Ordnungsgesetze des Lebens*, or *Laws of Life*; 1999). Antonovsky's principle of salutogenesis also continues aspects or ordering therapy.

Ordering therapy includes the levels of dispersing information, changing consciousness and behaviour. It has rules on nutrition, life economy, life rhythm and the ordering of the spiritual life. Only a few of the rules have so far been scientifically evaluated. However, there are large Anglo-American studies that show that changes in lifestyle can have positive effects on health. This also applies of course to overcoming chronic myofascial pain.

23.3.7 Detoxifying/cleansing procedures

Detoxifying procedures are considered part of naturopathic remedies in the wider sense. Distinctions:

- external procedures: e.g. cupping, leech therapy, blood letting, cantharide plaster, baunscheidt therapy;
- internal procedures: e.g. the administration of laxatives, purgatives, sudorifics, bile stimulants, diuretics and medicines to promote menstruation.

The following describes cupping and leech therapy, but we cannot recommend treatment for the other procedures for back pain.

Cupping

Cupping over mTrPs, tenderpoints, connective tissue swelling and segmental function disorders can have an analgesic and relaxing effect on acute and chronic myofascial pain. The cups can usually be placed directly over the trigger point or on the known Abele cupping zones (see Fig. 13.8).

Practical course of action: the cup is placed either over the affected area or paravertebrally in the affected segment and is left for 5–20 min, depending on the reaction of the patient (see Fig. 23.4). After a positive test this treatment can then be carried out independently by the patient. Cupping should also be used on the basis of reflectory and cutivisceral associations as a segmental treatment (e.g. also contralaterally) or in accordance with the Abele cupping zones.

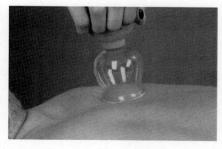

Fig. 23.4 Cupping treatment for segmental function disorder of the thoracic spine. For muscular tension the cup can be pushed over the whole paravertebral vertebral column muscles with the help of massage oil (cupping massage).

For acute muscular strain, a cupping massage three to five finger widths paravertebrally along the whole back extensor muscles can bring some relief and relaxation. This massage can be carried out by a partner.

Leech therapy

The effectiveness of leeches for acute tissue injury with haematoma has been shown. The effect is based on local unblocking and haematocrit-lowering effects and on the effect of hirudin, eglin, hyaluronic acid and enzymes. This procedure has already found a place in all care sectors but is only used for acute pain caused by trauma or massive myogeloses. The prerequisite for application is a knowledge of handling leeches, careful explanation to the patient and using the leeches only once. Leech therapy is not indicated for chronic pain.

23.3.8 Acupuncture

For a detailed explanation of acupuncture see Ch. 22.

23.3.9 Qigong

Qigong is a traditional method in Chinese medicine which has the aim of preventing and treating diseases. The life power of 'Qi' is mobilised and trained by body posture, exercise, breathing and concentration exercises. According to TCM, Qi unfolds to strengthen body, mind and soul and help to relieve pain permanently. The basic principle of Qigong is consistent practice. Tai chi is a related form characterised by more complex movement processes and is somewhat closer to the Chinese martial arts. A number of different styles have been described for both procedures. They are enjoying increasing popularity with patients and can be integrated as group exercise into multimodal pain programmes with the aim of improving the mental and physical capacity to relax, discipline and body perception.

There are numerous studies on both procedures from the Chinese-speaking world. However, in most cases, where they are available, these do not meet the quality standards required so there is no evidence available of the efficacy of Qigong or Tai chi for back pain (for details of the method see Ch. 24).

23.3.10 Tuina

Tuina is an umbrella term for the manual techniques of TCM. The TCM system of disease forms the theoretical basis. The basic techniques comprise squeezing, kneading, pushing, grasping and pinching, rolling, rubbing, rotating, traction, shaking and exercising. The therapy is based on the meridians and acupuncture points. These are predominantly massage techniques which can easily be combined with other physiotherapy procedures or acupuncture.

However, manipulative techniques are also described. These should be used with caution as they do not correspond to the latest biomechanical knowledge (medical or physiotherapy checks). There is evidence that Tuina is more effective for back pain than conventional (Western) massage. However, there is not yet any evidence of long-term efficacy (Furlan et al. 2002) (details of the method see Section 22.8).

23.3.11 Chinese pharmacotherapy

Chinese pharmacotherapy is based on TCM models of explanation. It is the most frequently used procedure in TCM. Similarly to Western phytotherapy, the pharmaceutical products are attributed to various qualities ('free the surface', 'draw out moisture', 'strengthening', etc.) Mastering the rules of Chinese pharmacotherapy requires a much more intense examination of the theoretical basis of Chinese medicine than acupuncture. There are very few non-Chinese physicians and therapists who can devote themselves to the long training period.

Efforts are being made on standardisation and quality control of the medicinal products and formulae (e.g. Association of German TCM Pharmacists). There are potential threats from recurrent grey imports and imports of ready-to-use medicinal products for which it is very difficult to check the individual content. There are monographs for individual medicinal herbs but the use of Chinese pharmacotherapy cannot be recommended at this time.

23.3.12 Chinese nutritional therapy (*Ordnungstherapie*)

Chinese nutritional therapy is a preventative and therapeutic measure based on TCM. Foodstuffs are divided according to temperature behaviour (cold, cool, neutral, warm, hot), taste (sweet, sharp, salty, sour, bitter, neutral), their relationship to the circle of function of TCM and accepted direction of effect (rising, swaying, lowering, falling). For example, for back pain with deterioration of motion and cold symptoms, warming and strengthening foods are recommended, such as chicken soup, duck with walnuts, cooked pigs' kidneys, lamb and chestnut. Chinese nutritional therapy has not yet been the object of scientific studies.

Similar to the ordering therapy of Western naturopathic remedies, there are TCM rules for a healthy lifestyle for the prevention of disease. They cover all the areas of life. For the prevention of back pain, an appropriate alternation between exercise and resting phases, and protection from external climatic factors such as wind, cold and moisture by suitable clothing are recommended, as is avoidance of sexual excess and eating seasonal foods with the emphasis on fortifying foodstuffs.

23.3.13 Homeopathy

Homeopathy is a treatment system which uses the tiniest doses in accordance with the principle of healing like with like. Homeopathy is one of the most commonly used alternative therapies. In Europe, between 28 and 56% of the population uses homeopathic treatment for a variety of diseases (Fisher, Ward 1994). The scientific basis must be interpreted with caution. Many of the trials examined non-representative indications and problems with the methods used have made it difficult to draw conclusions. There is currently insufficient evidence of the efficacy of homeopathy for chronic pain. Because of positive tendencies from clinical trials and analyses (Gmunder, Kissling 2002), the low rate of side effects, low costs and lack of interaction with other procedures mean that it may be appropriate depending on the patient's wish for concomitant homeopathic medicine for acute reduction of chronic pain. However, treatment cannot be recommended based on the current data.

23.3.14 Neural therapy

Huneke neural therapy uses the injection of LA for therapeutic purposes. It consists of segment therapy and disrupted field therapy. The more modern term 'therapeutic LA' for LA injections is sometimes also used as a synonym for neural therapy. The main difference lies in neural therapy's own theory and treatment of the disrupted field.

Segment therapy comprises an intracutaneous injection (stimulating spot) and deeper injections into the muscles, tendons, ligaments and bones, which can be painful. This field of neural therapy shows some short-term efficacy on pain. There has so far not been any evidence of long-term effects. As part of neural therapy, LAs are also injected peridurally, at the nerve roots, at the sympathic ganglia and at peripheral nerves. An evaluation of these injections can be found in Ch. 21.

The basis of the Störfeld (disturbed field) theory is the acceptance that any disease can be caused by a Störfeld and that any part of the body can be a Störfeld, which can restrict the body's own regulatory capacity. The teeth, tonsils, paranasal sinuses and scar tissue are regarded as susceptible to the formation of interference fields. The theoretical basis used is the Pischinger 'cell milieu system', which cites the significance of the unity of cell, interstitium with capillaries and nerve endings and sees in a repolarisation disorder the morphological functional correlate for the occurrence of interference fields. This is then switched off by the injection of LA at or into the affected structure. There are plenty of case reports that support these theories but there is as yet no scientific evidence for the existence of interference fields.

The preferred LA for neural therapy injections is 1 or 2% procaine hydrochloride solution. This recommendation is based more on the acceptance of specific effects of procaine in the 'cell milieu system' than on scientifically reproduced tests on the theory, so other LAs can be used as well (for the choice of LAs see also Ch. 25).

The described long-term regulatory effects of neural therapy injections have so far not been covered by any scientific studies.

Procedure: neural therapy injections can be helpful for the treatment of acute back pain if they are used for segmental spot treatment and injections at myofascial and ligamentary mTrPs.

- For intracutaneous injection 0.2–0.5 ml of LA are injected into the area of the affected segment over the main pain points. Optimum success is achieved by using several injections in the reflected segments of the skin of the hyperalgesic zones. The spot treatment can be carried out on one side only or on both sides if pain is severe. For diffuse symptoms, a series of spot treatments is recommended on both sides over the transverse processes of the affected segments.
- The injection of LA into mTrPs has proved a reliable neural therapy technique for back pain. It has found a place in conventional pain therapy and is carried out according to the recommendations of Simons and Travell and after manual and functional anatomical examinations (Travell, Simons 1992).
- The injections at the small vertebral joints and the iliosacral joint should be carried out according to the appropriate manual examination findings and their confirmation by imaging procedures initially for diagnosis under X-ray or CT guidance.
- More invasive techniques such as injections into the epidural space or sympathetic ganglia blockades, which are also described as neural therapy techniques, are only performed under appropriate safety conditions with sufficient indication and by an experienced therapist.
- LA injections into scars, teeth or other structures which may be hyperalgesic or hyperaesthetic (see discussion of interference fields, above) may in individual cases lead to the relief of pain. There are reports of associations between sensitive incisors (including the relevant mucosa) according to Kramer and retromolar points according to Gleditsch, with functional symptoms in the area of the lumbar spine and it is worth trying to switch them off with LA if findings are abnormal. As with all test and diagnostic injections, this should lead to a definite reproducible relief of pain.
- Hyperalgesic scars in the area of the vertebral column can be test-infiltrated relatively without risk.

23.3.15 Autohaemotherapy

Autologous blood injection is performed with or without processing (including haemolysis, short-wave radiation, UV radiation, addition of certain medicinal products) of the removed blood. The theoretical concept is based on the stimulation–reaction principle and the triggering of an 'autonomic change'. It is a widespread complementary procedure, including among chronic pain patients. Beyond individual case reports and observations of use there are no studies, so it cannot be recommended for myofascial pain.

23.3.16 Ozone and oxygen therapy

Ozone and oxygen are used in various forms. Widespread among pain patients are von Ardenne's multi-stage oxygen therapy, ozone injections (intracutaneous, subcutaneous, intramuscular, intra-articular) and the enrichment of autologous blood with ozone or oxygen. There is no scientific basis for any of the procedures which go beyond the known physiological effects of oxygen. There are no clinical trials, so the treatment cannot be recommended.

23.3.17 Magnetic field therapy

The use of magnets for therapy has a very long tradition. Magnetic field devices (mats), magnetic coils and various magnetic objects are used. The stronger the field, the greater the evidence of *in vitro* effects on the cell organism. However, no effects relevant to disease have been shown and most of the theories lack a scientific basis. Clinical studies are of insufficient quantity and quality, so patients are often advised not to purchase the equipment.

23.3.18 Manual medicine, chiropractice and osteopathy

All three procedures can be classified as CAM, but they have found a place to varying degrees in conventional medicine. Manual medicine and physiotherapeutic methods are therefore discussed in Chapter 18.

Osteopathy was developed in the USA at the end of the 19th century and is a widely used method of manual therapy there. It involves complex treatment of the whole body and its homeostasis. Some of the underlying theories, however, do not stand up to scientific testing. Osteopathy indicates functional disorders and diseases as a limitation of synovial joint surfaces/connective tissue articular surfaces and changes in tissue tension. Structural and functional changes to the skeleton, especially the vertebral column, are of particular significance. There are three different systems for the diagnosis and therapy, in which tissue blockages can occur:

- the parietal system, the real skeletal system with posture and support function and the associated joints, muscles, tendons and fascia,
- the visceral system with the visceral organs and the associated vascular, lymphatic, fascial and neuronal structures,

- the craniosacral system with skull, spinal canal and sacrum as well as the associated sutures, meninges, membranes and fascia.

The osteopath uses various manual techniques to release tissue blockages. The aim is to restore normal tissue mobility and tension.

In practice there is an increasing clientele for osteopathic treatment. Besides numerous case reports there has been an increase in research in the last few years. The first randomised studies showed evidence of positive effects for osteopathy for back pain (Williams et al. 2003), although the evidence of superiority over manual medicine and chiropraxis has not been produced as yet. There is insufficient evidence of the efficacy of osteopathy for myofascial pain. Based on positive experiences, the treatment of the muscles and their fascia with specific techniques, some of which are classified as osteopathy, are described in the section on fascial techniques (see Section 18.4).

23.3.19 Kinesiology

Kinesiology is a relatively new procedure which brings together elements of manual therapy, chiropractice, acupuncture, homoeopathy and other complementary medicine methods. It is an holistic system for diagnosis and treatment and consists of various variations (applied kinesiology, behavioural kinesiology, touch for health, etc.)

The most common variation is applied kinesiology (AK). The muscle test is the diagnostic basis during which muscular reaction patterns are observed after diagnostic provocation in a mechanical, (bio)chemical or psychological manner and the history and examination also provides information on the areas of disorder and their cause.

There are in fact a series of clinical studies on AK, but weaknesses in method and the individualised therapeutic procedure do not lend themselves to a scientific assessment of AK, so we must assume there is insufficient evidence of the efficacy of AK for myofascial pain.

23.3.20 Reflex zone therapy

The most well-known reflex zone is the foot, but reflex zones have also been described on the hands, the skull and other body parts such as the nose, ear and mouth (Gleditsch 2002, and Section 22.4). Common to all is the assumption that an effect can be caused on the whole organism from a small area of the body. The system is based on the somatotopic structure of the body. There are some interesting physiological explanations for individual connections but there is as yet no conclusive evidence of the existence and function of the reflex zones and the efficacy of the treatment based on scientific knowledge.

The patient may be prompted to self-massage or partner massage of the foot reflex zones as complementary treatment for myofascial pain.

23.4 INTEGRATING CAM INTO MULTIMODAL PAIN PROGRAMMES

23.4.1 Integration of individual methods

Some CAM methods can be integrated with appropriate prerequisites in multimodal pain programmes. These include acupuncture, acupressure, reflex therapies, Qigong/ Tai chi, yoga, naturopathic hydrotherapy, thermotherapy, breathing therapy, exercise therapy and regulatory therapy and osteopathy. They have already found a place at the national and international levels in a range of specialised treatments.

If a CAM procedure is chosen as a component of a multimodal programme, the following items should be noted:

- the therapists and leaders should be highly trained (possibly obtaining certification by a recognised institution),
- therapists and leaders should be experienced and competent in the handling of pain patients,
- for adaptation to the underlying plan, i.e. for programmes which work exclusively with activity-promoting elements, do not choose passive methods or else adapt these (acupuncture could be adapted to instructions for autonomic acupressure),
- avoid competition between 'conventional medicine' and 'naturopathic' procedures by mutual exchange of information between therapists about the characteristics of the methods used,
- no mystification of the cause of the pain through CAM,
- avoid overlap between methods.

23.4.2 Naturopathically based multimodal pain programme: three-stage plan

The combination of a naturopathically based multimodal pain programme appears possible and promising under certain conditions. However, the essential and reliable elements of a conventional pain programme should not in any way be sacrificed. These include important educative elements such as patient seminars and training, the back-pain-specific elements of ergotherapy and training therapy and psychological pain elements.

Naturopathic elements such as the pursuance of aspects of regulatory therapy and an holistic view of the diseases from the naturopathic point of view, explanation of nutritional therapy and Eastern or Western naturopathic exercise therapy can be added to these tried and tested programme parts and supplement them.

An appropriate 4-week pain programme, partly as an inpatient, has been developed and tried out at the Munich

University Hospital Pain Centre. It is now a fixed component of a three-stage long-term programme for chronic pain patients (Munich naturopathic pain programme, three-stage plan) (Irnich et al. 2005).

Stage 1: 4-week intensive programme (partly in-patient)

A group of eight patients was treated for 5 days a week using an interdisciplinary approach following a fixed treatment plan. Besides the individual treatments there was an emphasis on group work. Participation requires active participation and a willingness to come to terms with different aspects of chronic pain.

The aim of the holistic plan is to encourage the patient as far as possible to take on the responsibility of managing the pain and its effects. The wide range on offer also allows the individual identification of effective therapeutic approaches.

The in-patient intensive group programme is divided as follows.

Motivation and information
1. Seminar: chronic pain as an holistic biological, psychological and social event.
2. Seminar: medical and non-medical treatments.
3. Seminar: naturopathic treatments: theory, possibilities and limits.
4. Seminar: diet awareness as the basis of maintenance of health.
5. Seminar: overcoming stress, pain in work and family.

Activities and exercises for overcoming pain
1. Meditation and imagination.
2. Art therapy.
3. Glaser psychotonics (communicative exercise therapy).
4. Breathing therapy.
5. Qigong.
6. Exercise – coordination – play.
7. Rhythmics.

Naturopathic treatments
1. Acupuncture (traditional Chinese, microsystems, trigger point acupuncture), moxibustion and related techniques.
2. Neural therapy/therapeutic local anaesthesia.
3. TENS with detailed individual search for optimum location and optimum stimulation parameters.
4. Introduction and instructions on baths, wraps and drenches.
5. Naturopathic autotherapy.

Stage 2: open groups

Stage 2 of the Munich naturopathic intensive pain programme builds on the first stage. The experiences of the 4-week programme are intensified in open groups. These are composed entirely of participants from prior intensive pain programmes. Open groups mean that the group structure of the 4-week programme is preserved and that

it is not compulsory to take part but the opportunity is there at any time (even after a lengthy pause).

This second phase allows patients to continue their individual positive experiences. The open groups are led by the same lecturer as stage 1. This makes sure the build-up of trust is maintained and specific needs of patients are taken into account.

Deepening their knowledge of the procedures learned enables the patients to become more secure and independent in the chosen procedures in the long term. The aim is to integrate these experiences into their everyday lives and help to change the pain experience and lead to an increase in their feeling of wellbeing.

A small financial contribution is requested for open groups, depending on the course they are on.

Stage 3: long-term support

Stage 3 includes regular group meetings, sometimes in the absence of a physician or therapist, with discussions. These meetings help to maintain the group dynamic developed during the intensive programme and includes an exchange of experiences, mutual support, motivation for self-help and social involvement.

This part makes use of the benefits offered by participation in a self-help group. Involvement in the prescribed plan should, however, avoid any potential disadvantage of self-help groups. Lectures on various topics to do with pain therapy are also offered within this framework once a fortnight.

This plan was awarded first place out of 40 submitted projects in the national hospital promotion prize 2002 from the Bayerischen Landesbank.

23.4.3 A vision of integrated medicine

The word integration (Latin *integer*; Greek *entagros* = unspoilt, undamaged, whole) means in English the creation of a whole. In sociology, integration means the holding together of parts in a systemic whole and a delimitation from an unstructured surrounding.

In medicine, 'integrated medicine' means the synthesis of various healing procedures and opinions to form an holistic form of therapy.

For further discussion, please note that the term integrated therapy was defined and reserved in the 1970s as a specific form of human therapy in German and Switzerland by Petzold et al. They combined exercise therapy, sociotherapy and psychotherapeutic approaches and developed a unique metatheory. The main psychotherapeutic sources of integrative therapy are psychodrama, Gestalt therapy, active Ferenczi psychoanalysis and aspects of behavioural therapy. The most significant philosophers who influenced the development of integrative therapy were Merleau-Ponty, Gabriel Marcel and later Hermann Schmitz.

> The above definitions show that the unstructured and voluntary stringing together or placing next to each other of various therapies, which is sometimes dependent only on chance or personal or economic interests, cannot be described as integration as long as there is not supporting 'whole'.

However, this aspect is not always taken into account if you look at the frequently all-too-often inflationary use of the terms integration and integrative in medicine. An analysis of the many plans offered under the heading 'integrative' shows that different methods are just offered next to each other with there being any synthesis.

What theoretical demands should now be attached to the term integrative medicine?

- The roots of a medicine which can be described as integrative must stem from various treatments and various therapies and opinions.
- A new whole must arise from these roots by definition.

- A parallel range of various therapies cannot be described as an integrative concept of medicine.
- It should be clear from the description which therapies have been brought together (e.g. Eastern or Western traditional medical systems).
- Plans which do not take into account the knowledge of Western naturopathic medicine are hardly integrative, as they overlook the prevailing opinion.

The following practical consequences help to fulfil these demands:

- there must be a close physical, structural and spiritual connection between the participants,
- doctors and therapists from the different systems must be able to work together,
- a prerequisite is that they are all highly trained, have many years of experience and be able to critically examine themselves in order to grasp the possibilities and limits of their own methods and procedures,
- another prerequisite is the development together of the continuing plan, this is only possible outside everyday hospital or practice life,
- all participants must get to know the peculiarities of the procedures that have been integrated in order to work together,
- it is particularly important for the use of an integrated plan that feedback from patients and particularly the course of treatment is discussed in regular team meetings.

Chapter 24

Relaxation techniques: body and mind

Christine Irnich

24.1 PRELIMINARY REMARKS

Systematic relaxation techniques are used in many areas of application by doctors, psychologists and sports and exercise therapists, both preventatively and for rehabilitation. As part of the treatment of myofascial pain, with or without restricted movement, relaxation techniques and body and mind therapy initially play a secondary role. For chronic MPSs with biological, psychological and social consequences, relaxation techniques can be a valuable component of a multimodal treatment plan and play a key part in successful healing.

What these techniques all have in common is that they all lead to a definite reduction in muscle tension if successfully practised. This supports the patient's ability to master the pain. There are as yet no studies available on specific MFSs.

24.1.1 Forms of relaxation technique

Western relaxation techniques	• Autogenic training (AT) • Jacobsen progressive muscle relaxation (PMR) • Imagination techniques (catathymic image experience, active imagination, fantasising, hypnosis, etc.) • Biofeedback
Eastern relaxation techniques	• Meditation • Qigong • Yoga

Systematic methods of physical and psychological relaxation are distinct from individual forms of relaxation and recuperation (such as 'having a rest', listening to pleasant relaxing music or individual activities where you can 'switch off') in that they are empirically researched and scientifically validated as standardised, more or less generally applicable techniques.

They are based on the systematic practising of psychomotor relaxation routines. With sufficient training or experience the desired effects can be quickly and voluntarily achieved with some stability and regularity. This applies particularly to applications during and after stressful situations where unsystematic relaxation techniques more often fail.

All systematic relaxation techniques allow experiences of the systematic, deliberate switching from sympathetic stimulation (performance and activation reaction) of the autonomic nervous system to parasympathetic stimulation (relaxation and recuperation reaction).

24.1.2 Use for myofascial pain

Preventative use	• Reduction of susceptibility to stress factors • Capacity of a person to maintain and improve his or her mental and physical health • Shortening duration of disease • Improvement in disease management
Rehabilitative use	• Reduction of risk of relapse • Active influence on own development • Self build up • Self regulation

http://dx.doi.org/10.1016/B978-0-7020-4312-3.00024-6

Relaxation techniques are useful adjuvant therapy for:

- chronic myofascial pain caused by:
  - strains,
  - continued use of the muscles on one side,
  - being forced into an awkward position,
  - blockade of segments of the vertebral column,
  - lack of coordination/poor exercise technique,
  - poor posture;
- change in muscle tension of psychological or emotional cause such as:
  - stress,
  - anxiety,
  - anger and annoyance,
  - depressive mood.

Relaxation techniques have a basic concept in common:

- They contribute to a reduction in muscle tension.
- Individual muscle groups and muscle function chains can be identified and relaxed by training in body awareness and this can lead to a reduction in pain.

24.2 WESTERN RELAXATION TECHNIQUES

24.2.1 Autogenic training

Definition

Autogenic training is a method of autosuggestion which teaches a clearly structured process where the patient concentrates on relaxing. The aim is to transform oneself into a state of relaxation. The patient influences themself using formulae and statements spoken in their thoughts.

Physiological principles

Involuntary body reactions are influenced by stabilisation and changing the autonomic nervous system and encouraging parasympathetic reactions.

Theoretical basis

Autogenic training was developed in the 1920s from the systematic observation of hypnotised patients by neurologist I.H. Schultz, but in contrast to hypnosis it is based exclusively on autosuggestion. In the early stages, physical processes are influenced by basic exercises. Weight, warmth, breathing, abdominal, heart and forehead exercises (see below) are used. After concentrating on the feelings generated by these exercises for some time, the patient actually senses them and the body reacts. The more advanced levels of autogenic training are based on the use of imaginative techniques.

Indications

Muscle tension, stress, mental unrest, pain, migraine, asthma, sleep disorders, cardiovascular symptoms, hypertension and gastric symptoms are all indications for autogenic training.

Contraindications

Severe anxiety state, depression and delusions are contraindications for autogenic training.

Practical procedure for myofascial pain

The advantage of autogenic training is that it can be used at any time and anywhere. In the early stages, it is mostly the physical processes that are influenced. The patient tries to concentrate exclusively on the body. The patient lies relaxed on the back or seated like a rag doll.

The basic exercises include the following.

- **Weight exercise:** the patient initially concentrates on a specific part of the body, usually an arm or a leg. The therapist may say: 'My arm is very heavy'. The heaviness can later be extended to other parts of the body and the whole body.
- **Warmth exercise:** as for the weight exercise, it is initially suggested that a certain part of the body is feeling very warm, then the pleasant feeling of warmth is spread across the whole body.
- **Breathing exercise:** the formula repeated by the therapist may be: 'My breathing is very quiet'.
- **Abdominal exercise:** concentration is on the upper abdomen and the patient attempts to guide warmth into this area of the body.
- **Heart exercise:** the heart is influenced by concentrating on an even and quiet heartbeat.
- **Forehead exercise:** the formula repeated by the therapist may be: 'My head is light'.

The patient is guided through the exercises by an experienced therapist and after several practice sessions the patient actually feels that the body react to the suggested sensation.

> The statements must be spoken in a quiet and gentle voice and must always be positive: a negative should not occur. Thus 'My arm is very heavy', not 'My arm is not light'.

The exercises last about an hour and it is important that the relaxed condition at the end of the session is revoked again, or else the patient will want to sleep directly afterwards. After about 10 therapy sessions most patients are able to carry out the lower-level exercises for themselves. Audio aids (CDs, etc.) can be used to support independent training.

At the higher levels of autogenic training, images and self-selected situations are imagined. Patients can put themselves in a scene and experience it as if it were real. This offers an opportunity for new solutions to problems. Self-knowledge and conscious consideration are practised and encouraged. Regular practice is sensible in order to accustom the body and mind to a rhythm. After practising for some time, the relaxed conditional can be achieved faster and faster.

24.2.2 Jacobsen's progressive muscle relaxation

Definition

Jacobsen's progressive muscle relaxation (PMR) (Jacobsen 1938) is a procedure for achieving a condition of deep relaxation of the whole body through the voluntary and conscious tensing and relaxing of specific muscle groups. The individual muscle parts are initially tensed in a specific order, the muscle tension is held for a brief time and then released. The main aim is the deliberate, continuous reduction in tension in the individual muscle groups of the locomotor apparatus.

Physiological principles

The principle of PMR is based on relaxation of the affected region after strong tensing of the muscles. Repeated use leads to a 'cultivation of muscle sense'; the patient consciously learns to be sensitive to the body and perceive the tiniest tension in order to know where to relax.

Theoretical basis

The physiologist Edmund Jacobsen worked on the assumption that a condition of rest or relaxation can most reliably be established by a reduction in neuromuscular tension and that inversely activity in the CNS can be reduced through a reduction in muscle tension (the premise of reciprocity). He began to gather empirical evidence of this interplay between the central nervous, mental processes and peripheral muscle changes in a series of studies in 1920. Jacobsen investigated the startle reaction after a sudden loud noise and ascertained that people who have learned to relax their muscles are not startled.

The level of muscle tension also affects the extent of the reflex. Jacobsen also ascertained that mental visualisation, especially if associated with exercise, led to slight but measurable muscular activity. For example, he showed that imagining specific arm movements was associated with an increase in EMG activity of the biceps muscles.

Appropriate eye movements could also be recorded by visualising images (e.g. following the zigzag movements of a rabbit). Empirical evidence for the effect of the power of the imagination on the muscles or on various body functions was provided in a series of later investigations.

Indications

Muscle tension, stress, mental unrest, pain, migraine, asthma, sleep disorders and cardiovascular symptoms are all indicated.

Contraindications

Acute and/or decompensated diseases or conditions are contraindicated.

Procedure

The procedure builds on the principle of tension (for 1–2 min) and then relaxation (for 3–4 min) for each muscle group. The tension phase does not depend on contracting the muscle as far as possible but on learning to perceive the most subtle tension in individual muscle groups. The patient should concentrate on the relevant sensations in the tension and relaxation phases. They thus learn to distinguish ever weaker contractions and even to break down minimal tension. All the muscle groups of the locomotor apparatus from the head to the toes are successively tensed and then relaxed.

Jacobsen described several individual training units for seven practice areas in the following series:

- arm exercises (for upper arm, forearm and finger muscles),
- leg exercises (for hip flexors, buttock, thigh, lower leg, calf and toe muscles),
- trunk exercises (for abdomen, back, rib, diaphragm, chest and shoulder muscles),
- neck exercises (for neck muscles),
- exercises of the eye region (for forehead, face and eye muscles),
- visualisation exercises (perception of even weak contractions of the eye muscles),
- exercises for the tools of speech (for muscles of mastication, floor of the mouth, face and tongue).

The individual exercises can be carried out either seated or lying down. Here are three examples of part-exercises to illustrate the method.

- **Arm exercise:** the patient is lying down with eyes closed. The lift the forearm at a right angle to the bed and close the fist (1–2 min). Meanwhile they note the feeling of tension in the whole arm. They then let the arm fall and concentrate on loosening the arm (3–4 min). The exercise is repeated after a rest.
- **Neck exercise:** in a seated position, the head is first pressed back and then forward against external resistance. The head is finally pressed to the left and then to the right. Between these four tension phases are relaxation phases.
- **Visualisation exercise:** to perceive even weak contractions of the eye muscles the patient is seated or lying down with eyes closed and initially imagines,

e.g., a train moving past for about 1 min. This causes horizontal eye movements. After a pause the patient imagines, for example, looking to the top of a tree. This causes vertical eye movements. Finally, complex eye movements can be caused by, e.g., imagining a rabbit zigzaging while running away. The exercise is repeated after a rest (with the eyes open).

According to the original version of PMR, daily exercise times of an hour and over 50 training sessions (about three muscle groups per session) were envisaged. That means that it could take 3–6 months before the patient has mastered the relaxation technique.

After mastering the basic exercises, the so-called 'differentiated relaxation' could be added. This includes implementing PMR in everyday life (e.g. when reading and writing at work or when driving a car). The necessary movements should be carried out economically and any muscle groups not required should remain as relaxed as possible. Jacobsen suggested inducing relaxation in stages for learning differentiated relaxation, for example from lying down to seated to simple seated tasks.

24.2.3 Imagination techniques

Definition

With imagination techniques the human power of imagination is used to support self-healing. With imagination it is possible to reach a state of changed consciousness which can cause or heal diseases. Imagination encourages mental perception to reactivate the patient's own resources.

Physiological principles

Imaginative techniques allow experiences of the systematic, deliberate switching from sympathic stimulation (performance and activation reaction) of the autonomic nervous system to parasympathetic stimulation (relaxation and recuperation reaction).

Theoretical basis

Catathymic imaging developed by Leuner (1994) is the basis of analytical therapy. This is a psychodynamic, i.e. deep psychologically based, procedure in which mental images in the form of imagination play a key role. In contrast to PMR, which is practised in training sessions and then carried out independently, the company of a therapist plays a big part in catathymic imaging.

In the literature there are also a number of different fantasy journeys and imaginative procedures which predominantly serve positive images (pictures from nature, a place where you feel good, etc.) to contribute to physical and mental relaxation. It is also possible to focus on the pain with the aid of the imagination in pain therapy and work out what could lead to further relaxation.

Imagination can:

- make it possible to experience positive emotions,
- offer variety in relaxation,
- distract from the pain by means of imaginative images,
- help one learn to perceive an imaginative transformation of the experience of pain,
- increase motivation for overcoming the disease,
- make it possible to process the imaginings which occur during therapy.

Indications

Imaginative techniques can have a supportive effect in the processing of acute and chronic attacks of pain in the presence of chronic pain disease with biological psychological and social consequences and myofascial pain components. It can increase motivation for the patient to overcome the pain and provide an impulse for surmounting the disease.

24.2.4 Biofeedback methods

Definition

Biofeedback is a method for creating visible or audible signals from one's own body functions, using unconscious physical regulatory processes such as the heartbeat, to later learn to influence them deliberately.

Indications

- Diseases caused by stress, which are associated with increased muscle tension. This is frequently the case with back pain or headaches. Increased muscle tension can be visualised in, e.g., the form of a curve on a computer monitor. If muscle tension changes, the image of the curve also changes. The patient therefore gains direct feedback of any changes in muscle tension. Even the tiniest changes can be perceived and can be consciously controlled in the end.
- Migraine or tinnitus can be treated with biofeedback.
- Whatever applies to muscle activity, for example, can also be transferred to other functions such as respiration, skin temperature, skin conductivity, brain activity, blood pressure and pulse.
- Biofeedback is often used within the framework of psychotherapy and can help patients to break the vicious circle of stress, tension and physical symptoms. The patient can see the direct connection between thoughts, moods, feeling, tension and relaxation, and the body processes. The patient learns which behaviour most quickly achieves the desired relaxation and how willpower influences health problems.

After successful training, these skills can be used without imaging monitors or loudspeakers. However, to maintain the effect, further regular practice is desirable.

Theoretical basis

Biofeedback is based on the idea that people are, in principle, in a position to influence their body to make it relax. Continuous feedback on progress in the appropriate relaxation allows the patient to affect their state of tension or relaxation until a predefined level is reached. Biofeedback is based on three scientific pillars:

- learning theory,
- psychophysiology,
- experimental analysis of behaviour.

Benefits of biofeedback:
- conscious perception of difficult to access body processes,
- objective data for feeding back the state of relaxation in each case,
- possibility of staged shaping procedures, especially for specific symptoms,
- experience of control and autoefficacy,
- positive support from changed feedback on successful relaxation processes.

Disadvantages of biofeedback:
- some of the costs for the technical equipment are high,
- high staffing costs as one-to-one sessions are usually used,
- some patient associations are critical of medicine that involves the use of mechanical apparatus,
- because of the high cost, it is doubtful whether it is more effective than the learning of relaxation techniques.

In spite of the disadvantages, there is currently a series of indications for the use of biofeedback to justify its use.

Measuring prerequisites

- Measuring equipment with artefact-free, continuous, sensitive feedback on the measured body processes.
- Possibility of a successive approach to the desired target behaviour within the framework of the overall exercise programme. The threshold from when positive relaxation is fed back to the patient must be successively changed during the programme.
- 'Translation' of the measured signals suitable for the patient (technical and complicated feedback systems using graphs which are part of the everyday life of therapists and diagnosticians are usually not suitable).
- Minimal standard in feedback: simple bar charts or cessation of acoustic signals when the desired threshold is reached (modern and costly biofeedback procedures rely on (photo)graphic feedback systems as well, such as smiling faces, surfboarders riding the waves or similar).

Examples of individual derivations which are used for biofeedback

- **Electroencephalographic (EEG) feedback:** mostly alpha activity in the EEG is used as feedback on the state of relaxation, occasionally also theta activity (few empirical studies). A high component of alpha waves means an increased state of relaxation or relaxed mood.
- **EMG feedback:** biofeedback using surface electrodes is used to feed back a relaxed state. For clinical use, a 'frontal feedback' with a lead on the forehead muscles is frequently used. Other possible lead points are the forearms or the back and shoulder areas. EMG feedback is highly specific, i.e. the feedback on the state of tension or relaxation of the relevant muscle groups is reliable but there are no generalisation effects. Relaxation using biofeedback in the frontal area does not automatically mean that the forearm or neck areas are also in a relaxed state.
- **Vasomotor feedback:** the temperature of the hands or fingers is recorded using temperature sensors or – for cephalic vasomotor feedback – using pressure sensors, photocells or Doppler ultrasound to record the perfusion and tension of the blood vessels. Vasomotor feedback is frequently characterised by positive effects after a short period of practice, which then remains constant for a long time, although further training periods do not produce any more positive effects after the initial experience.
- **Cardiovascular feedback:** the heart rate is recorded using an ECG or pulse recording using pressure sensors.
- **Other leads:** these record the body condition, such as skin temperature, skin resistance measurements, rate of respiration. They are often used for specific indications.

24.3 EASTERN RELAXATION TECHNIQUES

24.3.1 Meditation

Definition

Meditation (Latin *meditatio* = thinking about, or *medius* = middle) is a concentration exercise with the aim of achieving a changed state of consciousness or even enlightenment. In a former use of the term, 'meditation' means simply thinking about a topic or the results of this thought process.

Meditation can mean any unintentional concentration on an activity or an object. Concentration is not controlled by understanding but is produced as a consequence of contemplation. The activity can be actively manipulated although it can also be about the inner contemplation of an object or an idea. The key in every case is a state of 'relaxed awareness', requiring surroundings with no stimuli and the capacity to allow the mind to rest. Neurologically, a meditative state is often associated with a change in the pattern of the brainwaves.

Theoretical basis

The term mediation is used as a description of a state and also as the technique of meditating. The object of meditation can be chosen almost at will, so playing music or carrying out simple work which does not demand attention can be performed in a meditative manner. Some of the most well-known meditation techniques rely on breathing and an awareness of breathing (Zen meditation techniques, yoga, Qigong). Others are anchored in the Christian tradition of 'walking' (e.g. St. James' Way in Spain) or working (ora et labora). Meditation can be carried out alone or in a group under guidance.

Types of meditation are listed below.

Praying to Jesus	Tai chi chuan
Mantra	Transcendental meditation
Qigong	Vipassana
Samatha	Zazen
Tables of Chartres	Contemplation

The different meditation techniques can roughly be divided into two groups:

- passive (contemplative) meditation,
- active meditation.

In general usage, only the passive form without external stimulus is meant by the word meditation, while other forms are usually described as rituals, exercises or similar. Meditation is a key component of many religions where contemplation is understood to be an exercise in approaching a higher being ('God') or a higher state of consciousness.

Silent meditation

- Praying and reciting the Eucharist, praying and concentration exercises as techniques in the Christian tradition.
- In Hinduism and Buddhism as well as Daoism: passive, contemplative meditation.
- In Western countries it has been used for decades as a means of counteracting the consequences of civilisation such as noise, hectic pace, pressure to perform and other stress.
- Therapeutic meditation as a route to hypnotherapy (gaining in importance in Western countries).
- Autogenic training helps with relaxation and control of consciousness but is usually not understood as meditation because suggestions have a bigger role here than in traditional forms of meditating.

Musical meditation

Many schools use rhythmic sounds and music to make meditation easier.

- in the Christian tradition, chants and saying the rosary can be similarly meditative to a mantra,
- in Hinduism and Buddhism, mantras can be either silent or spoken quietly or chanted.

Christian Gospels are usually not musical meditations as they include singing, but they mainly serve to confirm one's own belief and contribute to a lightened mood. In some forms, gospel singing can lead to a trance state.

Active meditation

- 'Meditation' supported by dancing can be found, mainly in the oriental tradition (e.g. Dhikr in Sufism, the Islamic mystic) and in many primitive peoples. Very monotonous dance movements are usually performed over a long period, often supported by a fast drumbeat or by bells or rattles carried by the dancers themselves. This technique can lead to a trance-like state of consciousness. Whether these techniques still come under the term of meditation is not clear.
- Often, a physical activity is used to give focus to meditation. The simplest activity is probably walking, which is used in Christian culture (in various orders of monks, etc.) and in the culture of the Far East.
- In the tradition of yoga, various body posture and exercises, as well as fasting and other types of asceticism, are used to support meditation.
- In Zen Buddhism on the other hand, very varied activities can be the object of meditation such as flower arranging (Ikebana), calligraphy (Shodō) and archery (Kyūdō).
- Martial arts can also be the object and vehicle of meditation: in the Daoistic traditions of the inner martial arts in particular (e.g. Tai chi chuan) the meditative aspect plays a large part. In some styles the martial arts origin almost disappears (Qigong). Meditative practices are also used in many of the external martial arts.
- In more recent times (since the end of the 1970s), Bhagwan Shree Rajneesh also developed meditation techniques geared to 'Westerners' in his Ashram in Poona. These include dynamic meditation, Kundalini, Nataraj and Nadabrahma meditation.
- Another school of meditation known in the West is transcendental meditation. Organisations which run courses on meditation are controversial.

Entheogenic meditation

Some cultures rely on entheogenic substances (consciousness-extending drugs) for meditation. It should be noted, however, that the use of a drug on its own does not usually lead to a meditative state: the appropriate mental techniques are required as well. It is also uncertain with many of these practices whether they are still covered by the term meditation. Substances used can be:

- mild stimulants such as incense as used in Catholicism,
- psychotropic substances such as hashish which is mainly used by Rastafarians for religious and meditative purposes,
- psychoactive plants, used among the Native Americans for sweat lodge rituals,
- strong hallucinogenics, used particularly in shamanistic culture usually in combination with dancing or similar ritual to achieve a trance state.

24.3.2 Qigong

Definition

Qigong is an umbrella term for a variety of exercise methods which deal in various ways with the power of life (Qi). Qigong is often described as the active part of Chinese medicine, away of using one's own effort to health and healing. Postures, movement, breathing exercises and mental exercises for concentration and imagination are associated with Qigong.

Physiological principles

The slow flowing movements of Qigong lead to vagotonia, breathing is deepened and the muscles are relaxed.

Theoretical basis

Qigong has a long history as a movement art for health and healing. Ancient manuscripts show how the ancient Chinese practised mental exercises, breathing exercises and motion exercises of Qigong. Qigong is based on a thousand years of a system of empirical medicine. The underlying concepts of TCM are reflected in Qigong: the teaching of Yin and Yang, the circle of function (Zang-fu), the system of the meridians (jingluo), the sites of influence and acupuncture points and body areas with specific function as a gathering place of Qi (dantian). In accordance with an understanding of health as a dynamic balance between the polarities of Yin and Yang, all Qigong exercises are intended to bring Yin and Yang in harmony.

Yin and Yang teaching includes instructions on exercises, breathing and dealing with tension and relaxation.

Indications

- Maintaining health and strengthening.
- Treatment of chronic diseases.
- Relief of pain and other symptoms.

Effects

- Relaxing effect.
- Affects breathing.
- Influence on the locomotor system and posture.
- Strengthens the physical constitution.
- Increases the body's resistance.
- Supports the healing of various complaints and diseases.
- Spiritual balance and mental stability based on unity of mind, body and soul.

By adapting the exercises to the individual conditions, Qigong can be learned and practised at any age and largely independently of the state of health. Suitable exercise methods must be selected according to the physical constitution, the clinical picture and the phase of the disease so that they do not produce any undesirable effects.

Contraindications and undesirable effects

Qigong therapy is not suitable for the most seriously ill patients with mental illness. Exercises where the preservation and control of the powers of the imagination play a big part are not suitable for people emotional state is not stable or are very easily excitable. These people should choose exercises where physical movement forms the main aspect.

Undesirable effects mostly occur if the following key points for Qigong are not adhered to:

- relaxation, rest, naturalness,
- the power of imagination and Qi follow each other,
- movement and rest belong together,
- above 'empty', below 'firm',
- adaptation of level of exercise,
- practise stage by stage.

Abnormal effects (e.g. dizziness, head fullness, head tension, catching the breath) only occur if training is carried out against the requirements of the exercise. To prevent these abnormal effects, the beginner should practise under the guidance of an experienced teacher.

Procedure

In spite of the many different methods, Qigong exercises are all divided into exercises in body posture, breathing and the power of imagination:

- exercises at rest.
- exercises in motion.

Gentle movement exercises are most suitable for trigger point therapy: these exercises gently extend and strengthen the muscles. The gentle flowing movements lead to improved perfusion of the muscles and a reduction in muscle tension.

24.3.3 Yoga

Definition

The term yoga (from Sanskrit *yuga*: yoke, for tensioning, harnessing, yoking) describes an Indian philosophical teaching which frees people from being bound to the burden of the physical using specific mental and physical exercises (e.g. meditation or asceticism). Yoga is one of the six classical schools (Darshanas) of Indian philosophy. Yoga is used to unify the individual self with the infinite universal self.

Physiological principles

The most important effect of yoga is relaxation; the breathing rate is slowed down, and the heart rate, blood pressure and muscle tension are lowered.

Theoretical basis

There are many different forms of yoga and all have their own philosophy and practices. Some meditative forms of yoga focus on mental concentration, while others concentrate on physical exercises and positions (asanas) or asceticism. The theoretical and philosophical principles of yoga go back to the Vedas, the oldest Indian holy scriptures from about 1500 BCE.

Four ways of yoga are described in the classical Indian scriptures. These include not just physical exercises but different religious and spiritual ways:

- Raja yoga (also known as Ashtanga yoga; Patanjali eight part yoga),
- Jnana yoga (yoga of discovery; intellectual direction),
- Karma yoga (yoga of deed/acting selflessly),
- Bhakti yoga (yoga of veneration/devotion),

The following terms are associated with the practice of yoga:

- Hatha yoga (yoga of physical and spiritual balance),
- Sahaja yoga (spontaneous self-realisation),
- Marma yoga (yoga of linking of biological rhythms).

In the West (i.e. USA/Europe) Hatha yoga, Marma yoga and Kundalini yoga are the most common forms of yoga.

Procedure

Yoga exercises basically pursue a holistic approach to bring the body, mind and soul into harmony. In a typical teaching unit (series of exercises) there are:

- both static and dynamic asanas,
- a phase of deep relaxation,
- meditation.

An example from Kundalini yoga: through a combination of body postures, movement sequences, mental concentration points, controlled breathing and the use of mantras (words for meditation) and mudras (hand positions; finger yoga), Kundalini energy is stimulated so that it begins to rise though the chakras (energy centres).

Chapter | 25 |

Systemic pharmacotherapy

Philip Lang, Dominik Irnich

25.1 INTRODUCTION

Pain relief, muscle relaxation, sleep encouragement and the prevention of depression resulting from long-term pain are the aims of the use of pharmacotherapy in MPSs. The analgesic efficacy depends on the specific effect of a product and its non-specific effect or objective and subjective factors (see Fig. 25.1).

In principle, systemic pharmacotherapy should not be dispensed with if the patient is in acute pain, unless the pain can be quickly and effectively reduced by other means. One of the key factors in the chronification of pain is the lack of suppression of the nociceptive stimulation and its continuation, with the subsequent consequence of neuroplastic change at the central level.

With increasing chronification drug treatment fades further and further into the background, as the profile of effect is usually unfavourable compared to the drug's undesirable effects and the cost–benefit ratio. If an effective drug for treatment of acute cases is identified there should be no delay in prescribing it in the short term for the acute exacerbation of chronic symptoms.

Overall, it must be stated that the scientific evidence for various analgesics, co-analgesics and muscle relaxants is weaker than frequently believed.

> The exclusive and long-term use of pharmacotherapy for myofascial pain should be critically assessed.

25.2 SUBSTANCE GROUPS

25.2.1 Overview of drugs for pain therapy: classification of analgesics

Non-opioids	Acid anti-inflammatory and antipyretic analgesics Non-acid antipyretic analgesics Other
Opioids	Weak-acting opioids Strong-acting opioids (narcotics)
Muscle relaxants	Centrally effective myolytics Centrally effective muscle relaxants with and without tranquillising properties Benzodiazepines
Co-analgesics	Tricyclic antidepressants Corticosteroids Antihistamines

25.2.2 Non-opioid analgesics with antipyretic effect

Derivatives of weak carbonic acid

Acetylsalicylic acid (ASA)

Acid anti-inflammatory and antipyretic analgesic

Trade names: include Aspirin®, Acesal®, ASS-CT®, ASS-ratiopharm®, Godamed®. Also commonly known as aspirin.

http://dx.doi.org/10.1016/B978-0-7020-4312-3.00025-8

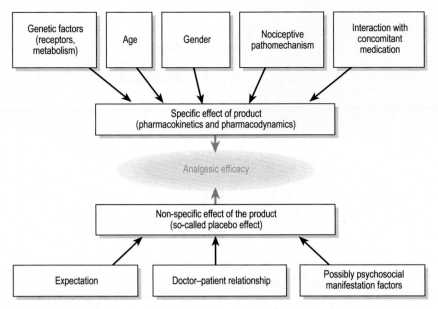

Fig. 25.1 Factors influencing analgesic efficacy.

Mechanism of effect: inhibition of prostaglandin synthesis.
Dosage: single dose 500 (–1000) mg, daily dose 2500 (–4000) mg.
Side effects: gastrointestinal symptoms, tendency to bleeding (irreversible acetylisation of platelets), pseudoallergic reactions, 'analgesic asthma', Reye's syndrome (children before puberty with viral infection).
Interactions with other drugs: strengthens effect of indirect coagulants (coumarin derivatives) with >5 g/day.
Contraindications: gastric and duodenal ulcers, increased tendency to bleeding, bronchial asthma.

Diclofenac

Acid anti-inflammatory and antipyretic analgesic

Trade names: include Diclofenac-ratiopharm®, Diclofenac-Sandoz®, Diclofenac-STADA®, Diclac®, Diclo®, Effekton®, Rewodina®, Voltaren®.
Mechanism of effect: inhibition of prostaglandin synthesis, inhibits the COX-2 isoform more than the COX-1 enzyme.
Dosage: single dose 50–100 mg, maximum 200 mg/day.
Side effects: gastrointestinal events (nausea, vomiting, gastritis, bleeding), dizziness, headaches, (usually temporary) increase in transaminases.
Contraindications: gastric and duodenal ulcers, blood formation disorders, severe heart failure, pregnancy and breast feeding.

Ibuprofen

Acid anti-inflammatory and antipyretic analgesic

Trade names: include Aktren®, Anco®, Dolgit®, Ibuprofen-CT®, Ibuprofen-Heumann®, Ibuprofen-STADA®, Ibuprofen-CT®, Urem®, Neurofen®.
Mechanism of effect: inhibition of prostaglandin synthesis.
Dosage: single dose 400 mg, maximum daily dose 2400 mg.
Side effects: gastrointestinal symptoms and risk of bleeding is smaller than with ASA, pseudotumor cerebri, headaches, visual disturbances, meningitis (usually patients with lupus erythematodes).
Interactions with other drugs: retention of lithium, reduced renal elimination of methotrexate.
Contraindications: as for diclofenac.

Pyrazolone derivatives

Metamizol

Non-acid analgesic with high antipyretic potency

Trade names: include Novalgin®, Novaminsulfon®.
Mechanism of effect: analgesic, antipyretic and spasmolytic properties (mechanism of effect not fully explained, supposedly central and peripheral).
Dosage: 1–4 times 500–1000 mg per day, maximum daily dose 4000 (–5000) mg
Side effects: shock reactions after too-rapid intravenous injection, allergic agranulocytosis, rarely allergic skin diseases or drop in blood pressure.
Contraindications: blood formation disorders, hepatic porphyria, glucose-6-phosphate-dehydrogenase deficiency, dose reduction for liver and kidney function disorders.

Aniline derivatives

Paracetamol

Non-acid antipyretic analgesic

Frequently used in pain therapy for children and for mild to moderate pain in adults.

Trade names: include Ben-u-ron®, Captin®, Paracetamol-ratiopharm®, Perfalgan®.

Mechanism of effect: analgesic and antipyretic mechanisms of effect have not been definitively explained but a central and peripheral effect is probable. There is evidence of pronounced inhibition of cerebral prostaglandin synthesis.

Dosage: single dose 500–1000 mg, maximum daily dose 4000 mg.

Side effects: liver damage with overdose (>6–8 g/day) and/or prior liver damage as a result of exhaustion of hepatic glutathione reserves.

Contraindications: liver disease, alcoholism.

Cyclo-oxygenase 2 inhibitors

Celecoxib

Anti-inflammatory effect analgesic

Trade names: include Celebrex®, Onsenal®.

Mechanism of effect: selective COX-2 inhibition, discussion of specific deposit in the 'side pocket' in the hydrophobic tunnel of the COX-2 isoform; 375-fold higher affinity for COX-2 than for COX-1.

Dosage: single dose 100–200 mg, maximum daily dose 400 mg.

Side effects: diarrhoea, nausea, abdominal pain, flatulence, water and electrolyte retention (oedema), rash, sinusitis, anaemia, hyperkalaemia, sleep disorders, anxiety states, dizziness, hypertension, tinnitus.

Contraindications: coronary heart disease, cerebrovascular disease, cardiac insufficiency (New York Heart Association classification II–IV), pregnancy and breast feeding, severe liver and kidney function disorders, chronic inflammatory bowel disease, gastric and duodenal ulcers.

Etoricoxib

Anti-inflammatory effect analgesic

Trade names: Arcoxia®.

Mechanism of effect: selective COX-2 inhibition.

Dosage: single dose 60–90 mg, maximum for short term 120 mg/day.

Side effects: as for celecoxib, dose reduction for liver and kidney failure.

Contraindications: as for celecoxib.

25.2.3 Non-opioid analgesics without antipyretic effect

(See also Table 25.1)

Pyridyl carbamate

Flupirtine

Non-opioid analgesic without antipyretic and anti-inflammatory effect

Trade names: include Katadolon®, Trancolong®, Trancopal dolo®.

Table 25.1 Pharmacokinetic non-opioid analgesics

ACTIVE SUBSTANCE	ELIMINATION HALF-LIFE ($t_{1/2}$, H)	MAXIMUM PLASMA CONCENTRATION (t_{MAX}, H)	BIOAVAILABILITY (% DOSE)	PROTEIN BINDING (%)
ASA (anti-inflammatory effect)	≈0.25	≈0.25	50–70	50–70
ASA (analgesic effect)	2.5–4.5	0.5–2	80–100	80–95
Diclofenac	1–2	1–12 (high variability)	30–80 (first pass)	99.5
Ibuprofen	1.5–2.5	0.5–2	80–100	99.5
Metamizol	2–4	1–2	≈100	58
Paracetamol	1.5–2.5	0.5–1.5	70–100	5–50
Celecoxib	11–16	2–4	60–80	94–98
Etoricoxib	19–32	1–2	≈100	92
Flupirtine	≈10	1.5–2.5	90	≈84

Mechanism of effect: activation of tension-controlled potassium channels (stabilisation of the resting membrane potential of nerve cells).
Dosage: single dose 100 (–200) mg, daily dose 300 (–600) mg.
Side effects: tiredness, reduced capacity to concentrate, unrest, dizziness, gastric symptoms.
Interactions with other drugs: enhances the sedative effect of diazepam and the hypothrombinaemic effect of warfarin by displacement from plasma protein binding.

25.2.4 Opioid analgesics

(See also Table 25.2)

Codeine

Weak-acting opioid analgesic

Trade names: include Codeinsaft-CT®, Codeintropfen-CT®, Codipront mono®, Tyrasol®.
Mechanism of effect: pure opioid receptor agonist: activation of encephalinergic receptors with increase in potassium outflow with concomitant inhibition of calcium inflow and therefore reduced excitability of the neurons participating in the pain event.
Dosage: single dose 30–60 (–100) mg, maximum daily dose 300 mg.
Side effects: constipation (contraction of smooth muscle; also urinary retention, biliary colic) cough suppression (even at doses of 10 mg), sedation, nausea, vomiting, miosis, low blood pressure, bradycardia, itching and reddening of the skin (release of histamine).
Contraindications: central suppression of respiration, obstruction of the respiratory tract (e.g. status asthmaticus).

Tramadol

Weak-acting opioid analgesic

Trade names: include Tramadol-CT®, Tramadol-ratiopharm®, Tramadol-Sandoz®, Tramadolor®, Tramal®, Tramundin®.

Table 25.2 Dosages of weak-acting opioid analgesics		
ACTIVE SUBSTANCE	**DOSE (MG)**	**DURATION OF EFFECT (H), DOSAGE INTERVAL**
Codeine	60–100	3–4
Tramadol	50 from 100 (retard form)	2–48–12
Tilidine combined with naloxone	50/4–100/8 from 100/8 (retard form)	2–38–12

Mechanism of effect: opioid receptor agonist, inhibition of the neuronal reuptake of noradrenaline, increased serotonin release.
Dosage: up to 4 times 50–100 mg, 1–2 times 100–200 mg retard form, maximum 400 (–600) mg/day.
Side effects: occasionally constipation, sedation, nausea and vomiting, especially in the retard form.
Contraindications: patients taking monoamine oxidase (MAO) inhibitors, insufficiently controlled epilepsy, central respiratory suppression, asthma, massively reduced liver function, circulatory shock, prostate hypertrophy, myasthenia gravis, pregnancy and breast feeding.

Tilidine combined with naloxone

Weak-acting opioid analgesic in combination with a morphine antagonist

Trade name: Valoron N®.
Mechanism of effect: tilidine is a prodrug with a weak opioid effect; the actual active substance is nortilidine. The combination with a morphine antagonist is to prevent misuse.
Dosage: up to 4 times 50/4–100/8 mg, twice 50/4–150/12 mg retard, maximum 400 (–600) mg/day.
Side effects: nausea, dizziness, hardly any constipation because of the addition of naloxone.
Contraindications: opiate dependency (danger of withdrawal symptoms), massively limited liver function, pregnancy and breast feeding.

25.2.5 Muscle relaxants

Tolperisone

Centrally effective myolytic

Trade names: Mydocalm®, Viveo®.
Mechanism of effect: structural similarity to lidocaine, membrane-stabilising effect on peripheral nerves and on a spinal and central and reticular level.
Dosage: daily dose 3 times 50–150 mg.
Side effects: tiredness, dizziness, nausea, mouth dryness, increase in liver enzymes.
Contraindications: myasthenia gravis, pregnancy, breast feeding.

Baclofen

Centrally effective muscle relaxant without tranquillising properties

Trade names: include Baclofen AWD®, Baclofen-ratiopharm®, Lioresal®.

Mechanism of effect: binding to the gamma-aminobutyric acid B (GABA$_B$) receptor in the spinal cord, which prevents the release of the stimulants glutamate and aspartate. Enhancement of presynaptic inhibition, which leads to dulling of excitability transfer and thus to a reduction in spastic muscle tension.

Dosage: initially 3 times 5 mg; gradually increasing the individual dose by 5 mg should be carried out every third day at the earliest, optimum daily dose usually 30–75 mg/day in 3 single doses, discontinue gradually, otherwise rebound effect, maximum daily dose 75 mg.

Side effects: nausea, vomiting, sedation, dizziness, muzziness, confusion, headaches, depressed respiration, cramp, liver function disorders.

Contraindications: epilepsy, terminal renal failure, gastric and duodenal ulcers, obstruction of the respiratory tract, psychosis, Parkinson's disease, syringomyelia.

Benzodiazepines

Diazepam

Centrally effective muscle relaxant with tranquilising properties

Trade names: include Diazepam-CT®, Diazepam-ratiopharm®, Faustan®, Valocordin-diazepam®, Valium®.

Mechanism of effect: binding to the benzodiazepine receptor, strengthening the effect of the inhibitory transmitters GABA.

Dosage: 5–15 mg/day.

Side effects: tiredness, sedation, dependency, ending a long treatment with high doses can lead to sleeplessness, agitation, depressive or psychotic conditions, muscle twitches or cramp.

Contraindications: alcohol or soporific drug intoxication, myasthenia gravis, severe liver damage, respiratory failure, sleep apnoea syndrome, ataxia, pregnancy, breast feeding.

Tetrazepam

Centrally effective muscle relaxant with tranquillising properties

Trade names: include Musapam®, Musaril®, Tetrazepam-ratiopharm®, Tetrazepam-Sandoz®, Tetrazepam-STADA®, Rilex®, Tetramdura®.

Dosage: 50–200 mg/day.

Side effects: as for diazepam.

Contraindications: as for diazepam.

25.2.6 Co-analgesics

Tricyclic antidepressants

Amitriptyline

Trade names: include Amineurin®, Amitriptylin-CT®, Amitriptylin-dura®, Amitriptylin-Sandoz®, Novoprotect®, Saroten®.

Mechanism of effect: increase in the function of inhibitory monoaminergic transmitters by inhibition of their reuptake in neurons.

Dosage: for analgesia: 20–100 mg/day, as antidepressant: 50–150 mg/day.

Side effects: mouth dryness, accommodation disorders, mydriasis, tachycardia, micturition disorders, constipation, orthostatic regulatory disorders, conduction disturbance, sedation, headaches, dizziness, reduction in cramp threshold.

Contraindications: glaucoma, prostate hypertrophy, acute myocardial infarction, cardiovascular disorders, bradycardia, long QT syndrome, hypokalaemia, increased tendency to spasms, psychosis, disorders of liver and renal function, patients taking MAO inhibitors.

Clomipramine

Trade names: include Anafranil®, Hydiphen®.

Mechanism of effect: as for amitriptyline.

Dosage: for analgesia: 20–100 mg/day, as antidepressant: 50–150 mg/day.

Side effects: as for amitriptyline.

Contraindications: as for amitriptyline.

Doxepin

Trade names: include Aponal®, Espadox®, Mareen®.

Mechanism of effect: as for amitriptyline.

Dosage: for analgesia: 30–150 mg/day, as antidepressant: 75–150 mg/day.

Side effects: as for amitriptyline.

Contraindications: as for amitriptyline.

Corticosteroids

Prednisone

No analgesic properties but reduction in pain as a result of effect on tissue reaction

Trade names: include Decortin®, Prednisone-ratiopharm®, Rectodelt® (Supp.).

Mechanism of effect: inhibition of the formation of inflammatory cytokines such as IL-1, IL-6, TNF and interferon-γ as well as the formation of leukotrienes and prostaglandins. Anti-inflammatory and anti-oedematous effect; indirect analgesic effect.

Dosage: begin with 60 mg daily, then reduce within a week (every other day) to 10 mg/day (in the morning).

Side effects: adrenal failure, iatrogenic Cushing's syndrome, type 1 diabetes, increased risk of infection, wound-healing disorders, gastrointestinal ulcers, osteoporosis, psychological disorders, hypertension.

Contraindications: infection (acute viral infection, HbsAG-positive chronic active hepatitis, 8 weeks before and up to 2 weeks after vaccinations, lymphadenitis following BCG vaccination), glaucoma, cataracts, gastrointestinal ulcers, type 1 diabetes, difficult to control hypertension, severe osteoporosis.

Interactions with other drugs: numerous interactions; combined with ASA or other NSAIDs risk of reactivation of ulcers and bleeding in the gastrointestinal tract.

Antihistamines

Dimenhydrinate

Water-soluble salt: antihistamine and antiemetic

Trade names: include Dimen®, Vertigo-Vomex®, Vomex A®.

Dosage: 50 mg.

Mechanism of effect: H1 receptor antagonist, anticholinergic, central sedation, antiemetic, LA.

Side effects: central suppression (positive), antiemetic (positive), effect similar to atropine (e.g. mouth dryness, constipation, micturition disorders).

Interactions: alcohol taken at the same time increases the effect of suppression of the CNS.

Contraindications: acute asthma attack, glaucoma, pheochromocytoma, porphyria, epilepsy, prostate hyperplasia, limited liver function, hypokalaemia, hypomagnesaemia, bradycardia, long QT syndrome.

Diphenhydramine

Antihistamine, sedative and antiemetic

Trade names: include Dolestan®, Emesan®, Sediat®, Vivinox®.

Dosage: 25 mg.

Mechanism of effect: H1 receptor antagonist, anticholinergic, central sedation, antiemetic, LA.

Side effects: similar to atropine (see dimenhydrate).

Interactions: as for dimenhydrate.

Contraindications: acute asthma attack, glaucoma, pheochromocytoma, porphyria, epilepsy, prostate hyperplasia, hypokalaemia, hypomagnesaemia, limited liver function, bradycardia, long QT syndrome, taking MAO inhibitors, pregnancy and breast feeding.

Promethazine

Neuroleptic, sedative at low dosage

Trade names: include Atosil®, Eusedon mono®, Promethazin-neuraxpharm®, Prothazin®, Soporil®.

Dosage: 12.5 mg.

Mechanism of effect: H1 antihistamine, anticholinergic, antiserotonergic and membrane stabilising.

Side effects: similar to atropine (see dimenhydrate); hypotension.

Interactions: as for dimenhydrate.

Contraindications: acute intoxication with central suppression drugs or alcohol, severe blood cell or bone marrow damage, circulatory shock or coma.

25.3 TREATMENT PLAN

A 'reflex-like' prescription of analgesics should stop unless no other possibilities can be considered. The choice should usually be made from an individual assessment of findings, previous diseases, body weight, expected behaviour, general toleration of medicines, patient preference, organ function and individual strain imposed by suffering. The rules of standard medical treatment of pain should be adhered to (see Fig. 25.2).

If the long-term administration of analgesics is not checked regularly it can lead to permanent negative consequences. Remember that after taking NSAIDs for 2 months the risk of dying from gastrointestinal bleeding is on average 1 in 1220 (Tramèr et al. 2000).

25.3.1 Basic principles of medical treatment for pain

- By the clock: taking analgesics at regular intervals.
- By mouth: if possible.
- By the ladder: the order of analgesics selected follows a staged plan.
- By the individual: basic medication with retarded preparation in individually adjusted doses; prescribe medicine on demand for peaks of pain.

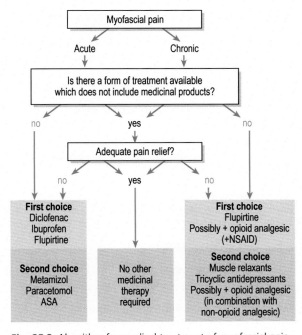

Fig. 25.2 Algorithm for medical treatment of myofascial pain.

- Attention to detail: note the manner and effect of prior medication; combination of analgesics, co-analgesics and adjuvant substances as required.
- Discuss likely side effects and possibly initiate prophylaxis.
- Give precise written instruction on taking the drugs to the patient and, if necessary, to relatives as well.
- Ensure regular follow-ups and checks of the documentation, possibly with adjustment of the pain therapy (by a physician).

25.3.2 Pain-specific procedure for medical treatment

If the patient needs acute pain reduction and other options to provide rapid relief are not available (or the patient declines them), it is appropriate to begin medical treatment. For longer-lasting pain also consider whether non-medical procedures can be used and possibly supported by pharmacological solutions.

Acute myofascial pain

- *First choice*: diclofenac; ibuprofen, flupirtine.
- *Second choice*: metamizol; paracetamol (first-choice drug for children); ASA.

- If insufficient analgesia combination with opioid analgesic, begin with a weak-acting opioid (tramadol or tilidine/naloxone).

Longer-term myofascial pain

- *First choice*: flupirtine, NSAIDs (short term as a bridge for acute exacerbation of chronic pain),
  - or severe pain conditions: opioid analgesics (in combination with non-opioid analgesic), begin with a weak-acting opioid (tramadol or tilidine/naloxone).
- *Second choice*: muscle relaxants; tricyclic antidepressants,
  - for severe pain conditions: opioid analgesics (in combination with non-opioid analgesic), begin with a weak-acting opioid (tramadol or tilidine/naloxone),
  - for sleep disorders (caused by myofascial pain):
    – first choice: antihistamines,
    – second choice: benzodiazepines.

Adjuvant pharmacotherapy

- Massage: muscle relaxants; flupirtine.
- Acupuncture, dry needling, trigger point injection: muscle relaxants; flupirtine.

Warning: non-opioid analgesics such as ASA can lead to increased tendency for bleeding.

Section | 3 |

Muscles and trigger points

With the collaboration of: Reinhard Putz (anatomy), Johannes Fleckenstein (trigger points and acupuncture points), Roland Gautschi (instructions for manual trigger point therapy), Armin Slugocki (stretching), Jochen Gleditsch (microsystem acupuncture), David Euler (Kiiko Matsumoto acupuncture),

Florian Pfab (introductory text for Chapters 27 and 29–34).

Representation of muscle anatomy and anatomical texts: Modified from Sobotta Atlas of Human Anatomy, Putz, R. (ed.), Papst, R. (ed.), 22nd edition Elsevier Urban & Fischer, Munich 2006.

Chapter | 26 |

Head

Dominik Irnich, Jean-Marc Pho Duc, Kathrin Spiegl

26.1 HEADACHES

Dominik Irnich

26.1.1 Functional context

Headaches can be a relevant health problem but also occur as part of everyday life. Their lifetime prevalence is 71%, of which 38% are tension headaches, 27% migraine and 6% rare forms of headache. In Germany, 54 million people suffer from acute or chronic headaches, including 21 million people who suffer from migraine and 29 million who suffer from episodic tension headaches. More than 100 000 people suffer from permanent headaches caused by analgesic medicines.

If a patient goes to a doctor with headaches, they usually need treatment. The basis of treatment is appropriate diagnosis. The patient's history plays a significant role, as the routinely available technical test procedures do not provide definitive findings that explain the pain in 90% of primary headaches. The underlying warning symptoms for the presence of secondary (symptomatic) headaches are:

- violent headaches occurring for the first time,
- definite progression,
- focal neurological signs,
- signs of cranial pressure, meningism,
- fever and disturbance of consciousness.

These symptoms must be investigated by a specialist.

There is no agreement on the involvement and valency of myofascial findings. We must assume, however, that – if you regard headaches as a disorder in the processing of stimulation with increased sensitivity to stimulation and reduced

adaptation and habituation to repetitive stimulation – mTrPs can quite reasonably play a part. Particularly with tension headaches, a connection has been described between increased pericranial muscle activity and stress load and the development of headaches.

Some theories also assume that an intermittent headache initially caused by pathological afferent signals from the pericranial muscles can become chronic and truly central as a result of central sensitisation. The early treatment of painful mTrP in the head area may therefore be of particular significance.

26.1.2 Diagnostic and therapeutic considerations

The diagnosis of headaches rests initially on the characteristic clinical picture and normal physical and neurological findings. The total duration of the headaches, pain frequency, intensity, duration and quality, accompanying symptoms such as visual disturbances, triggers, causes, trauma, hormones, diet, the taking of painkillers, family problems, emotional factors and social history should all be investigated. Any psychological findings should be immediately investigated. A headache diary can both serve as a diagnostic tool and provide a valuable check on treatment. Keeping a diary for several months should be avoided, as this can also contribute to the headaches becoming chronic (as a result of focusing attention on the headaches).

As far as therapy goes, the recommendations of the International Headache Society and other relevant guidelines should be applied. However, treatment exclusively with drugs is to be avoided and mere reference to 'relaxation techniques' is insufficient. Competently performed acupuncture is, from a scientific point of view at least, as

http://dx.doi.org/10.1016/B978-0-7020-4312-3.00026-X

effective as prophylactic drugs, even though the physiological mechanism of effect has been insufficiently explained.

The use of a multimodal therapy concept with investigation, psychological pain therapy, motivation and the competent use of individually suited relaxation, exercise and physical perception techniques, gentle stamina training and stress management are prerequisites for a long-term improvement in headaches.

26.1.3 Investigation of function for mTrP identification

The examination of mTrPs should form part of a detailed physical examination. The site of the pain indicates localisation of the mTrP. A migrating headache is rarely purely myofascial in origin.

The M. trapezius (Section 27.12), M. temporalis (Section 26.4) and the short suboccipital muscles (Section 27.9) are of particular significance in the development of relevant headaches. If the latter are affected, there are frequently also functional disorders of the atlanto-occipital joint. These have a functional connection with the trigeminovascular reflexes and the trigeminoautonomic system, which in their turn are connected with the development of chronic headaches. A completely isolated myofascial headache is seldom found. Nevertheless, we have repeatedly been successful in definitely improving acute or chronic headaches by means of treatment of active mTrPs.

If a mTrP is found, it should immediately be treated if there are headaches. Usually, the affected muscles are easily accessed for infiltration (M. temporalis (Section 26.4), M. trapezius (Section 27.12)) or dry needling (suboccipital muscles (Section 27.9)).

Where there are headaches, the following muscles should be examined no matter what.

HEADACHE LOCALISATION	SEARCH FOR mTrPs IN
Temporal headache	M. trapezius (27.12), M. sternocleidomastoideus (27.10), M. temporalis (26.4), M. splenius cervicis (27.7)
Occipital headache	M. trapezius (27.12), M. temporalis (26.4), Mm. semispinalis capitis and cervicis (27.8), suboccipital muscles (27.9), M. splenius capitis (27.6), M. sternocleidomastoideus (27.10)
Frontal headache	M. frontalis, M. sternocleidomastoideus (27.10), M. semispinalis capitis (27.8), M. orbicularis oculi
Headache focused on the crown of the head	M. splenius capitis (27.6), M. sternocleidomastoideus (27.10), suboccipital muscles (27.9)
Peri-auricular pain	M. pterygoideus (26.5 and 26.6), M. masseter (26.3), M. sternocleidomastoideus (27.10)

26.2 STOMATOGNATHIC SYSTEM

Jean-Marc Pho Duc, Kathrin Spiegl

Disorders of the stomatognathic system used to be bundled together under the term 'myoarthropathy' but are now attributed to the umbrella term of 'craniomandibular dysfunction' (CMD). The stomatognathic system represents an extremely complex system and involves the temporomandibular joint, the teeth and the muscles of mastication, and is influenced and controlled via the neuromuscular regulatory circuit. Disorders in one part of the system will frequently have an effect on one or more of the muscles involved in the movements of mastication. A pathological change in the area of the mandible signifies a changed situation for the muscles of mastication, which can, as a result, be subject to painful adaptation processes. Conversely, however, muscle pathology can also lead, for example, to arthropathy of the mandibular joints as a result of a parafunction such as bruxism (teeth grinding). The patient's bite can thus have a causative function and can also experience a change caused by the altered interplay between the joints and the muscles, which is displayed as an occlusion disorder from a dental point of view.

It is therefore important for the therapist to get an overview of the condition of the whole stomatognathic system in order to provide therapy if necessary for the causative factors, as well as to treat the muscular components, if necessary in cooperation with other disciplines.

Changes in the muscles caused by parafunction are predominantly found in the area of the large muscles which close the jaw, as described below.

- The M. temporalis (Section 26.4) is mostly affected in the anterior and medial segment, while the M. masseter (Section 26.3) is affected over all parts of the muscle from the origin to the insertion. These muscles are most easily accessible to extraoral palpation and represent the first indicator.
- The M. pterygoideus medialis (26.5) is found inside the mouth and forms a loop of muscle with the M. masseter.

- Other frequently affected muscles are the M. pterygoideus lateralis (26.6), which is active in laterotrusion and the posterior and anterior parts of the M. digastricus (Section 26.7) and the M. mylohyoideus (Section 26.9). which belong to the muscles in the floor of the mouth and are accessory muscles of mastication

After examination by the doctor, the patient's first question is frequently about the cause of the problems. Both the clinical findings and the history are of great significance here. Parafunctions such as gnashing and grinding can have quite simple causes.

- For example, a change in the bite can be the result of a recently fitted false tooth. Fitting a new false tooth always assumes that the patient is able to adjust to some extent. This ability to adjust can be significantly reduced by stress factors, psychological factors or chronic pain.
- However, it can also happen because the patient may have had CMD for years and until now this has been compensated for by other systems in the body.

As soon as an additional stimulus has an effect on the stomatognathic regulatory circuit, caused by the dentist or even by a traumatic event, the whole structure decompensates. However, if the occurrence of the symptoms and the external stimulus (dental intervention) are closely connected in time, this assumed cause can lead to the actual cause being disregarded. Both physical and psychological factors can be the underlying reason for the disease in the CMD system.

- Among the physical factors, the interaction between posture and position of the jaw is of significance. There is scientific evidence of this dependence, which is why if a connection is suspected the interdisciplinary cooperation of dentistry, ear, nose and throat, orthopaedics, physiotherapy and physical medicine is needed.
- If a psychological illness or psychosomatic disorder are suspected, we should strive for cooperation with psychosomatic disorders or psychiatric specialists.

> We cannot emphasise enough that, because of the complexity of mastication and the ever-present interaction with a person's psyche, only an interdisciplinary approach will provide a successful cure, based not only on the symptoms but also on the cause; this should be taken into account in practice.

26.2.1 Muscle overview

The following overview shows the significance of individual muscles of mastication in movements of the jaw and the restrictions to which they can lead.

Muscles that close the mouth			
Retrusion	M. temporalis	M. masseter M. pterygoideus medialis	Protrusion
	Suprahyoid muscles	M. pterygoideus lateralis	
Muscles that open the mouth			

26.2.2 Clinical functional analysis of the stomatognathic system

This chapter demonstrates the clinical examination of the masticatory system, oriented towards the diagnosis of CMD. The physical examination of the craniomandibular system includes essentially an analysis of the bite, palpation of the individual muscles of mastication and the mandibular joints as well as an assessment of the movements of the mandibular joints in three planes (e.g. opening the mouth). This examination is also described as a clinical functional analysis.

The examination is divided into:

- history, with particular emphasis on the teeth,
- localisation of the pain,
- myogenetic components,
- arthrogenous components,
- occlusal factors.

The objectives of the physical examination of the masticatory system are:

- the formation of a diagnosis and differential diagnosis,
- identification of co-factors,
- need for interdisciplinary cooperation,
- need for additional diagnostic tests such as imaging procedures of the mandibular joints.

The analysis of function should be repeated after each course of therapy is concluded. Follow-ups may be carried out during therapy using visual analogue scales, measurement of mobility of the lower jaw and palpation of mTrPs.

The water-butt model is also a very good aid in CMD for understanding the complex combination of different factors in the occurrence of the disease. The advantage of a diagrammatic protocol is that it is a standardised procedure, which is always followed in the same order, contains all the important clinical findings and prevents any significant factors relating to the water-butt model being overlooked.

In most cases, the clinical functional analysis produces the diagnosis and the relevant therapeutic measures. If the findings and the way the patient feels do not match, or the patient demonstrates signs of a psychosomatic pain disorder (e.g. repeated unsuccessful interventions, doctor hopping, etc.), we must suspect a chronic orofacial pain syndrome or an atypical facial pain. Pain referral pattern and affected muscles in the area of the head are shown in Fig. 26.1.

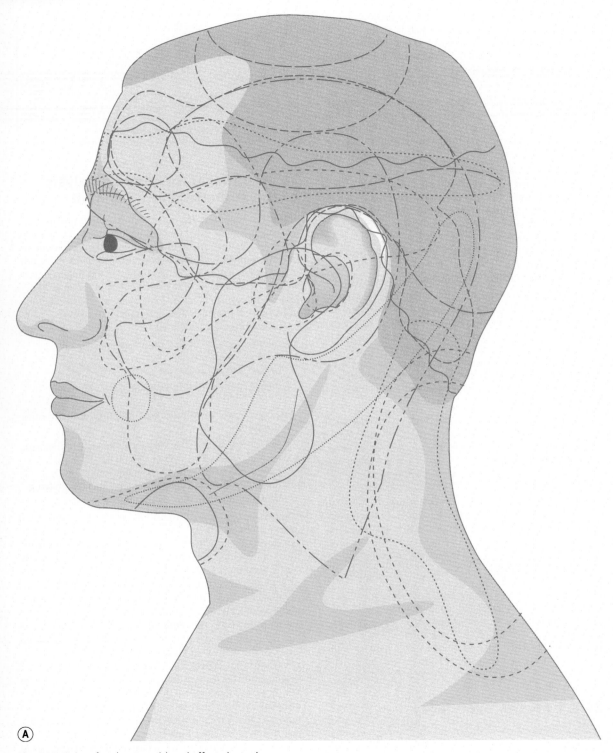

Ⓐ

Fig. 26.1 Pain referral pattern (a) and affected muscles

Continued

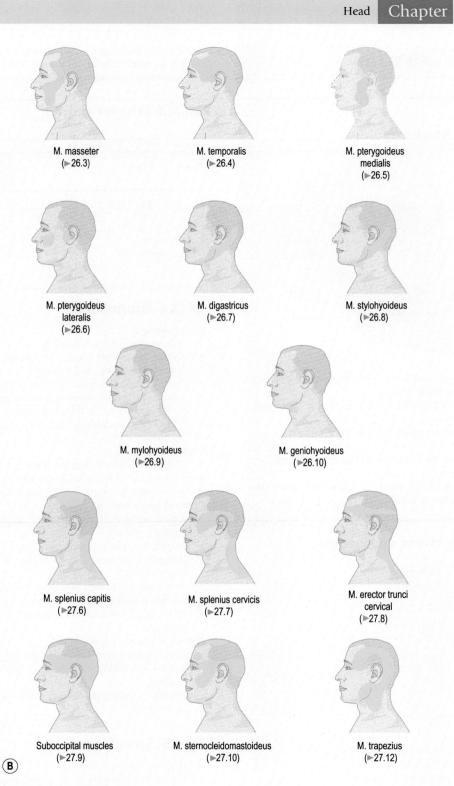

M. masseter
(▶26.3)

M. temporalis
(▶26.4)

M. pterygoideus
medialis
(▶26.5)

M. pterygoideus
lateralis
(▶26.6)

M. digastricus
(▶26.7)

M. stylohyoideus
(▶26.8)

M. mylohyoideus
(▶26.9)

M. geniohyoideus
(▶26.10)

M. splenius capitis
(▶27.6)

M. splenius cervicis
(▶27.7)

M. erector trunci
cervical
(▶27.8)

Suboccipital muscles
(▶27.9)

M. sternocleidomastoideus
(▶27.10)

M. trapezius
(▶27.12)

Fig. 26.1—cont'd (b) in the area of the head.

26.3 M. MASSETER

Dominik Irnich

26.3.1 Anatomy

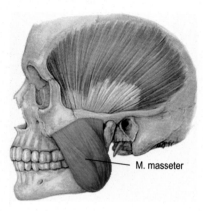

M. masseter

Innervation: masseteric nerve (mandibular nerve (V/3)).
Origin: zygomatic arch:
* *superficial part*: distal margin, anterior two-thirds (sinewy),
* *deep part*: posterior third, medial surface.
Insertion:
* *superficial part*: mandibular angle, masseteric tuberosity,
* *deep part*: lateral surface of the mandibular branch.
Function: closing the jaw.

26.3.2 Patient symptoms

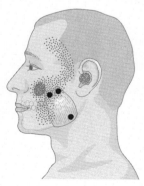

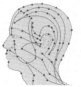

* Pain in the area of the ears or cheeks.
* Periorbital facial pain.
* Frontal pain (complex picture).
* Radiation into the teeth.

* Possible diagnoses: atypical facial pain, temporomandibular syndrome (CMD), Costen's syndrome, chronic toothache of unknown cause.

26.3.3 Trigger points

mTrP	LOCALIS-ATION	RADIATION	mTrP→ACUPUNCTURE POINT
1, 3	Superficial part	Cheeks, upper jaw, premolars	ST 6, ST 5 (also superior and inferior)
2	Deep part	Ear, periauricular area, cheeks	ST 7

26.3.4 Diagnosis

Questioning
* Pain quality and localisation.
* Dental treatment? Toothache on one side with resultant chewing on one side?
* Teeth grinding at night (bruxism)? Ask life partner.
* Frequent masseter tension (chewing gum), e.g. pressing teeth together when thinking (stress)?
* Click in the mandibular joint? (not necessarily pathological)

Inspection
* Occasional muscle hypertrophy.
* Asymmetry when opening the mouth.
* Asymmetrical mouth movements when speaking.

Physical examination
* Examination while sitting on a stool on a couch or in a supine position.
* Mouth opening less than two finger widths of the patient's finger is usually pathological (<40 mm, 'two-finger rule').
* Asymmetrical mouth closure or opening movement.
* Surface palpation for the superficial part.
* Index finger intraoral and thumb extraoral for the deep part.

Technical examination
* For suspected involvement of the maxillary joint → functional tests with a dentist with advanced training.
* Possibly imaging procedures (MRI with maxillary joint spool).

26.3.5 Specific aspects

* Principal sphincter muscle.
* Extremely powerful muscle, strong enough to break the zygomatic arch, this strength would not be introduced

through the tough fascia above the insertion of the temporalis into the skull.
- This can create what feels like a ring of pressure in the sense of a tension headache.
- With chronic symptoms frequently affected together with the temporomandibular joint and is often the cause of temporomandibular joint problems.
- Frequently overused with parafunctions or excessive chewing of chewing gum.
- Above it lies the parotid gland, insertion at SI 18 (=anterior margin of the masseter muscle), meaningful below the zygomatic bone.
- Cooperation with a dentist experienced in gnathology (treatment with a brace or splint and if necessary correction of the bite after resolution of muscle tension).
- Relaxation possible using a TENS machine.

26.3.6 Therapy

Instructions on manual trigger point therapy
- Extraorally with slightly opened mouth (more easily palpable with forward/prior extension of the myogenic fibres/taut bands).
- Intraoral with pinch grip (thumb intraoral and index/middle finger extraoral).
- Gentle, pain free mobilisation of the temporomandibular joint.

Extension

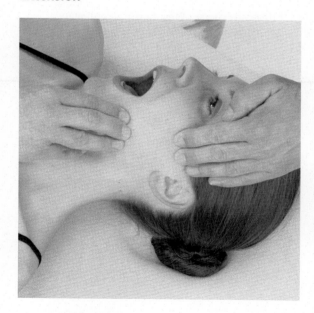

- Open the mouth.
- Extension as illustrated from extraoral or from intraoral, pulling forward and down.

- Anterior traction on the mandible:
  - grasp the bottom teeth and the lower jaw in the middle (incisors) with the fingers (thumb on the floor of the mouth, index and middle finger intraoral),
  - anterior traction.
- Caudal traction on the mandible:
  - as for anterior traction,
  - just pull the lower jaw cautiously in a slightly anterior direction,
  - then pull it cautiously in a caudal direction.

Physical therapy procedures

Application of heat or cold, at the correct temperature (hot or cold packs, wrapped in a towel).

Infiltration techniques/dry needling

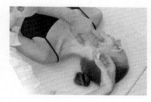 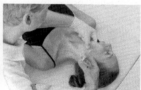

- Supine position or sitting on the bed.
- Mouth slightly open (using a mouth wedge if necessary).
- Insert needle flat and posterior at SI 18 or vertically at ST 5 (anterior margin).
- Finger protection technique (see Fig. left) or index finger intraoral as support (see Fig. right)
- Deep part up to 4 cm deep.
- Multiple stimulations, as many small mTrPs, some obstinate.
- **Warning:** pterygopalatine ganglion (paraesthesia!).
- Supporting irritable spot at paravertebral level C2.

Classical Chinese acupuncture

Local and locoregional points (also contralateral): ST 5, ST 6, ST 7, SI 18.
Distal points: SP 6, ST 36, SI 3, TH 5, GB 20, BL 20.
Control points/symptomatic points: ST 43, ST 44, SI 2, CV 21, KI 27.

Microsystem acupuncture

Ear: temporomandibular joint, upper jaw, lower jaw, Jérôme point.
YNSA: A zone, mouth point, forehead.
Mouth: intraoral retromolar and vestibulum points.

Hand line V: area at the fifth metacarpal, corresponds to SI 2 (or surroundings).

Kiiko Matsumoto acupuncture

- If there is a neurological cause of the muscle symptoms: CV 12 and CV 10.
- If there is tenderness in the area of the stomach meridian: ST 44 and ST 45 (metal and water).
- A point about 1 cm below GB 21 very effective, vertical needling to the course of the fibres from above to below.

Psychosomatic treatment/relaxation

- Overcoming stress.
- Topics: 'worry episodes', problem-solving.
- The first muscle to demonstrate increased tone as a result of emotional stress.
- Pushes the jaw forward: the topics of 'asserting oneself' and 'struggling through'.
- Worries about the future.
- Digestion in the physiological and the transferred sense (overcoming problems).
- Anxiety.

26.3.7 Recommendations for the patient

Self-extension

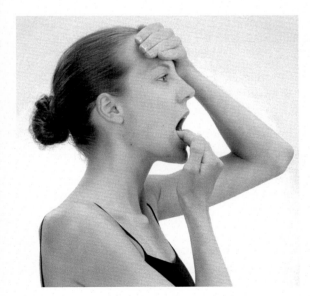

As depicted. When doing this, it is important that the mouth is not 'torn apart' but that gentle traction is exercised in an anterior and caudal direction.

Self-massage

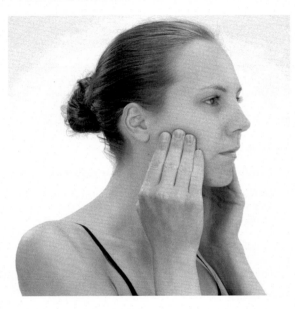

- Palpate the course of the muscle according to instructions from the therapist.
- Circular massage, kneading movement along the course of the muscle.
- Additional 'slight squashing' of the muscle belly (one finger intraoral, one extraoral).
- Move gently to the pain margin.
- Twice daily 5–10 min (overall massage time).

Coordination exercise

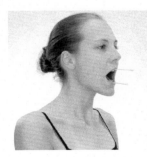
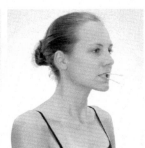

The following exercise can contribute to training mouth opening coordination:

- The patient clenches a wooden dental hygiene stick between the upper and lower middle incisors.
- When opening the mouth, the lower wood should move in a vertical line parallel to the upper wood.

If clenching the wood is not possible, alternatively, a coloured dot on the tip of the nose and the chin can serve as reference points. The mouth should be opened without demonstrating any visible deviation.

Lateral movements can also be trained in the same manner. In this case, the reference point moves evenly towards the lower right or lower left.

The coordination exercise trains the interplay of the muscles of mastication and promotes perception of one's own jaw position.

Coordination and spatula exercise can be applied to all muscles of mastication.

Spatula exercise

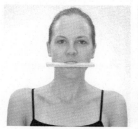 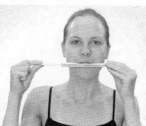

The spatula exercise is indicated if there is largely pain-free shortening of the muscles. During this exercise, individual wooden spatulas are pushed one after the other between the teeth of the upper and lower jaw and the shortened muscles are extended for a few minutes as follows:

- At first, as many wooden spatulas as possible are inserted over each other, corresponding to the current mouth opening.
- After this number is reached, an additional wooden spatula is inserted and the extension of the sphincter muscles maintained.
- This exercise can be repeated several times a day.

Usually, mouth opening can be increased in stages to an acceptable extent over several days or a few weeks.

An indication of restricted mouth opening is the two-finger rule. If the patient cannot manage to insert the index and middle fingers at the same time above each other between the cutting surfaces of the front teeth, this is an indication of restricted mouth opening.

Additional measures

- Bite splint/brace.
- Relax the lower jaw for 60 s and allow it to hang down, then tighten it briefly (repeat five times, three times daily).
- Avoid perpetuating factors and factors which cause the problem (habitual chewing of gum, chewing on one side, biting the nails, bruxism).
- Loosely chewing gum (maximum 5 min) (applies to all the muscles of mastication).
- Self-monitoring by the patient, e.g. with small post-it notes on the computer screen or in the car, to control jaw clenching during the day.
- Relaxation techniques such as Jacobsen progressive muscle relaxation, autogenic training, Feldenkrais technique, yoga.
- Overcoming stress, communication training.
- Relaxation using hot flannels.
- Functional 'jaw gymnastics'.

26.4 M. TEMPORALIS

Kathrin Spiegl, Jean-Marc Pho Duc

26.4.1 Anatomy

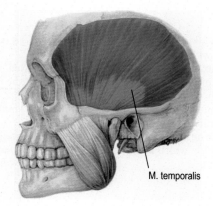

M. temporalis

Innervation: deep temporal nerves (mandibular nerve (V/3)).
Origin: temporal bone below the inferior temporal line and the deep blade of the temporal fascia.
Insertion: tip and medial surface of the coronoid process of the mandible.
Function: closing the jaws, posterior portion: retrusion of the lower jaw.

26.4.2 Patient symptoms

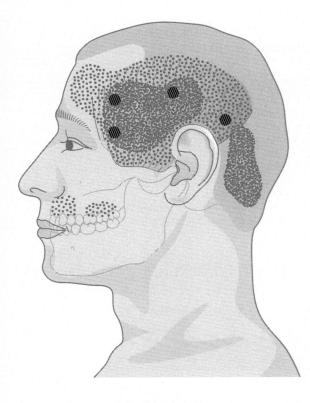

- Pain all along the temples, the eyebrows and behind the eye.
- If the anterior region of the muscle is stressed, this can produce pain which is projected to all the upper teeth.
- Frequently accompanied by limitation of mouth opening.
- If the head is pushed forward, this can encourage a jaw position which leads to overload of the temporalis muscle.

26.4.3 Trigger points

mTrP	LOCALIS-ATION	RADIATION	mTrP↔ ACUPUNCTURE POINT
1, 2	Anterior part	Eyebrows, periorbital area, fascia of the upper jaw	Ex-KH 5 (Taiyang), ST 8
3	Medial part	Upper jaw: side teeth, infraorbital and inferior areas	GB 8
4	Posterior part	Occipital, dorsocranial areas	GB 9

26.4.4 Diagnosis

Questioning
- Pain quality and localisation.
- Headaches radiating into the forehead, temples and eyes.
- Grinding the teeth at night, unconscious jaw clenching and grinding.
- Ask about preceding teeth treatment of change in dental situation.
- Pain in the area of the front teeth of the upper jaw, over the eye (mTrP anterior part).
- Pain radiating in the area of the maxillary sinus or the side teeth of the upper jaw (mTrP medial part).

Inspection
- Is the head extended forwards?
- Mouth opening.

Physical examination
- Examination while sitting on a couch or in a supine position.
- Mouth opening (maximum cutting edge distance).
- Asymmetrical mouth opening.
- Palpation of the anterior, medial and posterior section.
- Palpation is separated into the anterior, medial and posterior parts.
- mTrP anterior part in the area of the temples (mTrP 1 and 2).
- mTrP medial part over the ear (mTrP 3).
- mTrP posterior part at the back of the skull behind the ear (mTrP 4).

Technical examination: If involvement of the temporomandibular joint is suspected → function tests with a dentist with specialised training and possibly imaging procedure (MRI with temporomandibular spool!).

26.4.5 Specific aspects

- Together with the main sphincter muscle, the masseter muscle.
- Frequently overused with parafunctions or excessive chewing of gum.
- Tension in this area typically causes tension headaches.
- The muscle lies below a tough fascia which introduces the strength of the masseter muscles from the

zygomatic bone into the vault of the skull: there is some strong resistance when needling!
- Pain following therapy is often helpful: it makes the patient aware when they are pressing the teeth together.
- Ask the patient to keep a diary: access to psychosomatic disorder.

26.4.6 Therapy

Instructions for manual trigger point therapy

- mTrP treatment: (a) temporal region of origin, (b) region of insertion coronoid process:
  - extraoral: through the skin of the cheek with the mouth wide open (this makes palpation accessible to parts of the M. temporalis, which are otherwise concealed by the zygomatic branch); or
  - intraoral: the index finger can easily reach the insertion zone, which frequently demonstrates definite tenderness (coronoid process and attachment area of the mandibular branch).
- Gentle mobilisation of the temporomandibular joint.

Massage

Stroking, rubbing, kneading, effleurage and vibration; acupressure.

Extension

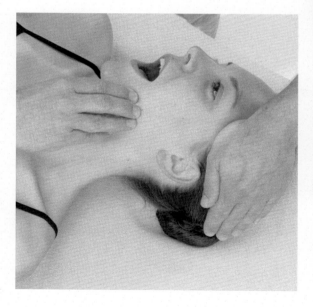

- Open the mouth.
- Extension, as illustrated, extraorally or intraorally, pulling forward and down (similar to extension with the M. masseter).

- Anterior traction on the mandible: grasp the bottom teeth and the lower jaw in the middle (incisors) with the fingers (thumb on the floor of the mouth, index and middle finger intraoral), anterior traction.
- Caudal traction: as for anterior traction but with the lower jaw a little further forward and then cautious traction downwards.
- Soft tissue toning M. temporalis.

Physical therapy exercises

- Bite splint; heat or cold therapy (chronic/acute) with hot or cold gel compresses; local laser treatment extraorally.

Infiltration techniques/dry needling

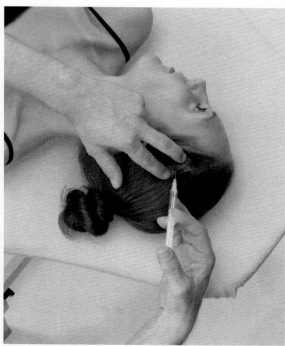

- Treatment in the supine position or sitting on the bed.
- Single infiltration or dry needling with the aid of two-finger protection technique with the mouth slightly open.
- A short (2 cm) needle is usually sufficient.

Classical Chinese acupuncture

Local and locoregional points (also contralateral): GB 7, GB 8, GB 9, TH 20, ST 8, Ex-KH 5 (Taiyang).

Distal points: SI 2, SI 3, ST 44.
Control points/symptomatic points: LR 3, SP 6 (for dull spreading pressure headache).

Microsystem acupuncture

Ear: temporomandibular joint, upper jaw, lower jaw, Jérôme point.
YNSA: A zone.
Hand line V: area at the fifth metacarpal, corresponds to SI 2 (or surrounding area).

Kiiko Matsumoto acupuncture

- If there is a neurological cause of the muscle symptoms: CV 12 and CV 10.
- For tenderness in the area of GB 39: GB 43 and GB 44.
- Additional points: GB 1, TH 1 and TH 2 (particularly if palpation in the area of TH 4 is painful), TH 9 or TH 5 to relieve tenderness in the area of the Mm. sternocleidomastoideus and temporalis (TH 9 or TH 5 are effective if there is pain on the contralateral side), ST 9, LR 17 for the M. sternocleidomastoideus.

Psychosomatic treatment/relaxation

- Overcoming stress (see above).
- Relaxation techniques such as yoga, Feldenkrais technique, autogenic training.
- Topics: 'worry episodes', problem-solving.
- Try to avoid parafunctions (jaw clenching, chewing fingernails, excessive gum chewing) on the day.
- Psychosomatic disorder: worries about the future, digestion in the physiological and the transferred sense (overcoming problems), anxiety, stress.
- Following mTrP therapy there is often a feeling of relief and widening of determined narrow thinking.

26.4.7 Recommendations for the patient

Self-massage

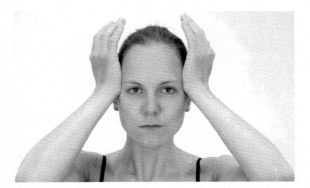

- Patient sits at a table with the elbows supported.
- Use the balls of the hands to exert pressure and massage in circles in a fan shape along the course of the muscle (isometric power transmission).

Additional measures

- Relax the lower jaw for 60 s and allow it to hang down, then tighten it briefly (repeat five times, three times daily).
- Avoid chewing on one side.
- Avoid perpetuating factors and factors which cause the problem (habitual chewing of gum, chewing on one side, biting the nails, bruxism).
- Self-monitoring by the patient e.g. with small post-it notes on the computer screen or in the car, to control jaw clenching during the day.
- Possibly a bite splint for bruxism.
- Coordination and spatula exercises (Section 26.3.7).
- Application of heat (muscle relaxation using hot flannels).
- Self-monitoring (clenching the teeth) → relax.
- Functional 'jaw gymnastics'.

26.5 M. PTERYGOIDEUS MEDIALIS

Kathrin Spiegl, Jean-Marc Pho Duc

26.5.1 Anatomy

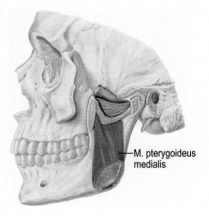

M. pterygoideus medialis

Innervation: N. pterygoideus medialis (N. mandibularis (V/3)).
Origin: pterygoid fossa and lateral lamina of the pterygoid process, part of the pyramidal process of the palatine bone.

Insertion: medial surface of the mandibular angle, pterygoid tuberosity.
Function: closing the jaw.

26.5.2 Patient symptoms

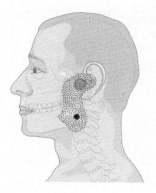
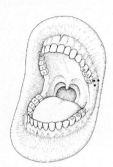

- Pain in the area of regions which are difficult to delineate (tongue, throat and hard palate) below and behind the temporomandibular joint and deep in the ear.
- Transfer of pain to the retromandibular and infra-auricular area, including the base of the nose and throat ('neck pain').
- Diffuse pain, dull feeling in the ear can be a symptom for mTrPs in the M. pterygoideus medialis.
- Difficulties swallowing, restricted mouth opening.

26.5.3 Trigger points

mTrP	LOCALIS-ATION	RADIATION	mTrP⟶ Acupuncture point
1	Muscle body at the medial side of the mandible	Retromandibular area, temporomandibular joint area, 'ear'	Mouth acupuncture 'retromolar area'

26.5.4 Diagnosis

Questioning
- Pain quality and localisation.
- Grinding the teeth at night (bruxism)? Ask the life partner.

Inspection: usually no perceivable changes outside or inside the mouth.

Physical examination
- Extraoral: medially at the mandibular angle from the floor of the mouth outwards, the patient should turn the head slightly to the side palpated so that the tissue slackens and the muscle is better accessible.
- Intraoral palpation: as a result the gag reflex in the area of the throat mucosa is barely possible.

Technical examination
- Measurement of mouth opening.
- Lateral movements of the lower jaw.

26.5.5 Specific aspects

- With chronic symptoms frequently affected together with the temporomandibular joint.
- Together with the masseter muscle forms the muscle loop of the lower jaw, therefore it is frequently also involved if the sphincter muscles M. masseter and M. temporalis are affected.

26.5.6 Therapy

Instructions for manual trigger point therapy

- Slowly open the jaw against slight resistance from the therapist.
- mTrP treatment:
  - extraoral: mouth opened slightly, finger pressure at the mandibular angle from the medial side of the mandible against the bony resistance of the mandible;
  - intraoral: index finger palpates inside the mouth along the body of the mandible as far as possible in a caudal direction and then slowly in the direction of the mandibular angle in a dorsal direction.

Extension/relaxation

- Extension together with the masseter muscle (Section 26.3).

Physical therapy

- The application of heat is preferable because with cold application there is the danger of irritating the parotid gland.

Infiltration techniques

- No infiltration treatment because of the tight anatomical conditions (watch out for the parotid gland).

Classical Chinese acupuncture

Local and locoregional points (also contralateral): ST 7, TH 17, ST 9.
Distal points: CV 21 (relaxation of floor of mouth; lymph system, suspected mandibular angle; stress), KI 27.
Control points/symptomatic points: ST 36.

Microsystem acupuncture

Mouth: inside the mouth retromolar points lower jaw lingual ('retromolar area').
Ear: Jérôme point (relaxation point), Shenmen; soothing analgesia point, thalamus point; analgesia point.
Hand line V: area at the fifth metacarpal, corresponds to SI 2 (or surrounding area).

Kiiko Matsumoto acupuncture

- ST 41 painful on palpation: ST 44 and ST 45 ipsilateral.
- Point between GB 21 and SI 13 ipsilateral for pain relief in the muscle; needling at an angle of 15° in the direction of SI 13.

Psychosomatic treatment/relaxation

- Overcoming stress.

26.5.7 Recommendations for the patient

Self-extension

As for masseter muscle (Section 26.3).

Self-massage

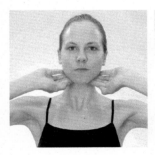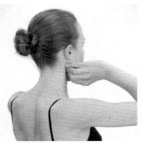

Because of the anatomical course, the patient can only massage the muscle in the insertion area.

- With the pads of the index, middle and ring fingers grasp the hollow in the medial mandibular angle.
- Exercise gentle circular pressure over the muscle.

Additional measures

- Mouth-opening exercise with the therapist can also be carried out as an exercise at home (slowly open the jaw against slight resistance caused by the patient).
- For bruxism bite a splint if necessary.
- Spatula and coordination exercise (Section 26.3.7).
- Self-monitoring (teeth clenching) → release.
- Functional 'jaw gymnastics'.
- Avoid factors which cause the problem (habitual chewing of gum, chewing on one side, biting the nails, bruxism).

26.6 M. PTERYGOIDEUS LATERALIS

Kathrin Spiegl, Jean-Marc Pho Duc

26.6.1 Anatomy

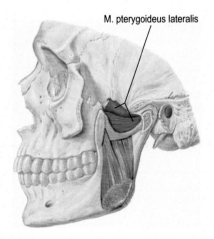

M. pterygoideus lateralis

Innervation: N. pterygoideus medialis (N. mandibularis (V/3)).
Origin:
- *superior head*: external surfaces of the lateral lamina of the pterygoid process, maxillary tubercle,
- *inferior head (accessory)*: temporal fascia of the greater wing of the sphenoid bone.

Insertion: pterygoid fossa of the mandibulocondylar process, disc and capsule of the temporomandibular joint.
Function:
- *superficial head*: closing the jaw and forward movement (=protrusion) of the lower jaw,
- *inferior head*: opening the jaw.

26.6.2 Patient symptoms

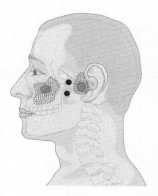
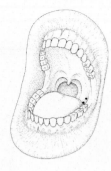

- Symptoms when chewing, particularly when eating hard foods.
- Pain in the region of the temporomandibular joint, some malocclusion (premature contact of the front teeth), can be confused with inflammation of the temporomandibular joint.
- Pain in the area of the maxillary sinus.

26.6.3 Trigger points

mTrP	LOCALIS-ATION	RADIATION	mTrP→ ACUPUNCTURE POINT
1	Superficial part	Pain in the area of the temporoman-dibular joint; maxillary sinus	Mouth acupuncture 'retromolar area'
2	Inferior part	Pain in the area of the upper jaw	

26.6.4 Diagnosis

Questioning
- Restricted mouth opening.
- Pain quality and localisation.
- Pain in the temporomandibular joint.
- Grinding the teeth at night, unconscious jaw clenching and grinding.
- Pain radiating into the area of the maxillary sinus, not the upper teeth (differential diagnosis: M. temporalis).

Inspection: usually no perceivable changes outside or inside the mouth.

Physical examination
- Difficult to palpate; area dorsal from the upper wisdom teeth in a medial direction, palpation is mostly unpleasant to painful, even for muscles not affected.
- Isometric testing, lateral movement of the slightly opened jaw against resistance by the therapist's hand.
- With stress on the M. pterygoideus lateralis the lateral pressure against resistance is painful.

Technical examination
- Function tests with a dentist with advanced training.
- Possibly imaging procedures (MRI with temporomandibular joint spool!) if differential diagnosis is uncertain to find out whether the joint is involved.

26.6.5 Specific aspects

- Bruxism, particularly in the area of the canine teeth, can be the cause and consequence of mTrPs in the M. pterygoideus lateralis.
- Various habits/activities can lead to severe strain on the muscle: extreme gum chewing, biting the nails, sucking the thumb in children.
- **Warning:** musicians playing wind instruments with the lower jaw pushed forward (e.g. transverse flute), persistent pressure of the mandible against a violin.
- mTrPs in the M. pterygoideus lateralis is also listed as a cause of tinnitus in the literature.

26.6.6 Therapy

Instructions for manual trigger point therapy

- mTrP treatment:
  - extraorally with the mouth slightly open, (a) palpation of the mandibular notch, treatment through the masseter muscle (and the anterior part through the M. temporalis), (b) also treat the insertion area of the superior part in the dorsal joint space of the disc;
  - intraoral: with the little finger with maximum laterotrusion (access not always possible).

Extension/relaxing the muscle

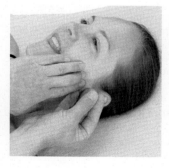
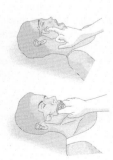

- Postisometric relaxation.
- With a gloved finger grasp the region of the M. pterygoideus.
- Slide gradually upwards at the margin of the lower jaw.
- The region is situated between the rising branch of the mandible and the zygomatic arch.
- Pressure to the pain limit.
- Advise the patient that the palpation can be unpleasant.

Physical therapy procedures

- Bite splint; hot or cold therapy (chronic/acute condition?).

Dry needling

Warning: infiltration because of danger of injury (parotids, facial nerve). Cautious dry needling possible as acupuncture needles are less traumatic.

Classical Chinese acupuncture

Local and locoregional points (also contralateral): ST 7, TH 17, ST 9.
Distal points: CV 21 (relaxation of floor of mouth; lymph system, suspected mandibular angle; stress).
Control points/symptomatic points: ST 36.

Microsystem acupuncture

Mouth: intraoral retromolar points upper jaw buccal ('retromolar area').
Ear: Jérôme point (relaxation point), Shenmen point: soothing analgesia point, thalamus point: analgesia point.
Hand line V: area at the fifth metacarpal, corresponds to SI 2 (or surrounding area).

Kiiko Matsumoto acupuncture

- As for Section 26.5.
- Also KI 9 for tenderness at the superior anterior iliac spine and the medial pterygoid muscle; exact localisation and needling angle.
- Needling of KI 27 on both sides at an angle of 10° in the direction of the sternoclavicular joint.

Psychosomatic treatment/relaxation

- Overcoming stress.

26.6.7 Recommendations for the patient

Self-extension

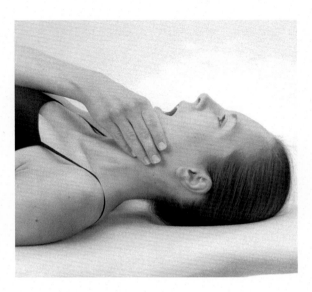

Self-extension by shortening the muscle (muscularly limited mouth opening), but not for acute inflammation of the muscles and/or arthrogenic cause of the limitation.

- The patient should lean the head to take on a relaxed basic posture for the jaw (in the supine position).
- In a seated position the forehead should also be held in place with a hand.
- Firmly grasp the chin with the hand to be used for the extension and slowly extend the lower jaw in a caudal direction (alternatively the thumb and index finger).
- Maintain the open position for several seconds and then slowly release.
- This exercise can be repeated several times a day.
- Self-monitoring (teeth clenching) → release.
- Functional 'jaw gymnastics'.
- Avoid perpetuating factors and factors which cause the problem (habitual chewing of gum, chewing on one side, biting the nails, bruxism).

Additional measures

- Exercises to coordinate the opening and closing movements of the lower jaw.
- For bruxism bite a splint if necessary.

26.7 M. DIGASTRICUS

Kathrin Spiegl, Jean-Marc Pho Duc

26.7.1 Anatomy

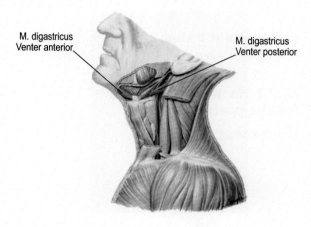

M. digastricus
Venter anterior

M. digastricus
Venter posterior

Innervation:
- *anterior belly*: N. mylohyoideus (N. mandibularis (V/3)).
- *posterior belly*: Ramus digastricus (N. facialis).

Origin: *posterior belly*: mastoid incisor of the temporal bone, intermediate tendon at the small horn of the hyoid bone.

Insertion: *anterior belly*: digastric fossa of the mandible.

Function: lowering of the lower jaw, lifting or fixing of the hyoid bone; supports the mylohyoid muscle.

26.7.2 Patient symptoms

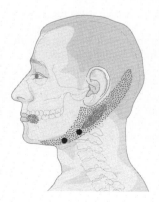

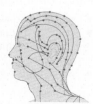

- Restricted mouth opening/pain on opening the mouth.
- Radiating pain at the insertion of the sternocleidomastoid muscle as far as the ear area.
- Pain in the area of the lower front teeth and the accompanying alveolar ridge.
- Pain dorsal to the mandibular angle.
- Swallowing difficulties, 'lump in the throat'.
- Grinding the molars (retral lower jaw).

26.7.3 Trigger points

mTrP	LOCALIS-ATION	RADIATION	mTrP↔ ACUPUNCTURE POINT
1	Posterior belly	Upper section of the sternocleido-mastoid muscle	TH 17
2	Anterior belly	Lower front teeth	–

26.7.4 Diagnosis

Questioning
- Pain quality and localisation.
- 'Earache'.
- Restricted mouth opening.
- 'Pseudosternocleidomastoid pain'.

Inspection: Under some circumstances there is slight swelling ('filling') ventral and posterior of the lower jaw.

Physical examination: extraoral palpation.
- *Anterior belly*: medial to the lower jaw connection submandibular.
- *Posterior belly*: retromandibular area and medial to the mandibular angle.

Technical examination: palpation within the framework of a function analysis by a dentist with advanced training.

26.7.5 Specific aspects

- Bordering on swollen lymph nodes, parotitis.
- Other suprahyoid muscles are also frequently affected.

26.7.6 Therapy

Instructions for manual trigger point therapy
- Release of mTrP through pressure.
- *Posterior belly*: directly below/medially to the mandibular angle in the direction of the mastoid process.

- *Anterior belly*: pinching around the lower jaw (thumb inside the mouth, index finger outside).

Physical therapy procedures

- Bite splint; heat therapy or cryotherapy (chronic/acute) with hot/cold gel compresses.

Infiltration techniques/dry needling

- Infiltration with cannula not recommended because of the risk of injury to the salivary gland ducts/tracts.
- Cautious dry needling possible as acupuncture needles are less traumatic.

Classic Chinese acupuncture

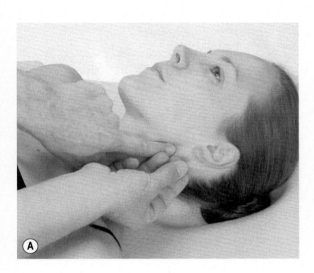

Local and locoregional points (also contralateral): TH 17, CV 23, SI 17.
Distal points: CV 21 (relaxation of floor of mouth; lymph system, suspected mandibular angle; stress), TH 4, TH 5.
Control points/symptomatic points: after TCM.

Microsystem acupuncture

Ear: temporomandibular joint, upper jaw, lower jaw, Jérôme point.
Lymph belt: specific sternal point CV 20/21.

Kiiko Matsumoto acupuncture

- ST 30 ipsilateral, needling (mostly at an angle of 45° in the direction of the pubic bone).
- If palpation of GB 38 is painful (fire point) needling of GB 43 and GB 44 (water and metal point); if toes are cold, moxa stimulation or indirect moxibustion for warming the toes.
- In some cases, the needling of TH 5 and GB 41 (for a rapid pulse) or TH 9 and GB 40 for improvement.

Psychosomatic therapy/relaxation

- Over KI 27 and CV 21 often good for relaxation.

26.7.7 Recommendations for the patient

Self-massage

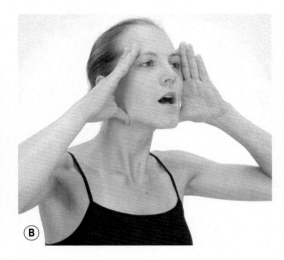

- Self-massage of the retromandibular and submandibular region by the patient using the pads of the fingers.
- Stroke along the course of the muscle or massage with the thumbs by opening and closing the mouth.

Additional measures

- Functional 'jaw gymnastics'.
- Avoid perpetuating factors and factors which cause the problem (habitual chewing of gum, chewing on one side).
- Stretching massages.

26.8 M. STYLOHYOIDEUS

Kathrin Spiegl, Jean-Marc Pho Duc

26.8.1 Anatomy

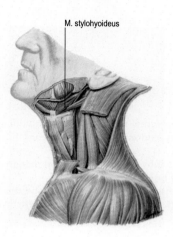

M. stylohyoideus

Innervation: ramus stylohyoideus (N. facialis (VII)).
Origin: processus stylohyoideus of the temporal bone.
Insertion: lateral margin of the body of the hyoid bone with two ends at the posterior and anterior perimeter; usually surrounds the intermediate tendon of the digastricus muscle.
Function: fixation of the hyoid bone, pulls it back in a superior direction during the act of swallowing.

26.8.2 Patient symptoms

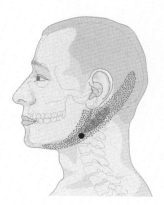

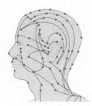

- Difficulties in swallowing.
- Pain in the upper neck area.
- Dizziness.

26.8.3 Trigger points

mTrP	LOCALIS-ATION	RADIATION	mTrP→ Acupuncture point
1	Somewhat deeper than the region of the styloid process	Area of the digastricus muscle, neck region, larynx	TH 17

26.8.4 Diagnosis

Questioning
- Pain quality and localisation.
- Difficulties in swallowing.
- Pain of uncertain cause in the upper lateral area of the neck.

Inspection: usually no visible changes outside the mouth.
Physical examination: checking maximum head rotation and inclination ('styloid syndrome').
Technical examination: radiographic investigations, possibly volume tomography to rule out 'styloid syndrome'.

26.8.5 Specific aspects

- The suprahyoid muscles form a functional unit which is frequently affected at the same time.
- Lengthening of the styloid process can induce mTrP in the stylohyoid and digastricus muscles.
- Treatment of styloid syndrome can make surgical intervention necessary.

26.8.6 Therapy

Instructions for manual trigger point therapy

- Treatment such as the posterior belly of the digastric muscle (from which it is difficult to distinguish on palpation): Directly below or medial to the mandibular angle in the direction of the styloid process.

Classic Chinese acupuncture

Local and locoregional points (also contralateral): TH 17, SI 17.
Distal points: CV 21 (relaxation of floor of mouth; lymph system, suspected mandibular angle; stress).
Control points/symptomatic points: in accordance with TCM.

Microsystem acupuncture

Ear: temporomandibular joint, upper jaw, lower jaw, Jérôme point.
Lymph belt: specific sternal point CV 20/21.

Kiiko Matsumoto acupuncture

- As for Section 26.7.
- For tenderness at the superior anterior iliac spine: KI 9 ipsilateral at the exact localisation and needling angle until tenderness at the superior anterior iliac spine and the pterygoid muscle is relieved.
- KI 27 on both sides, needling at an angle of 10° in the direction of the sternoclavicular joint.

Psychosomatic therapy/relaxation

- Over KI 27 and CV 21 often good for relaxation.

26.8.7 Recommendations for the patient

Self-massage

- The patient is not really in a position to reach the individual muscle areas such as the digastric muscle (Section 26.7).

Additional measures

- Relaxation exercises, self-monitoring for clenching the teeth (tongue thrust).
- M. mylohyoideus: styloid syndrome.
- M. geniohyoideus: as for M. digastricus.

26.9 M. MYLOHYOIDEUS

Kathrin Spiegl, Jean-Marc Pho Duc

26.9.1 Anatomy

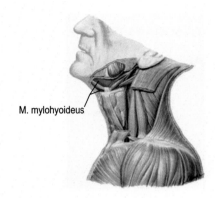

M. mylohyoideus

Innervation: N. mylohyoideus (N. mandibularis).
Origin: short tendon from the mylohyoid line of the mandible.
Insertion: mylohyoid raphe and upper margin of the body of the hyoid bone.
Function: lifts the floor of the mouth and the tongue (swallowing), lowers the lower jaw, lifts the hyoid bone.

26.9.2 Patient symptoms

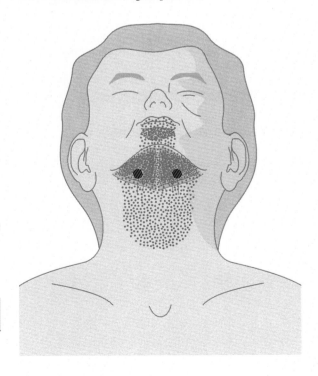

- Difficulties in swallowing.
- Pain in the upper neck area.

26.9.3 Trigger points

mTrP	LOCALIS-ATION	RADIATION	mTrP→ACUPUNCTURE POINT
1, 2	Whole floor of the mouth	Area of the larynx, anterior side of the neck, mouth area tongue, swallowing difficulties	CV 23

26.9.4 Diagnosis

Questioning
- Pain quality and localisation.
- Difficulty eating.

Inspection: hardening of the floor of the mouth.
Physical examination: the floor of the mouth is palpated between the index finger (intraoral) and the thumb (extraoral); if the floor of the mouth is soft, muscle tone is physiological.
Technical examination: palpation as part of the function analysis.

26.9.5 Specific aspects

- Suprahyoid muscles form a functional unit which is frequently affected as well and makes delineation into individual muscle parts difficult.
- Breathing through the mouth at night can lead to strain.

26.9.6 Therapy

Instructions for manual trigger point therapy

- Extraoral and intraoral treatment.

Extension

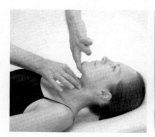
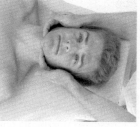

- Patient in supine position, head slightly elevated, reclined. Traction between the chin and the thyroid cartilage (left).
- Or spread and extend the course of the muscle with the fingers (right).

Physical therapy procedures

- Bite splint; heat or cold therapy (chronic/acute) with hot or cold gel compresses.

Infiltration techniques/dry needling

Suitable infiltration techniques are described in the literature. Because acupuncture (CV 21) and manual relaxation techniques are highly effective infiltration can be avoided, especially as this is stressful for the patient.

Classic Chinese acupuncture

Local and locoregional points (also contralateral): TH 17, CV 23, Ashi points (cautious needling).
Distal points: CV 21 (relaxation of floor of mouth; lymph system, suspected mandibular angle; stress).
Control points/symptomatic points: in accordance with TCM.

Microsystem acupuncture

Ear: temporomandibular joint, upper jaw, lower jaw, Jérôme point.
Lymph belt: specific sternal point CV 20/21.

Kiiko Matsumoto acupuncture

- If palpation of ST 41 is painful: ST 43 and ST 44.
- In some cases, pain can be relieved at ST 41 and the mylohyoid muscle by needling of KI 3 and KI 27 ipsilateral.
- For pain in the area of KI 2: Needling of KI 10 and KI 7 (instead of KI 3), adjust angle and depth of needle, until pain in the area of KI 2 and in the area of the muscle is reduced.
- In some cases KI 7, KI 27 and BL 11 on both sides; BL 11 vertically to the muscle fibre and downwards with the flow of the meridian; angle for KI 27 10° in the direction of the sternoclavicular joint.

Psychosomatic therapy/relaxation

- Relaxation exercises.
- Over KI 27 and CV 21 often good for relaxation.

26.9.7 Recommendations for the patient

Self-massage

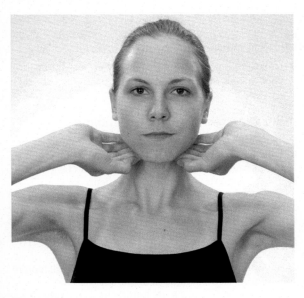

- Hands and palms of hands upwards.
- Pads of the fingers along the course of the muscle.
- Stretch out along the course of the fibres to the side.

Additional measures

- Reclination.
- Self-monitoring for clenching the teeth (tongue thrust).

26.10 M. GENIOHYOIDEUS

Kathrin Spiegl, Jean-Marc Pho Duc

26.10.1 Anatomy

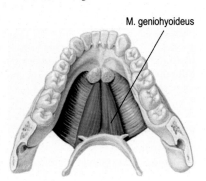

M. geniohyoideus

Innervation: ansa cervicalis (cervical loop).
Origin: mental spine of the mandible.
Insertion: body of hyoid bone.
Function: supports the digastrics muscles in retraction and lowering of the lower jaw, works together with the mylohyoid muscle to lift the tongue, lift or fix the hyoid bone.

26.10.2 Patient symptoms

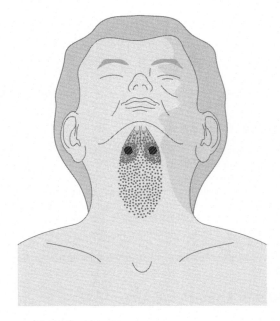

- Difficulties in swallowing.
- Pain in the upper neck area.
- Pain when retracting the lower jaw.
- Restricted mouth opening/pain on opening the mouth.

26.10.3 Trigger points

mTrP	LOCALIS-ATION	RADIATION	mTrP↔ ACUPUNCTURE POINT
1, 2	Each aligned centrally in the pairs of muscle bellies	Anterior neck region, swallowing difficulties	–

26.10.4 Diagnosis

Questioning
- Pain quality and localisation.
- Restricted mouth opening.
- Pain when swallowing?

Inspection: not possible because of the concealed anatomical position.
Physical examination: difficult to palpate because of the anatomical position above the mylohyoid muscle.
Technical examination: MRI in exceptional cases.

26.10.5 Specific aspects

- Other suprahyoid muscles are also frequently affected.

26.10.6 Therapy

Instructions for manual trigger point therapy

Treatment of the mylohyoid, digastrics and stylohyoid muscles.

- Intraoral access: tangible on the floor of the mouth during swallowing movements; treatment using pincer grip (thumb inside the mouth, index/middle finger outside).
- Extraoral access: treatment from the outside through the mylohyoid together with the anterior belly of the digastricus (with which it runs parallel).

Extension

- As for M. mylohyoideus (Section 26.9).

Physical therapy procedures

- Bite splint/brace.

Classic Chinese acupuncture

Local and locoregional points (also contralateral): CV 23, ST 9.

Distal points: CV 21 (relaxation of floor of mouth; lymph system, suspected mandibular angle; stress).
Control points/symptomatic points: in accordance with TCM.

Microsystem acupuncture

Ear: temporomandibular joint, upper jaw, lower jaw, Jérôme point.
Lymph belt: specific sternal point CV 20/21.

Kiiko Matsumoto acupuncture

- As for M. mylohyoideus (Section 26.9).

Psychosomatic therapy/relaxation

- Over KI 27 and CV 21 is often good for relaxation.

26.10.7 Recommendations for the patient

Self-massage

- No direct self-massage possible because the mylohyoid lies over it.
- Stretch out in the direction of the chin.

Additional measures

- Relaxation exercises.
- Self-monitoring for clenching the teeth (tongue thrust).

Chapter | 27 |

Neck and shoulder region

Nicolas Behrens, Dominik Irnich

27.1 FUNCTIONAL ASSOCIATIONS

The neck joins together the head and the torso. Feedback from the neck muscles is essential for orientation and for safe upright movement around a space, especially the muscle spindles of the short suboccipital muscles (see Section 27.9). Because of the high density of receptors with a variety of proprioceptors and nerve connections to trigeminal nuclei, the deep, short neck muscles are regarded as accessory sensory organs (the 'neck receptor field' of Scherer). This information is fed into these muscles from the balance organs and the eyes. Not until this is done are we able to perceive the effect of gravity on the head and especially the torso.

- We make the assumption that the afferent impulses from the upper cervical spine gain in significance as we get older, as they also compensate for a weakening of the sensory organs. In this situation, (asymmetrical) muscle tension and malafference are particularly unfavourable.
- Another close connection between the sensory organs of the head (the eyes) and the short, deep, suboccipital muscles is that, according to Putz, the latter act like an optomechanical image-stabilisation system, which keeps the head parallel to the horizon so that objects perceived by the eyes remain as unblurred as possible: undistorted optical/spatial orientation is essential (Putz, personal communication).

These neurophysiological aspects enable us to understand that shortening or tension disorders of the neck muscles can cause numerous symptoms, and can also make them worse and cause them to persist.

We see this also in the manual examination of the cervical spine, including the accessory muscles. These should be approached with caution, particularly in the elderly as they can cause or worsen a number of autonomic symptoms such as dizziness or visual disturbances. A differential diagnosis of atherosclerosis, particularly of the vertebral artery, should also be considered as a cause of such symptoms.

> Clinical experience shows that we can also make good use of these associations, independently of the various models of explanation from different schools of treatment, which may be more or less easily understandable. Many symptoms, including dizziness, uncertain gait, visual disorders and nasal dysfunction, as well as general symptoms such as poor concentration and tiredness, can be relieved through treatment of the cranial neck muscles and/or the atlanto-occipital joint.

The key role of the atlanto-occipital joint is well known and has long been described in manual medicine. That is why there is such a large number of treatment techniques for this area. It is interesting that there are also schools of treatment that prefer to treat the rest of the body via the atlanto-occipital joint, as well as others which by contrast focus on the lumbar region, pelvis and hips and their treatment. From clinical experience, both are effective: in our opinion there are two complementary approaches to the axial spine and the trunk. From experience, we can see the close association between the two 'problem regions' of the vertebral column, the cervical and lumbar spine and the transitions to the occiput and the sacrum. The relevant experience in acupuncture is known as the 'bladder meridian'.

http://dx.doi.org/10.1016/B978-0-7020-4312-3.00027-1

If there are problems in the area of the neck, the lumbar, pelvic and hip region should always be thoroughly examined and treated as well. If the basic stance is insecure (lack of stability when standing, difficulty standing up and sitting down), it is difficult for the upper body or neck to relax, and vice versa if there is 'neck tension' or 'flight mindset' as it is unlikely that the lumbar spine will be relaxed.

Experience of acupuncture also shows that the topmost part of the cervical spine is of special therapeutic significance. The virtually unique points of the neck, to which is also attributed a special control function, are GB 20 and BL 10, which lie at the level of C0/C1 and C1/C2. Deep needling here can reach the short suboccipital neck muscles. They are not just effective for neck problems and tension headaches but also have a generalised effect on head symptoms including dysfunction of the sensory organs and on all the paravertebral muscles (bladder meridian).

Other therapy systems, such as neural therapy, recognise the association between the cervical spine and the head or sensory organs, in this case in the form of the paravertebral Adler–Langer pressure points (Langer 1977).

The Alexander technique is not so widespread but is used with the aim of improving personal development and an 'overall view' for chronic tiredness, strain, whole body tension and poor coordination; it was originally used to improve mood disorders by using subtle touch impulses, instructions on body awareness and posture and behaviour training, and it strives primarily to improve the whole attitude by releasing the neck muscles.

27.2 PSYCHOSOMATIC ASSOCIATIONS

The neck is a sensitive, easily injured region. Psychosomatically, anxiety can 'sit' in the neck, for example after a 'whiplash' injury, as well as in the form of the somatic aspect of post-traumatic stress disorder. Anger and annoyance can also lead to increased tension ('wanting to bang your head against a brick wall'). If there is a great deal of anxiety or annoyance, we often try to control our bodies and our emotions. The topic of control and reduced contact with oneself/one's body can also have an effect on the neck or be 'transferred' to the neck, which then functions like the 'neck of a bottle' between the head and the trunk, between thought and feeling. Stress 'breathing down your neck', which we 'carry on our shoulders' or fear of its consequences can lead to 'pulling in the head'. Poor posture often expresses the feeling that a patient is feeling like a 'whipping boy' and is drawing in his head to make it less likely to be injured.

Careful monitoring of body posture and physical expression by 'feeling your way' and showing empathy can help to understand the patient better. With chronic cervical spine symptoms it is important and indispensable – for the successful therapy of somatic approaches as well – to take note of any underlying stress situations and internal spiritual tension and maybe cause the patient to reflect on these.

However, a prerequisite for such integrated procedures is that the patient must not be confirmed in their somatic understanding of the illness based on one-sided, simplified or even highly complex biomechanical explanations. Luckily, the patient can often be reassured after the examination that this is a purely functional and reversible disorder, although it is easily understandable that this can cause the patient's symptoms. This is the reason why the findings from imaging procedures should never be overvalued (in the eyes of the patient); furthermore, multiple scientific tests indicate that the association between radiological findings and subjective symptoms is extremely slight. It is often even sensible in patients who are fixated on their X-ray findings ('iatrogenic somatisation' by unconscious hypnotherapy, the induction of a trance as a result of overvaluing X-ray images can also be described as the 'nocebo' or 'voodoo' effect) to try to put these in as much perspective as possible or to resolve them completely by providing a precise explanation of the findings and their harmlessness (e.g. 'more than 50% of people your age have this without symptoms'). The most convincing and effective treatment is then of course a persistent improvement in symptoms or even freedom from symptoms as a result of successful (trigger point) therapy: the 'de-hypnotherapeutic effect'. Then the 'osteophytes' (which in the X-ray mostly tend to be historic findings or expression of attempts by the body to repair itself) crumble away in the mind of the patient.

A first valuable route to the reconstruction of the trusting doctor–patient relationship is a detailed but precautionary functional anatomical examination of the cervical spine. The patient must be told to say immediately if there is any pain. Fear of chiropractice is fairly common, so patients should be reassured that no unexpected manipulation manoeuvres will be performed. Once trust has been gained, the patient's dependence on the therapist standing behind them during the examination can be an important therapeutic step.

27.3 SYMPTOMS

The possible symptoms of myofascial disorders of the cervical spine derive predominantly from the functional anatomy and the neurophysiological and partly also empirical associations (see above):

- painful tension of the neck and back muscles (pain quality often dull and oppressive);
- restricted mobility ('stiff neck'): common but not always a symptom; if there is any asymmetry, the patient feels that the restriction is worse;
- sensitivity to wind/draughts and cold;
- head and face pain, some of it difficult to attribute, so-called upper cervical spine syndrome; pain is transferred from the suboccipital muscles (Mm. rectus

capitis posterior minor and major and obliquus capitis superior and inferior, see Section 27.9) and the M. sternocleidomastoideus (see Section 27.10), the M. splenius (see Sections 27.6 and 27.7) and M. semispinalis capitis (see Section 27.8); less commonly, mTrPs also project into the M. trapezius descendens (see Section 27.12) and into the middle to lower cervical spine muscles to the head and into the face;

- cervicobrachialgia as the pattern radiation of mTrPs of the paravertebral muscles of the lower cervical spine (also the upper and middle thoracic spine; so-called lower cervical spine syndrome) but also as a co-reaction with the arm muscles with the formation of additional mTrPs with longer existing disorders of the cervical spine and the pectoral girdle muscles;

- the most variable autonomic symptoms: coordination disorders, any kind and severity of dizziness, difficulty concentrating, (apparent) dysfunction of the balance system, and lack of stability when standing or uncertain gait, which is particularly associated with a dysfunction and mTrPs in the deep suboccipital muscles (M. obliquus capitis superior and inferior, see Section 27.9);

Warning: other causes of these symptoms must first be ruled out!

- various disorders of the sensory organs of the head, the paranasal sinuses and even the muscles of mastication can be associated with mTrPs in the area of the cervical spine muscles.

If an individual mTrP is the probable cause of the symptoms, the only evidence of an association can be that the therapy is successful.

27.4 DIAGNOSTIC AND THERAPEUTIC CONSIDERATIONS

The neck region is particularly suitable for testing function. If therapists are not very experienced in diagnosis or functional anatomy, or if the functional examination does not produce a definitive result, it is sufficient to proceed in accordance with the findings on palpation and the information from the patient. 'Diagnostic treatment' with loosening of the frequently fixed neck is usually painful. This particularly applies if the therapist finds some hardening, in which case it is also most appropriate if the patient will tolerate this. If needling between the occiput and the spinous process of C2 is no deeper than 3 cm, there is no risk. The vertebral artery is not reached at this depth. The spinous process of C2 is the first palpable bone in a inferior direction in the midline from the occiput. Below

this, needling can be 4–5 cm deep, approximately one finger width laterally to the midline with vertical insertion, depending on the constitution; with inferolateral needling it is still safer: this is where contact is regularly made with the laminae of the cervical spine at 5–6 cm.

Recognising and treating muscle disorders with targeted testing, however, brings even better results if treatment is continued.

If movement is painful and/or passive mobility is restricted (with the exception of extension), with or without pain on extension at the end of the range of movement, and there is a definite improvement in the pain and/or mobility through the passive lifting of the shoulder girdle if you push the patient's arm up on the side you believe to be affected and painful, it is sensible to first palpate and treat the M. trapezius descendens (see Section 27.12) and the M. levator scapulae (see Section 27.13; nickname 'stiff neck'). The test manoeuvre of moving the scapula in a superior direction leads to relaxation of the above two muscles which apply traction from the scapula to the occiput and to the upper cervical spine. However, the patient should not raise their own shoulders during this manoeuvre, otherwise the evidence is not definitive.

If dizziness (see above) is definitively not neurogenic/caused by the labyrinth, it is sensible to examine and treat the suboccipital muscles if findings are positive and when the patient is suffering head and facial pain or even chronic sinusitis. Needling up to 3 cm deep is often sufficient. In the area of acupuncture points GB 20 and BL 10 the needle then reaches as far as the M. semispinalis capitis (see Section 27.8).

The insertions need to be deeper to reach the short suboccipital muscles. If there is dizziness or pain in the head or face, the M. sternocleidomastoideus (see Section 27.10) should also be palpated.

Segmental function disorders which also demonstrate degenerative radiological changes may be present, especially if the disorder has existed for a long time (osteochondrosis, facet joint arthritis); in this case, treatment of the immediately paravertebral deep-lying short muscles attributable to the segment (Mm. multifidii, rotatores breves, see Section 27.8) is indicated. Take care that the spinous processes of the cervical spine are up to two finger widths deeper than the vertebral bodies, depending on the lordosis of the cervical spine; i.e. palpate and possibly treat a good deal further in a superior direction!

If there is interscapular pain in addition to mTrPs of those muscles (caudal part of the M. levator scapulae (see Section 27.13), M. trapezius ascendens (see Section 27.12) and the Mm. rhomboidei (see Section 28.13)) a differential diagnosis should also involve a consideration of the Mm. scaleni and the deep paravertebral muscles at the level of C5–C7.

If there are symptoms of unknown cause, most likely in the form of otitis externa, but without local findings, mTrPs in the M. sternocleidomastoideus (see Section 27.10) or in the deep part of the M. masseter (see Section 26.3) should be sought.

Consider possible influences from other usually neighbouring regions, especially if there is resistance to treatment. For the cervical spine, the stomatognathic system is particularly interesting here. However, shortening of the Mm. pectoralis major and minor (Sections 30.7 and 30.8), with poor posture and kyphosis of the thoracic spine and then compensatory hyperlordosis of the cervical spine, can also be relevant. The lumbar, pelvic and hip region and the overall static equilibrium should immediately be taken into account (see above).

From the acupuncture point of view, an approach or access via the distal points and microsystems has, in general, proved its worth (see Sections 22.2 and 22.4). This is indispensible if the tissue structures are highly irritated, as they are with irritated conditions of the cervical spine, when they may appear almost like Sudeck's atrophy, e.g. after several whiplash injuries to the cervical spine. With such irritated conditions (Schöps/Senn classification), characterised by a persistent deterioration following minor stress ('repeat damage'), a differential diagnosis of a somatoform pain disorder or pain components should be considered, where acupuncture represents a sensible way in, albeit as complementary treatment.

As part of a differentiated acupuncture therapy, local mTrP needling oriented to the actual findings naturally represents an important pillar of treatment. Myofascial (residual) symptoms which are associated with palpable hardening with identifiable mTrP can be well eased or completely eliminated. The distal points can relieve the pain of treatment somewhat and often help afterwards so that the patient suffers less subsequent pain.

27.5 FUNCTIONAL TESTING FOR mTrP IDENTIFICATION

After muscles have been shortened regularly with mTrPs they can usually be easily identified based on the limited mobility found when normal function is tested. The following table offers reliable, practical help in this. During examination, ask the patient where it 'pulls' every time there is limited or painful movement, then palpate this area (Figure 27.1).

Limited function	Search for mTrPs using passively assisted examination (the main muscles are printed in italics)
Rotation in flexion	*M. levator scapulae** (c + i) *M. trapezius descendens** (i + c) *M. splenius capitis and cervicis* (c) M. semispinalis capitis (i) Suboccipital muscles (M. obliquus capitis inferior, M. rectus capitis posterior major and minor; all c)

Rotation in normal/neutral position	As for rotation in flexion M. sternocleidomastoideus (i) M. splenius cervicis (c) Mm. multifidii (i) Mm. rotatores (i) M. scalenus anterior
Flexion	*M. trapezius descendens** *M. levator scapulae** All the *dorsal paravertebral muscles* (lateral and medial tract depending on palpation findings including M. splenius, suboccipital muscles)
Lateral flexion, especially under slight flexion	*M. trapezius descendens** *M. levator scapulae** All the *paravertebral muscles* (lateral > medial tract; all c)
Lateral flexion, especially under slight extension	M. scalenus medialis and posterior M. sternocleidomastoideus
Extension	M. sternocleidomastoideus M. scalenus anterior Anterior neck muscles (M. sternohyoideus)
Retraction	Suboccipital muscles (M. obliquus capitis superior, Mm. recti capitis posteriores) M. sternocleidomastoideus Paravertebral muscles

*Improvement by passive elevation of the shoulder on the painful side.
c, contralateral; i, ipsilateral.

Example of the use of this table

If there is limited left rotation in flexion, the patient reports pulling in the left dorsolateral area radiating into the shoulder:

- if the extent and/or (extension) pain during this movement is improved by passive lifting of the patient's left elbow (and thus the left shoulder girdle) by the therapist, it may safely be assumed that the left M. trapezius descendens is involved;
- if lifting both sides of the shoulder girdle does not produce any effect or only a small effect, the right M. splenius capitis is the most likely 'guilty party', especially if the patient spontaneously or on palpation reports pain there (GB 20 or rather medial and inferior from there).

With ipsilateral (concave side) pain with cervical spine lateral flexion, because of simple biomechanical considerations it is sensible to check whether the facet compression probably causing the pain is associated because of shortening of the contralateral, convex side muscles (e.g. Mm. scaleni or M. trapezius descendens) with corresponding disturbance of the course of the movement.

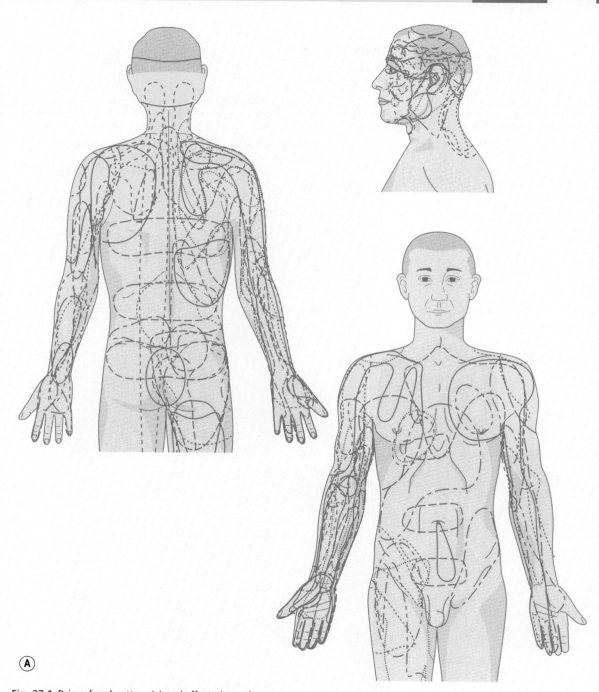

Fig. 27.1 Pain referral pattern (a) and affected muscles

Continued

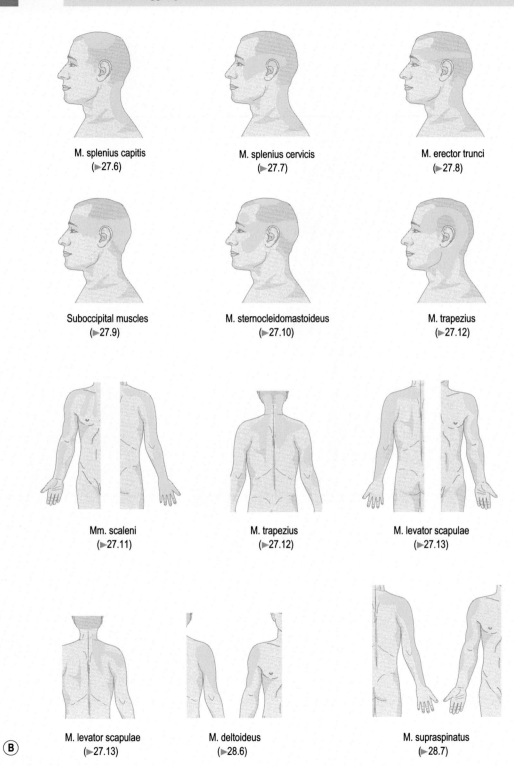

M. splenius capitis
(►27.6)

M. splenius cervicis
(►27.7)

M. erector trunci
(►27.8)

Suboccipital muscles
(►27.9)

M. sternocleidomastoideus
(►27.10)

M. trapezius
(►27.12)

Mm. scaleni
(►27.11)

M. trapezius
(►27.12)

M. levator scapulae
(►27.13)

M. levator scapulae
(►27.13)

M. deltoideus
(►28.6)

M. supraspinatus
(►28.7)

Fig. 27.1—cont'd (b) of the neck and shoulder region.

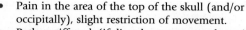

27.6 M. SPLENIUS CAPITIS

Nicolas Behrens

27.6.1 Anatomy

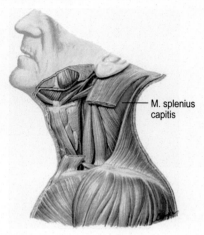

M. splenius capitis

Innervation: posterior branches of the cervical nerves.
Origin: spinous process approximately C4 to T3 including the supraspinous ligaments.
Insertion: mastoid process including bordering occipital bone, superior nuchal line, below the insertion of the M. sternocleidomastoideus.
Function:

- *one-sided action:* theoretically lateral flexion (but an EMG does not show any activity in this movement), rotation of the head (and thus the cervical spine) to the same side;
- *two-sided action:* extension of the cervical spine.

27.6.2 Patient symptoms

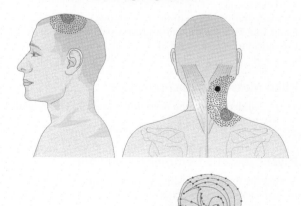

- Pain in the area of the top of the skull (and/or occipitally), slight restriction of movement.
- Rather stiff neck (if disorder occurs together with the levator scapulae muscle: almost total stiffening of the cervical spine).

27.6.3 Trigger points

mTrP	LOCATION	RADIATION	mTrP ↔ ACUPUNC-TURE POINT
1	At the level of the spinous process at C2 laterally to the descending trapezius muscle/cord of the autochthonal neck muscles	To the scalp	TH 16

27.6.4 Diagnosis

Questioning: 'pressure cooker valve' pain: possibly bridge to the topic 'of being steamed up'.
Inspection

- Head protraction.
- Postural problems and asymmetry.

Physical examination

- Turning to the opposite side restricted when in a flexed position.
- In contrast to the levator scapulae muscle no improvement from passive lifting of the shoulder blade.
- Limited opening of the cervical spine during flexion.
- Always examine the levator scapulae, sternocleidomastoideus and deep neck muscles as well.

27.6.5 Specific aspects

Frequently overlaid by the levator scapulae muscle initially: treat the latter first (see Section 27.13) and then examine again for residual restriction of movement by the splenius capitis (and cervicis) muscles

27.6.6 Therapy

Instructions for manual trigger point therapy

- Thin, flat muscle.
- The middle course of the splenius capitis muscle between the dorsal margin of the sternocleidomastoideus muscle and the anterior margin of the descending part of the trapezius muscle are directly accessible for palpation and treatment.

293

- Treatment of the inferior part of the muscle through the descending part of the trapezius muscle.
- Treatment of the superior part of the muscle inferior and posterior the sternocleidomastoideus muscle.
- Fascia separation technique between the M. splenius capitis and M. trapezius.

Extension/stretching

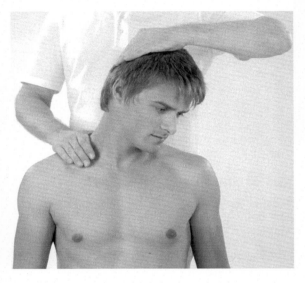

- The patient is seated, with the therapist standing behind.
- Head position: maximum flexion, rotation and lateral inclination of the cervical spine to the opposite side.
- The therapist's hand lies on the top of the shoulder.
- The thumb can also be placed if necessary on the taut band or mTrP with gentle massage or to palpate the muscle tone.
- Exercise slight pressure against the direction of movement with the hand in the parieto-occipital position.

Physical procedures

- Compresses, cushions.

Infiltration techniques/dry needling

- The patient should lie in the prone position (bed with breathe hole) or seated.
- Depending on the findings on palpation, the simplest way is with moderate extension: insert the needle suboccipitally between the origins of the descending part of the trapezius muscle and the sternocleidomastoideus muscle (GB 20).
- Guide the needle to the palpated taut band/mTrP.

- Shallow search through the muscle in the sector using the long needle like a fan from lateral to inferior.
- Needle length up to 5 cm.

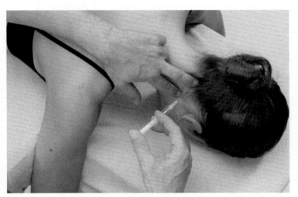

Classical Chinese acupuncture

Local and locoregional points (also contralateral): the mTrP corresponds to the TH 16: association of the triple warmer meridian to rotation movement; GB 20 (for injection technique see above).
Distal points: TH 5, SI 3 zone from Gleditsch, GB 39, Ex-AH 8.
Control points/symptomatic points: LR 3, ST 36.

Microsystem acupuncture

Ear: vertebral column, sympathic ganglia, Shenmen, Jérôme point; pressure-sensitive points like a helix close to the area of representation of the cervical spine on the antihelix margin.
YNSA: A and/or B area of the base points.
Hand line V: area at the fifth metacarpal, between SI 2 (or surrounding area) and SI 3.

Kiiko Matsumoto acupuncture

- For tenderness on the right in the area of the occipital insertion ST 26 or ST 27.

Psychosomatic treatment/relaxation

Anxiety in the neck, feeling under pressure. The muscle is activated by hyperextension of the cervical spine with head protraction and increased kyphosis of the thoracic spine, such as when reading in a slumped, seated position.

27.6.7 Recommendations for the patient

Autostretching

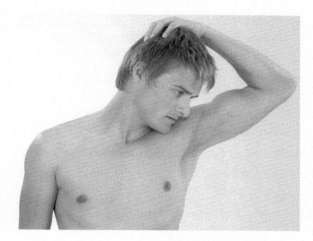

- Maximum flexion of the head or cervical spine, lateral flexion and rotation to the other side.
- Grasp the head with the hand from the side not affected and if necessary use breathing and postisometric relaxation to extend further.
- Make sure that the shoulders are not lifted and if necessary hold on to the chair or couch (M. splenius cervicis, see Section 27.7).

Additional measures

- Shower the neck with hot water and use hot, moist compresses.
- Wear a scarf: the muscle is particularly sensitive to draught and cooling.
- When driving push against the head rest as an exercise or against your own folded hands used as resistance: training of head retraction.
- Avoid sitting incorrectly: it is better to rest the head.

27.7 M. SPLENIUS CERVICIS

Nicolas Behrens

27.7.1 Anatomy

Innervation: posterior branches of the cervical nerves.
Origin: spinous process of T3–T6 including the supraspinous ligaments.

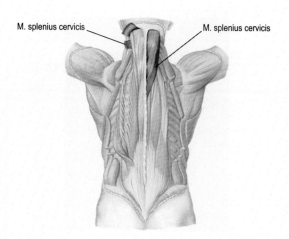

M. splenius cervicis   M. splenius cervicis

Insertion: posterior tubercle of the transverse process of C2–C1 (C3).
Function:
- one-sided action: lateral flexion, rotation of the cervical spine to the same side;
- two-sided action: extension of the cervical spine.

27.7.2 Patient symptoms

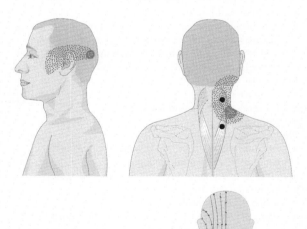

- Deep diffuse pain in the skull radiating from the back of the head, sometimes to the back of the eyes.
- Blurred vision on one side.
- Less commonly radiation of pain to the shoulder/neck area.

27.7.3 Trigger points

mTrP LOCATION	RADIATION	mTrP ↔ ACUPUNCTURE POINT
1 Paravertebrally at the level of the spinous process at C3/C4	Ring-shaped or diffusely over the skull at the level of the eyes, particularly behind the eyeball	BL '10½'
2 Paravertebrally at the level of the spinous process at C7 (vertebra prominens)	Angle of the shoulder and neck below the middle of the descending part of the trapezius muscle	BL 11 needled diagonally in a superior direction

27.7.4 Diagnosis

Questioning
- Acute or repetitive strain, especially when sitting or working with head protraction?
- Trauma? Cold, draughts?
- For chronic back pain and predominantly somatic disease make a careful psychological evaluation: profession, feeling of stress: 'everything is too much', 'left in the lurch', relationships, neck tension.

Inspection
- Head protraction.
- Postural problems and asymmetry.
- Scoliosis.

Physical examination
- Painful limitation of movement, especially with rotation in maximum flexion.
- Limited opening of the cervical spine during flexion.
- Segmental function examination.
- Kibler fold (skin-rolling test).
- Palpation: the M. splenius cervicis lies predominantly under the Mm. trapezius (dorsal) and levator scapulae (lateral):
  - the upper mTrPs can be palpated between the descending trapezius muscle and the levator scapulae muscle, directly behind the transverse processes at C3 and C4; during this, the cervical spine should be leaned towards the side examined in order to relax the Mm. trapezius and levator scapulae get to the side;
  - the lower mTrPs can be palpated through the overlying M. trapezius. By pre-tensing the M. splenius cervicis (slight flexion and rotation to

the opposite side) the taut bands/mTrPs are more easily palpable.
  - Always examine the levator scapulae, sternoclei-domastoideus and deep neck muscles as well.

27.7.5 Specific aspects

- Often co-activated with whiplash injuries; examine as well, especially where there is diffuse, changeable visual disturbance.
- The suboccipital muscles may also be affected if there is retro-orbital pain.

27.7.6 Therapy

Instructions for manual trigger point therapy

- Treatment of the inferior part of the muscle through the descending part and transverse part of the trapezius muscle.
- Treatment of the superior part of the muscle below or behind the sternocleidomastoideus muscle.
- Fascia separation technique between the M. splenius capitis and M. trapezius.

Stretching

As for M. splenius capitis (Section 27.6).

- The patient is seated, with the therapist standing behind.
- Head position: maximum flexion, rotation and lateral inclination of the cervical spine to the opposite side.
- The therapist's hand lies on the top of the shoulder.
- Exercise slight pressure against the direction of movement with the other hand in the parieto-occipital position.

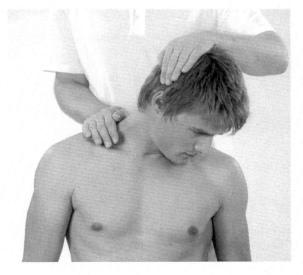

Physical procedures

- Compresses, cushions.

Infiltration techniques/dry needling

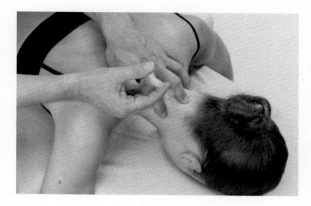

- Treatment in prone position: vertical injection approximately 2.5 finger widths laterally to the spinous process. This technique can easily be used to treat more superficial mTrPs in the area of the upper and middle cervical spine.
- Treat deeper-lying mTrPs in the lateral decubitus with a pillow under the head.
- Upper mTrPs:
  - injection just dorsal to the transverse processes C3 or C4,
  - guide the needle from the lateral to the medial direction in a fan shape using palpation by the other hand in the frontal plane,
  - needle length 4–5 cm,
  - as you move forward, mTrPs of the M. levator scapulae covering the lateral M. splenius cervicis can also be affected, which is usually makes sense.
- Lower mTrPs:
  - analogous to the needling for the upper mTrPs,
  - injection just dorsal to the transverse process of C7,
  - guide the needle through the M. trapezius,
  - needling in the frontal plane is safer in regard to a pneumothorax. However, it is also possible to needle from a dorsal direction (injection approximately 3 finger widths lateral to the spinous process of C7) in an anterior or medial direction to the lamina of C7,
  - needle length approximately 5 cm.

Classical Chinese acupuncture

Local and locoregional points (also contralateral): BL 11, Ashi points superficially in the segment (Very Point technique of Gleditsch).

Distal points: SI 3 including satellite points (see microsystem acupuncture below), TH 5, GB 39, SI 6, GB 34 and/or GB 41, Ex-AH 8, Ex-AH 7 ('Yaotongdian').
Control points/symptomatic points: LR 3, ST 36.

Microsystem acupuncture

Ear: vertebral column, sympathic ganglia, Shenmen, Jérôme point; pressure-sensitive points towards the helix close to the area of representation of the cervical spine on the antihelix margin.
YNSA: A and/or B area of the base points.
Hand line V: area at the fifth metacarpal, between SI 2 and SI 3.

Kiiko Matsumoto acupuncture

- One or two points on the liver meridian on the medial side of the thigh to relieve tenderness in the neck in the area of the muscle; location: imaginary line on the liver meridian between LR 8 and LR 11, divide the section into three; the 'Hashimoto eye point' lies in the third distal to LR 11 and one third proximally from LR 8.
- Treatment: these points should be palpated at the medial side of the thigh in the direction of the spleen and stomach meridian (from medial to ventral); a tenderpoint must correlate with the symptoms.
- 'Basilar artery' treatment: needling ventrally from LR 8, KI 10 and TH 9 on the affected side, dorsally BL 60 (against the flow of the meridian), BL 58 and BL 40 (with the flow of the meridian).

Psychosomatic treatment/relaxation

- Anxiety/anxiety-avoidance behaviour.
- Professional and/or social stress.

27.7.7 Recommendations for the patient

Autostretching

- Maximum flexion of the head or cervical spine, lateral flexion and rotation to the other side.
- Grasp the head with the hand from the side not affected and if necessary use breathing and postisometric relaxation to extend further in the direction of rotation (look in the direction of the armpit).
- Make sure that the shoulders are not lifted and if necessary hold on to the chair or couch using the hand from the side to be extended.

Additional measures

- The mTrPs can be squeezed by lying on a tennis ball on both sides of the relevant spinous processes.

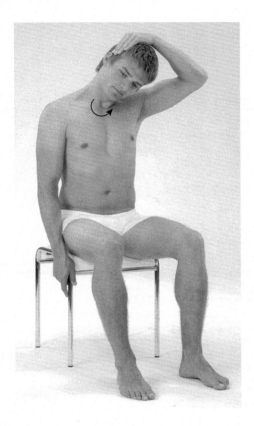

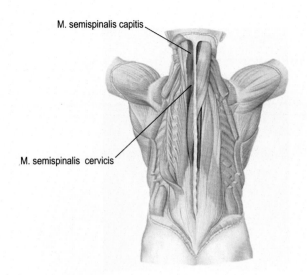

M. semispinalis capitis

M. semispinalis cervicis

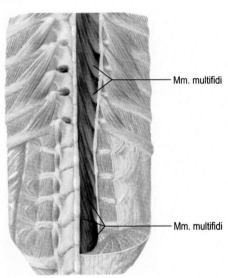

Mm. multifidi

Mm. multifidi

- Shower the neck with hot water on the maximally flexed neck or use hot, moist compresses.
- Wear a scarf.
- See also M. splenius capitis (see Section 27.6).

27.8 MUSCLES OF THE CERVICAL M. ERECTOR TRUNCI

Nicolas Behrens

27.8.1 Anatomy

The cervical M. erector trunci comprises:

- the lateral tract: M. iliocostalis cervicis, M. longissimus cervicis, M. longissimus capitis,
- the medial tract: Mm. multifidi, cervical part; Mm. interspinales cervicis, M. spinalis cervicis, M. spinalis capitis, M. semispinalis capitis, M. semispinalis cervicis.

Innervation: posterior branches of the spinal nerves:

- the lateral tract: posterior branches of the spinal nerves (M. longissimus cervicis, M. longissimus capitis),

- the medial tract: posterior branches of the spinal nerves C3–C6 (Mm. interspinales cervicis, M. spinalis cervicis, M. spinalis capitis); posterior branches of the spinal nerves C1–C5 (M. semispinalis capitis); posterior branches of the spinal nerves C3–C6 (M. semispinalis cervicis).

Origin

- The lateral tract:
  - M. iliocostalis cervicis: 7.–(4.) 3, rib medial to the costal angle,
  - M. longissimus cervicis: transverse processes of T6–T1 and C7–C3,
  - M. longissimus capitis: transverse processes of T3–C3,

- The medial tract:
  - Mm. multifidi, cervical part: inferior articular processes of C7–C4,
  - Mm. interspinales cervicis: spinous processes of C7–C2,
  - M. spinalis cervicis: spinous processes of (4.) T3–T1 and C7–C6,
  - M. spinalis capitis: spinous processes of T3–T1 and C7–C6,
  - M. semispinalis capitis: transverse processes of (8.) T7 to C3,
  - M. semispinalis cervicis: transverse processes of (7.) T6 to C7.

Insertion
- The lateral tract:
  - M. iliocostalis cervicis: posterior tubercle of the transverse process of C6–(4.)C3,
  - M. longissimus cervicis: posterior tuberculum of the transverse process of C5–C2,
  - M. longissimus capitis: posterior margin of the mastoid process.
- The medial tract:
  - Mm. multifidi, cervical part: spinous processes of C7–C2,
  - Mm. interspinales cervicis: spinous processes of T1 to C3,
  - M. spinalis cervicis: spinous processes of (6.) C5–C2,
  - M. spinalis capitis: squamous parts of the occipital bone between the highest nuchal line and the superior nuchal line close to the external occipital protuberance,
  - M. semispinalis capitis: squamous parts of the occipital bone (between the highest nuchal line and the superior nuchal line, medial area),
  - M. semispinalis cervicis: spinous processes of C6–C3.

Course
- Mm. semispinalis capitis and cervicis: approximately parallel to the cervical spine between the superficial Mm. splenius capitis and cervicis and the deeper Mm. multifidi and the even deeper Mm. rotatores (provided that there is little rotatory effect, as far as the predetermined slight 'forced rotation' of the vertebral bodies on the same side caused by lateral flexion as a result of the shape of the vertebral joints).
- Mm. multifidi: cervical part crossing vertebrae C2–C4 diagonally from caudolateral to craniomedial; the fibres of both sides together form the shape of a house gable, similar to the M. trapezius descendens, but less steep.
- Mm. rotatores: flatter course, 'segmentally' from one vertebra to the next or crossing a vertebra.

Function
- Mm. iliocostalis cervicis, longissimus cervicis and capitis:
  - one-sided action: lateral flexion,
  - two-sided action: extension.

- Mm. multifidi:
  - one-sided action: segmental lateral flexion, rotation to the opposite side and slight extension,
  - two-sided action: extension (and stabilisation). As the deepest neck muscles they are important for the perception and regulation of the position of the individual vertebral bodies in relation to each other.
- Mm. semispinalis capitis and cervicis: segmental extension:
  - one-sided action: lateral flexion,
  - two-sided action: extension.
- Mm. semispinalis capitis and cervicis: according to EMG tests predominantly for balancing the head, stabilising effect; one-sided action: lateral flexion to the same side and questionable rotation of vertebral column and head to the opposite side. Two-sided action: extension only of the head (M. semispinalis capitis) and the cervical spine (M. semispinalis cervicis).

27.8.2 Patient symptoms

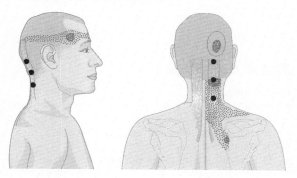

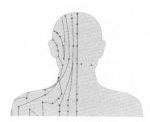

- Neck pain, limited (occasionally painful) flexion (and rotation, to some extent also extension).
- Headaches radiating from the neck.
- Sensitive to local pressure (pillow).
- If there is irritation of the major occipital nerve as a result of entrapment: tingling or even numbness and (burning) pain in the occipital region.
- Non-specific preliminary diagnosis: degenerative ('upper' and/or 'lower' cervical/thoracic spine) syndrome, segmental function disorder 'blocking'/'intervertebral disc'; cervicogenic cephalgia, post-traumatic cephalgia, occipital neuralgia.

27.8.3 Trigger points

mTrP	LOCATION	RADIATION	mTrP→ ACUPUNCTURE POINT
1	M. semispinalis capitis: just suboccipital, approximately two finger widths lateral to the midline	Ring-shaped around the biggest circumference of the skull, especially the region of the temples	GB 20, needled towards medial or BL 10, needled in a superior direction
2	M. semispinalis cervicis (and capitis) 2–4 cm below the occiput, at the level of the second spinous process*, approximately two finger widths lateral to the midline	Superiorly to the occiput	BL 10
3	Predominantly Mm. multifidi with deep needling, but also local twitch response of the superficial M. semispinalis cervicis (and capitis) Usually at the level of C4/C5, approximately two finger widths lateral to the midline; also search further in a superior and inferior direction	Suboccipital, neck, interscapular and mediocranial margin of the scapula Most frequently correlated with the three mTrPs with an entrapment of the major occipital nerve	BL '10½'

*The spinous process of C2 (axis) is the first palpable bony prominence when you palpate the loosely flexed neck in the midline from the occiput in a inferior direction.

27.8.4 Diagnosis

Questioning
- Acute or repetitive stress, particularly through working for lengthy periods with the neck flexed, such as reading or working overhead (e.g. electrician)?
- Trauma? Cold, draughts?
- Where neck pain is chronic, also go through a psychological evaluation, neck stress, feeling under pressure, making an effort, perfectionism, 'setbacks', 'obstinacy'.

Inspection
- Weak posture, head protraction ('vulture posture').
- Sitting with poor posture: spectacles vertically adjusted?

Physical examination
- (Painful) limitation of movement, especially during flexion and/or rotation (typically, where there is limited rotation by the cervical erector trunci muscles so that they are not affected by lifting the shoulder on the painful side).
- Inharmonious relaxation of the neck during flexion.
- Segmental function examination.
- Strong paravertebral palpation.
- Almost no local twitch responses are triggered during palpation.

Technical examination: X-rays and/or CT/MRI scans are not usually required if there is no nerve root compression; if available, however, they can provide advice: at the level of particular degenerative segmental changes there are usually also particularly hardened deep neck muscles.

27.8.5 Specific aspects

- Most 'non-specific' neck pain is caused by mTrPs. Watch out: patients are often, even iatrogenically, set on the concept 'intervertebral disc'; possibly address and use 'de-hypnotherapy'. Many unnecessary X-rays and (subsequent) costs can be avoided through targeted palpation and therapy.
- For chronic neck pain, physiotherapy possibly accompanied by psychological support.
- If the patient is under great and chronic strain refer to a specialised interdisciplinary treatment unit.
- Watch out also for (radiologically still little evidence of degeneration) stressed/hypermobile to unstable segments (functional X-rays in maximum, flexion and extension may be required) and treat them at their level as well; this can make these muscle segments more dynamically stable. If there is any doubt, explorative treatment/needling or infiltration of the whole cervical spine, as it is often difficult to palpate hardening of the deep muscles.

- The relatively little amount of pain found on palpation does not always correlate with the powerful symptoms (or the pronounced reaction to mTrP infiltration or needling).
- Treat both sides as far as possible as disorders of one side will soon have an effect on the other side as well; untreated mTrP on the opposite side can easily lead to recurrence.
- Entrapment of the major occipital nerve ('occipital neuralgia') possible: the major occipital nerve emerging from the medial branch of the dorsal branch of the second cervical nerve can be irritated and possibly also compressed as it passes through the M. semispinalis capitis (and M. trapezius descendens) each about one finger width lateral to the median line and below the occiput, medial to the mTrP 1, as a result of tension bands. Typically, local application of heat no longer helps, although the application of cold compresses by the patient may relieving the burning pain of neuralgia. Directly suboccipitally performed superficial nerve blocks then help only for as long as the LA remains effective. Long-term improvement can often be achieved by treatment of the above mTrP, when surprisingly the mTrP 3 lying distinctly inferiorly to the crossing site ('Mm. multifidi', where fibres of the Mm. semispinalis capitis and cervicis are also affected) often brings the best effect. Treat until the whole cord of the neck muscles is as relaxed as possible and the cervical spine can be flexed forward harmoniously.
- Often combined with mTrPs in other synergistic and antagonistic neck muscles, secondarily also mTrP development along the muscle function chain of the thoracic and later also lumbar parts of the M. erector trunci.

- If symptoms persist (rather laterally) at the back of the head, look for mTrPs in the M. digastricus, venter dorsalis and M. infraspinatus.
- The muscles of the cervical M. erector trunci have a tendency to form satellite mTrPs (e.g. from the ascending part of the trapezius muscle) → treat primary mTrPs.

27.8.6 Therapy

Instructions for manual trigger point therapy

- Patient in prone position or lateral decubitus.
- M. semispinalis can be handled on one or both sides using a flat grasp.
- Mm. multifidi and rotatores:
  - access from a lateral direction (fascia separation technique to the M. semispinalis cervicis),
  - access from a dorsal direction (finger pressure through the M. trapezius, M. splenius and M. semispinalis capitis).

Stretching

- Mm. semispinalis capitis and cervicis: maximum flexion of the cervical spine, possibly with slight lateral flexion to the opposite side (not illustrated).
- Mm. multifidi, cervical part: flexion of the cervical spine with slight lateral flexion to the opposite side and rotation to the affected side (left).
- The patient is asked to let the head hang forward, hunch the back and stretch against the therapist's hand, which is placed at the top or in the middle of the neck (centre and right).

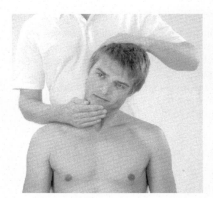
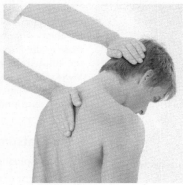
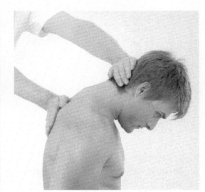

Physical procedures

- Neck pillow, hot shower on the flexed neck, aromatherapy pack, laser.

Infiltration techniques/dry needling

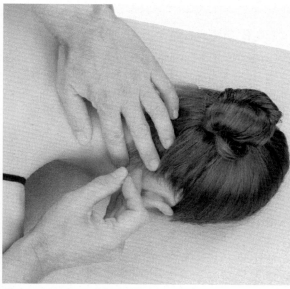

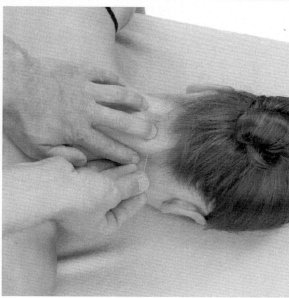

- Treatment in a prone position on a couch with a breathe hole or possibly in lateral decubitus with straight cervical spine (pillow).
- With severe tension first contralateral, superficial needling to relax and reduce pain (consensual reaction).

- Insertion for all mTrPs approximately one or two finger widths laterally to the nuchal line.
- mTrP 1:
  - insertion approximately one finger width suboccipitally; guide the needle diagonally in a superior direction over the occiput;
  - insertion into the vertebral artery is often feared but is not possible until a depth of at least 4 cm has been reached. During infiltration aspirate if necessary.
- mTrP 2 and 3:
  - guide the needle vertically or slightly in a inferior direction until bone contact with the lamina of C2 or C4; then gently search medially and laterally like a horizontal fan within the hardened area;
  - it is also possible to needle from a lateral direction if this is definitely performed dorsally to the transverse process; this also allows mTrPs of the Mm. splenius capitis and cervicis to be treated at the same time;
  - remove the needle quickly once the mTrP is encountered: the taut bands can react violently and powerfully and may grasp the needle until it bends; this can cause severe pain.
- Gentle segmental mobilisation following needling.
- Needle length at least 2 cm: for mTrP 1 it can be 4 cm; for mTrP 2 and 3 up to 6 cm.

Classical Chinese acupuncture

Local and locoregional points (also contralateral): BL 10 (TrP 2), GB 20 (medial needling in the direction mTrP 1), Ashi points, Ex-R 1 ('Hua tuo jiaji on the cervical spine', one finger width lateral to the midline); segmental search paramedially with the Gleditsch Very Point technique is sensible.
Distal points: BL 40, BL 60, BL 62, SI 3, SI 6, GB 41, KI 3, Extra-AH 7 ('Yaotongdian'), SI 26.
Control points/symptomatic points: KI 3 for anxiety symptoms, LR 3 for build-up of emotions, particularly annoyance and for visual disorders or retro-orbital pressure.

Microsystem acupuncture

Ear: vertebral column, sympathic ganglia, Shenmen, Jérôme point; pressure-sensitive points towards the helix close to the area of representation of the cervical spine on the antihelix margin.
YNSA: D zone; A and/or B area of the base points.
Hand line V: area at the fifth metacarpal, corresponds to SI 3 (or surrounding area).

Kiiko Matsumoto acupuncture

Mm. semispinalis capitis, cervicis and multifidii:

- treatment of the basilar arteries (see Section 27.7.6),
- for tenderness on the right at the level of C3: LR 1 on the right,

- for tenderness on the left at the level of C3: SP 1 on the left,
- for tenderness on the right at the level of the occipital insertion: ST 26 and ST 27 (only M. semispinalis and cervicis).

Psychosomatic treatment/relaxation

- Anxiety (neck stress), anxiety avoidance behaviour (control, excessive thinking/brooding).
- Professional and/or social stress (putting up with it/seeing it through), bullying, being under pressure, knots in the neck, refusal to cooperate, stiff neck.
- mTrP 2 (BL 10) is described as the turtle point→pulling in the head in the face of danger.
- Relaxation exercises or meditation with the head up straight.
- Exercise: when is my head directly centred over the spine and feeling light?

27.8.7 Recommendations for the patient

Autostretching

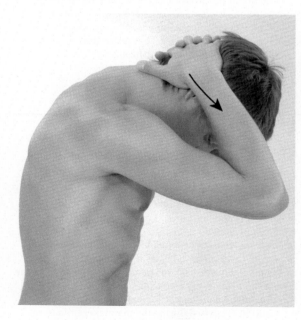

- Patient sits on the front of a chair or stool seat.
- The patient lets the head hang down loosely and places interlaced hands on the occiput.
- Push the head down (= forwards) using the weight of the arms and pull the head forward at the axis (= lengthening the spine).

- Increase traction on the thoracic spine by bending the trunk forwards.
- The patient should 'breathe in' through the neck and allow it to protrude outwards, like a cat pressing against a table leg.
- Ideally, this should be carried out under a hot fixed shower or with a hot damp towel on the neck.

Additional measures

- When reading or working at a desk, use an angled work surface.
- Adjust the frame of (reading) glasses so that the lenses are at an angle of about 30° to the frontal plane.
- Encourage the patient to mobilise by retracting the head (dorsal translation): feel it suboccipitally with the fingers and then push the upper neck into these fingers.

27.9 SUBOCCIPITAL MUSCLES

Dominik Irnich

27.9.1 Anatomy

Innervation
- Mm. obliquus capitis inferior and superior: N. suboccipitalis (dorsal branch of the N. cervicalis (C1)).
- Mm. rectus capitis posterior major and minor: N. suboccipitalis (dorsal branch of the N. cervicalis (C1)).

Origin
- Mm. obliquus capitis superior: posterior tuberculum of the transverse process of the atlas.
- Mm. obliquus capitis inferior: spinous process of the axis.
- Mm. rectus capitis posterior major: spinous process of the axis.
- Mm. rectus capitis posterior minor: posterior tuberculum of the posterior arch of the atlas.

Insertion
- Mm. obliquus capitis inferior and superior: inferior nuchal line (lateral third).
- Mm. obliquus capitis inferior: transverse process of the atlas (posterior margin).
- Mm. rectus capitis posterior major: inferior nuchal line (middle third).
- Mm. rectus capitis posterior minor: inferior nuchal line (medial third).

M. rectus capitis posterior major   M. rectus capitis posterior minor

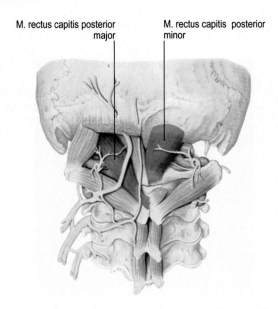

M. obliquus capitis superior

M. obliquus capitis inferior

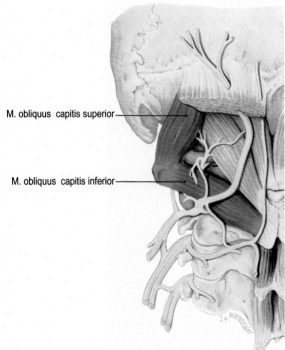

27.9.2 Patient symptoms

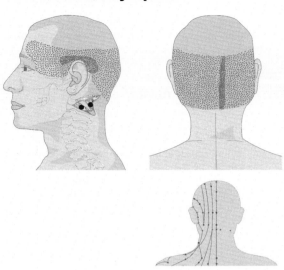

- Dull, dragging headache, from the cervical spine over the scalp or the side of the head to the forehead.
- Limitation of rotation.
- Feeling of dizziness, uncertain gait, visual disturbances, functional disorders of the nose, but also general symptoms such as lack of concentration and tiredness.
- Possible preliminary diagnoses: tension headaches, cervical neuralgia, cervical spine syndrome, cervical spine block, post-traumatic headache.

27.9.3 Trigger points

27.9.4 Diagnosis

Questioning
- Trauma?
- Remain in the same position for a long time with the head extended (painting the ceiling, watching a film at the cinema, poor eyesight)?
- Exposure to wind or cold (driving a convertible)?
- Sleep position?

Inspection: when questioned about the locality of the headache, the patient indicates this with a sweeping movement from the back of the neck over the scalp or the side of the head to the forehead.

Physical examination
- Caution is advised during the manual examination, especially with elderly patients, because neurological symptoms can quickly be triggered.
- Small circles of the head: the therapist places the palms of the hands (wrist superior) on the parietal skull and the middle finger extended in a inferior direction on the transverse process of the atlas → slight hypomobility,

Function
- Mm. obliquus capitis inferior and superior: work together in the fine determination of position and the kinematics of the atlanto-occipital joint.
- Mm. rectus capitis posterior major and minor: work together in the fine determination of position and the kinematics of the atlanto-occipital joint.

mTrP	LOCATION	RADIATION	mTrP ↔ ACUPUNCTURE POINT
1	Suboccipitally at the lateral margin of the trapezius muscle M. rectus capitis minor	From the cervical spine over the scalp to the forehead	–
2	Suboccipitally between the trapezius muscle and the posterior margin of the sternocleidomastoideus muscle (close to the insertion) M. obliquus capitis superior M. rectus capitis minor	From the cervical spine over the side of the head to the forehead	GB 20
3	Two finger widths lateral to the spinous process C2 suboccipitally at the lateral margin of the trapezius muscle M. obliquus capitis inferior	From the cervical spine over the scalp to the forehead	BL 10

slight limitation of rotation in flexion (still remains when the M. levator scapulae and M. trapezius are released by passive lifting of the shoulders).

- Tenderness predominantly in the area of the 'gap' palpable suboccipitally between the trapezius muscle and the posterior margin of the sterno-cleidomastoideus muscle (close to the insertion).
- Additional symptoms, e.g. dizziness are occasionally caused by lengthy pressure (>10 s).
- Tenderness just superiorly (M. obliquus capitis superior) or dorsocaudally (M. obliquus capitis inferior) to the transverse process of the atlas.
- Direct palpation of the mTrP is not usually possible.
- Examine the M. sternocleidomastoideus at the same time.

Technical examination: further imaging if there is clinical evidence of structural damage, e.g. image of the cervical spine if the situation follows a whiplash injury.

27.9.5 Specific aspects

- mTrPs in the suboccipital muscles frequently occur together with segmental functional disorders of the upper cervical spine and hypomobility in the atlanto-occipital joint.
- Because of the high density of receptors with a variety of proprioceptors and nerve connections to trigeminal nuclei, the deep, short neck muscles become accessory sensory organs ('neck receptor field' from Scherer).
- Close connection between sensory function and function of the suboccipital muscles (Putz's 'steady shot mechanism'). This causes the suboccipital muscles to act like an optical mechanical image stabilisation system.
- Following whiplash injury, mTrPs frequently occur. They particularly play a role if no other pathological findings can be found.
- The problems may spread to the temporomandibular joint with the development of a relevant mTrPs in the masseter muscle.

- The suboccipital muscles have a tendency to form satellite mTrPs (e.g. from the ascending part of the trapezius muscle) → treat primary mTrPs.

27.9.6 Therapy

Instructions on manual trigger point therapy

- The M. obliquus capitis inferior can be easily differentiated on palpation.
- Identify the reference points during palpation (spinous process C2 to transverse process C1, the connecting line between these reference points corresponds to the course of the fibres of the M. obliquus capitis inferior.
- The taut bands of the mTrPs are easily palpable.

Stretching

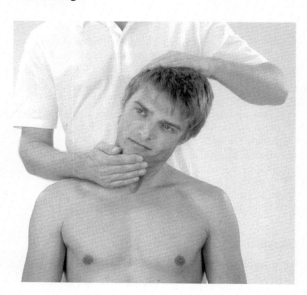

- Patient sits or stands.
- Maximum head retraction (double chin), then flexion and depending on sensation slight to moderate rotation and lateral flexion.
- Gentle guidance of the head and slight pressure at the end of the range of movement (stop if it feels hard at the end of the range of movement).

Physical procedure

Laser, cautious application of other physical procedures because of slight likelihood of causing neurological symptoms (gradual increase in strength depending on individual constitution).

Infiltration techniques/dry needling

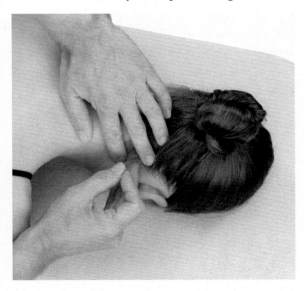

As the suboccipital muscles lie deep (below the M. semispinalis capitis) next to neuronal structures and vessels, dry needling is preferable.

- Needling in the prone position or while seated, the head must be kept straight (no flexion).
- Palpation of the 'gap' between the trapezius muscle and the posterior margin of the sternocleidomastoideus muscle (close to the insertion).
- Attempt to displace the M. semispinalis capitis with rotating finger movements.
- Needle insertion slightly medial, possibly gentle correction in a superior or inferior direction.
- No laterocaudal needling (vertebral artery).

Classical Chinese acupuncture

Local and locoregional points (also contralateral): GB 20, BL 10, GV 15, GV 16, ST 9 (M. sternocleidomastoideus), TH 17, Ex-KH 14, Ex-KH 15, other points on the bladder or gallbladder meridian in the area of the head, depending on sensitivity or radiation of pain.
Distal points: SI 3, Ex-AH 8, BL 60, BL 62, with lateral radiation: GB 41 and TH 3.
Control points/symptomatic points: GB 34, oriented to the symptoms in accordance with TCM: KI 3 (+BL 23) for cold, dizziness, sounds in the ears, KI 6 for tiredness.

Microsystem acupuncture

Ear: pressure-sensitive points towards the helix close to the area of representation of the cervical spine on the antihelix margin.
YNSA: A and/or B area of the base points.
Hand line V: area at the fifth metacarpal, corresponds to SI 3 (or surrounding area).

Kiiko Matsumoto acupuncture

Mm. rectus capitis posterior major, capitis posterior minor, obliquus, capitis superior:

- basilar artery treatment (see Section 27.7.6).
- for tenderness on the right at the level of the occipital insertion: ST 26 and ST 27.
- for ipsilateral atlas shift (or subluxation): Yaotongxue (N-UE-19 lumbar pain points).

M. obliquus capitis inferior: for ipsilateral atlas shift (or subluxation) Yaotongxue (N-UE-19 lumbar pain points).

Psychosomatics/relaxation

- The upper cervical spine area is a particularly sensitive, easily injured area ('breaking your neck') and a region of the body which receives anxiety ('anxiety in the neck'), anger and annoyance ('banging your head against a brick wall').
- Relaxation exercises keeping the head straight (e.g. meditation, Qigong).

27.9.7 Recommendations for the patient

Autostretching

- It is important that the patient keeps the head retracted (double chin) and holds the retraction during the various extensions.
- For self-extension of the straight running suboccipital muscles, the cervical spine is flexed in the retraction position and gently supported by the hands placed on the occiput (left and centre).
- Self-extension of the diagonally running occipital muscles is performed in a seated position with fixed arm on the affected side and head rotated to the affected side (right).

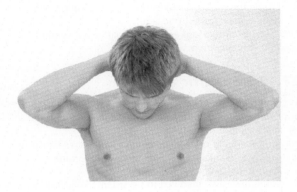 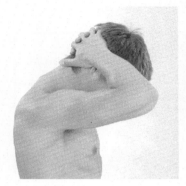 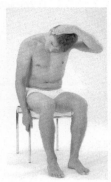

- Here, too, it is important to maintain head retraction. Otherwise it is predominantly the M. levator scapulae and M. trapezius which are extended.

Additional measures

- Concomitant gentle mobilisation of the atlanto-occipital joint.
- Posture training (regular head retraction).
- Adjustment of visual aids.
- Work place ergonomics.
- No cervical collar.

27.10 M. STERNOCLEIDOMASTOIDEUS

Dominik Irnich

27.10.1 Anatomy

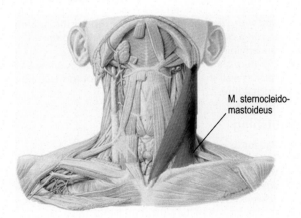

M. sternocleido-mastoideus

Innervation: N. accessorius (XI), plexus cervicalis.
Origin:
- caput sternale: along the tendon from the anterior surface of the sternum,

- caput claviculare: short tendon from the sternal third of the clavicle.

Insertion: posterior range of the mastoid process and lateral half of the superior nuchal line.
Function: holds the head still, turns the head up; flexes the inferior cervical spine and extends the superior cervical spine and the atlanto-occipital joint; innervated on one side it bends the head forwards and turns it to the opposite side, helps to hold the head still during inspiration.

27.10.2 Patient symptoms

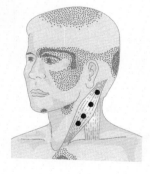 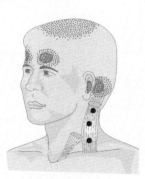

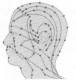

- Pain around the ears, cheeks, periorbital facial pain, frontal headache (complex picture).
- Visual disturbance (blurring) and non-specific one-sided eye symptoms (e.g. tears), globus pharyngis, dizziness.
- Possible preliminary diagnoses: atypical facial pain, chronic otitis or sinusitis, tension headache, blockade of the sternoclavicular joint.

27.10.3 Trigger points

mTrP	LOCATION	RADIATION	mTrP→ ACUPUNCTURE POINT
1	Sternal part, several mTrPs along its course, especially at the level of the larynx and superiorly from there	Retroauricular, periorbital, cheek, upper jaw	LI 17, LI 18, SI 17ST 10
2	Clavicular part, several mTrPs along its course, especially at the level of the larynx and superiorly from there	Ear, retroauricular, ipsilateral forehead, rarely contralateral	TH 16, LI 17, LI 18, SI 17
Other	Irregular distribution along the muscle and close to the insertion		–

27.10.4 Diagnosis

Questioning
- Worse after reading, especially if the head is rotated?
- Badly adjusted spectacles?
- Several pillows for sleeping (or no pillow) for other reasons?
- Strain when working overhead (e.g. painting the ceiling)?
- Sports strain, especially tennis, golf?
- Strain as accessory respiratory muscle (e.g. bronchial asthma, chronic obstructive pulmonary disease)?

Inspection
- Crooked neck.
- Head protraction.

Physical examination
- Examination while seated on a couch, therapist stands behind the patient.
- Palpation on one side with pincer grip with slight rotation to the other side (note: glomus caroticum!).
- Cervical spine extension limited, makes symptoms worse (test on both sides).
- Head protraction from retraction position (test on both sides).

- Lifting the rotated head in the supine position when lying down (test on one side).

Technical examination: eye, ear, throat or jaw symptoms: specialist investigation.

27.10.5 Specific aspects

- Complex pattern of symptoms.
- Frequently mTrPs at the origin and insertion of the sternocleidomastoideus.
- If the sternal muscle is present this can also radiate into the chest and the arm (pseudo angina pectoris symptoms).
- Sometimes also involved in persistent cervical spine syndrome (muscular imbalance).
- Pay careful attention to this muscle following previous whiplash injury.

27.10.6 Therapy

Warning: glomus caroticum! Take special care when treating the middle part of the muscle. Avoid concomitant treatment on both sides!

Instructions for manual trigger point therapy
- It is helpful if the patient is in the supine position or lateral decubitus, as strong pressure can cause short-term dizziness, oscillopsia or autonomic symptoms (nausea).
- Pinch grip.
- Fascia separation technique to the Mm. scaleni: grasp the sternocleidomastoideus muscles with a pinch grip and with a turning movement (like turning the ignition key in a car) move the muscle in relation to the underlying Mm. scaleni.
- Insertion site at the mastoid process and examine and treat as well the bordering two-thirds of the superior nuchal line.

Stretching
- Patient in supine position.
- The head should be free if possible, but it is important that the patient can reliably put the head down. It is an advantage if the required retraction of the head can be achieved through gravity.
- Ipsilateral arm of the patient under the thigh, shoulder lowered.
- The therapist holds the head with one hand and places the other hand on the clavicle (or over the sternoclavicular joint, if the sternal part is to be extended).

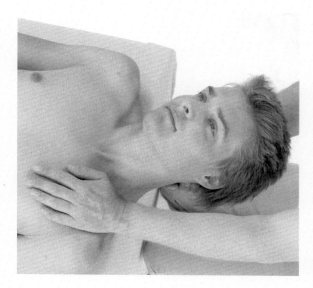

- The head position should then be in rotation and lateral flexion in order to visualise the muscle.
- Extension is now performed by dorsal extension and rotation to the affected side.

Physical procedure

- Local laser treatment.

Infiltration techniques/dry needling

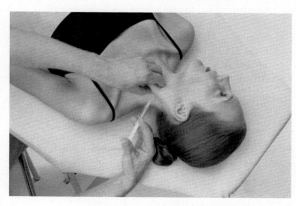

The mTrP is usually easily palpable. The local invasive treatment is frequently felt as unpleasant by anxious patients, so treatment should be commenced with non-invasive procedures in this area. Local invasive measures should only be used for these patients if symptoms persist.

- Supine position, head slightly elevated (thin pillow) and rotated in the opposite direction.
- The therapist sits on the affected side.

- Mobilise the muscle (pinch grip).
- Inject into the pinch grip.
- Intracutaneous injection close to the insertion and origin.

Classical Chinese acupuncture

Local and locoregional points (also contralateral): LI 17, LI 18, ST 9 (note: carotid artery), ST 10, SI 17, TH 16.
Distal points: LI 4 (generally effective analgesia), LU 7 (confluence point of the ren mai), GB 20 (point close to insertion with good analgesic effect), ST 36 (important analgesic point, associated with meridian).
Control points/symptomatic points: LR 3 (relaxes muscle), SP 6 (FK stomach/spleen), TH 17 (for dizziness), CV 22 (for lump in the throat), depending on pain quality (see Section 13.1), in accordance with TCM diagnosis (see Ch. 22).

Microsystem acupuncture

Ear: lower cervical spine, upper thoracic spine (muscular), mastoid, stellate ganglion, Jérôme point; pressure sensitive points in the direction of the helix close to the area of representation of the cervical spine on the margin of the antihelix.
YNSA: A and/or B area of the base points.
Hand line V: area at the fifth metacarpal, corresponds to SI 3 (or surrounding area).

Kiiko Matsumoto acupuncture

Shao Yang treatment if the muscle on one side is hard, thickened and tender; main points for loosening the muscle: TH 5 and GB 41 or TH 8 and GB 40 contralateral.

Psychosomatics/relaxation

- Unusual protraction or retraction in contact with the opposite side, stress muscle, suppressed aggression.
- Partner exercises.
- Role play.
- Overcoming stress.
- Topics: 'making contact', 'give and take', sometimes ambivalence between keeping your head down and banging it against a wall.

27.10.7 Recommendations for the patient

Autostretching

- Retraction of the head and then rotate the head gently to the opposite side.
- Now the patient should use the hand on the non-affected side to feel the muscle, and to feel where it runs.
- The patient must find their own optimum head position.
- Keep the arm on the affected side fixed on the edge of the chair or use traction in a inferior direction.

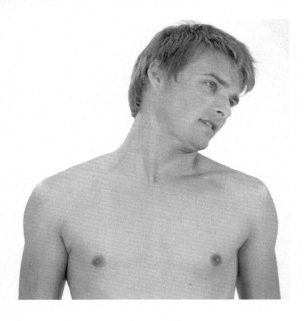

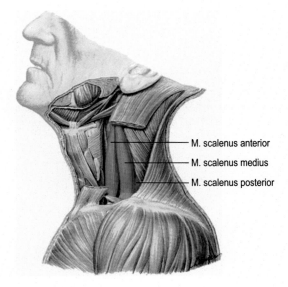

M. scalenus anterior
M. scalenus medius
M. scalenus posterior

- Extension is now performed by extension and rotation of the head by 90° in the direction of the affected side.
- This movement extends the sternal and clavicular parts to a variable extent.
- The patient must find for themself the position which actually leads to extension.
- For support, the contralateral arm may be placed over the head and slight pressure exercised; the disadvantage is that the patient frequently cancels the necessary retraction by these measures (therefore not illustrated).

Additional measures

- Pillow advice: adjust the pillow, the head should be in a neutral position (note: fixed position).
- Frequent change of work posture.
- Reading position: cervical spine in neutral position and look straight ahead.

27.11 MM. SCALENI

Dominik Irnich

27.11.1 Anatomy

Innervation: direct branches of the cervical plexus and the brachial plexus
Origin:
- anterior: anterior tubercle of the transverse process of C3 (C4) to C6,

- medius: anterior tubercle of the transverse processes of the whole cervical spine,
- posterior: posterior tubercle of the transverse process of C5 and C6.

Insertion:
- anterior: short tendon at the tuberculum musculi scaleni anterioris of the first rib,
- medius: short tendon at the first rib, lateral to the anterior scalene muscle behind the groove for subclavian artery,
- posterior: short, flat tendon at the upper margin of the second (third) rib.

Function:
- thorax: lifting the two superior ribs (respiratory muscles: inspiration),
- vertebral column: lateral flexion of the cervical spine.

27.11.2 Patient symptoms

- Pain in the area of the shoulder, medial shoulder blade, chest and arm, radiating radially and/or ulnarly into the fingers.
- Ipsilateral pain in the face or forehead.
- Numbness or paraesthesia of the arms.
- Upper thoracic back pain, predominantly the medial margin of the shoulder blade.
- Occasionally pain similar to angina pectoris.
- Breathing problems, even to the extent of symptoms of asthma, as a result of shallow or clavicular breathing.
- Possible preliminary diagnoses/syndromes: shoulder–arm syndrome, first-rib syndrome, thoracic outlet syndrome, radiculopathy C5, C6 or C7.

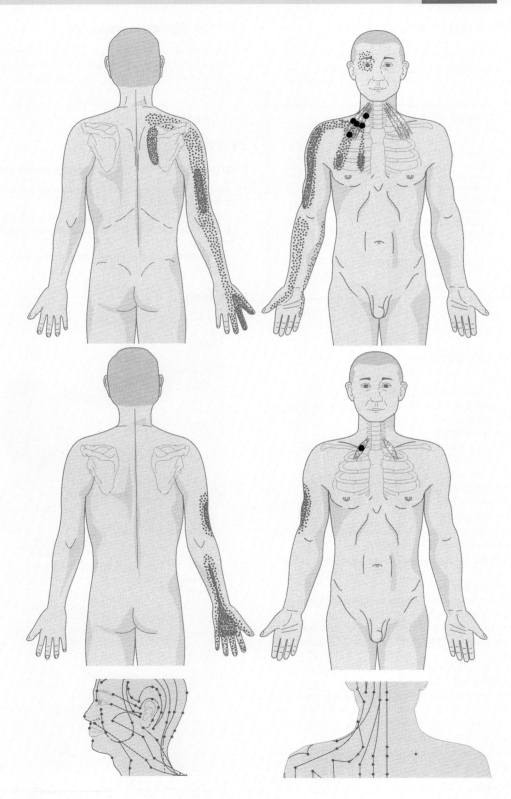

27.11.3 Trigger points

mTrP	LOCATION	RADIATION	mTrP→ ACUPUNCTURE POINT
1–2	M. scalenus anterior	Back, shoulder, chest	SI 16
3	M. scalenus medius	Arm shoulder, head	–
4	M. scalenus posterior	Arm shoulder, head	(SI 14)
5	M. scalenus minimus	Arm, shoulder as far as the thumb, particularly the back of the hand and the ulnar area	–

27.11.4 Diagnosis

Questioning
- Cervical spine (whiplash) trauma?
- Falling asleep in an incorrect position, i.e. with the head hanging down heavily?
- Asthma bronchiale?
- Lifting heavy object while holding one's breath?
- Riding?
- Head on one side, e.g. playing certain musical instruments, reading?

Inspection: usually normal, occasionally torticollis.

Physical examination

- Limited lateral movement, but frequently only slightly limited mobility of the cervical spine.
- Examine the M. sternocleidomastoideus at the same time.
- Scalene cramp test:
  - chin in the supraclavicular fossa on the opposite side → positive with local pain,
  - with radiation into the arm → differential diagnosis: compression of the vessel nerve cords in the scalene gap,
  - relief of mTrPs by lifting and anteversion of the shoulder and arm elevation.

The scalene muscles basically have higher tone and can be felt as relatively hard, therefore comparison of sides and longer compression (approximately 10 s) at sites where mTrPs are considered likely → radiation.

Technical examination: exclusion of neurogenic or vascular disorders.

27.11.5 Specific aspects

- Thoracic outlet syndrome as a result of the vessel and nerve cords in the scalene gap between the middle and anterior scalene muscles (veins not affected).
- Phrenic nerve runs diagonally over the anterior scalene muscle; it is possible for needling to cause irritation of the diaphragm (rare).

27.11.6 Therapy

Instructions for manual trigger point therapy

- Suitable starting positions: patient in prone position or lateral decubitus.
- Fascia separation technique to the descending part of the trapezius muscle and the M. levator scapulae.
- Fascia separation technique to the sternocleidomastoid muscle.

Stretching

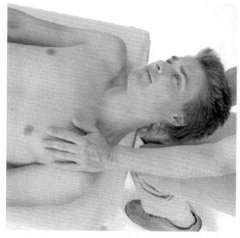

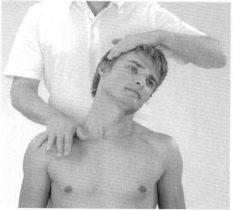

- Patient in supine position.
- The head should be free if possible, but it is important that the patient can reliably put his head down. It is an advantage if the required retraction of the head can be achieved through gravity.
- Ipsilateral arm of the patient under the thigh, shoulder lowered.
- The therapist holds the head with one hand and places the other hand on the lateral half of the clavicle.
- Extension by lateral flexion and traction and then rotation.
- Extension synchronised with breathing.
- Extension can also be performed if the patient is seated.

Physical procedure

- Local laser treatment.

Infiltration techniques/dry needling

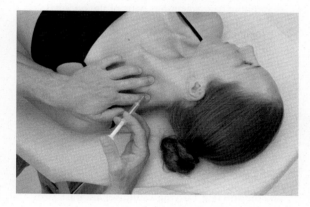

- Deeper-lying mTrPs should be treated using dry needling because of the neighbouring nerve and vessel structures.
- Two finger protection technique, look out for and delineate the large vessels.
- Injection and needling requires a particularly good relationship between the doctor and patient.
- The Mm. scalenus anterior, medius and posterior may be well mobilised or fixed in each case.
- **Warning:** pneumothorax when treating the inferior parts of the muscles close to the ribs.
- **Warning:** pneumothorax when attempting needling of the scalene muscle via SI 14 from a dorsal direction.

Classical Chinese acupuncture

Local and locoregional points (also contralateral): ST 9, ST 10, ST 11, LI 17, LI 18, Ex-KH 14, SI 14, BL 11, SI 9, LU 1.
Distal points: SI 3, SI 6, SI 8, PC 6, for headaches additional distal points depending on the affected meridian.

Control points/symptomatic points: with anxiety and/or angina similar symptoms KI, PC or HT points following TCM differentiation, for the treatment of breathing disorders e.g. LU 1, BL 13, LU 5 or LU 7 depending on TCM.

Microsystem acupuncture

Ear: pressure-sensitive points towards the helix close to the area of representation of the cervical spine on the antihelix margin.
YNSA: A and/or B area of the base points.
Hand line V: area at the fifth metacarpal, corresponds to SI 3 (or surrounding area).

Kiiko Matsumoto acupuncture

- LU 7 ipsilateral (needle-insertion angle 10–15° in the direction of LU 8).
- Point between CV 15 and CV 16 (needle-insertion angle 10–15° with the flow of the meridian).
- KI 16 ipsilateral (needle-insertion angle 45° in the direction of the navel).
- HT 3 ipsilateral (needle-insertion angle 15–45° with the flow of the meridian).
- Master Nagano's SP 3.2 (diagonally or at an angle of 45° with the flow of the meridian).

Psychosomatics/relaxation

- Frequently affected with shallow or clavicular breathing by tension disorder of the abdominal/back muscles, anxiety and excessive thinking/brooding/self-control.
- Also as a result of incorrect back posture ('I must keep my back straight').

27.11.7 Recommendations for the patient

Autostretching

- Patient seated, shoulders lowered.
- Hand of the affected side grasps underneath the chair surface to fix the upper thoracic aperture as far as possible.
- Contralateral hand grasps the head and pulls it in a lateral direction while breathing out at the same time, possibly slight reclination and/or rotation.
- Similar procedure as for the M. trapezius (see Section 27.12).

Additional measures

- Correction of poor posture and poor load bearing are essential for long-term success of treatment.

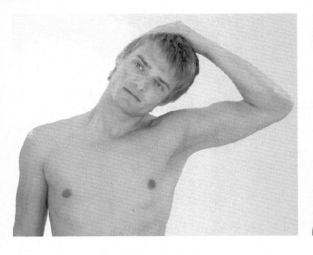
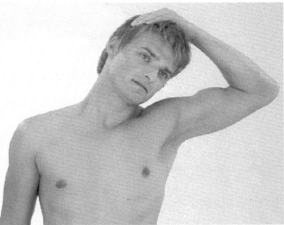

- Support the elbows when working at a table.
- Make sure the head is straight when reading.
- Middendorf breathwork.
- Practise deep abdominal breathing.

27.12 M. TRAPEZIUS

Dominik Irnich

27.12.1 Anatomy

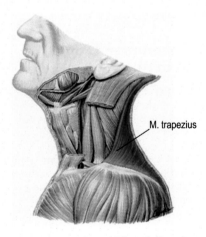

M. trapezius

Innervation: accessory nerve (XI) and direct branches of the cervical plexus. In the area of origin between the middle and lower thoracic spine a characteristic tendon pattern has formed.

Origin:
- descending part: squamous parts of the occipital bone (between the highest and the superior nuchal line), spinous processes of the upper cervical vertebrae (via the nuchal ligament),
- transverse part: spinous process of the lower cervical and upper thoracic vertebrae,
- ascending part: spinous processes of the middle and lower thoracic vertebrae.

Insertion:
- descending part: clavicle (acromial third),
- transverse part: acromion,
- ascending part: spine of scapula.

Function: pectoral girdle:
- descending part: hold onto the shoulder girdle and the arm (e.g. carrying a suitcase), lift the scapula (e.g. inspiration) and rotation upwards (to elevate the arm beyond the horizontal: M. serratus anterior), with the shoulder established rotation of the head to the opposite side, with bilateral action extension of the cervical spine,
- transverse part: adduction of the scapula,
- ascending part: lowering of the scapula and rotation downwards.

27.12.2 Patient symptoms

- Cervical spine symptoms with lateral pain.
- Limitation of lateral flexion on the opposite side and/or rotation.
- Both sides are often affected, even if symptoms are only on one side.
- Occipital and parietal headache.
- Possible preliminary diagnoses: acute or chronic cervical spine syndrome, occipital neuralgia, cervicobrachialgia, 'cervical migraine', shoulder arm syndrome, tension headache.

27.12.3 Trigger points

mTrP	LOCATION	RADIATION	mTrP→ ACUPUNCTURE POINT
1	Ascending part, middle of the acromion	Cervical spine, mastoid, temples	GB 21
2	Horizontal part, laterally over the M. supraspinatus	Occipital ipsilateral	TH 15, LI 16
3	Ascending part, between the shoulder blade and T8 and T9	Predominantly locoregional, rarely occipital, shoulder region	BL 44, BL 45
4	Horizontal part, between the shoulder blade and C7/T2	Locoregional	BL 41, BL 42, BL 43

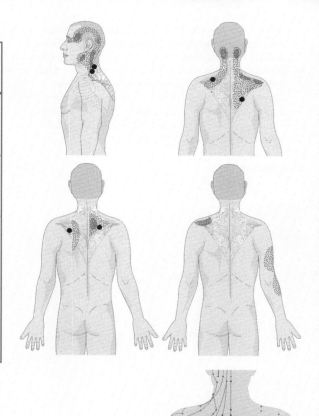

27.12.4 Diagnosis

Questioning
- Pain quality: dull pressure?
- Deterioration in wind and cold?
- Abrupt combination movement of arm extension and lateral flexion of the cervical spine on the other side?
- Work posture, e.g. workplace with computer?

Inspection: one-sided or bilateral shoulder elevation.

Physical examination
- Descending part: rotation and rotation in anteflexion (ipsilateral) ↓, lateral flexion (contralateral) ↓, anteflexion (ipsi- and contralateral) ↓.
- Horizontal part: scapula hypermobile with restriction of the humeroglenoidal articulation, non-fixed habitual shoulder elevation.
- Traction of the cervical spine is found to be pleasant.
- For passive lifting of the shoulders (= relief of the Mm. trapezius and levator scapulae) reduction of rotation pain (ipsilateral) and increase of lateral flexion (contralateral).
- Taut bands and mTrP, especially in the ascending part.
- Sensitivity (C2–T2), motor function (M. deltoideus, C5), strength.

Technical examination:
- If polymyalgia is suspected → laboratory results: ESR, C-reactive protein, full blood count.
- If degenerative cervical spine syndrome is suspected (e.g. facet joint arthritis) → imaging.

- If radiculopathy is suspected → nerve conduction speed, imaging.
- With suspected shoulder joint capsule lesion → ultrasound.

27.12.5 Specific aspects

- The most common mTrP in adults.
- In patients with 'bull neck' (short neck, very hypertensive muscles) give intensive physiotherapy initially.
- Psychosomatic disorder: carrying a burden (on the shoulders, for others too); anxiety; 'head drawn in like a dog which has been beaten'.

27.12.6 Therapy

Instructions for manual trigger point therapy

- M. trapezius pars descendens: treatment with pinch grip (it is helpful if the patient is in the prone or supine position or lateral decubitus, as short term dizziness or autonomic symptoms (nausea) can occur).

- M. trapezius pars transversa: based on the course of the fibres of the taut bands, it is possible to differentiate whether a mTrP lies in the M. trapezius pars transversa or in the underlying Mm. rhomboidei or the erector trunci.
- M. trapezius pars ascendens: can be treated in isolation with the pinch grip (patient in lateral decubitus, scapula passively guided in retroversion/depression) or finger pressure treatment (patient in prone position).
- Fascia separation technique to the Mm. scaleni, M. levator scapulae and Mm. splenii.

Stretching

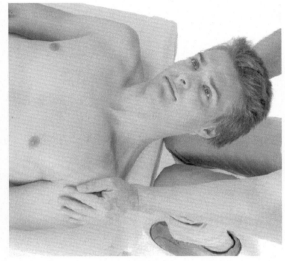

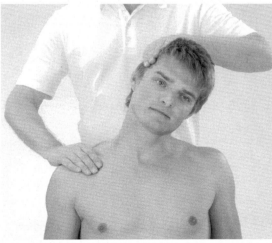

- Patient in supine position, therapist stands or sits facing the head.
- With the contralateral hand therapist holds the overhanging head occipitally.

- Therapist's ipsilateral hand grasps the shoulders with the acromion below the ball of the thumb.
- Extension by lateral flexion; depending on the affected muscle parts, slight flexion and rotation (ipsilateral) may be necessary.
- All movements under slight traction.
- Pushing the scapula in a inferior direction can also be necessary for extension (ascending part).
- Extension also possible in a seated position.

Physical procedure

Application of warmth (natural peat) better than heat (volcanic mud can be too hot), hay bag on the cervical spine and shoulder region; local application of TENS to mTrP; laser treatment if mTrP is superficial.

Infiltration techniques/dry needling

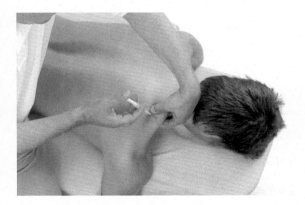

- Patient in prone position (or sitting on the couch).
- Dorsal pinch grip.
- Vertical needle insertion.
- With mTrPs 2–4 additional two-finger protection technique and tangential insertion (**warning:** pneumothorax).
- Maximum depth 2 cm (tangential maximum 3 cm).
- Good release of local twitch response, especially at GB 21 and TH 14.
- Consider the underlying muscles if radiation is untypical!
- Occipital, paravertebral or scapular cupping over the muscle insertion.

Classical Chinese acupuncture

Local and locoregional points (also contralateral): GB 21 (common predilection site for mTrP!), TH 14, TH 15, BL 10, BL 11, BL 15, BL 43, BL 46, BL 47, Ashi points.
Distal points:
- SI 3 (master point of the du mai, has a relation to the meridian), TH 5 (relation to meridian), BL 60 (relation

to meridian, for pain close to the vertebral column), BL 62 (relation to meridian, for pain close to vertebral column), TH 14 (common predilection site for mTrP).
- Ventral points in the cervical spine-shoulder region: LU 1 (forward back rule), LU 2 (forward back rule), Ren 22 (for extension pain), Gleditsch lymph belt (locoregional, forward back rule).

Control points/symptomatic points: LR 3 (source point, relaxing, analgesic), GB 34 (master point); for dizziness: TH 17, depending on pain quality (see Section 14.2.1), in accordance with TCM diagnosis (see Ch. 22).

Microsystem acupuncture

Ear: pressure-sensitive points towards the helix close to the area of representation of the cervical spine on the antihelix margin.
YNSA: A and/or B area of the base points.
Hand line V: area at the fifth metacarpal, corresponds to SI 3 (or surrounding area).

Kiiko Matsumoto acupuncture

- One or two points in the area of the medial thigh on the liver meridian.
- Hua tuo jiaji points on both sides of the spine between T10 and T12, needle with an angle of 45° angle in the direction of the vertebral column.

Psychosomatics/relaxation

- Burden on the shoulders: allow the patient to say repeatedly 'it is too much' and ask what is happening.
- Sometimes also build-up of anger, here 'frozen'.
- All exercises and relaxation techniques which lead to lowering of the shoulders and practise these.
- Learn strategies to overcome stress and watch head position.
- Role plays with the aim of self-assertion.
- All exercises and relaxation techniques which lead to lowering of the shoulders and practise these.
- Qigong: 'the condor spreads his wings' (sixth exercise from the 15 forms of expression).

27.12.7 Recommendations for the patient

Autostretching
Pars ascendens:
- sitting or lying down,
- the patient's contralateral hand reaches over the head and gently presses it to the opposite side (lateral flexion),
- while lying down, the ipsilateral hand under the ipsilateral thigh (trunk to back of hand), when seated fixation to leg of chair or chair seat, when standing fixation to desk (or similar) or pull with the contralateral hand to the other side with the arm fully extended and the shoulders lowered.

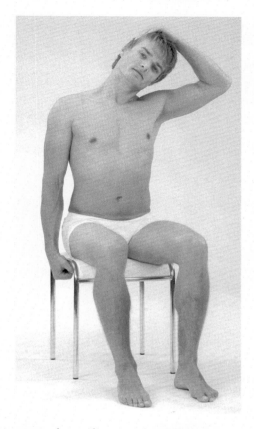

Transverse and ascending parts (complex movement!):
- in the supine position or while standing, bring the forearm (hand to elbow) in front of the trunk,
- in this position, lift the arms over the head,
- then stretch the arms with the palms of the hands forwards,
- afterwards, guide the arms down to the sides until the hands are extended alongside the body,
- exhale deeply, relax and breathe in during the first part of the exercise,
- 10–20 slow repetitions and pay attention to breathing.

Additional measures
- Lying and rolling on a tennis ball (mTrPs in the horizontal and ascending parts): ischaemic compression.
- Clasp a thick book between the elbows and the trunk for 5 min several times a day: to lower the shoulders.
- Swimming, skipping, no jogging.
- At the work station, the chair should have adjustable arm rests or if the arm rests are fixed adjust using seat cushion or similar: lower shoulders, upper arm parallel to trunk, forearm at a right angle.

27.13 M. LEVATOR SCAPULAE

Dominik Irnich

27.13.1 Anatomy

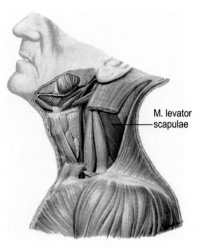

M. levator scapulae

Innervation: N. dorsalis scapulae, plexus cervicalis (fibres from C3 and C4).
Origin: posterior tubercle of the transverse processes of C1–C4.
Insertion: cranial segment of the medial border of the scapula (margo medialis scapulae).
Function: lifts and slightly turns the shoulder blade, extends the cervical spine.

27.13.2 Patient symptoms

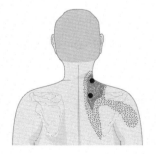
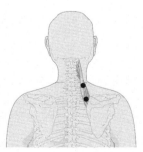
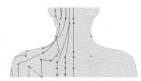

- Pain in the neck with limited rotation.
- Stiff neck.
- Severe pain possible at rest.

27.13.3 Trigger points

mTrP	LOCATION	RADIATION	mTrP→ ACUPUNCTURE POINT
1	At the muscle insertion on the upper angle of the shoulder blade	Predominantly locally at the upper angle of the shoulder blade and lateral cervical spine	SI 14
2	At the level of C6	Lateral cervical spine	Caudal SI 16

27.13.4 Diagnosis

Questioning
- Cervical spine injury with rotated head?
- Walking aids, e.g. using a walking stick or crutches for too long?
- Working at a desk with the table too high and/or head rotated?
- Talking on the telephone for long periods with telephone clasped between the shoulder and the cervical spine?
- Exposure to wind and cold?

Inspection
- Shoulders raised.
- Neck turned slightly to the affected side.

Physical examination
- Examination while seated or in lateral decubitus (non-affected side).
- Rotation ipsilateral ↓, rotation in flexion ↓.
- Slight pain during abduction in the shoulder joint.
- Shoulder blade mobility ↓.

27.13.5 Specific aspects

- Very frequently affected with cervical spine syndrome.
- Shortening leads to malposition of the scapula with possible strain of the supraspinatus muscle.
- Travell and Simons' 'stiff neck'. Instructions on treatment: often definite improvement by loosening the lumbar pelvis region (up-down association, particularly familiar in acupuncture and used therapeutically).
- May accompany infections of the upper respiratory tract.

27.13.6 Therapy

Instructions for manual trigger point therapy

- Patient in lateral decubitus, prone position or seated.
- Insertion sites (superior angle of the scapula and transverse processes C1–C4), if tender, treat as well.
- Fascia separation technique to M. trapezius.

Stretching

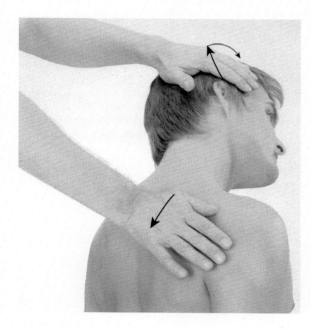

- Possible lying down or seated.
- Therapist's hand on the temples.
- Cervical spine flexion, lateral flexion to the same side and rotation to the other side.
- With the other hand, inferior push of the shoulder blade, balls of the thumbs in the supraspinatus fossa.

Physical procedure

- Laser therapy; heat treatment

Infiltration techniques/dry needling

- Treatment while seated or in prone position with the head in neutral position.

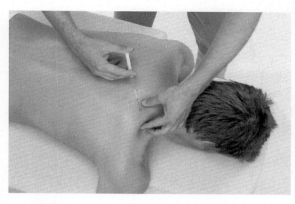

- mTrP 1:
  - mobilise and fix muscle bulge at the upper angle of the shoulder blade with pinch grip,
  - needling in the mobilised and fixed muscle bulge from inferior to superior and lateral (direction GB 21) as parallel as possible to the skin layer = encounter the mTrP from lateral and strictly tangentially,
  - **warning:** no vertical needling because of the risk of pneumothorax.
- mTrP 2: needling in the shoulder–neck angle from lateral in the direction of C6 ventral to the trapezius muscle.

Classical Chinese acupuncture

Local and locoregional points (also contralateral): SI 14, SI 15, SI 16.
Distal points: SI 3, SI 6, TH 5, BL 60, BL 62.

Microsystem acupuncture

Ear: cervical and thoracic spine zone, shoulders, Jérôme point; pressure-sensitive points towards the helix close to the area of representation of the cervical spine on the antihelix margin.
YNSA: A and/or B area of the base points.
Hand line V: area at the fifth metacarpal, corresponds to SI 3 (or surrounding area).

Kiiko Matsumoto acupuncture

Ipsilateral Master Nagano immune point in the area between LI 10 and LI 11; find the point: patient in supine position, arms with dorsal side uppermost and placed at the elbow gently flexed on the body; palpation between LI and TH meridians at the level LI 10 and LI 11; geloses to be found in the area of the radius.

Psychosomatics/relaxation

- 'Neck worries': the shoulders are lifted as protection; standing is also unstable and the back tensed so shoulders are raised for balance.

27.13.7 Recommendations for the patient

Autostretching

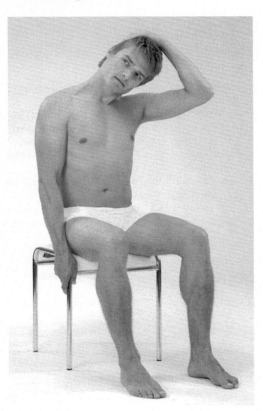

- Cervical spine flexion, lateral flexion to the same side and rotation to the other side.
- The extended arm on the affected side grasps the chair seat and pulls the shoulder girdle down (shoulder depression).
- The other hand surrounds the head (hand in front of the ear) and presses in a lateral direction.
- Extension can also be supported with the appropriate eye movements (look directly upwards to the right).

Additional measures

- Lie in the supine position with mTrP 1 on a tennis ball and roll or 'squeeze' this over the mTrP.
- Any exercises which train the patient to lower the shoulders.
- Clasp a thick book between the elbows and the trunk for 5 min several times a day; this leads to lowering of the shoulders.
- At the work station, the chair should have adjustable arm rests or if the arm rests are fixed adjust using seat cushion or similar: lower shoulders, upper arm parallel to trunk, forearm at a right angle.

Chapter | 28 |

Shoulder and upper arm

Nicolas Behrens

28.1 FUNCTIONAL ASSOCIATIONS

With chronic shoulder conditions, the symptoms frequently radiate from the soft tissue coat. This applies not only to predominant humeroscapular periarthropathy including impingement (see below), but also to the less common degenerative changes such as omarthritis/inflammation of the shoulder joint. The interplay of several, or all, of the muscles of the shoulder girdle is usually disturbed. This is not just a consequence but an essential co-cause of functional disorders and the resulting degenerative changes.

The coordinated, concomitant activity of various muscles is essential for physiological movements. The glenohumeral joint in particular, with its relatively small socket, is sensitive to a disorder of intermuscular coordination. Any shortened or weakened muscle can have an effect on the whole movement and can be a cause of mTrPs in the other shoulder muscles.

- For all movements of the arm, particularly abduction, the scapula must also move appropriately on the thorax and be stabilised at the same time (scapulohumeral rhythm) so that the shoulder socket is optimally positioned for the arm.
- In the transverse plane, the infraspinatus and subscapularis muscles in particular centre the head of the humerus in the shoulder socket as the most important and closest to the joint lateral and medial rotators.
- In the frontal plane during abduction the adductors are the cocontractors which make sure that the head of the humerus does not rise superiorly against the roof of the shoulder (acromion and especially the coracoacromial ligament), but remains centred in the shoulder socket. In this role abduction is performed by the supraspinatus muscle and up to 60° by the acromial part of the deltoid

muscle. Dorsally the Mm. infraspinatus, teres minor and major, and latissimus dorsi (and as far as 60° the pars spinalis of the M. deltoideus) and ventrally (inferior part) the Mm. subscapularis and pectoralis major (and up to 60° the pars clavicularis of the M. deltoideus) are involved in adduction.

Disturbance of the latter interplay can lead to impingement, a functional narrowing of the subacromial space, with irritation or strain on the structures there, such as the subacromial bursa and the tendons of the 'rotator cuff'. However, a shortened supraspinatus muscle can also disturb the normal rolling movement of the humerus in the socket during abduction, preventing inferior articulation because of increased compression of the joint, so that the head of the humerus rolls further and 'lifts itself up'. Narrowing of the subacromial space can also arise at rest with the arm hanging down (often visible in an X-ray) with the head of the humerus in an elevated position, as a result of long-term shortening of the deltoid muscle. This can be emphasised by too much tension in the biceps and/or triceps brachii.

If there is impingement, the supraspinatus tendon in particular is in danger of (partial) rupture. This is not just overload caused by the pressure of the head of the humerus as it rises in a superior direction. The disturbed trophism of the tendon also plays a key role and itself continues to encourage a poor tendency to healing when the strain is relieved. This reduced trophism arises because the tendon is predominantly supplied by the supraspinatus, which is regularly hardened, leading to reduced perfusion.

Because of these complex associations it is sensible if the symptoms have existed for some time, to palpate not only the active mTrPs causing the pain (isometric examination) and/or the latent mTrPs limiting mobility (passive examination), but (in further treatments) all the major shoulder muscles (see below) and to treat all the taut bands found if

http://dx.doi.org/10.1016/B978-0-7020-4312-3.00028-3

possible. If the patient is not responding sufficiently to the treatment the mobility of the scapula on the thorax (i.e. the whole shoulder girdle including the sternoclavicular and acromioclavicular joints and the relevant muscles) should be tested.

It is also appropriate to examine and possibly treat the cervical spine (including the Mm. scaleni) and the thoracic spine at the same time. The cervical spine is not just interesting because of its segmental associations; the shoulder levators which insert there are also regularly strained by compensatory movements. There are also associations which go beyond the segment in the thoracic spine: This is why, in our experience, therapy of paravertebral mTrPs at the level of the middle thoracic spine often has a very positive influence on shoulder problems.

> It is essential to take into account the whole bearing and state of tension of the lower back, because if this is not resolved it is also difficult for the shoulder girdle to rest calmly on the thorax (see Ch. 27).

28.2 PSYCHOSOMATIC ASSOCIATIONS

The shoulder region is an area with manifold functions:

- movement of the arms to affect, control and handle the environment,
- carry loads,
- protection by elevating the shoulders,
- make space.

For symptoms and muscular tension disorders of the whole shoulder and neck area, the effort, the inner demands on oneself and the resulting tendency to endeavour – which shows itself in chronically raised shoulders – is typical. Anxiety and uncertainty can play a role or emphasise this as well. In other words, if the patient has a good sense of self-worth, is at peace and feels satisfied both personally and with the world, the shoulders rarely become tense and the rest of the body is also relaxed.

> With mTrPs that have become chronic in patients who have been too tense for a long time, treatment is rarely successful in the long term unless this basic attitude is changed and is sensible only as complementary therapy. Unfortunately it is often difficult and requires physical and/or behavioural/ psychotherapeutic competence to bring the patient to a place where this pattern of behaviour can change, to properly and comprehensively treat the causes (use of multimodal therapy).

28.3 SYMPTOMS

The symptoms can vary greatly, depending on the structures affected.

- Typically the pain is during active exercise and frequently leads to a protective posture and the development of evasive movements.
- Abduction is particularly frequently affected, with a painful arc (severe pain in the area of about 60–120°, over which relatively low-pain movement is again possible).
- If abduction is painful, the affected shoulder may be raised to compensate, resulting in strain of the Mm. trapezius descendens and levator scapulae and secondary neck pain, as well as hunched shoulders.
- Pain at rest is usually dull and dragging, with movement also shooting or stabbing, even raging.
- Patients often report pain at night when lying on the shoulder.
- Crepitation occurs increasingly as the pain becomes chronic: this can be explained by incorrect centring of the shoulder joint (and increased pressure on the head of the humerus), but can also radiate from the scapula because of disturbed articulation on the thorax or adhesions.
- Restriction of passive movement is less common.
- There can be sensitivity to cold and wind/draft (although this is not often reported spontaneously).
- Radiation may occur into the upper arm, to the radial elbow and in some cases as far as the hand. If there is paraesthesia and a feeling of coldness in the hands, the scalene muscles – thoracic outlet syndrome – should also be considered, as well as segmental associations including radicular radiation of pain.

28.4 DIAGNOSTIC AND THERAPEUTIC CONSIDERATIONS

Surgical widening of the subacromial space is becoming ever more common (Neer's operation) but without preliminary normalisation of muscle disorders it is not pathogenetically oriented and is not successful in many cases. As with operations on the rotator cuff, particularly the supraspinatus tendon, concomitant mTrP therapy can remove tension from the muscle and improve the movement that has caused the problem, thus hastening healing by improving the tropism.

As an example, the following represents an example of an overall therapeutic concept oriented to the phase and findings for acute and chronic pain as well as function disorders of the shoulders. With modifications, the plan can be adapted to other regions as well:

Acute painfulness/severe tenderness (e.g. bursitis/irritation)

Sufficient pain therapy	NSAIDs, TENS, therapeutic LA
Physiotherapy	Relaxing massages, gentle mobilisation, soft tissue massage
Physical procedures	Cold applications, laser treatment, compresses, cushions
Acupuncture	Distal points (meridian, microsystem, contralateral)
Aim of treatment	Pain reduction, improvement in mobility, reduction in muscle-tone disorder

After reduction of acute pain

Pain therapy	NSAIDs as required, possibly muscle relaxants
Physiotherapy	Increasingly intensive with mobilisation of the shoulder/shoulder girdle
Acupuncture	Use reliable distal points, increasingly more local points corresponding to the palpation and function findings; dry needling or infiltration of mTrPs
Physical therapy	Adjust cold or heat treatment depending on effect! Shock wave therapy, compresses, support cushions, cupping
Aim of treatment	Completely pain-free unlimited mobility without protective posture

If there are residual contractures

Physiotherapy	Regular (manual medicine) mobilisation, possibly whole-body treatment (posture, training)
Acupuncture	Distal points (stimulate at the beginning or end of treatment); focus on intensive dry needling especially of the shortened antagonists
Physical therapy	Learn procedures for self-treatment, e.g. mTrP massage
General	Take into account functional associations up to the lumbar spine and muscles of mastication, etc. as well as psychological and emotional aspects (see above)

If there is an increasing tendency to chronification

Take into account
- Psychosocial stress factors
- Segmental associations (cervical/thoracic spine) and posture

If posture is weak, initiate training and body perception training with kinesiotape using traction both sides of the thoracic spine

For scapular rotation use stretched kinesiotape from the acromion to about T7 to activate scapular retractors (after relaxation of the major and minor pectoral muscles)

Intensive mTrP treatment

Aim of treatment: improvement of (tenderness,) pain and mobility, optimisation of local tone regulation and loosening of the muscles as well as improvement in tropism (rotator cuff) (medium- to long-term effect)

TIP FOR IMPINGEMENT

As often as possible, clasp a heavy book under the armpit, between the upper arm and trunk, to train the adductors during abduction.

28.5 EXAMINATION TO IDENTIFY mTrPs

When examining the shoulders for mTrPs, it has proved worthwhile to test isometrically (actively against resistance) for pain on straining before palpation. While the cervical spine is primarily examined for shortening and the mTrPs sought in the antagonists of the passively examined movements, the mTrPs are found in the agonists in this type of diagnosis of the shoulder (Figure 28.1).

FINDINGS ON INSPECTION	POSSIBLE MUSCLES TO BE TREATED
Shoulders raised	M. trapezius descendens, M. levator scapulae, possibly Mm. scalenii (and M. sternocleidomastoideus pars clavicularis)
Shoulder protraction	M. pectoralis major and minor, M. trapezius descendens, M. serratus anterior

Pain during active movement

Abduction in the sense of impingement (especially painful arc)	M. supraspinatus → Jobe test[1], M. deltoideus pars acromialis (depending on palpation findings) Teres group[2] as 'co-contracting antagonists' M. biceps brachii caput longum, M. deltoideus pars clavicularis and spinalis if abduction >60°
Elevation– abduction beyond the horizontal plane	Abduction and mobility for scapula: M. serratus anterior pars inferior, M. trapezius descendens, Mm. rhomboidei, M. levator scapulae
Medial rotation clasping hands behind the back	M. subscapularis, M. latissimus dorsi, M. teres major, M. pectoralis major, M. deltoideus pars clavicularis
Lateral rotation	M. infraspinatus, M. teres minor, M. deltoideus pars spinalis, M. supraspinatus
Anteversion	M. deltoideus pars clavicularis, M. pectoralis major pars clavicularis, M. coracobrachialis, M. biceps brachii
Retroversion	M. deltoideus pars spinalis, M. latissimus dorsi, M. teres major
Adduction	M. pectoralis major, M. latissimus dorsi, Teres group, M. deltoideus pars clavicularis and spinalis (if abduction <60°), M. coracobrachialis, M. triceps caput longum

Restricted movement, pain with passive movement or extension at the end of the range of movement: mTrPs in the antagonists

Abduction	Teres group, M. pectoralis major and M. trapezius ascendens, M. latissimus dorsi M. deltoideus pars clavicularis and spinalis (with initial abduction up to <60°)
Lateral rotation (also for frozen shoulder)	M. subscapularis, M. latissimus dorsi, M. teres major, M. pectoralis major, M. deltoideus pars clavicularis
Medial rotation	M. infraspinatus, M. teres minor, M. supraspinatus, M. deltoideus pars spinalis
Articulation of the scapula in a ventral direction: Half Nelson test[3] limited	M. levator scapulae, M. trapezius all parts, Mm. rhomboidei, M. latissimus dorsi, (M. pectoralis minor)

Articulation of the scapula in a dorsal direction	Mm. pectoralis major and minor, M. serratus anterior
Cervical spine involvement: thoracic spine	Particularly consider the Mm. scaleni

[1]Jobe test is isometric abduction at 90° abduction in maximum medial rotation; testing by pressure on both wrists (comparison of sides) against resistance below, the arm is held gently horizontally and forwards to lengthen the scapular spine with the thumb extended downwards: targeted provocation of the supraspinatus muscle including tendon.
[2]Teres group: muscles predominantly of the posterior axillary fold which together adduct the humerus = Mm. latissimus dorsi, teres major, teres minor, inferior parts of the infraspinatus.
[3]'Half Nelson test: patient lies on their abdomen, the therapist places (one after the other to compare to two sides) the wrist of the shoulder to be examined on the middle lumbar spine and assesses how far the elbow drops against the couch. With reduced mobility/ reduced articulation of the scapula in a lateral/anterior direction, then examination and treatment if necessary of the Mm. trapezius (all parts), levator scapulae, rhomboidei and latissimus dorsi are sensible.

Palpation: suggested sequence for surveying all the shoulder muscles:
Posterior axillary fold: Teres group (= M. latissimus dorsi, Mm. teres major and minor) → M. infraspinatus → M. supraspinatus → M. levator scapulae (for acupuncturists: up to here follow the small intestine meridian) → M. trapezius descendens → interscapular muscles (Mm. rhomboidei, M. trapezius ascendens and horizontalis) → paravertebral muscles cervical spine to middle thoracic spine → M. deltoideus with all segments → M. pectoralis major and minor → M. serratus anterior → Mm. scaleni → M. biceps and triceps brachii

Treatment of shoulder symptoms following this procedure is usually very effective. Many patients can quickly be helped to significant and usually permanent improvement, often even freedom from symptoms, and sometimes avoid invasive, more expensive, measures. Furthermore, if an operation should be absolutely necessary, the results are definitely better as a result of concomitant mTrP treatment.

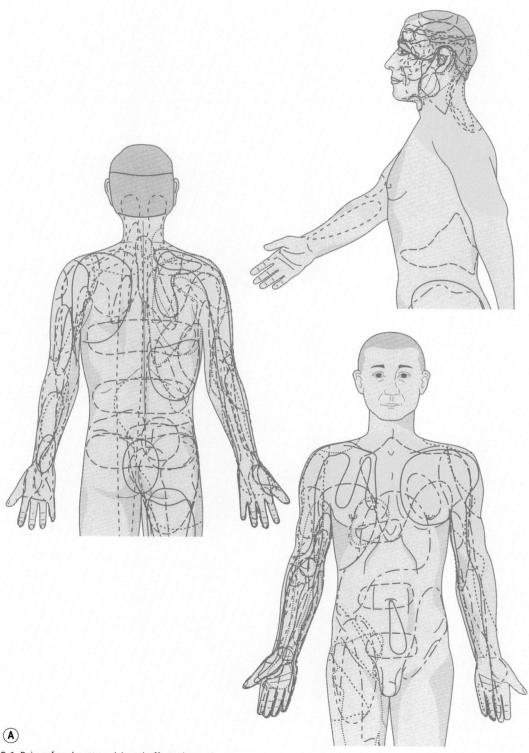

Continued

Fig. 28.1 Pain referral pattern (a) and affected muscles

Ⓐ

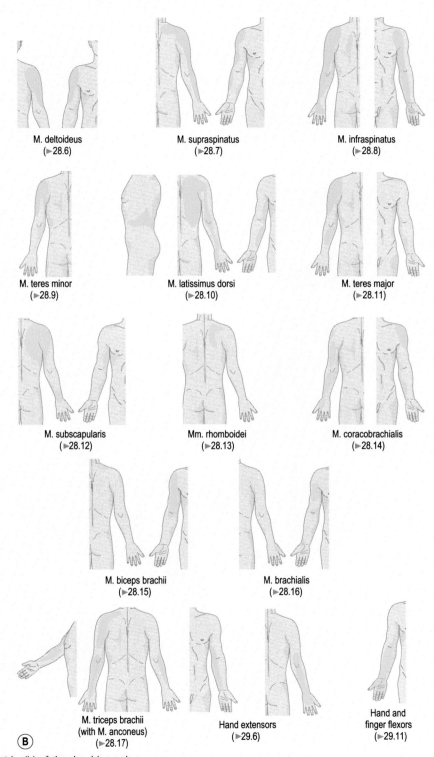

M. deltoideus
(▶28.6)

M. supraspinatus
(▶28.7)

M. infraspinatus
(▶28.8)

M. teres minor
(▶28.9)

M. latissimus dorsi
(▶28.10)

M. teres major
(▶28.11)

M. subscapularis
(▶28.12)

Mm. rhomboidei
(▶28.13)

M. coracobrachialis
(▶28.14)

M. biceps brachii
(▶28.15)

M. brachialis
(▶28.16)

M. triceps brachii
(with M. anconeus)
(▶28.17)

Hand extensors
(▶29.6)

Hand and
finger flexors
(▶29.11)

Fig. 28.1—cont'd (b) of the shoulder and upper arm.

28.6 M. DELTOIDEUS

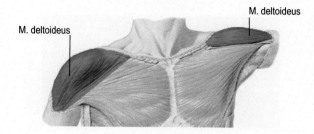

M. deltoideus

M. deltoideus

28.6.1 Anatomy

Innervation: axillary nerve (brachial plexus, infraclavicular part).
Origin:
- clavicular part: acromial third of the clavicle,
- acromial part: acromion,
- spinal part: lower margin of the spine of scapula.

Insertion: deltoid tuberosity (subdeltoid bursa between muscle and greater tubercle).
Function: shoulder joint.
- clavicular part: adduction (from about 60° increasingly abduction), anteversion, medial rotation (depending on initial position),
- acromial part: abduction as far as the horizontal,
- spinal part: adduction (from about 60° increasingly abduction), retroversion, lateral rotation (depending on initial position),
- all parts: support the weight of the arm and traction of the humerus in a superior direction (compensated by the weight of the arm and during abduction by the adductors).

28.6.2 Patient symptoms

- Chronic shoulder pain, locoregionally sensed; only rarely radiation from mTrPs over the deltoid muscle into the forearm.
- Possible preliminary diagnoses: subdeltoid bursitis, tendovaginitis of the long biceps tendon (with mTrPs in the clavicular part).

28.6.3 Trigger points

mTrP	LOCALISATION	RADIATION	mTrP→ ACUPUNCTURE POINT
1	Multiple localisations possible in the clavicular, acromial and spinal parts	Predominantly locally (little radiation)	LI 15, LU 1, LI 14, TH 14, SI 10 (LU 1)

28.6.4 Diagnosis

Questioning
- Duration of symptoms.
- Direct sports injury (collision injury).

Inspection
- Shoulders raised.
- Pronounced contours of the deltoid muscle (body building?).

Physical examination: limited inferior movement of the head of the humerus (inferior articulation in the glenohumeral joint under slight traction)?

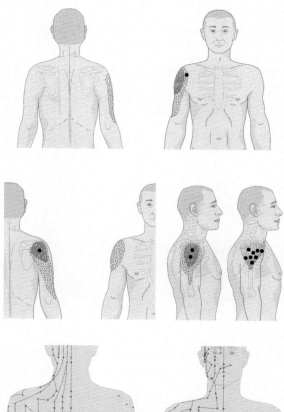

Technical examination
- X-ray of the elevated head of the humerus (in relation to the scapula/glenoid)?
- Ultrasound if subdeltoid bursitis is suspected.

28.6.5 Specific aspects

- To loosen the deltoid muscle it is necessary to palpate the whole muscle and loosen all the taut bands over each mTrP (the more chronic the symptoms, the more numerous the taut bands).

327

- The deltoid muscle is also considered a 'posing' muscle. It is a muscle that typically develops mTrPs if tensed too greatly. Suitable terms for making its attitude more definite are: 'I must', 'I am strong', 'I'll get through this'.
- The insertion of the deltoid muscle at the shaft of the humerus (deltoid tuberosity = acupuncture point LI 14) is painful at an early stage in the presence of impingement syndrome.

28.6.6 Therapy

Instructions for manual trigger point therapy

- Referred pain pattern is usually relatively locally restricted (mTrPs are embedded in the area of radiation) → local pain treatment is required.
- mTrPs are particularly common in the most ventral and dorsal parts.
- Fascia separation technique applied to the pectoralis major muscle is valuable.

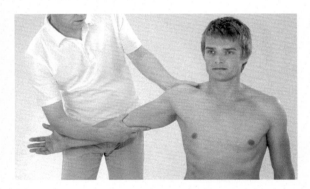

Extension

Extension of the clavicular part (ventral section, see photo).

- With the hand lying dorsally on the shoulder, exercise a slight ventral push.
- The second hand grasps the lower part of the upper arm and the elbow and provides contra-extension in the direction of retroversion.
- In this position the pectoralis major muscle is also extended.

Extension of the spinal part:

- 45° anteversion of the arm,
- maximum arm adduction and medial rotation of the shoulder (see autostretching).

Physical procedures

- Ultrasound; laser acupuncture.

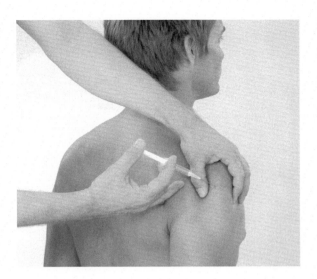

Infiltration techniques/dry needling

If this area is recommended for intramuscular injections, the risk for invasive mTrP therapy is very slight. It is sensible to search the whole muscle for taut bands or mTrPs and treat them.

- The taut bands are superficial and easily palpable and can easily be fixed between the fingers of the palpation hand.
- In the superior area of the muscle belly, two or three finger widths inferiorly from the clavicle, acromion or spine of scapula, where most mTrPs are to be found, it is easier and safer (avoids puncturing the joint capsule) to use flat needling from a superior to an inferior direction. Multiple mTrPs are usually to be found here with pronounced muscle twitch reactions.
- At the insertion of the humerus (acupuncture point LI 14) needle in a fan shape with a long needle in a superior direction into the muscle belly: good relaxation of the muscle is often already achieved with relief of the subacromial space.
- Autotraction is then sensible while that patient, for example, carries a bucket of water and consciously allows the weight to pull down the humerus.

Classical Chinese acupuncture

Local and locoregional points (also contralateral): there are four or five classical acupuncture points in the deltoid muscle, representing great clinical significance: without wide radiation of the mTrPs. Relatively distant in the inferior part of the muscle in each case lies:

- ventrally in the clavicular part of LI 15,
- laterally in the acromial part of TH 14,
- dorsally in the spinal part of SI 10 (which also has a relationship to the underlying infraspinatus muscle),
- inferiorly at the insertion at the humerus of LI 14.

Distal points: depending on localisation of the symptoms (and the findings) distal points on the affected axis:
- anterior axis: LI–ST; ST 38,
- lateral axis: GB 34 or GB 30/31,
- dorsal axis: Most likely BL 39.

The area of the buttocks (GB 34) is the logical corresponding region to the shoulder at the lower extremity. It is more usual, however (superficial and more easily reachable), to use distal points on the lower leg or knee area.

Microsystem acupuncture

Ear: points of the muscle zone of the thoracic spine representation (next to the antihelix margin in the direction of the helix).
YNSA: E zone on the forehead, C zone (angle of the hairline).
Hand line V: area between SI 3 and one finger width proximally along the course of the small intestine meridian.

Kiiko Matsumoto acupuncture

For pain in the area of the:

- anterior part: LR 5 and LU 9 ipsilaterally, insertion angle 10–45° with the flow of the meridian,
- lateral part: TH 5 and PC 7 ipsilaterally, insertion angle 10–45° with the flow of the meridian,
- posterior part: SI 5 and HT 7 ipsilaterally, insertion angle 10–45° with the flow of the meridian.

Psychosomatic treatment/relaxation

Upper body relaxation exercises, perception of strain (e.g. progressive muscle relaxation).

28.6.7 Recommendations for the patient

Autostretching

Clavicular part (left):
- extend the affected arm behind the back,
- with the other hand pull in a dorsocaudal direction,
- in a standing position, holding on to a bar or similar with the hand and leaning forwards.

Spinal part (right):
- extend and lift the affected arm in medial rotation in front of the chest,
- pull on the arm with the other hand and extend in the direction of the shoulder not affected,

activation of various fibres depending on whether the arm is guided above at the level or below (axillary area) the shoulder not affected,

full extension may not be possible if the infraspinatus muscle is shortened.

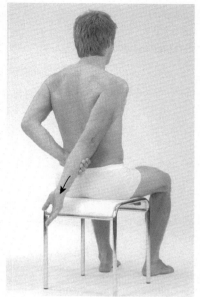

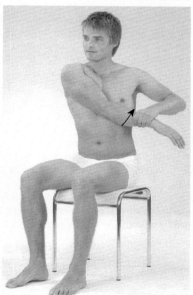

Additional measures

- To improve perception of the muscle with subsequent relaxation or release. Pull the arm (with and without a weight in the hand) up by only 1 cm and then slowly lower again by the same distance. On the next occasion move, e.g. 2 cm up and then 3 cm down: the image of an elevator is helpful (first floor – ground floor – second floor – basement – second floor – cellar...).
- Allow the arm to hang with a weight in the hand.

28.7 M. SUPRASPINATUS

28.7.1 Anatomy

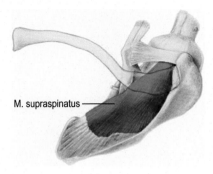

M. supraspinatus

Innervations: suprascapularis nerve (brachial plexus, supraclavicular part).
Origin: fossa supraspinata, fascia supraspinata.
Insertion: proximal facet of the greater tubercle.
Function: shoulder joint. Abduction in the scapular plane as far as the horizontal, slight lateral rotation, capsule stretcher, important function for maintaining scapulohumeral balance.

28.7.2 Patient symptoms

- Pain deep in the shoulder joint and in the area of the lateral shoulder.
- Little pain in the area of the muscle belly.
- Combing your hair, shaving and cleaning your teeth is painful; all movements in the horizontal as far as the painful arc.
- Possible preliminary diagnoses: impingement syndrome, chronic subdeltoid bursitis, humeroscapularis periarthropathy, shoulder arm syndrome.

28.7.3 Trigger points

mTrP	LOCALISATION	RADIATION	mTrP → ACUPUNCTURE POINT
1	In the middle of the supraspinata fossa	Deep shoulder joint pain, lateral shoulder and radiation on the radial side as far as the forearm	SI 12
2	At the medial end of the supraspinata fossa	Deep shoulder joint pain, lateral shoulder	SI 13
3	At the lateral end of the supraspinata fossa, below the acromion, transition from the muscle belly to the tendon	Deep shoulder joint pain, top of the shoulder	LI 16

28.7.4 Diagnosis

Questioning
- Prolonged working with elevated arm?
- Carrying heavy objects with arm hanging down?
- Frequently having a big dog on a lead?

Inspection: muscle atrophy: sunken fossa supraspinata.

Physical examination
- Abduction between about 60 and 120° painful (painful arc).
- Painful palpation of the insertion tendon at the humerus below the acromion with medial rotation (e.g. hand of the examined arm on lumbar spine so that the greater tubercle is easier to palpate through retroversion or medial rotation).
- Jobe test (also empty can test) positive: isometric strain of the largely shortened muscle (abduction of both arms up to 90°, anteversion approximately 30°, arms extended, thumbs pointing downwards) with resistance test through pressure down on both wrists → provocation of pain and/or reduced strength of one side compared to the other.

Technical examination
- If symptoms persist: ultrasound to assess the rotator cuff, more precisely the supraspinatus tendon.
- X-ray: visualisation of the subacromial space to rule out relative impingement, e.g. using a hook (bone spur rising from the acromion into the subacromial space). Possibly indication for an operation, although suitability disputed.

28.7.5 Specific aspects

- Always examine the 'antagonists' Mm. latissimus dorsi and teres major as well and treat if necessary: co-contraction.
- Shortening of the levator scapulae muscle can lead to strain of the supraspinatus muscle, so should be treated at the same time!

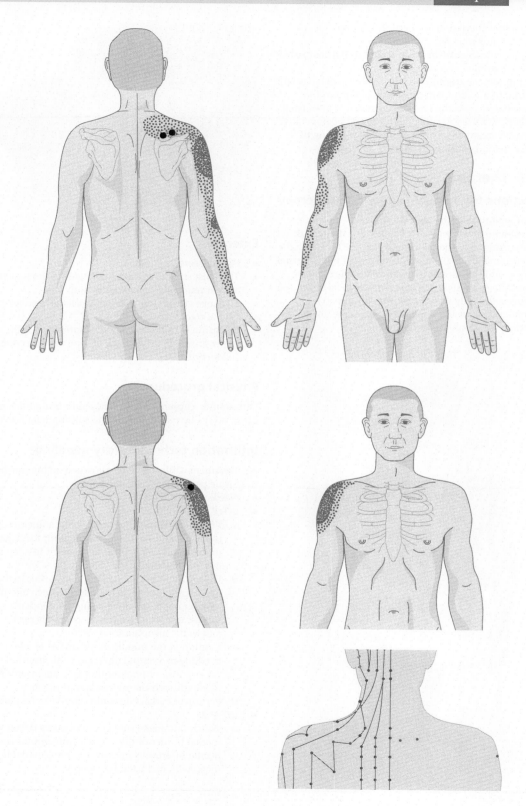

- Frequently affected in connection with the infraspinatus muscle.
- Frequent presence of insertion tendinitis if it has existed for a long time.
- To improve the trophism of the tendon with (partial) rupture of a rotator cuff or supraspinatus tendon immediately relax the taut bands, possibly also using intraoperative dry needling and pre- and postoperative intensive treatment. This requires the planning of longer periods during therapy!

28.7.6 Therapy

Instructions for manual trigger point therapy

- Treatment usually through the trapezius muscle.
- The anterior fibre segments can be directly treated: access using technique IV (see Chapter 18) between the anterior margin of the descending part of the trapezius muscle and the supraspinatus muscle (fibres of the descending part of the trapezius muscle must be relaxed as this is the only way to reach the deep part).
- If tender, also treat the insertion site at the greater tubercle (most superior portion).

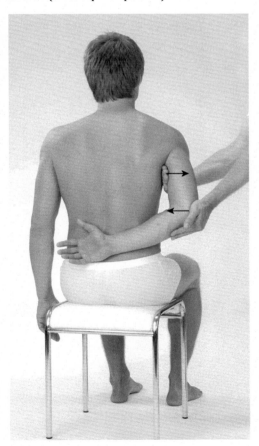

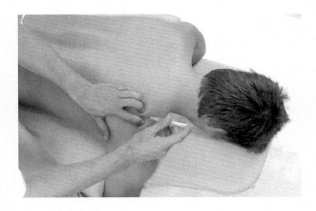

Extension

- Patient seated.
- Therapist stands beside patient, guides the patient's arm in retroversion and adduction.
- Therapist's hand close to head in axilla as hypomochlion.
- Lateral traction.
- Extension with the hand far from the head at the distal upper arm behind the back in a medial direction (adduction).

Physical procedures

Ultrasound; cupping, TENS frequently not sufficient because mTrPs lie partly deep in the supraspinata fossa.

Infiltration techniques/dry needling

- Treatment while the patient is seated on the couch or in prone position or lateral decubitus.
- Needle length 5–6 cm.
- mTrP 1 (see photo)
  - Vertical insertion superiorly to the spine of scapula in the direction of the supraspinatous fossa, parallel to the vertebral column, then search in a fan shape in a medial and lateral direction.
  - During infiltration at mTrP 1 it is sensible in the case of acute shoulder pain to perform a deep injection of a bigger depot of a long-acting LA: blockade of the suprascapularis nerve which sensitively treats a large part of the glenohumoral joint.
  - Caution at the middle mTrP (mTrP 1) when needling in a ventral direction if the insertion depth >4 cm. Risk of pneumothorax if the insertion is made through the suprascapular notch.
  - Periosteal contact does not usually cause pain.
- mTrP 2
  - Watch out: make sure you stay safely lateral to the medial border of the scapula (pneumothorax!), needle insertion vertically and predominantly diagonally in a lateral direction.

- mTrP 3 can be reached either with an needle of at least 6 cm in length by insertion of mTrP 1 flat in a lateral direction and slightly ventrally in a subacromial direction (2 in 1 technique) or from the laterodorsal direction through the deltoid muscle with the arm maximally adducted (purse/apron grip).
- **mTrP 3**
  - During infiltration of mTrP 3, a depot of LA at the muscle tendon transition is also sensible, particularly if there is a local inflammatory reaction or subacromial bursitis.

Classical Chinese acupuncture

Local and locoregional points (also contralateral): SI 12, SI 13, SI 16.
Distal points: TH 5, GB 34, ST 38, SI 3, SI 6.

Microsystem acupuncture

Ear: shoulder region; points of the muscle zone of the cervical spine representation (next to the antihelix margin in the direction of the helix).
YNSA: B zone, E zone on the forehead, C zone (angle of the hairline).
Hand line V: area between SI 3 and one finger width proximally with the flow of the meridian.

Kiiko Matsumoto acupuncture

- TH 5 and PC 7 ipsilaterally, insertion angle 10–45° with the flow of the meridian.
- For pain in the area of SI 5: SI 1 and SI 2 ipsilaterally.

Psychosomatic treatment/relaxation

- Latently suppressed aggression, tension, excessive demands ('it is all too much').
- Possibly wanting to elbow space for oneself.
- 'Elevator' exercise (see Section 28.6.7).

28.7.7 Recommendations for the patient

Autostretching

Standing
- Arm in adduction.
- 90° flexion in the elbow.
- Hold onto a door frame or hand rail with the hand.
- Push the buttocks to the opposite side for extension.

Seated position (apron/purse grip)
- Place affected arm in medial rotation behind the back at the lumbar spine.
- Grasp the wrist with the hand not affected.
- Traction in a medial or inferior–medial direction.

Additional measures

- Self-treatment ('linking' with the tips of the fingers of the hand on the opposite side).
- To train the antagonists and the muscles which centre the head of the humerus (Mm. latissimus dorsi and teres major) have the patient clasp a heavy book under the armpit.
- Regular extension at the workplace.

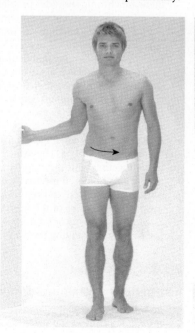
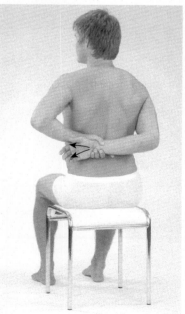

28.8 M. INFRASPINATUS

28.8.1 Anatomy

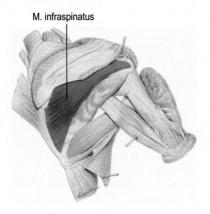

M. infraspinatus

Innervation: N. suprascapularis.
Origin: fossa infraspinata.
Insertion: middle area of the greater tubercle, distal to the insertion of the supraspinatus muscle.
Function
- Lateral rotation.
- Depending on the abduction position, use the inferior part as the adductor.
- Keeps the head of the humerus in the joint capsule.
- Possibly involved in anteversion.

28.8.2 Patient symptoms

- Pain in the area of the ventral shoulder.
- Painful and restricted movement reaching the back pocket of the trousers or undoing the bra (medial rotation).
- Restricted movement when combing the hair or cleaning the teeth (anteversion).
- Possible preliminary diagnoses: chronic tendinitis of the biceps tendon, shoulder arm syndrome, humeroscapular periarthropathy.

28.8.3 Trigger points

mTrP	LOCALI-SATION	RADIATION	mTrP→ ACUPUNCTURE POINT
1	Superior part of the muscle below the spine	Shoulder joint, anterior shoulder, anterior upper arm as far as the forearm	Approximately SI 11
2	At the edge of the medial border in the lower third	Between the vertebral column and the medial border of the scapula	–

Further mTrPs are frequently found irregularly distributed over the whole muscle, particularly in the medial area.

28.8.4 Diagnosis

Questioning
- Pain when sleeping on the affected side?
- Pain during active lateral rotation (reaching out when hitting a ball)?
- Pain during medial rotation at the end of the range of movement?

Inspection
- Muscle atrophy?
- Visible cords during isometric tension?

Physical examination
- Medial rotation passively and lateral rotation actively/ isometrically restricted and painful (especially with concomitant adduction movement).
- Anteversion painful.

28.8.5 Specific aspects

- Frequent concomitant causes of shoulder pain.
- The M. infraspinatus is frequently affected as well if there are chronic shoulder problems.
- Occasionally in patients with chronic obstructive pulmonary disease who try to improve breathing with lateral rotation of the shoulders.
- Functionally the infraspinatus muscle together with the M. subscapularis leads the head of the humerus into the joint socket in the transverse/horizontal plane through fine concomitant contractions they have a neat centring effect which is essential with small joint surfaces.
- Also occasionally after 'back training' during extreme training using sit-ups. The infraspinatus muscle is partly together with the scapular retractors (Mm. rhomboidei, trapezius ascending, latissimus dorsi, etc.) 'misused' to keep up straight ('chest out') in spite of weakness of the thoracic spine muscles.
- The infraspinatus is not a muscle for posture but is responsible for moving the arms.

28.8.6 Therapy

Instructions for manual trigger point therapy
- Access easy.
- If tender, also treat the insertion site at the greater tubercle (middle portion).

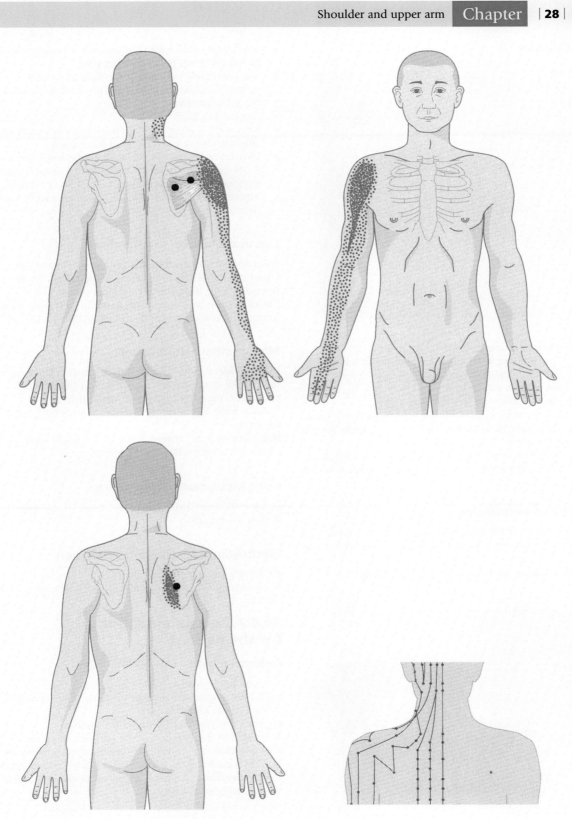

Extension

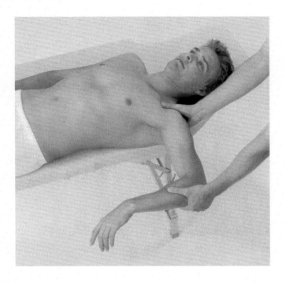

- Patient in supine position.
- The shoulder as far as the scapula should hang freely over the edge of the couch.
- Shoulder in 90° abduction.
- Elbow flexed.
- The therapist stands to the side of the patient's head.
- The hand next to the patient holds the scapula over the acromion.
- The hand away from the patient grasps the forearm close to the elbow and brings it into the medial rotation position.

Physical procedures

Cupping; laser therapy; shock waves; thermotherapy, if heat is found to ease the pain, with natural mud or hay bag.

Infiltration techniques/dry needling

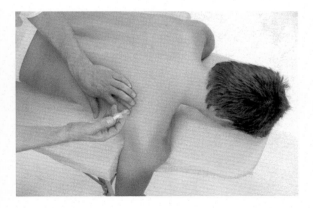

- Treatment while seated, in the prone position or in lateral decubitus on the healthy side.
- The taut bands/mTrPs are superficial and easily palpable and can easily be fixed between the fingers of the palpation hand.
- Vertical needling.
- Safe needling, as the scapula protects from pneumothorax, although take care at the edge of the scapula.
- Depending on muscle thickness needle length from 4 cm; with a longer needle, a bigger area can be reached with just one fan-shaped insertion, although several insertions are often technically easier and can be less painful for the patient.

Classical Chinese acupuncture

Local and locoregional points (also contralateral): SI 11.
Distal points: SI 3 (meridian), SI 6 (meridian), BL 40 (meridian), ST 38 (empirical shoulder point).
Control points/symptomatic points: GB 34 (master point tendons, dermal segmental treatment via LU 2 and KG 17).

Microsystem acupuncture

Ear: shoulder region, thoracic spine; points of the muscle zone of the thoracic spine representation (next to the antihelix margin in the direction of the helix).
YNSA: B zone, E zone on the forehead, C zone (angle of the hairline).
Hand line V: area between SI 3 and one finger width proximally with the flow of the meridian.

Kiiko Matsumoto acupuncture

SI 5 and HT 7 ipsilaterally, insertion angle 10–45° with the flow of the meridian.

Psychosomatic treatment/relaxation

- Staying upright (see Section 28.8.5).
- Breathing therapy with widening of the thorax.

28.8.7 Recommendations for the patient

Autostretching

- Standing or seated.
- Lift the medially rotated arm in front of the chest (90° abduction, elbow flexed).
- The hand not affected supports the elbow.
- Extend in the direction of the opposite shoulder.
- Activation of various fibres depending on whether the arm is guided above at the level or below (axillary area) the shoulder not affected (parts of the deltoid muscle are extended as well).

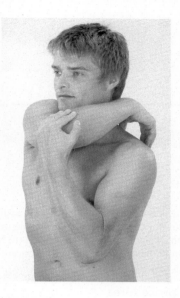

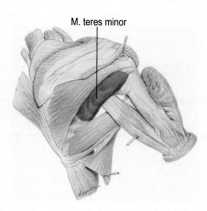

M. teres minor

Additional measures

- Self-treatment (with tennis ball).
- Regular extension at the workplace.

28.9 M. TERES MINOR

28.9.1 Anatomy

Innervation: axillary nerve (brachial plexus, infraclavicular part).

Origin: inferior section of the infraspinous fossa, middle third of the lateral border.
Insertion: distal facet of the greater tubercle.
Function: shoulder joint lateral rotation, adduction (in the scapular plane).

The teres minor muscle can also be regarded as (rather differently innervated) caudolateral part of the infraspinatus muscle (see Section 28.8).

28.9.2 Patient symptoms

- Painful and restricted movement reaching the back pocket of the trousers or undoing the bra (medial rotation).
- Restricted movement when combing the hair or cleaning the teeth (adduction).

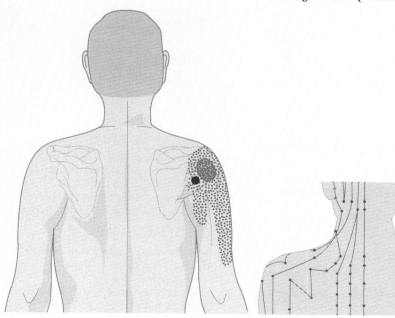

- Possible preliminary diagnoses: chronic tendinitis of the biceps tendon, shoulder arm syndrome, humeroscapular periarthropathy.

28.9.3 Trigger points

TrP	LOCALISATION	RADIATION	mTrP⟷ ACUPUNCTURE POINT
1	Medial and definitely superior to the lower end of the axillary fold	Upper arm, posterior shoulder	SI 9

28.9.4 Diagnosis

Questioning
- Pain when sleeping on the affected side?
- Pain during active lateral rotation (reaching out when hitting a ball) or medial rotation at the end of the range of movement?

Inspection: muscle atrophy?

Physical examination: medial rotation passively and lateral rotation actively/isometrically restricted and painful (especially with concomitant adduction movement).

28.9.5 Specific aspects

- This muscle is indeed usually easily delimited; although it can also be seen as inferior part of the infraspinatus muscle (see Section 28.8), its course and functions are largely identical. The teres minor muscle has more of an adductive effect because of its lateral course.
- As the inferior part of the infraspinatus muscle, the teres minor muscle is functionally important during abduction in the sense of a concomitant contraction with the supraspinatus to centre the head of the humerus in the relatively small joint socket.
- Frequently shortened following breast surgery with resulting lack of abduction capacity.

28.9.6 Therapy

Instructions for manual trigger point therapy

- Access easy.
- Fascia separation technique (technique IV; see Chapter 18) to the teres major muscle (rotation antagonist) important.
- If tender, also treat the insertion site at the greater tubercle (inferior position).

Extension

- Patient in supine position.
- Therapist guides the arm via abduction in maximum elevation.

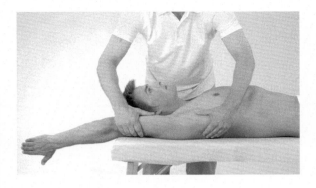

- Possibly additional extension through adduction.
- Rotation does not play a significant role in this position: possibly still guide the arm into lateral rotation (reverse the rotation in elevation).

Physical procedures

Axillary laser treatment.

Infiltration techniques/dry needling

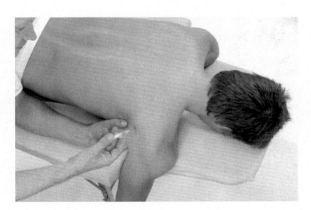

- Treatment while seated, in the prone position or also possible in lateral decubitus on the healthy side.
- Palpate the posterior axillary fold transversely, particularly close to the lateral border of the scapula.
- Needling or targeted infiltration with pinch grip technique.
- Insertion fairly close to the thorax and direction away from the thorax in a ventral or lateral direction into the 'pinch', in order to avoid a pneumothorax (risk of itself very low here).
- Needling length from 4 cm depending on muscle circumference.

Classical Chinese acupuncture

Local and locoregional points (also contralateral): SI 9 or TH 14 deep in each case (TH 14 lies over the insertion of the M. teres minor).
Distal points: SI 3, BL 58, ST 38.

Microsystem acupuncture

Ear: points of the muscle zone of the thoracic spine representation (next to the antihelix margin in the direction of the helix).
YNSA: E zone on the forehead, C zone (angle of the hairline).
Hand line V: area between SI 3 and one finger width proximally with the flow of the meridian.

Kiiko Matsumoto acupuncture

- SI 5 and HT 7 ipsilaterally, insertion angle 10–45° with the flow of the meridian.
- In some cases BL 2 and extra point Yuyao on both sides.

Psychosomatic treatment/relaxation

Release flank: possibly fear of vulnerability.

28.9.7 Recommendations for the patient

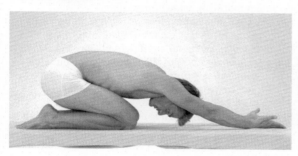

Autostretching

- As for M. infraspinatus (see Section 28.8):
  - standing or seated,
  - lift the medially rotated arm in front of the chest (90° abduction, elbow flexed),
  - the hand not affected supports the elbow,
  - extend in the direction of the opposite shoulder.
- Autostretching as illustrated together with the infraspinatus muscle (see Section 28.8) and the latissimus dorsi muscle (see Section 28.10).
- Additional extension is sensible together with all adductors and the whole flank:

- place the hand on the side to be extended as high as possible (over the head) on the wall or the doorframe,
- then press the pelvis away from the wall (side of body C-shaped convex).

Additional measures

- Self-treatment (with tennis ball).
- Regular extension at the workplace.

28.10 M. LATISSIMUS DORSI

28.10.1 Anatomy

Innervation: thoracodorsal nerve (brachial plexus, infraclavicular part).
Origin: over the thoracolumbar fascia of the spinous processes of the six lower thoracic vertebrae, the lumbar spine and from the dorsal fascia of the sacrum, the outer lip of the iliac crest (dorsal third), (9th rib), 10th–12th ribs; frequently further origin process from the inferior angle of the scapula.
Insertion: crest of lesser tubercle (with flat tendon surrounding the teres major muscle in a spiral; between them the subtendinous bursa of the latissimi dorsi muscles).
Function: shoulder joint: adduction, medial rotation, retroversion, depression of the scapula.

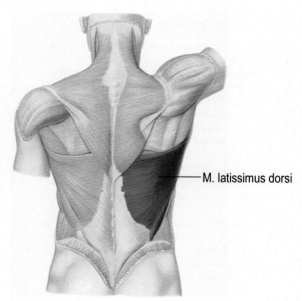

— M. latissimus dorsi

28.10.2 Patient symptoms

- Pain worse with apron grip.
- Extension pain and limited movement with stretching movements (e.g. hitting a tennis ball).

- Pain when lifting objects from the floor.
- Preliminary diagnosis: shoulder–arm syndrome, periarthropathy, thoracic spine syndrome, irritation of the ulnar nerve.

28.10.3 Trigger points

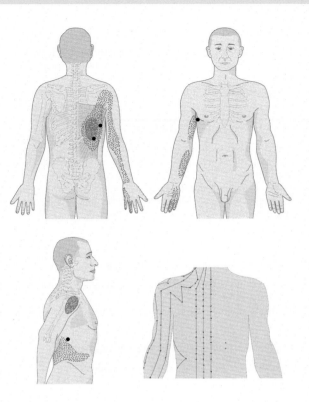

mTrP	LOCALI-SATION	RADIATION	mTrP→ ACUPUNCTURE POINT
1	Medial and inferior to the bottom end of the posterior axillary fold	Thoracic spine, ventral shoulder and ulnar side of the whole arm as far as the fingers	–
2	Varies between T9 and T12 inferiorly to the top of the scapula	Predominantly regional in the area of the thoracic and upper lumbar spine	BL 49, BL 50

28.10.4 Diagnosis

Questioning: symptoms when putting on a coat or similar or reaching up, working overhead, stretching movement; one-sided work load with the affected arm (craft work, musician).
Inspection: difference in development of the two sides.
Physical examination (seated)
- Active: the patient sits with the arm in an apron grip against resistance, keeping it further in adduction – medial rotation and retroversion – and then is guided in a inferior direction with targeted resistance. The therapist moves the patient's wrist forward and upwards, pushes outwards and asks the patient to resist.
- Passively: extension through abduction at the end of the range of movement, lateral flexion of the trunk on the other side (and lateral rotation: no longer plays such a big role with maximum abduction); palpation in this extended position

It is sensible to follow the course of the muscle further if the examination findings are positive and to include the common origin process on the scapula in the palpation.

28.10.5 Specific aspects

- Often following acute lifting injury.
- Like the other scapula retractors (Mm. rhomboidei, trapezius ascendens etc.) the latissimus dorsi is often 'misused' to maintain an upright posture ('chest out') in spite of weakness of the thoracic spine muscles, including after incorrect instruction in back training or if there are worries about a recurrence of an intervertebral disc prolapse.
- The M. latissimus dorsi is not a postural muscle but is responsible for movement of the shoulders and positioning of the scapula and thus the function of the arm.

28.10.6 Therapy

Instructions for manual trigger point therapy

- Treatment of the lateral fibres with pinch grip.
- Treatment of the dorsal fibres (vertebral and costal parts) with pressure directly against the thorax (muscle pre-extended).

Extension

- Patient in lateral decubitus:
  - maximum flexion of the hips and knees,

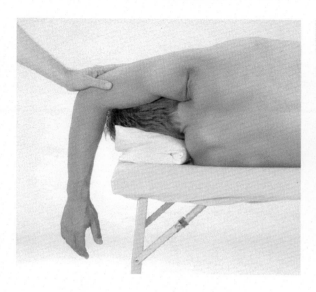
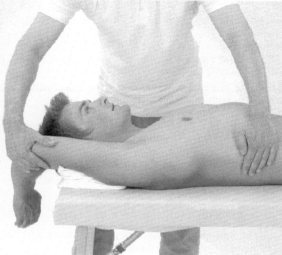

- therapist guides the arm on the side to be treated in elevation and flexed at the elbow behind the head,
- presses elbow towards the floor.
- Patient in supine position:
  - flexion of the hips and knees, feet together,
  - arm on the side to be treated flexed at the elbow,
  - therapist guides the arm at the level of the head,
  - medial pressure.

Physical procedures

Cupping suitable.

Infiltration techniques/dry needling

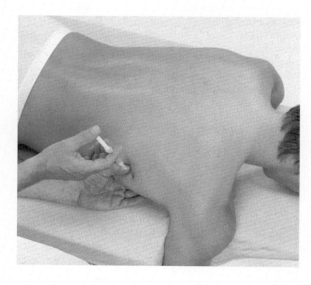

Infiltration as for teres major (see Sections 28.9 and 28.11) which is usually palpated and treated at the same time (common function as far as movement of scapula).

- Possible in prone or supine position or lateral decubitus.
- Infiltration/needling is performed predominantly in the area of the posterior axillary fold (SI 9 in acupuncture) using a pinch grip, where the latissimus dorsi lies in the most lateral position and is therefore the easiest to palpate.
- Search for and treat other mTrP in a more inferior direction, gently lifting the muscle using a pinch grip and articulating in a further inferior–medial direction.
- mTrPs in the process of origin can also be palpated and treated using a pinch grip.
- Needle length from 4 cm.
- Alternatively, if the mTrP is medial, flat (insertion angle <30°), needling parallel to the lateral margin of the scapula (and no deeper than this!).
- Guide the needle as much as possible from superior to inferior and across to the ribs in order to minimise the risk of pneumothorax.
- If the ribs are easily palpable, the two-finger protection technique is also possible: one palpation finger above and below each rib and then needle vertically between them

Classical Chinese acupuncture

Local and locoregional points (also contralateral): SI 9, BL 49, BL 50, GB 22.
Distal points: BL 57, BL 58, SI 3, ST 38 (shoulder), GB 39.
Control points/symptomatic points: GB 34, LR 3.

Microsystem acupuncture

Ear: points of the muscle zone of the thoracic spine representation (next to the antihelix margin in the direction of the helix).
YNSA: E zone on the forehead, C zone (angle of the hairline).
Hand line V: area between SI 3 and one finger width proximally with the flow of the meridian.

Kiiko Matsumoto acupuncture

- SI 5 and HT 7 ipsilaterally, insertion angle 10–45° with the flow of the meridian.
- In some cases TH 5 and GB 41 on both sides.

Psychosomatic treatment/relaxation

- As for infraspinatus: watch the posture, keep upright in spite of a feeling of weakness.
- Press the arms to the body: 'I am not taking up space, I am not ready to act'.

28.10.7 Recommendations for the patient

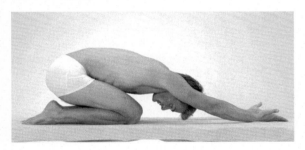

Autostretching

As for M. infraspinatus or M. teres minor (see Sections 28.8 and 28.9).

- If the patient has difficulty crouching (e.g. elderly people), the alternative is to kneel (with only 90° flexion).
- Place the forearms on a couch (or table).
- Move the upper body towards the floor for extension.

The extension is also possible in a seated position if the patient is very immobile, in which case the forearms should be placed on a piece of furniture with the palms facing upwards; extension by pressing the upper body towards the floor.
See also under M. teres minor (see 28.9).

Recommended additional measures

- Compression with pinch grip (upper part) or tennis ball (lower part).

- Cupping massage of the lower parts of the muscles by a partner.
- Ergonomic lifting of heavy objects.
- When sleeping place the cushion in the armpit between the elbow and the thorax.

28.11 M. TERES MAJOR

28.11.1 Anatomy

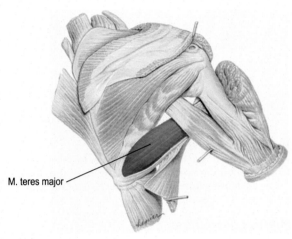

M. teres major

Innervation: subscapular nerve or thoracodorsalis nerve (brachial plexus, infraclavicular part).
Origin: inferior lateral border of the scapula as far as the inferior angle.
Insertion: crest of lesser tubercle (medially from the M. latissimus dorsi, separated from it by the subtendinous bursa of the latissimi dorsi muscles).
Function: shoulder joint; medial rotation, adduction in the scapular plane.

28.11.2 Patient symptoms

- Lateral shoulder pain.
- Similar to M. latissimus dorsi: pain with apron grip (active) and pain on extension during abduction at the end of the range of movement.
- Widen the ipsilateral side of the trunk or lateral flexion of the vertebral column to the opposite side has no influence in contrast to the latissimus muscle.

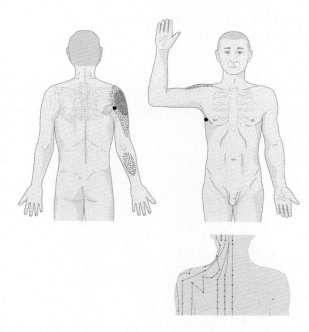

28.11.5 Specific aspects

- As with all the adductors, specifically during impingement/painful arc.
- If there are chronic shoulder symptoms, these must be taken into account and usually treated at the same time.

28.11.6 Therapy

Instructions for manual trigger point therapy

- Treatment with pinch grip (seated or in prone or supine position or lateral decubitus).
- Fascia separation technique (technique IV (see Chapter 18) important for the M. teres minor) to the teres major muscle (= rotation antagonist).

Extension

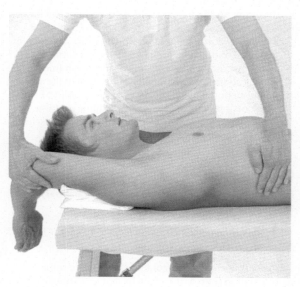

28.11.3 Trigger points

mTrP	LOCALISATION	RADIATION	mTrP→ ACUPUNCTURE POINT
1	Medial and above the axillary fold	Shoulder joint, lateral shoulder and upper arm, dorsal forearm	SI 9

28.11.4 Diagnosis

Questioning
- See also M. latissimus dorsi (see Section 28.10). Pain worse with apron grip (active).
- (Extension) pain on abduction at the end of the range of movement.

Inspection: no abnormalities.

Physical examination
- Pain with apron grip (active) and pain on passive extension during abduction at the end of the range of movement.
- Widening the ipsilateral side of the trunk or lateral flexion of the vertebral column to the opposite side has no influence in contrast to the latissimus muscle.

Technical examination: ultrasound (DD lymph nodes).

As for M. latissimus dorsi (see Section 28.10) as far as movement of the trunk.

- Patient in supine position.
- Maximum flexion of the hips and knees (avoid hollow back).
- Arm in elevation and elbow flexed behind the head.
- Therapist presses elbow in medial/superior direction (at maximum abduction the rotation no longer plays a role).

Physical procedures

Laser treatment, hot rolls.

Infiltration techniques/dry needling

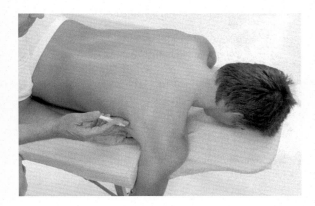

- Test in prone position.
- Finger as support during pinch grip.
- Push the needle forward in the direction of the finger.
- As for the Mm. teres minor (see Section 28.9) and latissimus dorsi (see Section 28.10) which are usually palpated and treated at the same time (common function). Adduction/centring of head of humerus during abduction: needling or infiltration in the area of the posterior axillary fold (acupuncture point SI 9) is also possible while seated or in the supine position. The teres major lies here between the two other muscles.
- Needle length at least 4 cm.

Classical Chinese acupuncture

Local and locoregional points (also contralateral): SI 9.
Distal points: SI 3, ST 38, BL 58.

Microsystem acupuncture

Ear: points of the muscle zone of the thoracic spine representation (next to the antihelix margin in the direction of the helix).
YNSA: E zone on the forehead, C zone (angle of the hairline).
Hand line V: area between SI 3 and one finger width proximally with the flow of the meridian.

Kiiko Matsumoto acupuncture

Generally muscle relaxing points such as SP 3 and ST 22 on the right, Hua tuo jiaji between T10 and T12.

Psychosomatic treatment/relaxation

Breathing exercises.

28.11.7 Recommendations for the patient

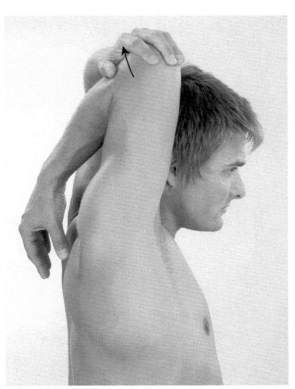

Autostretching

- Extension with traction at the elbow in a medial direction (behind the head).
- Elbow at the level of the shoulder or higher.
- Lumbar spine in hyperextension by means of a small step forward.
- Support with inspiration/expiration.
- This exercise extends parts of the Mm. pectoralis major, latissimus dorsi and subscapularis. The optimum position can only be carried out by careful testing.

Additional measures

- Self-massage of the muscles of the posterior axillary fold in pinch grip.
- Roll mTrPs on a tennis ball while lying down or in slight lateral decubitus.

28.12 M. SUBSCAPULARIS

28.12.1 Anatomy

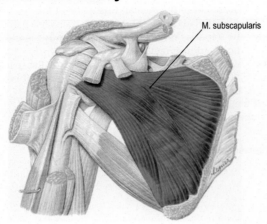

M. subscapularis

Innervation: subscapular nerve (brachial plexus, infraclavicular part).
Origin: costal surface, subscapular fossa.
Insertion: lesser tubercle and bordering part of the crest of the lesser tubercle (below the insertion lies the subtendinous bursa of the subscapularis muscles).
Function: shoulder joint – medial rotation, abduction (superior part), adduction in the scapular plane (inferior part).

28.12.2 Patient symptoms

- Posterior shoulder pain.

- Very similar to 'frozen shoulder': all lateral rotation (active and passive) hurts. To avoid this, keep the patient's arm held against the chest.
- If the mTrP is not so active, lifting the arm in the sense of lateral rotation is painful (e.g. playing tennis, but also passively).

28.12.3 Trigger points

mTrP	LOCALISATION	RADIATION	mTrP↔ ACUPUNCTURE POINT
1	Medially subscapular	Shoulder joint, shoulder blade	–
2	Lateral subscapular	Shoulder join, shoulder blade, thoracic spine	–

28.12.4 Diagnosis

Questioning
- As usual for the shoulders: ask specifically about pain during rotation movements and limited lateral rotation.
- Pain at night?
Inspection: arm held to chest?

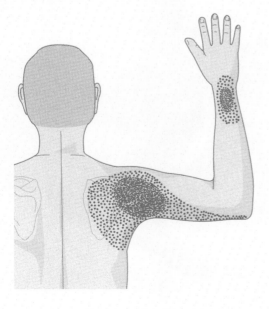

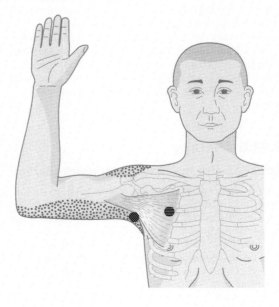

Physical examination

- Passive:
    - limited lateral rotation when comparing the sides in the neutral position and at 90° abduction. Typically, restriction in the neutral position is definitely pronounced,
    - limitation of lateral rotation can, however, also be caused by the teres major and latissimus dorsi muscles.
- Active: testing isometric medial rotation and comparing the sides.
    - the therapist stands behind the seated patient,
    - the patient places the upper arms on the chest and holds the elbows flexed at 90° forward,
    - the therapist presses the patient's wrists apart against this resistance: the therapist's own arm is supported on the patient's shoulders (saves energy!),
    - comparison of pain and energy.
- Provocation test of the already maximally shortened subscapularis muscle: from the apron grip the patient presses the wrist further in a dorsal direction against resistance, producing first resistance and then giving way so that first maximum contraction and then release are produced.

28.12.5 Specific aspects

- mTrPs of the subscapularis muscle are often overlooked. They are difficult to find because they lie deep in the muscle between the scapula and the dorsal thoracic wall.
- If needling treatment is used, there is also a relatively high risk of a pneumothorax, so this treatment should be reserved for experienced therapists after all less invasive measures have been exhausted.
- Functionally the subscapularis muscle together with the M. infraspinatus lead the head of the humerus into the joint socket in the transverse/horizontal plane, through fine concomitant contractions they have a neat centring effect which is essential with small joint surfaces.

28.12.6 Therapy

Instructions for manual trigger point therapy

- Access from lateral scapula margin (patient in supine position or lateral decubitus).
    - Initially careful and persistent release of adhesions (often pronounced) between the fascia of the subscapularis and anterior serratus muscles using manual fascia separation technique (important!).
    - Then direct treatment of the lateral and superior fibre parts of the subscapularis muscle.

- Access from the medial margin of scapula (patient in lateral decubitus or prone position).
    - The fingers of the therapist's hand slide from the medial margin of the scapula between the scapula and the thorax.
    - Treatment of the median fibre parts of the subscapularis muscle through the transverse part of the trapezius muscle, the rhomboid muscles and the anterior serratus muscle.
    - Mobilisation of the scapulothoracic articular space, lifting of the medial margin of the shoulder blade and the inferior angle of scapula.
- If tender, also treat the insertion site at the lesser tubercle.

Extension

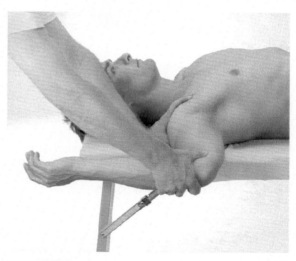

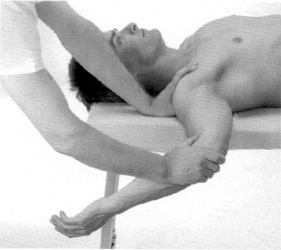

- Patient in supine position.
- Shoulder abduction, elbow flexed.
- Therapist stands sideways to the head.
- The hand next to the patient is on the acromion.
- The other hand is around the flexed elbow and brings the arm into lateral rotation.

Physical procedures

The medial part (subscapular) part of the muscle is very difficult to access; the lateral part is easily treated using laser acupuncture and hydrotherapy.

Infiltration techniques/dry needling

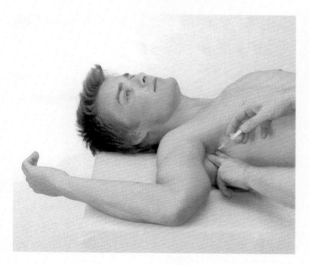

- There are three possible approaches. With all of them, it is important to make sure that the scapula is separated as far as possible from the thorax and the needle is guided as diagonally across to the ribs as possible, in order to keep the risk of pneumothorax as low as possible.
- In supine position over the armpit: best approach to the lateral and superior fibre parts. This is where the majority and the most important mTrPs are to be found.
  - Palpate precisely the lateral scapular margin and then the anterior surface of the scapula, on which needling is to be carried out from the depth of the armpit.
  - The position of the axillary artery is easy to locate.
  - Fix the mTrPs with the two-finger protection technique and then perform the needling.

- In the prone position or the lateral decubitus from the lateral inferior scapular margin, below the axilla: approach to the lateral inferior fibre parts.
  - Have an assistant draw the arm as far as possible from the thorax and separate the scapula from the thorax with the palpation hand.
- In the prone position with the shoulder blade raised from the medial margin of the scapula: treatment of the medial fibre parts.
- Long needles up to 9 cm are required. It may be sensible to use a thin spinal needle here, as it is more stable and easier to guide.

Classical Chinese acupuncture

Local and locoregional points: only via scapular dry needling, needling of points on the scapula; it is indeed sensible for mTrPs in the infraspinatus muscle (antagonist), but in our experience it only has a minor (segmental) effect on the subscapularis muscle.
Distal points: SI 3, BL 58, ST 38.
Control points/symptomatic points: PC 6 if there is a feeling of tightness in the chest.

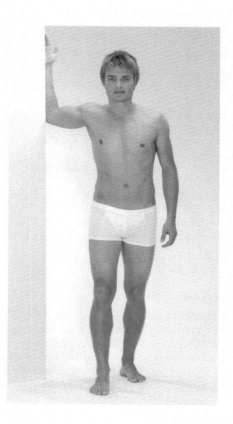

Microsystem acupuncture

Ear: points of the muscle zone of the thoracic spine representation (next to the antihelix margin in the direction of the helix).
YNSA: E zone on the forehead, C zone (angle of the hairline).
Hand line V: area between SI 3 and one finger width proximally with the flow of the meridian.

Kiiko Matsumoto acupuncture

- For pain in the area of TH 6 (fire point) needling of SI 5, PC 8 or HT 8 (metal and water points of the affected meridian).
- SI 5 and HT 7 ipsilaterally, insertion angle 10–45° with the flow of the meridian.

Psychosomatic treatment/relaxation

Similar to the serratus anterior muscle (the approach for needling is also similar) and the pectoralis major: narrowing of the anterior chest space, protective posture.

28.12.7 Recommendations for the patient

Autostretching

- Patient stands in door frame.
- Elbow at the level of the shoulder or supported higher on the door frame.
- Vertebral column in hyperextension by means of a small step forward.
- Do not turn the trunk too much so that the more shortened side is more extended.
- Support with inspiration/expiration: upper body forward while breathing out.
- Extend gently, otherwise irritation can be caused.
- This exercise extends parts of the Mm. pectoralis major, latissimus dorsi and subscapularis. The optimum position can only be carried out by careful testing.

Additional measures

- For chronic, therapy-resistant mTrP in the subscapularis muscle, the basis of successful therapy is the patient's motivation for daily extension over a defined period (about 4 weeks) and improvement in body perception away from the affected muscle (deflect attention)!
- Exercises to widen the thorax, e.g. breathing therapy.

28.13 MM. RHOMBOIDEI MAJOR AND MINOR

28.13.1 Anatomy

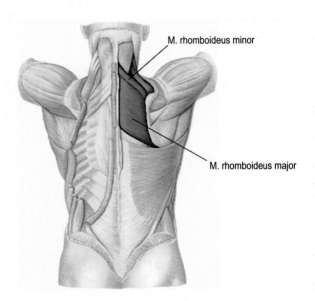

M. rhomboideus minor

M. rhomboideus major

Innervation: dorsalis scapulae nerve (brachial plexus, supraclavicular part).
Origin:
- M. rhomboideus major: spinous processes of the four upper thoracic vertebrae.
- M. rhomboideus minor: spinous processes of C6 and C7.

Insertion: medial border of the scapula (inferior to the scapular spine).
Function: adduction and lifting of the scapula; together with the serratus anterior muscle stabilisation of the scapula on the trunk.

28.13.2 Patient symptoms

- Interscapular, sometimes burning pain (tension under chronic strain leads to burning pain).
- Pain zone of the rhomboid muscles usually limited relatively locally on the interscapular space (mTrPs lie embedded in its area of radiation) in contrast to the referred pain pattern of the superior posterior serratus muscle, which very often radiates into the shoulder, arm and hand.

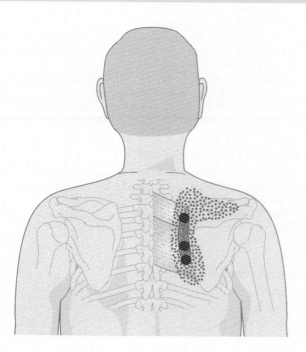

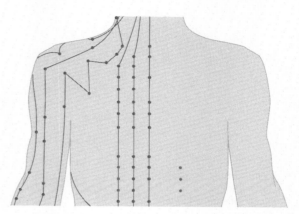

28.13.3 Trigger points

mTrP	LOCALISATION	RADIATION	mTrP→ ACUPUNCTURE POINT
1	Rh. minor	Shoulder, shoulder blade, thoracic spine	BL 42
2	Rh. major	Shoulder blade, thoracic spine	BL 44, BL 43

28.13.4 Diagnosis

Questioning
- Work activity with stressed posture.
- Burning pain between the shoulder blades, made worse when sitting or standing up straight for long periods?

Inspection
- Posture: especially sitting for long periods with rounded shoulders.
- Or does the patient try to force themself to stay upright?

Physical examination
- Examination of the pectoralis major and serratus anterior (antagonist) muscles and ability of the scapula to articulate on the thorax.

- Consider another two (myofascial) causes of interscapular pain: mTrPs in the scalene muscles (specifically the posterior scalene muscle) or disorders of the lower cervical spine segments or muscles.

28.13.5 Specific aspects

- Strain with formation of mTrPs with increased kyphosis of the thoracic spine: often an attempt to compensate for poor posture (spontaneously or incorrect posture instructions) by drawing the scapulae together.
- Another common cause of mTrP in the rhomboid muscles is shortening of the pectoralis major muscle with shoulder protraction, so the rhomboid muscles are always under the strain of traction. In this case, examine and treat the pectoralis major as well.
- Functionally, the rhomboid muscles belong to the pectoral girdle/arm muscles and serve to extend the working area of the hands and ensure or stabilise, but not keep upright.

28.13.6 Therapy

Instructions for manual trigger point therapy

- Treatment is carried out via the transverse part of the trapezius muscle.
- mTrPs in the rhomboid muscles are difficult to differentiate from mTrPs in the superior posterior serratus muscle (muscle fibres have the same course).

Extension

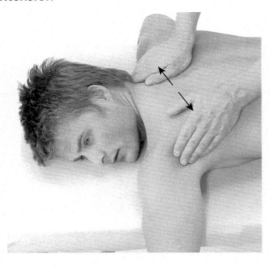

- Test in prone position.
- Arms hang down over the couch.
- Head rotated to the affected side.
- The therapist holds the vertebral column in place with the flat of the hand.
- The therapist's other hand lies flat on the medial border of the scapula.
- Extend the affected side by means of concomitant lateral and inferior thrust.

Physical procedures

Hydrotherapy; thermotherapy, natural healing (e.g. mustard powder, hay bag).

Infiltration techniques/dry needling

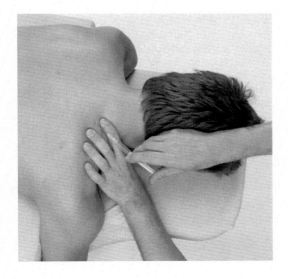

- **Warning:** pneumothorax!
- Maximum 1.5 cm vertically. It is better to insert a needle of about 5 cm in length 3 cm superiorly from the palpated mTrP.
- Push the needle forward to the mTrP in a flat tangential manner in a inferior direction.
- This makes it easier to control the depth of the insertion and the ribs form a protection (Venetian blind effect).

Classical Chinese acupuncture

Local and locoregional points (also contralateral): BL 42–BL 44. Particularly interesting is BL 43, also in reference to the ascending trapezius muscle.
Distal points: BL 57, BL 58, SI 6.
Control points/symptomatic points: P6 for tightness in the chest.

Microsystem acupuncture

Ear: points of the muscle zone of the thoracic spine representation (next to the antihelix margin in the direction of the helix).
YNSA: E zone on the forehead, C zone (angle of the hairline).
Hand line V: area between SI 3 and one finger width proximally with the flow of the meridian.

Kiiko Matsumoto acupuncture

- Find the most painful point under the ipsilateral scapular spine; direction of the pressure under the scapular spine either in the direction of the spine or the shoulder; when the right point is found, lessen the tension of the major and minor rhomboid muscles.
- Insert Japanese needle no. 2 or 3 exactly below the scapular spine (45° angle medially or laterally), after insertion of the needle examine the muscles between the shoulder blades; if there is no significant improvement, correct the angle of the needle until the muscles are more relaxed. Repeat the procedure until the right point is found (sometimes two or three needles are required).

Psychosomatic treatment/relaxation

- Good posture comes from the inside: from an interest in life and good breathing with well-toned abdominal space.
- I hold myself upright (avoid feelings of weakness/neediness), or with poor posture: 'I let myself go and let my wings drop – I don't feel well' (depression). However, this also applies to all the erector trunci.
- To improve posture consider supplementary breathing therapy and if possible tackle attitude to life ('no interest', 'I must', 'all too much').

28.13.7 Recommendations for the patient

Autostretching

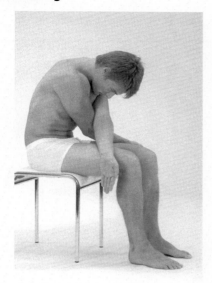

- Patient seated.
- Bends forward, arches the back.
- Arms in lateral rotation crossed in front of the chest, palms facing upwards.
- Extension by lowering the chest further while breathing out with additional adduction of the arms and press the palms outwards.

Additional measures

- Self-treatment (with tennis ball).
- Extension of frequently shortened pectoral muscles (and possibly the anterior serratus muscle, abdominal muscles, etc.) → treat mTrPs in the pectoral muscles, posture training.

28.14 M. CORACOBRACHIALIS

28.14.1 Anatomy

Innervation: musculocutaneous nerve (brachial plexus, infraclavicular part). The musculocutaneous nerve usually runs through the coracobrachialis muscle.
Origin: tip of the coracoids process (medial to the short head of the biceps brachii muscle).
Insertion: anterior facet of the humerus (medial, distal to the crest of lesser tubercle).
Function: shoulder joint: medial rotation, adduction, anteversion.

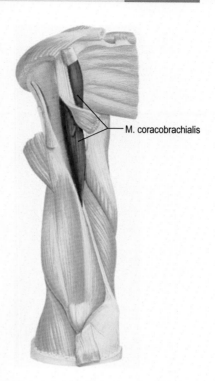

M. coracobrachialis

28.14.2 Patient symptoms

- Pain ventrolateral shoulder (deltoid area).
- Sensory disorders of the radial forearm (possible entrapment of the musculocutaneous muscle).
- Limited elevation.

28.14.3 Trigger points

mTrP	LOCALISATION	RADIATION	mTrP↔ ACUPUNCTURE POINT
1	Anterior shoulder	Ventrolateral shoulder, back of the arm as far as the middle finger	LU 1, LU 2

28.14.4 Diagnosis

Questioning: no relevant aspects.
Inspection: no specific findings.
Physical examination: compare the sides in a back scrub test (rubbing the back of the hand on the thoracic spine and the opposite side of the thorax → pain and limited mobility).

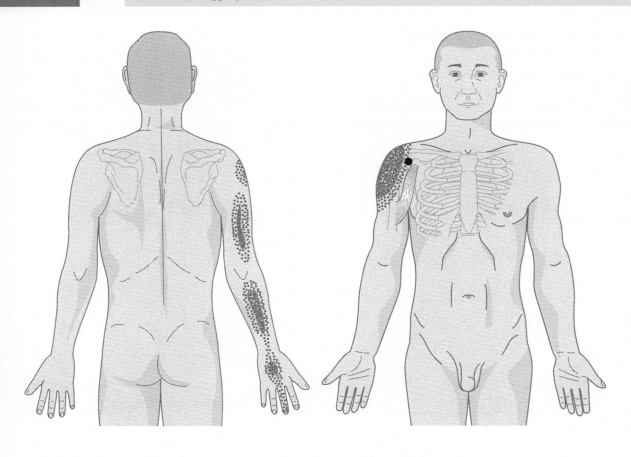

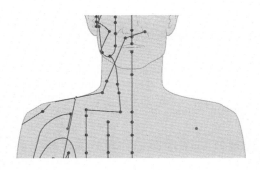

28.14.5 Specific aspects

- The clinical significance of this muscle is disputed. Some anatomists think it serves mainly to protect the vascular and nerve bundle which

supplies the arm (subclavian artery and brachial plexus).
- Can often only be identified if other mTrP at the shoulder have been sufficiently treated.

28.14.6 Therapy

Instructions for manual trigger point therapy

- Indirect treatment through the clavicular part of the major pectoralis muscle.
- Direct treatment: fascia separation technique between the major pectoralis muscle and the coracobrachialis muscle → can be tracked in the direction of the coracoid process and direct treatment of the coracobrachialis muscle.

Extension

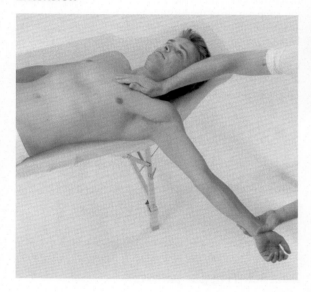

Two extension positions are possible depending on the position of the mTrP (note patient information during extension).

Position 1: supine.
- Lateral border of scapula on the edge of the bed.
- Shoulder in abduction, retroversion, slight lateral rotation: opposite arm in abduction (90°) and lateral rotation.
- Hand next to head on coracoids process and clavicle.
- Hand distant from head holds the wrist of the extended arm and increases retroversion (and to some extent abduction and lateral rotation).

Position 2: extension as for clavicular part of pectoralis major muscle (see Section 30.7).

Physical procedures

Heat application.

Infiltration techniques/dry needling

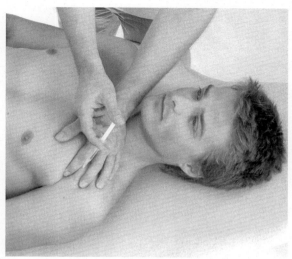

- Direct approach possible.
- Palpation of the coracoids process.
- Run the palpating fingers in a inferior direction.
- Ask the patient to abduct the arm, then adduct it again. A small cord should be palpable running to the coracoids process.
- **Warning:** vascular and nerve bundle between the coracobrachial and biceps muscles.

Classical Chinese acupuncture

Local and locoregional points (also contralateral): LU 1, LU 3, HT 2, PC 2 (**warning**: vascular and nerve bundle).
Distal points: LU 7, PC 6, ST 38.

Microsystem acupuncture

Ear: points of the muscle zone of the thoracic spine representation (next to the antihelix margin in the direction of the helix).
YNSA: E zone on the forehead, C zone (angle of the hairline).
Hand line V: area between SI 3 and one finger width proximally with the flow of the meridian.

Kiiko Matsumoto acupuncture

- If there is a neurological cause CV 12 and CV 10 as well.
- For pain in the area of the large intestine meridian: LI 5 and LU 9 (usually diagonally towards or with the flow of the meridian).
- For pain in the area of the TH meridian: TH 4 and PC 7 (usually diagonally towards or with the flow of the meridian).

Psychosomatic treatment/relaxation

No known special features.

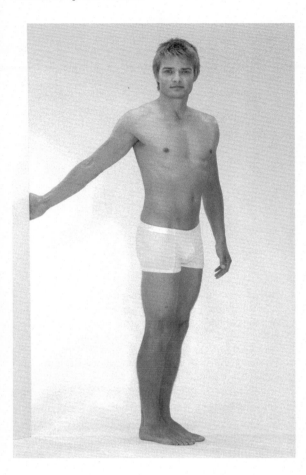

28.14.7 Recommendations for the patient

Autostretching

- Patient supported on the door frame with arm extended.
- Hand at the level of the hip.
- Extension by turning away from the door frame.
- The pectoral and deltoid muscles are extended at the same time.

Additional measures

As rarely affected on its own, depends on muscles also affected.

28.15.1 Anatomy

Innervation: musculocutaneous nerve (brachial plexus, infraclavicular part).
Origin
- Long head: supraglenoid tubercle, glenoid labrum (tendon runs freely through the shoulder joint).
- Short head: tip of the coracoids process (lateral to the coracobrachialis muscle).

Insertion: radial tuberosity (bicipitoradial bursa) and over the aponeurosis of the bicipitis brachii muscles on the antebrachial fossa.
Function: two-joint muscle, shoulder joint.
- Long head: abduction.
- Short head: adduction.
- Both parts: bearing the weight of the arm, anteversion, medial rotation.
- Elbow joint: flexion, supination.

28.15.2 Patient symptoms

- Pain in the anterior shoulder and upper arm, frequently easily locatable in the muscle.
- Pain with weakness in the sense of reduced innervation caused by pain such as with biceps tendon tendinitis in people who perform a great deal of holding work with the arms in sport (e.g. climbing) or professionally (hairdresser, waiter, call centre worker, etc.).

28.15.3 Trigger points

mTrP	LOCALISATION	RADIATION	mTrP→ ACUPUNCTURE POINT
1	Long head	Anterior region of the deltoid, elbow	LU 3
2	Short head	Anterior region of the deltoid, elbow	PC 4

28.15.4 Diagnosis

Questioning
- Strain in sport (using dumb-bells)/hobby or work?
- Pain on exertion or extension: limited extension of the elbow at the end of the range of movement.

Inspection
- Possibly difference between the sides in the upper arm flexion muscles.

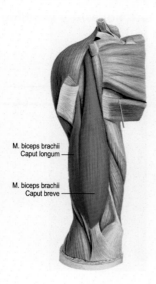

M. biceps brachii
Caput longum

M. biceps brachii
Caput breve

Physical examination

- Palpation of the insertions at the coracoids, radius and particularly in the area of the long biceps tendon in the channel between the greater and lesser tubercles, as well as palpation of the whole muscle belly for taut bands/mTrP.
- Isometric tension from the mid position, from extension and with submaximally shortened muscles, i.e. almost complete elbow flexion.
- Extension (comparison of sides) through maximum elbow extension first in anteversion. If this is already limited or painful, it is better to consider the brachialis muscle. An increase in symptoms of the extended and max. pronated arm through retroversion in the shoulder is characteristic of the biceps brachii as two joint muscle.

Technical examination: ultrasound for suspected rupture of a tendon.

- Affected side rather more slight.
- Real (protective posture caused by pain) or apparent atrophy (a contracted muscle with taut bands has the effect of atrophy).

28.15.5 Specific aspects

- 'Don't let yourself be led by the arm'.
- Biceps tendinitis often result of strain of the muscle with formation of mTrPs.

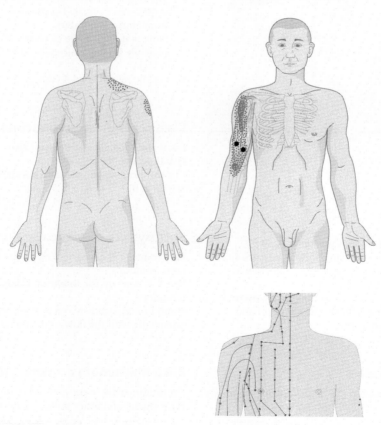

28.15.6 Therapy

Instructions for manual trigger point therapy

Treatment with pinch grip is straightforward.

Extension

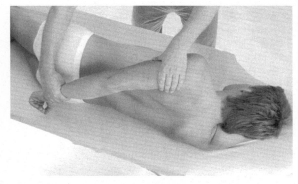

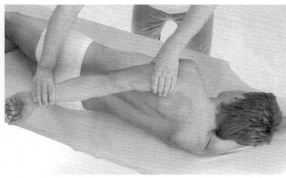

- Patient in lateral decubitus position.
- Therapist's hand by head holds the upper arm firm.
- Slight retroversion of the shoulder, adduction and lateral rotation.
- The hand away from the head holds the wrist and brings the forearm or elbow into extension and pronation at the same time.

Physical procedures

Heat, ultrasound and gentle massage of the mTrP are very suitable.

Infiltration techniques/dry needling

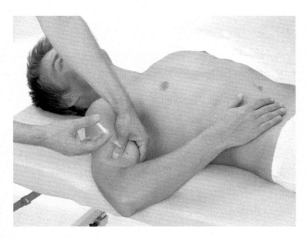

- This muscle is easy to examine and treat using a pinch grip.
- This succeeds in drawing the muscle away from the bundle of vessels and nerves.
- The frequently associated mTrPs of the brachialis muscle can be treated at the same time while needling from above (ventrally).
- Note that the bundle of vessels and nerves runs medially from the biceps brachii muscles or brachialis muscle.
- Needle length from 4 cm.

Classical Chinese acupuncture

Local and locoregional points (also contralateral): LU 3.
Distal points: SP 10, ST 34.
Control points/symptomatic points: for blood stasis SP 10, LR 2, BL 17.

Microsystem acupuncture

Ear: points of the muscle zone of the thoracic spine representation.
YNSA: E zone on the forehead, C zone (angle of the hairline).
Hand line V: area between SI 3 and one finger width proximally with the flow of the meridian.

Kiiko Matsumoto acupuncture

For pressure pain in the area of LU 10 (fire point): PC 8 or HT 8 (metal and water points of the affected meridian).

Psychosomatic treatment/relaxation

'Playing the strong man'.

28.15.7 Recommendations for the patient

Autostretching

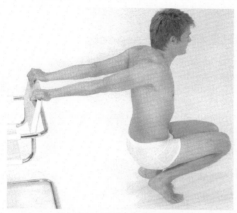

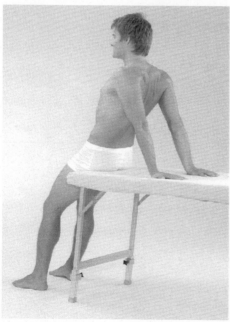

- Autostretching either on a chair squatting or supported on the bed or table.
- It is important that the forearm is pronated.
- Extension by means of inferior movement of the pelvis in the squatting position or move forward against the table or pushing the hands behind the back.

Additional measures

Those who use the telephone a lot: use a headset.

28.16 M. BRACHIALIS

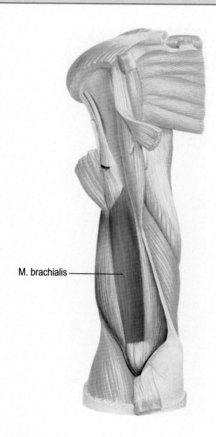

M. brachialis

28.16.1 Anatomy

Innervation: musculocutaneous nerve (brachial plexus, infraclavicular part).
Origin: anterior facet of the humerus (distal to the deltoid tuberosity, between the medial and lateral intermuscular septa).
Insertion: ulnar tuberosity.
Function: elbow joint flexion.

28.16.2 Patient symptoms

- Pain increased by lifting or carrying.
- Pain in the thumb.
- Sensory deficits are rare (compression of the radial nerve).
- Possible preliminary diagnoses: rhizarthrosis, epicondylopathia radialis humeri (tennis elbow).

28.16.3 Trigger points

mTrP	LOCALI-SATION	RADIATION	mTrP→ ACUPUNCTURE POINT
1	Several mTrP locations in the proximal part of the middle of the muscle belly	Medial arm, elbow, trapeziometacarpal joint of the thumb, radial part of wrist	LU 4, LI 13

28.16.4 Diagnosis

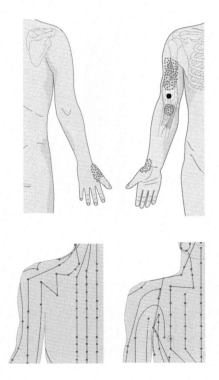

Questioning
- Pain corresponding to the characteristic areas of referred pain?
- Pain with active elbow flexion or extension at the end of the range of movement: is extension limited?

Inspection: difference between the sides in range of muscle or configuration?

Physical examination
- Palpation.
- Isometric tension from the mid position, from extension and during maximally shortened muscle, almost complete elbow flexion.
- Extension (compare sides) through maximum elbow extension; in contrast to the biceps brachii muscle no influence on the position in the shoulder joint as the brachialis muscle is a single joint muscle.

28.16.5 Specific aspects

- Principal arm flexor ('workhorse').
- Examine with any arm symptoms.
- Possible impingement syndrome (entrapment radial nerve).
- Frequently affected as a result of repetitive stress (elbow flexion) at work.

28.16.6 Therapy

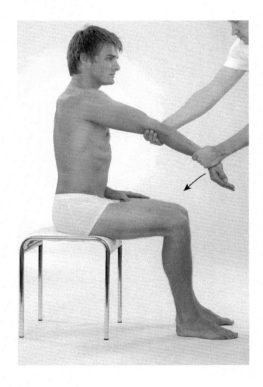

Instructions for manual trigger point-therapy

Treatment from lateral (and medial), below the biceps brachii.

Extension

- Patient seated.
- Affected arm in anteversion.
- One of the therapist's hands supports the elbow, the other guides the wrist to maximum elbow extension.
- **Warning:** elbow joint stress.

Physical procedures

Heat, cushions.

Infiltration techniques/dry needling

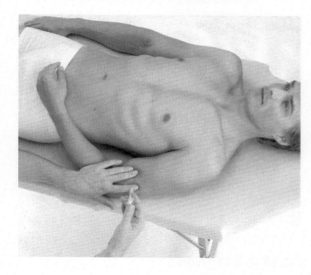

- If only mTrPs in the brachialis muscle are to be needled (without biceps brachii), the biceps brachii can be pressed down medially with the palpation hand in the distal area of the upper arm with the forearm relaxed and flexed.
- Then needling of the brachialis from above/ventrally or transversely from lateral.
- Infiltration is also possible through the biceps muscle (see Section 28.15).
- The vascular nerve bundle lies medial to the muscle: palpate the medial muscle border thoroughly and do not cross it, in order to avoid irritation or lesions.

Classical Chinese acupuncture

Local and locoregional points (also contralateral): LU 3, LU 4, LU 5, PC 3, PC 4, LI 13.
Distal points: PaM 145, ST 35, LU 7.
Control points/symptomatic points: ST 36, LR 3.

Microsystem acupuncture

Ear: points of the muscle zone of the thoracic spine representation (next to the antihelix margin in the direction of the helix).
YNSA: E zone on the forehead, C zone (angle of the hairline).
Hand line V: area between SI 3 and one finger width proximally with the flow of the meridian.

Kiiko Matsumoto acupuncture

For pain in the area of LU 10 (fire point): PC 8 or HT 8 (metal and water points of the affected meridian).

28.16.7 Recommendations for the patient

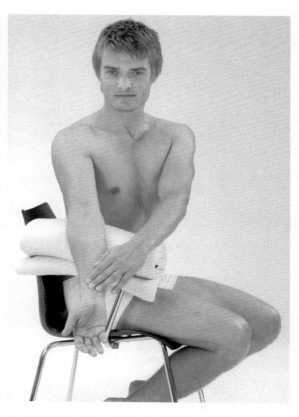

Autostretching

- Patient seated.
- Upper arm placed on a soft edge (e.g. rolled hand towel).
- Forearm in supination.

- With the other hand elbow extension or take the weight in your hand.
- Also extends the biceps brachii muscle.

Additional measures

These are needed for people with repetitive stress due to their workplace (poor ergonomics).

28.17 M. TRICEPS BRACHII (WITH M. ANCONEUS)

28.17.1 Anatomy

Innervation:
- M. biceps brachii: radial nerve (brachial plexus, infraclavicular part), long head: double joint; lateral head and medial head: single joint.
- M. anconeus: radial nerve (brachial plexus, infraclavicular part)

Origin:
- M.triceps brachii: long head: infraglenoid tubercle, lower circumference of glenoid labrum; medial head: posterior face of the humerus (medial, distal to the radial groove), intermuscular septum of the medial brachii; lateral head: posterior face of the humerus (lateral, proximal to the radial groove), proximal two-thirds of the intermuscular septum of the lateral brachii.
- M. anconeus: lateral epicondyle, adjacent to the lateral part of the medial head of the triceps brachii muscle.

Insertion:
- M. biceps brachii: olecranon (the fibres of the long head run longitudinally, those of the medial and lateral heads diagonally; together a wide tendon surface).
- M. anconeus: posterior surface of the ulna somewhat distal from the olecranon.

Function: shoulder joint: adduction (only long head), bears the weight of the arm.
Elbow joint: extension.

28.17.2 Patient symptoms

- Elbow joint pain.
- Dorsal shoulder pain.
- Pain when supported by the elbows, e.g. when sitting down on or standing up from a chair, but also when serving a tennis ball.
- If it has been present for a long time the whole of the back of the upper extremity.
- Can be involved in epicondylopathy.

28.17.3 Trigger points

mTrP	LOCALISATION	RADIATION	mTrP→ ACUPUNCTURE POINT
1	Long head, upper third	Shoulder, dorsal upper arm, occasionally dorsal forearm	TH 12
2	Lateral border of the medial head, 2–3 finger widths superior to the elbow	Lateral elbow	TH 11 (radial)
3	Lateral head, middle part	Dorsal upper arm, dorsal forearm, occasionally as far as fingers IV and V	Lateral to the connecting line LI 12 and LI 13
4	M. anconeus	Lateral epicondyle, but also the whole dorsal elbow	Lateral TH 10

28.17.4 Diagnosis

Questioning: symptoms when using the elbows for support?
Inspection: dorsal contour of upper arm.
Physical examination
- Palpation of the whole muscle belly for taut bands or mTrPs.
- Isometric tension from the mid position, from extension and during submaximally shortened muscle, almost complete elbow extension.
- Extension (compare the sides) by maximum elbow flexion first with arm hanging down If this is already limited or painful, consider instead the medial and/or lateral heads.
- For the double-jointed long head, maximum elevation of the arm in the shoulder and then flexion of the elbow behind the head are required for testing (= extension). Always compare both sides when making an assessment.

Technical examination
- X-ray elbow if loose bodies in the joint are suspected (hard feeling at the end of the range of movement with reduced flexion).
- Ultrasound if bursitis of the olecranon is suspected.

- The anconeus muscle and the triceps muscle can be therapeutically relevant in the case of chronic lateral epicondylopathy of the humerus.

28.17.6 Therapy

Instructions for manual trigger point therapy

- Long head: treatment with pinch grip. Fascia separation technique to the teres minor and teres major muscles important (with limited elevation in the shoulder joint at the end of the range of movement).
- Lateral head: treatment with pinch grip.
- Medial head: with lateral epicondylopathy, the active mTrPs are frequently very distal in the lateral part.
- **Warning:** the radial nerve should not be confused with a taut band and should not be subjected to intensive manual treatment. It is easy to differentiate the radial nerve by palpation: it winds around the humerus in a spiral and its course does not correspond to the course of the taut band in the triceps muscle.

Extension

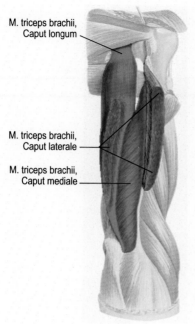

M. triceps brachii, Caput longum

M. triceps brachii, Caput laterale

M. triceps brachii, Caput mediale

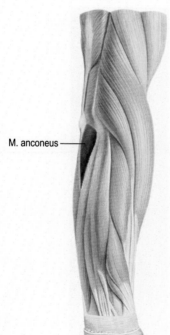

M. anconeus

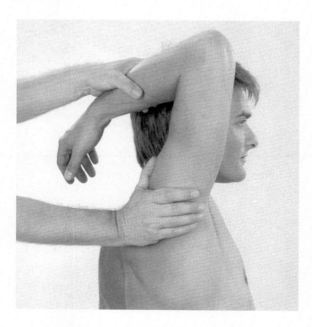

- The patient sits on a chair or a couch.
- Shoulder joint in elevation at the end of the range of movement.
- Elbow flexed.
- Hand by the patient supports the shoulder in elevation.
- The hand away from the patient extends over the forearm using additional flexion in the elbow and slight dorsal traction.

28.17.5 Specific aspects

- With chronic shoulder symptoms, shortening of the triceps muscle with its long head can also have an effect on narrowing the subacromial space.

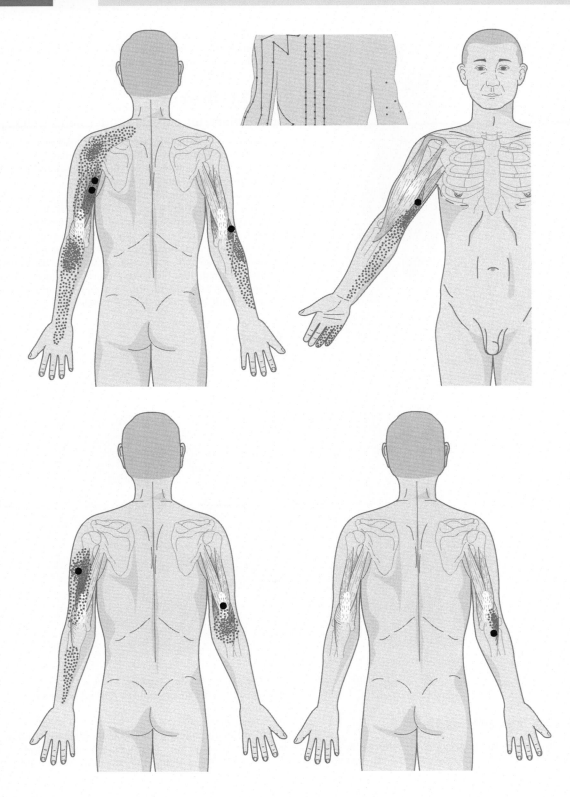

- **Warning:** frequent abnormal movement caused by hyperextension of the vertebral column (fix using the back of a chair or the therapist's body).

Physical procedures

Superficial, therefore most physical procedures are applicable.

Infiltration techniques/dry needling

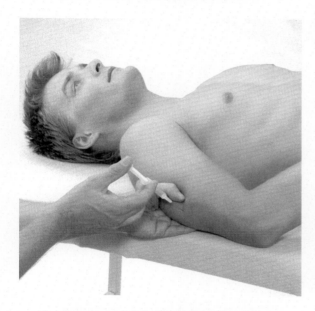

- The affected arm is lightly flexed on the patient's abdomen.
- Infiltration quite possible in pinch grip.
- Lateral insertion is better to avoid injury to the radial nerve, which winds in a spiral round the humerus.
- Needle length: 4 cm is usually sufficient.

Classical Chinese acupuncture

Local and locoregional points (also contralateral): TH 11, TH 12, TH 13, HT 2, LI 12, LI 13, LI 14 (in a inferior direction).
Distal points: SI 3, BL 39/BL 40 or palpate along the M. biceps femoris and needle sensitive points.

Microsystem acupuncture

Ear: points of the muscle zone of the thoracic spine representation (next to the antihelix margin in the direction of the helix).
YNSA: E zone on the forehead, C zone (angle of the hairline).
Hand line V: area between SI 3 and one finger width proximally with the flow of the meridian.

Kiiko Matsumoto acupuncture

- HT 3 ipsilateral.
- For pain in the area of TH 6, SI 5, PC 8 or HT 8 (metal and water points of affected meridian) for reduction of tenderness on the fire point and tenderness of the muscle.

Psychosomatic treatment/relaxation

Patient seated, shoulders maximally elevated, possibly withheld aggression in the sense of creating space for oneself – elbows – more precisely forearms/fists extended.

28.17.7 Recommendations for the patient

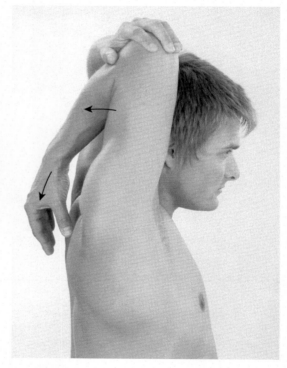

Autostretching

- The patient sits on a chair or a couch.
- Shoulder joint in elevation at the end of the range of movement.
- Elbow maximally flexed.
- Lateral and somewhat dorsal traction at the elbow with the hand not affected.
- Alternative: take belt in affected hand and pull the belt in a inferior direction with the other hand (behind the back).

Additional measures

Support elbow while working at a computer, arm rests on chair.

Chapter 29

Elbow, forearm and hand

Dominik Irnich

29.1 FUNCTIONAL ASSOCIATIONS

Finger, hand and forearm serve as a functional unit for grasping and moving objects. Their multiple functions are very complex, although their muscle movement is relatively simple. The thumb is capable of opposition, so plays a particular role. Strain and shortening of the muscles that move it can cause rhizarthrosis. The finger joints also bear a great load and are often the first to be affected by inflammatory/rheumatic and metabolic diseases and can be even more severely deformed than with polyarthrosis. The symptoms and progression can also be aggravated by the asymmetric traction of shortened muscles.

As a rotating hinge joint, the elbow allows both flexion and extension between the humerus and the bones of the forearm, as well as pronation and supination of the hand between the ulna and the radius, the latter together with the distal radioulnar joint.

The muscles of the forearm are divided into two groups: flexors and extensors. Predominantly the extensors are predisposed to functional strain. The individual muscles form relatively similar pain patterns, partly involving the tendons, in epicondylopathy.

> Even when only conditions (strain) but not the actual causes of the epicondylopathy humeri radialis are known, it is astounding how regularly so-called treatment-resistant patients respond to differentiated treatment of mTrPs in the extensors with improvement in terms of freedom from symptoms.

It is interesting that despite the relatively uniform course of these muscles one part is anatomically and histologically constructed for power (M. carpi radialis brevis, M. carpi ulnaris) and another part for speed and range of movement (M. extensor carpi radialis longus). If the functional disorder is more complex, both parts must be treated, even though primarily active mTrPs are not found.

> The close segmental and functional relationship of the upper arm, shoulder and cervical spine are important for diagnosis and treatment. These structures should therefore be included in the examination.

29.2 PSYCHOSOMATIC ASSOCIATIONS

Pathologies in the area of the elbow can be an indicator of assertive behaviour ('using your elbows'). Grasping difficulties can be an indication that the patient is trying to get a grip on something – life, a particular situation or a relationship – or wants to hold on to something or express an ambivalence between holding on and letting go. Here the patient must learn that even letting go (children, partner, loss) has to be an active and conscious process.

According to TCM, patients with epicondylopathy may have a functional disorder of the large intestine and/or lungs. This can also be expressed in concomitant diseases of the mucous membranes such as sinusitis or irritable bowel (especially constipation).

If the hands are cold and damp at the same time, as with autonomic dysregulation, it may be that the patient has withdrawn from their actions, refuses to take an active part in the world or is resigned to their fate.

You can get a great deal on information on the patient's regulation of tension by taking the patient's hand and gently moving the forearm.

29.3 SYMPTOMS

In the area of the elbow, forearm and hand, the locoregional symptoms are at the fore, with limited movement or weakness, pain, occasionally a feeling of numbness, dysaesthesia and feeling cold. Inflammatory and traumatic diseases in this area are usually easy to differentiate.

Entrapment syndrome with the development of neuropathic pain (burning, hypoaesthesia, dysaesthesia or paraesthesia) is not an uncommon secondary consequence of musculoligamentary disorders in this area.

29.4 DIAGNOSTIC AND THERAPEUTIC CONSIDERATIONS

Besides the regional muscles, muscle groups in the cervical spine and the shoulder area are frequently also involved in pain in the area of the forearm and hand: through direct pain radiation or influence of supplying nerves or blood vessels, pain radiating into the area of the hand can definitely be provoked by the proximal muscles (e.g. Mm. scaleni, brachialis, infraspinatus, pectoralis, latissimus dorsi, subclavius). mTrPs in the area of the hand, forearm and elbow can have their origin in the area itself (e.g. after trauma). However, a functional disorder in the cervical spine/shoulder area can lead to the deduction that symptoms are usually a consequence of incorrect posture of the whole body (examine the whole locomotor system if symptoms become chronic).

Good experiences are available for polyarthrosis in the area of the hand (particularly the distal interphalangeal joint of the fingers, Heberden type; see interosseus muscles) and rhizarthrosis (see M. adductor pollicis, M. flexor pollicis longus, DD referred pain from the Mm. brachialis or scaleni). Treatment of the interosseous muscles can also make a definite improvement in mobility of the fingers, particularly the spread, which is helpful for musicians, for example. Difficulties in grasping and holding, especially for climbers, are also a sensible indication.

For conservative treatment of carpal tunnel syndrome, or even for residual pain after an operation, mTrPs in the area of the shoulder girdle (scaleni muscles), the upper arm (M. brachialis) and forearm or hand (M. brachioradialis, radial extensors, Mm. palmaris longus, flexor carpi radialis, pronator teres, opponens pollicis and adductor pollicis) should be examined and treated if necessary.

As mentioned above, epicondylopathy as insertion tendinopathy is a good indication (see below) on the radial side of strain of the forearm extensors which insert there (tennis elbow), and on the ulnar side of the forearm flexors (golfer's elbow).

The most commonly affected muscles are the M. supinator and M. extensor carpi radialis longus. Also, with symptoms of strain of the upper arm muscles as a result of excessive work with a computer mouse ('repetitive strain injury syndrome') an attempt at mTrP therapy is sensible, with supplemental training of perception and improvement of sensing in and through the arm (e.g. Perfetti ergotherapy).

For mild Dupuytren's symptoms treatment via the M. palmaris longus can also be tried as stretcher of aponeurosis of the palm.

If there is insufficient improvement, it may be better to consider the possible protective function of myofascial changes (e.g. in a disorder of mobility of the carpus muscles against each other). However, the latter can also be caused by a muscular disorder as well.

29.5 FUNCTION EXAMINATION FOR mTrP IDENTIFICATION

FINDINGS ON INSPECTION	MUSCLES THAT MAY NEED TO BE TREATED
Elbow joint	
Flexion	M. triceps brachii and M. anconeus (see Section 28.17)
Extension	M. biceps brachii (see Section 28.15), M. brachialis (see Section 28.16), M. brachioradialis (see Section 29.7). Small circumference: M. flexor carpi radialis (see Section 29.11), M. palmaris longus (see Section 29.10), M. pronator teres (humeral head) (see Section 29.11).

Pronation from supination at the end of the range of movement	If there is hardening at the end of the range of movement consider loose body in the joint. M. biceps brachii (see Section 28.15), M. supinator (see Section 29.9), Mm. extensor indicis and extensor pollicis longus and brevis (see Section 29.8), M. abductor pollicis longus (see Section 29.12); depending on position M. brachioradialis (see Section 29.7)
Supination from pronation at end of the range of movement	Mm. pronator teres and quadratus (see Section 29.11), M. flexor carpi radialis (see Section 29.11), M. palmaris longus (see Section 29.10), M. extensor carpi radialis longus (see Section 29.6); depending on position M. brachioradialis (see Section 29.7)
Elbow flexed 90°	
Pronation from neutral position	M. pronator (see Section 29.11)
Supination from neutral position	M. supinator (see Section 29.9)
From pronation and supination position to normal neutral position	M. brachioradialis (see Section 29.7)

For active movement, isometric examination has proved reliable: classification is reversed.

For epicondylopathy of the radial humerus the following diagnostic procedure has proved reliable. From maximum palmar flexion, the patient should isometrically pull into dorsal extension:

- the wrist: resistance at the back of the hand (see M. extensor carpi radialis longus),
- the flexed fingers: resistance at the distal phalanges of the fingers (see M. extensor digitorum longus, especially of the ring finger),
- then give the patient your hand and turn it isometrically from the neutral position into supination (see M. supinator),

- then test the isometric elbow extension as well (see M. triceps brachii/M. anconeus).

Logically, the M. extensores digitorum should be examined if finger flexion is restricted.

If the patient has problems with the forearm and hand muscles, the patient should perform the painful movements and the therapist should palpate them to find which muscles are straining. For restricted movement, the opposite movement should be carried out and palpated (Figure 29.1).

29.6 HAND EXTENSORS

29.6.1 Anatomy

The hand extensors comprise the M. extensor carpi radialis longus, M. extensor carpi radialis brevis and M. extensor carpi ulnaris.

Innervation: N. radialis.
Origin
- M. extensor carpi radialis longus: lateral border of the humerus (distal end), lateral epicondyle, intermuscular septum brachii laterale.
- M. extensor carpi radialis brevis: lateral epicondyle of the humerus, annular ligament of radius.
- M. extensor carpi ulnaris: head of the humerus: lateral epicondyle of the humerus, collateral ligament of radius, ulnar head: posterior facet of the ulna (proximal two thirds), antebrachial fascia.

Insertion:
- M. extensor carpi radialis longus: dorsal aspect of the base of the second metacarpal bone.
- M. extensor carpi radialis brevis: dorsal aspect of the base of the third metacarpal bone.
- M. extensor carpi ulnaris dorsal aspect of the base of the fifth metacarpal bone.

Function: the extensors extend in the wrist and prevent concomitant flexion in the wrist during activity of the finger flexors (grip function).
- M. extensor carpi radialis longus: additional radial abduction.
- M. extensor carpi radialis brevis: additional radial abduction.
- M. extensor carpi ulnaris additional ulnar abduction.

29.6.2 Patient symptoms

- Lateral elbow pain.
- Weak grip.
- Possible preliminary diagnoses: lateral epicondyle of the humerus.

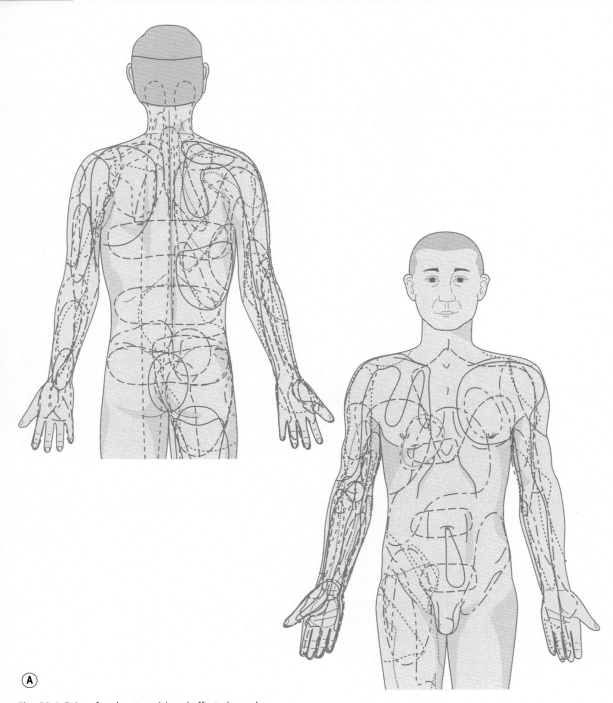

Fig. 29.1 Pain referral pattern (a) and affected muscles

Continued

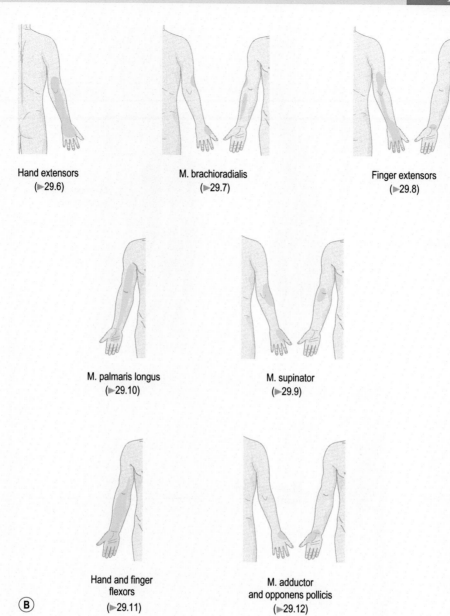

Hand extensors
(▶29.6)

M. brachioradialis
(▶29.7)

Finger extensors
(▶29.8)

M. palmaris longus
(▶29.10)

M. supinator
(▶29.9)

Ⓑ

Hand and finger
flexors
(▶29.11)

M. adductor
and opponens pollicis
(▶29.12)

Fig. 29.1—cont'd (b) of the elbow, forearm and hand.

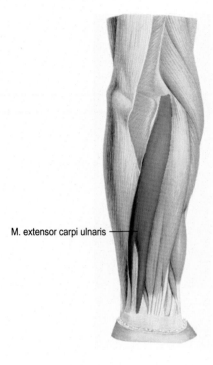

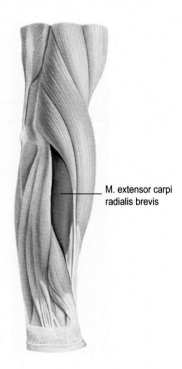

M. extensor carpi ulnaris

M. extensor carpi radialis brevis

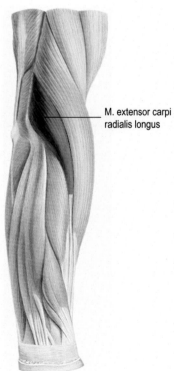

M. extensor carpi radialis longus

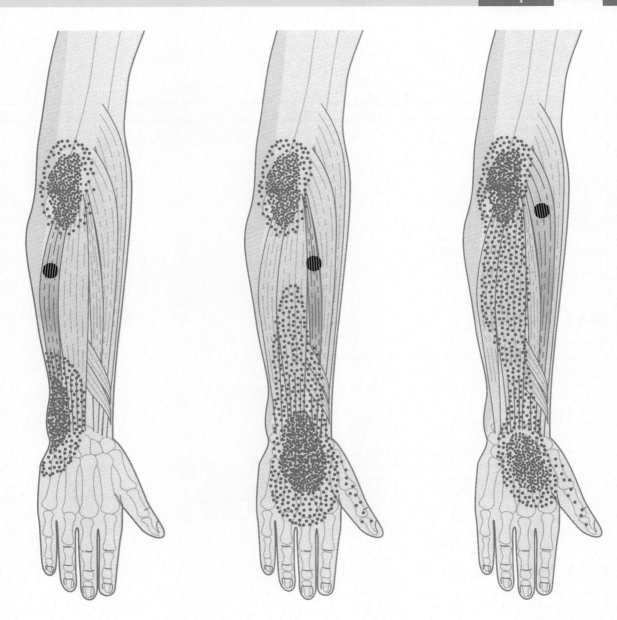

29.6.3 Trigger points

mTrP	LOCATION	RADIATION	mTrP→ ACUPUNCTURE POINT
1	In the M. extensor carpi radialis longus	Lateral epicondyle, back of hand, thumb	LI 10, LI 9
2	In the M. extensor carpi radialis brevis	Lateral epicondyle, back of hand, thumb	LI 8
3 (rarely)	In the M. extensor carpi ulnaris	Elbow, ulnar back of hand	TH 8

29.6.4 Diagnosis

Questioning
- Repetitive strain of grip function due to fixed wrist, e.g. working on an assembly line, playing tennis?
- Turning screwdriver? → M. extensor carpi radialis longus.

Physical examination
- Back of hand in different directions depending on direction of movement:
  - M. extensor carpi radialis longus and brevis: painful restriction of movement with extended elbow and flexed wrist, painful restriction of movement with extended elbow and ulnar abduction at wrist,
  - M. extensor carpi ulnaris: painful restriction of movement with extended elbow and radial abduction in wrist, careful palpation of muscle bellies with slightly flexed elbow.

29.6.5 Specific aspects

- mTrPs predominantly in upper third of forearm.
- The supinator and brachioradialis muscles are very commonly affected as well in cases of epicondylitis.

29.6.6 Therapy

Instructions for manual trigger point therapy

- M. extensor carpi radialis longus: treatment with pinch grip.
- M. extensor carpi radialis brevis: treatment with finger pressure technique.
- M. extensor carpi ulnaris: treatment with finger pressure technique.

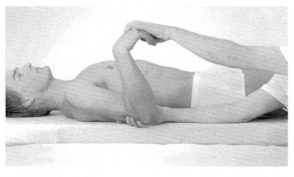

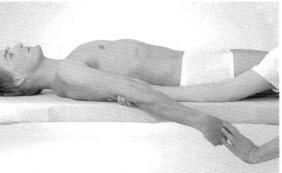

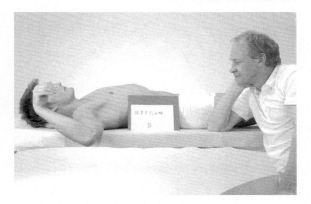

Extension

- Patient in supine position (also possible while seated).
- Therapist supports the elbow with one hand and guides the wrist into palmar flexion with the other.
- Important: before elbow extension (real extension movement) maximally flex the wrist and hold in flexion with resistance.
- The elbow should be supported so that it is not further overextended if hard resistance is encountered.
- M. extensor carpi ulnaris: additional radial abduction in the wrist.

Physical procedures

- Laser acupuncture, shock wave therapy, cupping.

Infiltration techniques/dry needling

- Patient places slightly flexed arm on the table or bed.
- Slightly flexed elbow and supported arm.
- Muscles in pinch grip.
- Needling/injection from the side.
- mTrPs are easily palpated and mobilised for the injection.

Classical Chinese acupuncture

Local and locoregional points (also contralateral): LI 4, LI 8, LI 9, LI 10, TH 5, TH 8, NP 67.
Distal points: ST 35 (Yang–Yang axis, joint analogy), ST 36 (Yang–Yang axis, joint analogy, analgesia), ST 40 (transformation of 'mucus').

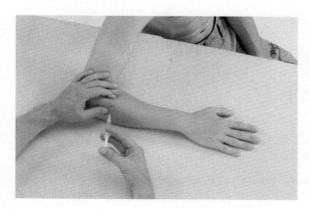

Microsystem acupuncture

Ear: elbow, cushion; representation of hand/wrist in the scapha.
YNSA: inferior area of the C zone (base point).

Kiiko Matsumoto acupuncture

General arm muscles:
- tenderness in the area of the arm muscles can usually be relieved by relieving the tenderness in the area of the scalene muscles,
- with involvement of the TNM: LR 8 ipsilateral and GB 34 on both sides, diagonal needling.

M. extensor carpi ulnaris: for tenderness in the area of TH 6: ipsilateral TH 1 and TH 2.
M. extensor carpi radialis longus: for tenderness in the area of LU 10: ipsilateral LU 5 and LU 8.

M. extensor carpi radialis brevis:
- in some cases, pain can be relieved by needling of TH 16 ipsilaterally and/or ST 26 on the right,
- for tenderness in the area of LI 5: ipsilateral LI 1 and LI 2.

Psychosomatics/relaxation

Difficulties in letting go in the transferred sense.

29.6.7 Recommendations for the patient

Autostretching

- M. extensor carpi radialis longus and brevis:
  - unaffected hand on the back of the hand on the affected side and with light pressure up to flexion at the end of range of movement in the wrist with flexed elbow (see photo, top left),
  - then extension in the elbow with pressure maintained on the flexed wrist (see photo, bottom).
- M. extensor digitorum: as above, but additional finger flexion.
- M. extensor carpi ulnaris: as above, possible additional radial abduction in the wrist.
- Alternatively can also be extended while standing with the aid of body weight (see photo, top right).

Additional measures

- Strengthen muscles and at same time train coordination (power ball, Qigong balls).
- Ergotherapy if there is a high level of resistance to treatment.

29.7 M. BRACHIORADIALIS

29.7.1 Anatomy

Innervation: N. radialis.
Origin: lateral border of the humerus, septum intermusculare brachii laterale.
Insertion: styloid process of radius.
Function: flexion in elbow, brings forearm in mid position from supination and pronation.

29.7.2 Patient symptoms

- Lateral elbow pain.
- No strength in grip.
- Possible preliminary diagnoses: epicondylitis humeri lateralis.

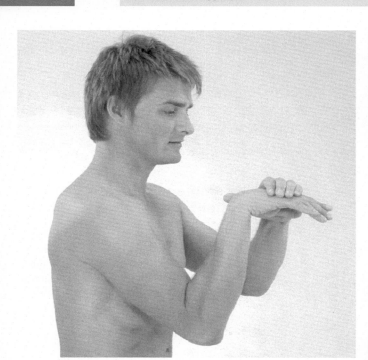

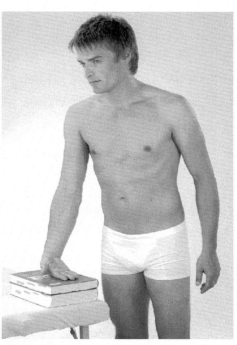

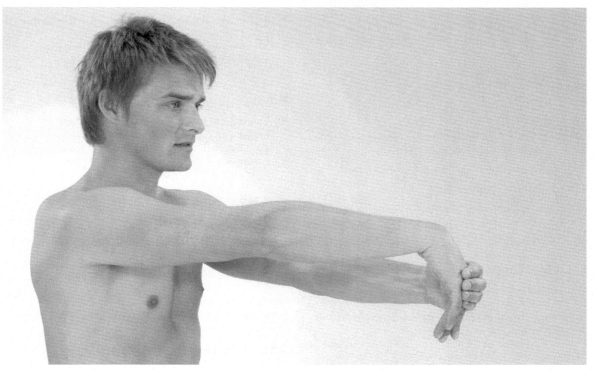

29.7.3 Trigger points

mTrP	LOCATION	RADIATION	mTrP→ ACUPUNCTURE POINT
1	Close to joint	Lateral epicondyle, radial forearm, elbow, back of hand and between metacarpals I and II	LI 10
2	Transition from upper to lower two-thirds	Forearm, back of hand and between metacarpals I and II	LI 9

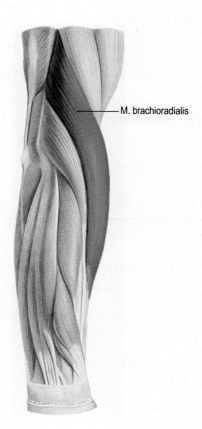

M. brachioradialis

29.7.4 Diagnosis

Questioning: repetitive strain of grip function with fixed wrist, e.g. working on assembly line, tennis, working in the garden (spade)?

Physical examination: press both hands for some time: watch out for loss of strength and pain at the lateral epicondyle when comparing sides (**warning:** difference depending on whether left or right handed).

29.7.5 Specific aspects

- mTrPs predominantly in the upper third of the forearm.
- With epicondylitis, the supinator and brachioradialis muscles are very frequently affected as well.
- Frequently secondary mTrPs or satellite TrPs.
- Patients with fibromyalgia syndrome frequently have mTrPs in the brachioradialis muscle.

29.7.6 Therapy

Instructions for manual trigger point therapy

Treatment with pinch grip.

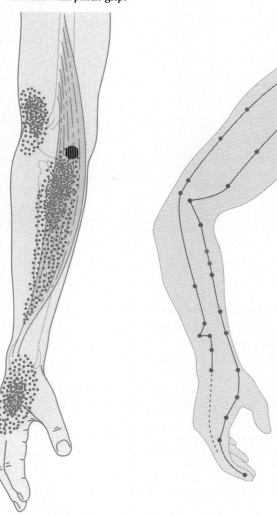

Extension

- Patient in supine position.
- Wrist in maximum palmar flexion.
- Forearm in pronation.
- Extension by extending the elbow.
- Also possible while seated.

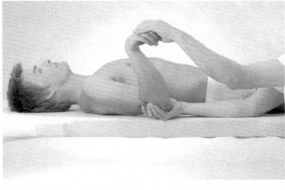

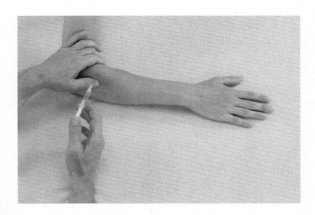

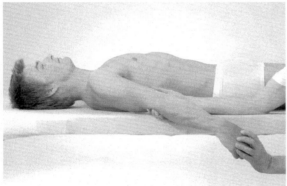

Classical Chinese acupuncture

Local and locoregional points (also contralateral): LI 4 (meridian and radiation zone), LI 9, LI 10, TH 5, NP 67.
Distal points: ST 35 (Yang–Yang-axis, joint analogy), ST 36 (Yang–Yang axis, joint analogy, analgesia), ST 40 (transformation of 'mucus').
Control points/symptomatic points: GB 34 (master point of the tendons).

Microsystem acupuncture

Ear: elbow, cushion; representation of hand/wrist in the scapha.
YNSA: inferior area of the C zone (base point).

Kiiko Matsumoto acupuncture

M. brachioradialis: for tenderness in the area of LU 10: ipsilateral LU 5 and LU 8.

Psychosomatics/relaxation

- Difficulties letting go in the transferred sense ('phase of cleaning and letting go').
- In combination with sinusitis and irritable bowel consider large intestine/lungs as in TCM.

Physical procedures

Cupping, shock wave therapy also in combination with direct treatment at the epicondyle; laser treatment, ultrasound.

29.7.7 Recommendations for the patient

Autostretching

- At first wrist in maximum palmar flexion by supporting on bed (keep vertebral column extended; see Section 29.6) or support from other hand.
- Forearm in pronation.
- Extension by extending the elbow.
- No extension if the wrist is not first maximally flexed and remains so during elbow extension.

Infiltration techniques/dry needling

- Patient places slightly flexed arm on the table or bed.
- Slightly flexed elbow and supported arm.
- Mid position in forearm.
- Muscles in pinch grip.
- Needling/injection from above.
- mTrPs are easily palpated and mobilised for the injection.

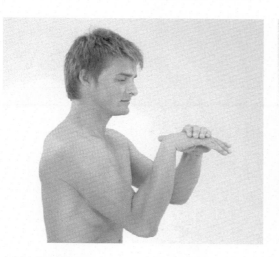

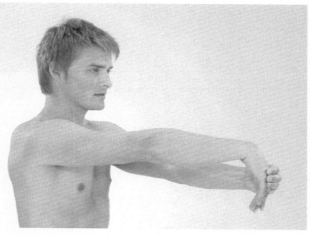

Additional measures

- Self-treatment with pinch grip.
- Ergotherapy if there is a high level of resistance to treatment.
- For tennis players: optimise technique and grip in direction of radial abduction, use a lighter or less top-heavy racket, advise tension and relaxation between ball changes in the sense of progressive muscle relaxation.

29.8 FINGER EXTENSORS

29.8.1 Anatomy

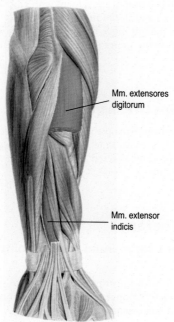

Mm. extensores digitorum

Mm. extensor indicis

Innervation:
- M. extensor indicis: radial nerve (brachial plexus, infraclavicular part).
- M. extensor digitorum (communis): radial nerve (brachial plexus, infraclavicular part).

Origin:
- M. extensor indicis: posterior facet of ulna (distal quarter), interosseous membrane.
- M. extensor digitorum (communis): lateral epicondyle of humerus, radial collateral ligament and radial ring, antebrachial fascia.

Insertion:
- M. extensor indicis: dorsal aponeurosis of index fingers.
- M. extensor digitorum (communis): dorsal aponeurosis of fingers 2–5.

Function:
- M. extensor indicis: wrist: dorsal flexion, radial abduction, proximal phalanx (II): extension, adduction, interphalangeal joint (II): extension.
- M. extensor digitorum (communis): elbow joint: extension, wrist: dorsal flexion, ulnar abduction, proximal phalanges (II–V)/phalanges (II–V): extension.

29.8.2 Patient symptoms

- Lateral elbow pain.
- No strength in grip.
- Wrist pain when flexing fingers.
- Stiffness of individual fingers or phalanges, especially interphalangeal joints.
- Possible preliminary diagnoses: epicondylitis of the lateral humerus, arthritis of the wrist, 'arthritis' of the interphalangeal joints.

377

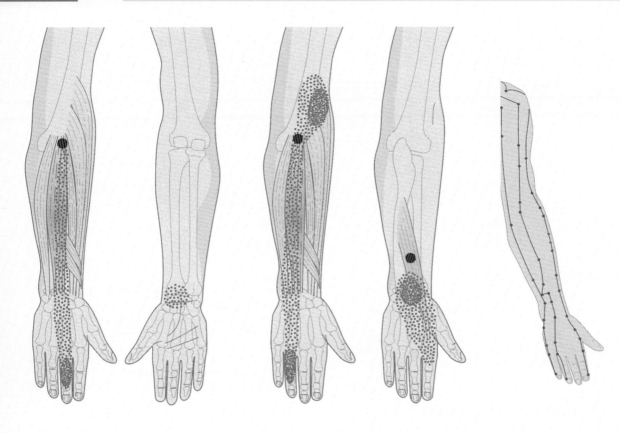

29.8.3 Trigger points

mTrP	LOCATION	RADIATION	mTrP↔ ACUPUNCTURE POINT
1	M. extensor digitorum longus in the upper third	Lateral epicondyle, back of hand, fingers	NP 67, LI 10
2	M. extensor indicis between the ulna and radius	Back of hand, index finger	TH 5

29.8.4 Diagnosis

Questioning
- Repetitive strain of grip function due to fixed wrist, e.g. working on an assembly line.
- Playing tennis? Golf (right-handed hitter with right-sided symptoms)?
- Turning screwdriver?

Physical examination
- Painful restriction of movement with elbow extended, flexed wrist and flexed finger.
- Have the patient move the painful fingers while you palpate the upper third of the M. extensor digitorum.

29.8.5 Specific aspects

- Crafts and sportspeople are frequently affected.
- The supinator and brachioradialis muscles are very commonly affected as well in the case of epicondylitis.

29.8.6 Therapy

Instructions for manual trigger point therapy

- Treatment with finger pressure technique.
- Local twitch response frequently obtainable at the middle finger extensor.

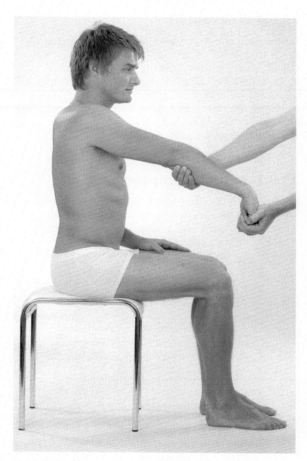

- Arm supported on table or couch.
- Slight flexion at the elbow.
- Muscles in pinch grip.
- Infiltration and dry needling using the two-finger protection technique.

Classical Chinese acupuncture

Local and locoregional points (also contralateral): LI 10, TH 4, TH 5, NP 67, SI 6.
Distal points: ST 36 (Yang–Yang axis, joint analogy, analgesia), LR 3 (muscle toning), analogous points at the lower leg and ankle depending on sensitivity (Very Point technique).
Control points/symptomatic points: ST 40 (move moisture and mucus), GB 34 (masterpoint of tendons).

Microsystem acupuncture

Ear: representation of the hand/wrist in the scapha.
YNSA: causal area of the C zone (base point).

Kiiko Matsumoto acupuncture

For tenderness in the area of TH 6: ipsilateral TH 1 and TH 2.

Psychosomatics/relaxation

Difficulties 'letting go' in the extended sense.

29.8.7 Recommendations for the patient

Autostretching

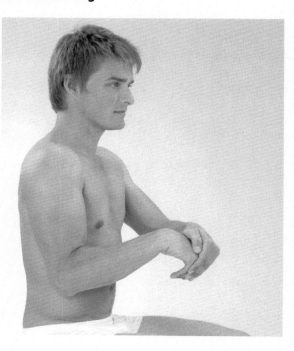

Extension

- Extension while lying down or seated.
- Do not hyperextend the elbow against hard resistance.
- Essential: fingers flexed throughout the whole extension phase (fist closed)!

Physical procedures

Shock wave therapy (2 bar), laser therapy, cupping (M. extensor digitorum).

Infiltration techniques/dry needling

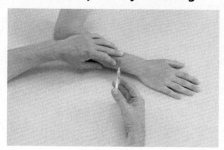

- Fingers flexed.
- The non-affected hand on the back of the hand on the affected side.
- Slight pressure as far as the end of the range of flexion movement in the wrist with flexed elbow.
- Then extension in the elbow with maintained pressure on the flexed wrist.
- Moving the individual fingers helps to identify the affected cord during self-palpation.

Additional measures

- Strengthens muscle and at the same time trains coordination (power ball, Qigong balls); ergotherapy if there is high resistance to therapy.
- 'Progressive muscle relaxation' in everyday life.

29.9 M. SUPINATOR

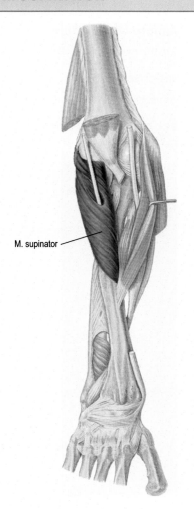

M. supinator

29.9.1 Anatomy

Innervation: radial nerve (brachial plexus, infraclavicular part).
Origin: lateral epicondyle of the humerus, collateral ligament of radius and radial rings, cistern of the supinator muscles of the ulna.
Insertion: anterior facet of the radius (proximal and distal to the radial tuberosity).
Function: radioulnar joints: supination.

29.9.2 Patient symptoms

- Symptoms of classic epicondylopathy of the radial humerus (tennis elbow) with pain at the radial epicondyle and occasional radiation as far as the thumb and index finger.
- Pain when carrying objects with extended elbow.

29.9.3 Trigger points

mTrP	LOCATION	RADIATION	mTrP→ ACUPUNCTURE POINT
1	On the radius 1–2 cm below the joint capsule (radial to the biceps tendon)	Lateral epicondyle, sometimes the whole radial part of the elbow, occasionally over the whole radial forearm as far as the thumb and index finger or its interdigital folds	LU 5, LI 11

29.9.4 Diagnosis

Questioning
- Supination strain, e.g. screwdriver, tennis (backhand)?
- Evidence of neuropathic pain, e.g. burning?
- Dysaesthesia or paraesthesia?

Inspection: protective posture when carrying objects in supination position.

Physical examination
- General examination of the elbow joint (loose body in the joint? pain in the olecranon? evidence of inflammation?).
- The therapist grasps the flexed elbow, wrist in neutral position.
- The therapist's other hand is placed on the back of the hand.

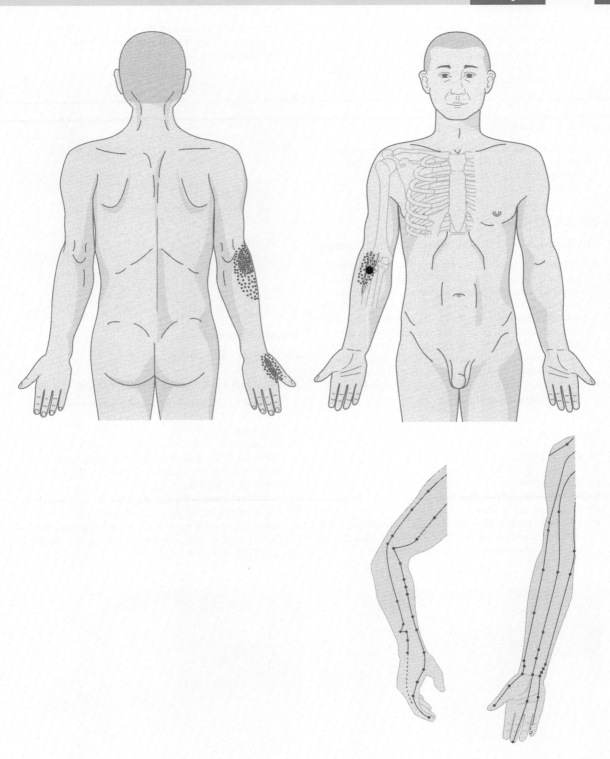

- The patient now supinates the forearm against resistance from the therapist.
- Pain provocation at the lateral epicondyle.
- Firm radial palpation of the biceps tendon one finger width distal from the elbow fold.
- Cervical spine examination.

29.9.5 Specific aspects

- The supinator is frequently the cause of treatment-resistant epicondylopathy of the radial humerus.
- Entrapment of the superficial branch of the radial nerve by the supinator muscle.

29.9.6 Therapy

Instructions for manual trigger point therapy

- **Approach 1:** treatment in the depth between the biceps tendon and the brachioradialis muscle, proximal and radial to the easily palpable pronator teres muscle. Alternating isometric activation and deactivation of the supinator muscle against resistance leads to palpable change of tension deep in the supinator muscle.
- **Approach 2:** treatment from lateral direction: distal to the head of the radius at the proximal third of the lateral radius (through the extensor carpi ulnaris).
- Very commonly the key muscle in the treatment of lateral epicondylopathy.

Extension

- Patient in supine position.
- Shoulder in 90° abduction.
- Elbow flexed.
- Hand in neutral position.
- One hand holds the elbow steady.
- The other hand grasps the wrist and extends the distal forearm in pronation (=rotation of the medial side of the palm of the hand in a lateral direction).

- Extension by rotation of the forearm in a lateral direction, i.e. the medial palm of the hand is turned 90° laterally.

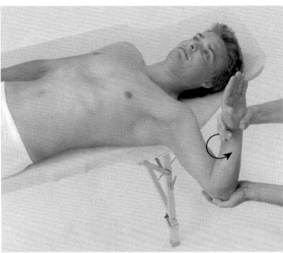

Physical procedures

Shock waves, laser acupuncture.

Infiltration techniques/dry needling

- Because of the nerve and vessel cord, first try dry needling.
- Palpation of the mTrP.
- Medial/ulnar shift of the vessel and nerve cord in the direction of the biceps tendon and at the same time press down on the brachioradialis with the second finger in a radial direction.
- Insertion between the two fingers.
- Slowly probe in the direction of the mTrP.
- After contact with the radius without encountering the mTrP withdraw the needle and probe again with slight change of direction (max. 5°).

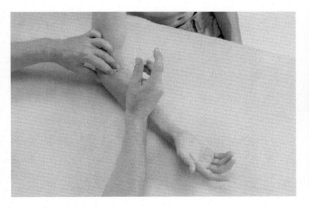

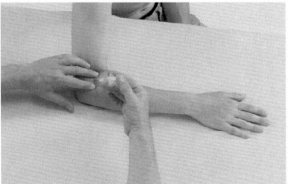

- a) Insertion in supination position (insertion one finger width radially and inferiorly from LU 5).
- b) Insertion in pronation position (orientation: one finger width LI 11).

Classical Chinese acupuncture

Local and locoregional points (also contralateral): LU 5, LI 11, LI 10, PC 3.
Distal points: Di 4 (meridian, analgesia), LU 7 (meridian, cervical spine).
Control points/symptomatic points: ST 36 (analgesia, joint analogy), GB 34 (master point of the tendons, joint analogy), LR 3 (muscle tone).

Microsystem acupuncture

Ear: representation of the hand/wrist in the scapha.
YNSA: inferior area of the C zone (base point).

Kiiko Matsumoto acupuncture

- Relief of pain in some cases with TH 16 ipsilaterally and/or ST 26 on the right.
- For pain in the area of LI 5: LI 1 and LI 2 ipsilaterally.

29.9.7 Recommendations for the patient

Autostretching

- Patient stands or sits.
- Elbow flexed, wrist extended in mid-position, the non-affected hand grasps the distal wrist and forearm.

- Movement of the distal forearm in pronation for extension (also some joint stress).
- Self-massage: pressure with thumb distal to the head of the radius at the proximal third of the lateral radius leads to forearm pronation and supination.

Additional measures

- Improvement of grip when playing tennis and hitting a backhand stroke.
- For craftspeople training to use the non-dominant hand.
- Carrying objects with slightly flexed elbow.

29.10 M. PALMARIS LONGUS

29.10.1 Anatomy

Innervation: median nerve (brachial plexus, infraclavicular part) (inconstant muscle).
Origin: medial epicondyle, antebrachial fascia.
Insertion: aponeurosis palmaris.
Function
- Elbow joint: flexion.
- Wrist: palmar flexion, tension of the palmar aponeurosis.

29.10.2 Patient symptoms

- Pain in the medial forearm and medial palm, location sensed predominantly on the surface.

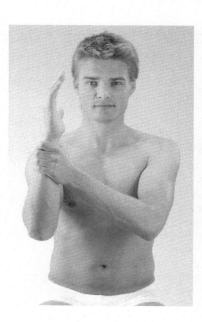 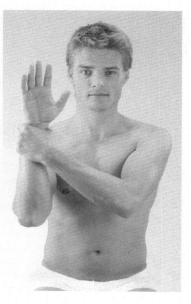 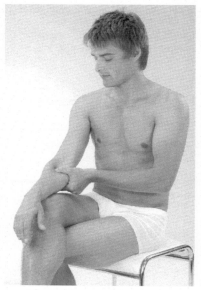

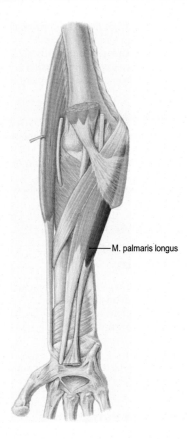

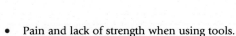
M. palmaris longus

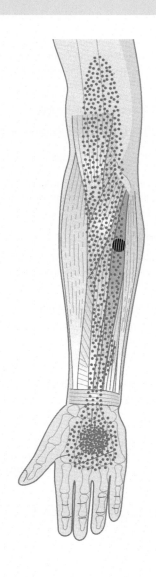

- Pain and lack of strength when using tools.
- If it has persisted for any length of time, symptoms may also be found in the upper arm along the muscle function chain.

29.10.3 Trigger points

mTrP	LOCATION	RADIATION	mTrP→ ACUPUNCTURE POINT
1	Usually in the upper third of the muscle	Palmar side of the forearm, palm of the hand, rarely radiating proximally into the upper arm	–

29.10.4 Diagnosis

Questioning
- Lack of strength when using tools?
- Fall on extended hand?

Inspection: evidence of Dupuytren's contracture?

Physical examination
- Identification of the muscle by forming a hollow with the hand and flexing the wrist slightly.
- Medial surface of the hand tender.
- Classical signs: sensitivity like '1000 needles'.

Technical examination: for suspected neuropathic pain: nerve conduction speed of the median nerve.

29.10.5 Specific aspects

- Muscle is 15–20% less than in the normal Western population.
- Frequently occurs at the same time as Dupuytren's contracture, but the mTrPs in the palmaris longus cannot be seen as a preliminary stage

29.10.6 Therapy

Instructions for manual trigger point therapy

- Direct treatment using finger pressure technique.
- The flexors and the palmaris longus run together close to the origin where there is hardly any possibility of differentiation.
- Concomitant mobilisation of the articular surface of the proximal root of the hand and/or mobilisation in the radiocarpal joint.

Extension

- The patient sits on a chair.

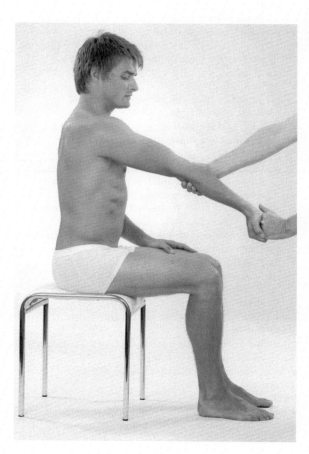

- Wrist maximally extended in a dorsal direction and kept in extension with resistance (important!).
- Metacarpophalangeal joint extended, distal interphalangeal joint and proximal interphalangeal joint remain free or slightly flexed.
- Than extension by extending the elbow.

Physical procedures

Laser therapy, shock waves.

Infiltration techniques/dry needling

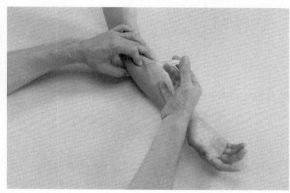

- Place forearm in supination.
- Easier, safer approach to the mTrPs in the middle part of the muscle.
- Caution with invasive procedure with mTrPs close to elbow (pain-sensitive tendon plate).
- **Warning:** median nerve with mTrPs in the middle part.
- No injections or deep needling into the palmar aponeurosis.

Classical Chinese acupuncture

Local and locoregional points (also contralateral): PC 4, PC 5, PC 6, PC 7, LU 5, Ex-AH 9 (Baxie), TH 9, Bizhong (at the proximal transition of the muscle belly to tension approximately 6 cm proximal to the fold of the wrist).
Distal points: LR 6 (meridian relation, to move Qi).
Control points/symptomatic points: SP 3 (function circle), SP 6 (function circle), GB 34 (master point of tendons).

Microsystem acupuncture

Ear: representation of the hand/wrist in the scapha.
YNSA: inferior area of the C zone (base point).

Kiiko Matsumoto acupuncture

- For pain in the area of HT 8: HT 3 and HT 4 ipsilaterally.
- For pain in the area of PC 8: PC3 and PC 5 ipsilaterally.

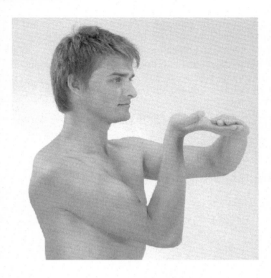
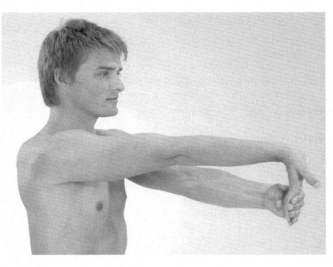

Psychosomatics/relaxation

Strain at work ('can't get hold of anything any more'), 'progressive muscle relaxation'.

29.10.7 Recommendations for the patient

Autostretching

- Maximum extension of wrist with flexed elbow and hold extension with resistance.
- Bring only the metacarpophalangeal joint in extension or hyperextension.
- Then extension by extending the elbow.

Additional measures

- Strengthening and at the same time trains coordination (power ball, Qigong balls).
- For craftspeople training to use the non-dominant hand.

29.11 HAND AND FINGER FLEXORS IN THE FOREARM

29.11.1 Anatomy

Innervation
- M. flexor carpi radialis: median nerve (brachial plexus, infraclavicular part).
- M. flexor carpi ulnaris: median nerve (brachial plexus, infraclavicular part).
- M. flexor digitorum superficialis: median nerve (brachial plexus, infraclavicular part).

- M. flexor digitorum profundus: ulnar nerve for the ulnar part, median nerve for the radial part (brachial plexus, infraclavicular part).
- M. flexor pollicis longus: median nerve (brachial plexus, infraclavicular part).
- M. pronator teres: anterior interosseus nerve (median nerve, brachial plexus, infraclavicular part).

Origin
- M. flexor carpi radialis: medial epicondyle of the humerus, antebrachial fascia.
- M. flexor carpi ulnaris:
  - head of the humerus: medial epicondyle of humerus, intermuscular septum of brachii mediale,
  - head of the ulna: olecranon, posterior border of the ulna (upper two-thirds), antebrachial fascia.
- M. flexor digitorum superficialis
- Humeroulnar head: medial epicondyle of the humerus, coronoid process.
- Head of the radius: anterior facet of radius (distal to the pronator teres muscle).
- M. flexor digitorum profundus: anterior face of the ulna (proximal two thirds), interosseous membrane.
- M. flexor pollicis longus:
  - head of the humerus: medial epicondyle of the humerus,
  - head of the radius: anterior facet of the radius (distal to the radial tuberosity).
- M. pronator teres: anterior border of the ulna (distal quarter).

Insertion
- M. flexor carpi radialis: palmar surface of the base of the second metacarpal bone (frequently III as well).

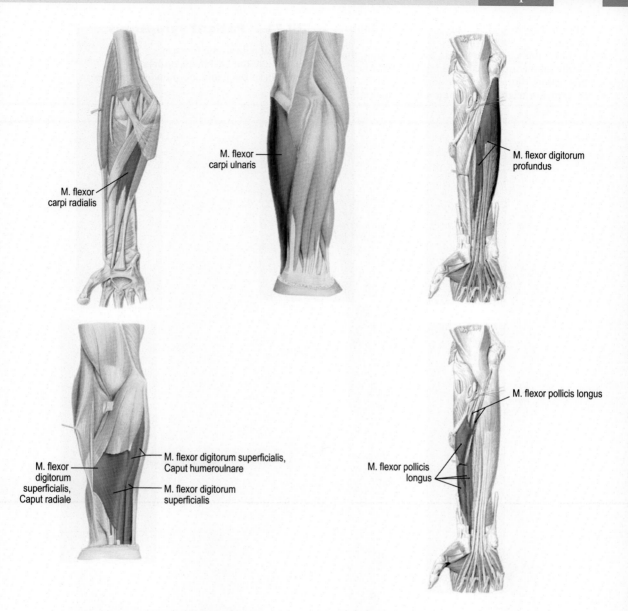

M. flexor carpi ulnaris

M. flexor carpi radialis

M. flexor digitorum profundus

M. flexor digitorum superficialis, Caput humeroulnare

M. flexor digitorum superficialis, Caput radiale

M. flexor digitorum superficialis

M. flexor pollicis longus

M. flexor pollicis longus

- M. flexor carpi ulnaris: pisiform bone, base of metacarpal bone V and hamate bone (over pisometacarpal and pisohamate ligament).
- M. flexor digitorum superficialis: with four long tendons at the bases of the middle phalanges of the second to fifth fingers.
- M. flexor digitorum profundus: base of the distal phalanx of second to fifth fingers.
- M. flexor pollicis longus: base of the distal phalanx of the thumb.
- M. pronator teres: border and anterior facet of the radius.

Function
- M. flexor carpi radialis: elbow joint: flexion, pronation, wrist: palmar flexion, radial abduction.
- M. flexor carpi ulnaris: elbow joint: flexion, wrist: palmar flexion, ulnar abduction.
- M. flexor digitorum superficialis: elbow joint: flexion, wrist: palmar flexion, ulnar abduction, proximal phalanges (second to fifth fingers): flexion, adduction, proximal phalanges (second to fifth): flexion.
- M. flexor digitorum profundus: wrist: palmar flexion, proximal phalanges (second to fifth): flexion,

387

adduction, proximal phalanges (second to fifth): flexion.

- M. flexor pollicis longus: wrist: palmar flexion, thumb saddle joint (carpometacarpal joint): adduction, opposition, thumb joints: flexion.
- M. pronator teres: radioulnar joints: pronation.

29.11.2 Patient symptoms

- Local pain in the forearm.
- Pain at the lateral epicondyle.
- Pain in the palm and individual fingers.

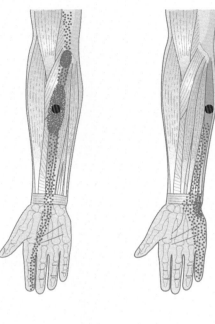

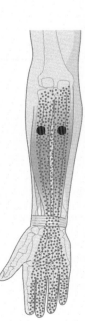
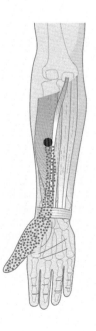
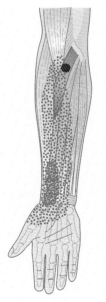
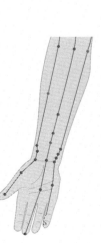

- Ulnar nerve signs of compression: M. flexor carpi ulnaris, M. flexor digitorum superficialis and profundus.
- Median nerve signs of compression: M. pronator teres, M. flexor digitorum superficialis.

29.11.3 Trigger points

mTrP	LOCATION	RADIATION	mTrP→ ACUPUNCTURE POINT
1	M. flexor carpi radialis	Local, palm, index finger, fold of wrist (radially pronounced), medial epicondyle, rarely upper arm towards the ulna	LU 6
2	M. flexor carpi ulnaris	Ulnar forearm, ulnar margin of hand and little finger V	–
3	M. flexor digitorum superficialis	Local, depending on affected muscle parts 1–2 fingers (second to fifth fingers), slight distal radiation	–
4	M. flexor digitorum profundus	Local, depending on affected muscle parts 1–2 fingers (second to fifth fingers), slight distal radiation	–
5	M. flexor pollicis longus	Local, radial forearm, ball of thumb, thumb	PC 6
6	M. pronator teres	Almost whole forearm as far as ball of hand	HT 3

mTrPs in the hand and finger flexors of the forearm lie predominantly in the middle area of the upper half of the forearm.

29.11.4 Diagnosis

Questioning: repetitive work with scissors (fabric, garden, etc.)?

Physical examination

- Elbow maximally flexed, forearm supinated, wrist and fingers extended, i.e. the patient looks at the medial surface of the hand in this position.
- Slowly extend elbow so that the therapist's hand remains on the medial surface of the hand and prevents lifting of the extension in the wrist and fingers.
- Finger extension test: patient places the fingertips of both hands together then brings the palms together so that the forearms are in a horizontal line.

Technical examination: if there is any evidence of neuropathy: nerve conduction speed.

29.11.5 Specific aspects

- Compression syndrome of ulnar nerve (M. flexor carpi ulnaris, M. flexor digitorum profundus) and median nerve (M. pronator teres).
- Examination of cervical spine for radiculopathy, function disorders in movement segment and muscle function chain.
- The scalene muscles radiate in a similar pattern.

29.11.6 Therapy

Instructions for manual trigger point therapy

- Direct treatment of the superficial finger and hand flexors.
- Indirect treatment of the deep layers of the finger flexors (part of the M. flexor digitorum superficialis and the M. flexor digitorum profundus) through the muscles of the superficial layer.
- The pronator teres muscle is the first definitely round muscle belly of the group of flexors distal to the biceps tendon; definitely perceptible during active pronation at the end of the range of movement.
- The median nerve runs between the ulnar and humeral head of the pronator teres muscle runs (can lead to entrapment, pronator teres syndrome).
- The ulnar nerve runs between the ulnar and humeral part of the M. flexor carpi ulnaris (can lead to entrapment, cubital tunnel syndrome).

Extension

- Patient in supine position (extension also possible while seated).
- Elbow flexed, wrist dorsally extended, fingers extended.
- The elbow is supported by one of the therapist's hands.
- The either hand holds the wrist in maximum dorsal extension.
- Extension by extending the elbow joint.

- During extension of the M. flexor digitorum superficialis and profundus hand in neutral position:
  - for extension of the M. flexor carpi ulnaris wrist in radial abduction,
  - for extension of the M. flexor carpi radialis extend in ulnar abduction.

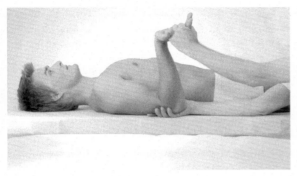

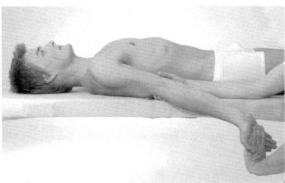

Physical procedures

Soft laser, shock waves, TENS contralaterally.

Infiltration techniques/dry needling

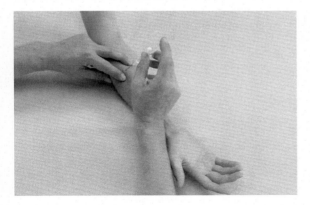

- Easy access with the two-finger protection technique.
- M. flexor digitorum and M. flexor pollicis lie deep.
- After treatment, spread and extend the muscles!

Classical Chinese acupuncture

Local and locoregional points (also contralateral): HT 4, SI 3, SI 5, SI 7, PC 4, PC 5, PC 6, PC 7, LU 5, Ex-AH 2, Ex-AH 9 (Baxie), TH 5, TH 9.
Distal points: LR 3, LR 6 (meridian relation, to move Qi).
Control points/symptomatic points: SP 3 (function circle), SP 6 (function circle), GB 34 (master point of tendons), ST 36 (move Qi).

Microsystem acupuncture

Ear: representation of the hand/wrist in the scapha.
YNSA: inferior area of the C zone (base point).

Kiiko Matsumoto acupuncture

M. flexor carpi ulnaris:
- if there is a neurological cause: CV 12 and CV 10,
- for tenderness in the area of HT 7: exact location and needling of KI 27, needling angle 10° in the direction of the sternoclavicular joint.

M. flexor carpi radialis:
- if there is a neurological cause: CV 12 and CV 10,
- for pressure pain in the area of ST 12 selection of following points: KI 16 (needling angle 45° in the direction of the navel), CV 15 (over the xiphoid at an angle of 10° in the direction of the sternum, sometimes also in the direction of the affected M. scalenus), LU 8 (needling angle 10–15° in the direction LU 9).

Mm. flexores digitorum superficialis and profundus:
- TH 16 ipsilateral and/or ST 26 on the right,
- TH 22 ipsilateral.

M. flexor pollicis longus (M. pronator teres): for tenderness in the area of LU 10: LU 5 and LU 8 ipsilaterally.

29.11.7 Recommendations for the patient

Autostretching

- Wrist maximally extended and kept in extension with resistance (above left).
- Then extension by extending the elbow (top left).
- Depending on whether the ulnar (below right) or radial part (below left) of the forearm flexors are to be extended, the position of the wrist can be altered.
- Carefully trying out of the optimum extension position is crucial.

Additional measures

- Strengthens and at the same time trains coordination (power ball, Qigong balls).

- Use arm rests to position the hand and forearm.
- Regular extension by the patient is easy and effective.
- Ergotherapy.

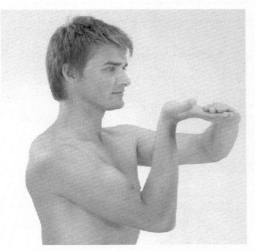
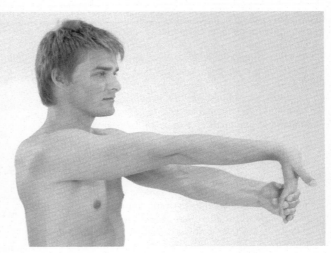

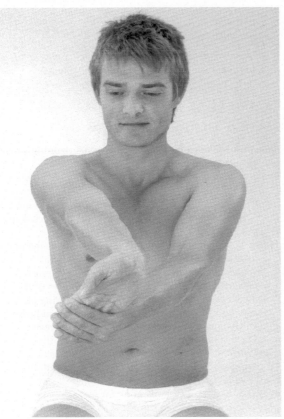
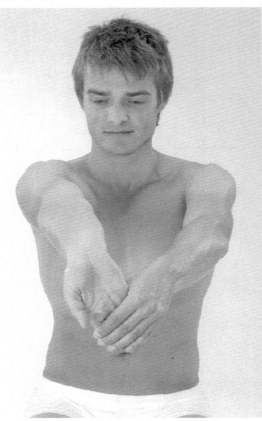

29.12 M. ADDUCTOR AND OPPONENS POLLICIS

29.12.1 Anatomy

Innervation
- M. adductor pollicis: deep branch of ulnar nerve (brachial plexus, infraclavicular part).
- M. opponens pollicis: median and ulnar nervea (brachial plexus, infraclavicular part).

Origin
- M. adductor pollicis: oblique head: capitate bone and base of the second metacarpal, radiate carpal ligament; transverse head: palmar surface of the base of the third metacarpal bone.
- M. opponens pollicis: flexor retinaculum, tubercle of trapezium bone.

Insertion
- M. adductor pollicis: ulnar sesamoid bone of the metacarpophalangeal joint of the thumb, ulnar border of the base of the proximal phalanx of the thumb radiating into the so-called dorsal aponeurosis of the thumb.

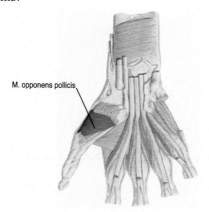

M. opponens pollicis

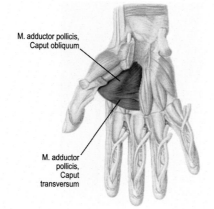

M. adductor pollicis, Caput obliquum

M. adductor pollicis, Caput transversum

- M. opponens pollicis: whole length of the radial border of the metacarpal bone.

Function
- M. adductor pollicis: palmar flexion, carpometacarpal joint of the thumb: adduction, opposition, metacarpophalangeal joint of the thumb: flexion.
- M. opponens pollicis: carpometacarpal joint of the thumb: adduction, opposition.

29.12.2 Patient symptoms

- Dull pain, predominantly due to strain.
- Fine motor function interplay disturbed between the thumb and the index finger.
- Preliminary diagnosis: rhizarthrosis, tendovaginitis stenosans (de Quérvain).

29.12.3 Trigger points

mTrP	LOCATION	RADIATION	mTrP→ ACUPUNCTURE POINT
1	In the M. adductor pollicis	Radial and volar side of the thumb	LI 4
2	In the M. opponens pollicis	Radial and volar side of the thumb, volar wrist	LU 10

29.12.4 Diagnosis

Questioning: thumb strain when writing, painting, sewing, gardening?

Physical examination
- Painful, clumsy pinch grip:
  - M. opponens pollicis; movement of the thumb in the direction of the fingertips 4 and 5 restricted and/or painful,
  - M. adductor pollicis: thumb adduction to the index finger painful against resistance.
- Palpation in relaxed pronation position in pinch grip: transverse course of fibres, lengthwise fibres of the interosseus dorsalis I muscle lie above during dorsal palpation, during ventral palpation of the adductor pollicis muscle and the M. flexor pollicis brevis.
- When examining both sides be aware that the dominant hand is always somewhat stronger.
- Snapping thumb: extension of the flexed thumb is difficult (blocking in flexion position).
- Examination of cervical spine for radiculopathy, function disorders in movement segment and muscle function chain.

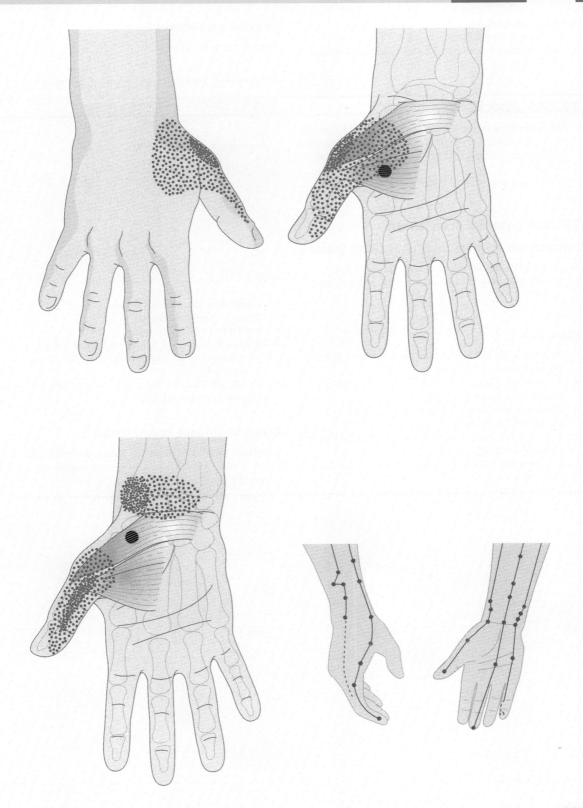

Technical examination

- Imaging if arthritis is suspected.
- Neurological examination if carpal tunnel syndrome is suspected.

29.12.5 Specific aspects

- M. scalenii, M. brachialis, M. supinator and M. extensor carpi radialis can also radiate into the radial wrist fold and the interdigital space between thumb and index finger.
- mTrPs are frequently linked to Heberden's nodes.

29.12.6 Special treatment

Instructions for manual trigger point therapy

- M. adductor pollicis: treatment with pinch grip.
- M. opponens pollicis: treatment with finger pressure technique.

Extension

- The therapist holds the four fingers of the patient's affected hand with one hand.
- The thumb of the other hand extends the patient's thumb in a dorsal direction.
- Extension also by spreading the index finger and thumb of the therapist's hand.
- For extension of the M. adductor pollicis radial traction (hyperabduction).
- For extension of the M. opponens pollicis dorsal traction.

Physical procedures

Laser therapy, shock waves.

Infiltration techniques/dry needling

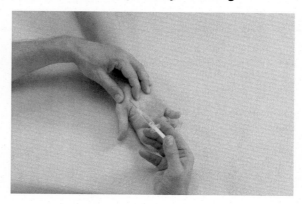

- Forearm lies on table or bench.
- Thumb slightly abducted.
- Muscles in pinch grip.
- Palmar approach for the M. opponens pollicis (needling close to acupuncture point LU 10; see photograph).
- Dorsal approach for the M. adductor pollicis (needling close to acupuncture point LI 4).

Classical Chinese acupuncture

Local and locoregional points (also contralateral): LI 3, LI 4, LI 5, LU 9, LU 10, Ex-AH 9 (Baxie), possible pericardial points (PC 4–PC 7).

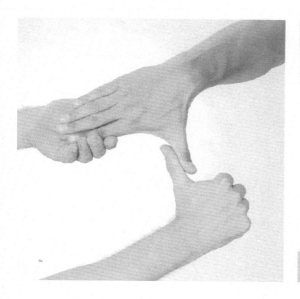

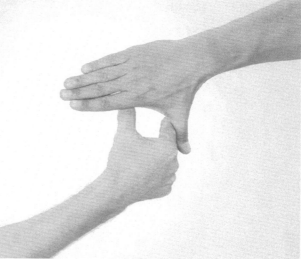

Distal points: segmental, paravertebral points in the area C6–T1 (two finger widths next to the spinous process as for the classical bladder points, medial branch), find analogous points in the area of the big toe (area LR 3 to SP 3).

Control points/symptomatic points: GB 34 (master point of the tendons), ST 36 (Qi move); spleen points if the function circle is affected e.g. SP 6, to move the blood in the case of blood stasis (localised stabbing pain): BL 17, BL 20, SP 6, SP 10, LR 2.

Microsystem acupuncture

Ear: representation of the hand/wrist in the scapha.
YNSA: inferior area of the C zone (base point).

Kiiko Matsumoto acupuncture

For tenderness at LU 10 (Japanese): LU 5 and LU 8 ipsilateral. If tendons are involved: LR 8 ipsilateral and GB 34 contralateral.

Psychosomatics/relaxation

'Tension in the detail', 'excessive hair-splitting' or 'holding at arm's length' (i.e. evaluation of to what extent compulsive behaviour could play a role in the stress).

29.12.7 Recommendations for the patient

Autostretching

- Self-treatment (also required for trigger point therapists!).
- Fingers extended.

- Thumb in extension.
- For M. adductor pollicis: radial traction with the other hand on the thumb (hyperabduction).
- For M. opponens pollicis: place thumbs and index finger pads of both hands against each other, then spread thumbs and index fingers to maximum and press against each other.

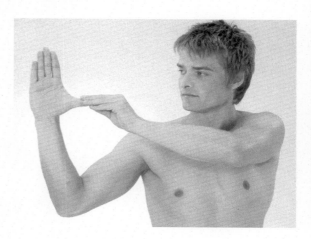

Additional measures

- Regularly have a break from fine motor function work (maximum 10 min); take a short break with extension and/or 'shake out the hands'.
- Coordination training of the hand and strengthen at the same time (e.g. Qigong balls, power ball).

Chapter | 30 |

Thoracic spine and thorax

Dominik Irnich

30.1 FUNCTIONAL ASSOCIATIONS

Compared to the neighbouring cervical spine and lumbar spine, the thoracic spine represents a less mobile, more stable structure. This is because the thoracic spine has a bony connection to the sternum via the ribs, to form the thorax. It encloses the thoracic cavity and because of the domed shape of the diaphragm, the upper part of the abdominal cavity as well.

The thorax and the thoracic spine form the stable part of the trunk (i.e. the more secure centre of the neighbouring areas of the vertebral column, allowing them great mobility). They also offer protection to the heart and lungs. Breathing would not be possible without the firmly delineated, but still mobile, bony framework of the thorax.

As the thoracic spine is built on the lumbar spine, it has to balance out any muscular malposition or bony deformities in order to create as good a base as possible for the cervical spine and the head, especially the level of the eyes.

- If there is pronounced lumbar lordosis, there is therefore appropriate compensatory thoracic kyphosis.
- If there is scoliosis or scoliotic malposture caused by a scoliotic pelvis and/or muscular imbalance in the lumbar spine area, there is normally an appropriate balancing contraconvex curvature in the thoracic spine area.

Because of the mechanics of the vertebral column, this also leads to a rotation component, visible in maximum flexion as one-sided buckling of the ribs.

These malpostures or deformities in the thoracic spine are transferred to the whole thorax, including the transitions from the ribs to the sternum, and lead to appropriate compensation here as well. These changes to the thoracic spine/thoracic space do not just directly affect the neighbouring structures such as the cervical spine, upper arms and lumbar spine:

- there is a direct connection to the pelvis via various muscles (Mm. latissimus dorsi, quadratus lumborum and abdominal muscles),
- via the M. psoas even to the thigh and via the muscles of the neck region (including Mm. trapezius and sternocleidomastoideus, both innervated by the accessory nerve) to the head region.

Respiration is the central function of the thorax and this means that all the thoracic muscles, including the so-called accessory respiratory muscles, have an essential function (the usually included Mm. scaleni are for example not accessory muscles but take part in normal respiration, as they initiate inspiration). As with all muscles, disorders are demonstrated in the form of taut bands, which are easily treated via the relevant mTrPs.

Shallow breathing is widespread (including in those with bronchial asthma) and is often partly caused by and exacerbated by contracted, overtaxed Mm. scaleni. As with contraction of the M. pectoralis minor, this can lead to thoracic outlet syndrome as a result of entrapment (see Section 30.3). Shallow breathing is often caused by chronic stress with strain and overtaxing ('holding your breath'), which also leads to tense abdominal muscles. The latter can also be caused by back pain. The restricted abdominal respiration also leads to shallow breathing.

30.2 PSYCHOSOMATIC ASSOCIATIONS

The thoracic spine/thoracic region is the human 'sensitive' centre. We feel our strongest sensations in the 'chest' – especially joy, inspiration and love ('my heart is open', 'I could embrace the whole world') – and, in contrast,

http://dx.doi.org/10.1016/B978-0-7020-4312-3.00030-1

anxiety (pressure on the chest, tightness, shutting down, protecting oneself). Rage can also create pressure here (rising from the abdomen), often with a sensation of internal pressure to 'bursting point' (see Ch. 12). However, it is usually expressed as sadness here.

The heart and lungs enable us to breathe and to distribute oxygenated blood throughout the body as far as each individual cell. In healthy people, the thoracic cavity feels wide. With deep breathing (e.g. Stanislav Grof's 'holotropic breathing', corresponding to hyperventilation) or at rest after intensive sport, a feeling of liveliness (Qi) flows like fresh oxygen through the whole body, and can even be sensed as a slight vibration. Instead of protecting ourselves by means of (partial) withdrawal, being mistrustful, we are 'in the moment', 'in the world' and 'open-hearted'. This can be seen in an upright, open posture: the thoracic spine and the thorax somatically have a key part in this, showing us the position of the person in their world. Because of its function as the respiratory centre, the thorax enables us to interact continuously with the environment and underlines its communicative component, along with body language.

In Eastern cultures (in the form of Chakras) as well as in the West a key position is allocated to the heart. Even in Western medicine, we have long known that pain in the heart is not just to do with reduced coronary perfusion. The symptoms often correlate more with things which affect the heart either acutely or chronically.

The thorax as centre of the body also expresses a great deal about the flexibility of a person, who may seem stiff and rigid or mobile and dynamic.

Notes on the association of posture with certain topics and patterns

Definite kyphosis of the thoracic spine, which reflects a physically 'depressed' posture, can be produced, for example, by psychological, or more commonly spiritual burdens, usually resting on the shoulders. The curvature can also resemble a protective shell expressing a kind of defence against kindness or a posture of frustration.

A collapsed posture, especially with drooping shoulders, usually suggests sorrow. Grief may be stored as a feeling of doubt or senselessness in mTrPs of the Mm. pectorales. In terms of body language, people with a slumped chest and who are withdrawn seldom appear sincere. This depressive, withdrawn posture can be associated with internal protest: 'switched off'.

An extended posture points upwards; that is, contact with the ground is more difficult. This 'elevated' state often reflects excessive self-confidence or arrogance, compensating for a feeling of insecurity or worthlessness.

An upright body posture reflects sociability, alertness, clarity and presence. It allows for flexible and fast reaction to appropriate external stimuli.

30.3 SYMPTOMS

The possible symptoms of myofascial disorders of the thoracic spine and thorax derive predominantly from functional anatomy and the neurophysiological and partly also empirical associations (see above), as follows.

- Painful tension of the trunk and back muscles (pain quality often dull and oppressive but sometimes stabbing).
- Limited mobility ('stiff chest') with effects on respiration and awareness of life: often affecting mobility of the shoulder and neck area. If there is any asymmetry, the patient feels that the restriction is worse.
- mTrPs of the muscles of the thoracic spine and the chest muscles usually have a locoregional referral pattern. The Mm. scaleni, subclavius and serratus posterior superior can, however, radiate well into the arms. Consider the functional and muscle associations behind and in front, beyond segmental referral.
- Radiation into the arms with position-dependent paraesthesia of unknown cause in the hands can be caused by entrapment of the fascicle of the brachial plexus (thoracic outlet syndrome) (Mm. scaleni and pectoralis minor).
- The rather loose posture with hyperkyphosis of the thoracic spine, retraction of the head with increased cervical spine lordosis and head hanging down in front of the shoulders (Brügger's 'sternosymphysal strain') is very common and can have wide-reaching effects on the whole body:
  - neck pain and headaches (including all the neck muscles including the suboccipital muscles, M. sternocleidomastoideus, M. scaleni; see Ch. 27),
  - shoulder pain – unfavourable spatial position of the scapula caused by contraction of the Mm. pectorales, etc. – leads to strain of the shoulder levators (M. trapezius pars descendens and M. levator scapulae) and the glenoid cavity (leading to strain of the shoulder muscles affecting all the arm muscles),
  - lumbar spine symptoms (including autochthonous back muscles, M. quadratus lumborum, M. psoas; see Ch. 32),
  - gluteal and iliosacral pain (gluteal muscles and referral to the Mm. longissimus thoracis, quadratus lumborum and rectus abdominis; iliosacral area and psoas muscle),
  - pubic bone symptoms (abdominal muscles, with the tuber pubicum as inferior insertion of the transverse abdominal muscles is an indicator: palpate for tenderness and possibly infiltrate and treat the mTrPs),
  - anterior/lateral thigh pain (M. iliopsoas, M. quadratus lumborum),

- posture-dependent chest pain (usually caused by the left M. pectoralis major: treat the thoracic spine as well),
- restricted respiration (affected by the accessory respiratory muscles).

Note: other causes of these symptoms must be ruled out, especially serious disorders of the organs of the chest such as a visceromuscular reflex arc.

Many symptoms that may be initially provoked in other regions can be indirectly caused by disorders in the thoracic spine or the chest area (for more precise distinction of vertebral column syndromes see Sections 14.1.4 and 14.2).

30.4 DIAGNOSTIC AND THERAPEUTIC CONSIDERATIONS

mTrPs in the area of the chest/thoracic spine can be found at least to some extent in everyone. The development of mTrPs in this area is predominantly caused by poor posture (see above).

mTrPs often occur as a reflex response. For example, diseases of the respiratory tract such as bronchial asthma or chronic bronchitis (especially autochthonous back muscles and accessory respiratory muscles), cardiac problems (especially in the area of the Mm. intercostales, rhomboidei and pectoralis) and gastrointestinal pain (especially the abdominal muscles) can provoke myofascial disorders via segmental or muscular associations. Structural changes in bordering areas can also affect the formation of mTrPs in the chest/thoracic spine; for example, the occurrence of a hernia in the abdominal area can provoke symptoms and mTrPs in the area of the lower ribs via a disorder of the abdominal muscles.

If symptoms occur in the area of the chest/thoracic spine, an appropriate functional examination of the whole vertebral column, pelvis and extremities is essential so that any causative or compensatory disorders are not overlooked. Treatment should also take the whole body into account.

Breathing can be positively affected by all mTrPs of the thoracic muscles: the M. pectoralis major is particularly interesting here. We have often found that patients spontaneously report that their breathing has improved after treatment of thoracic outlet syndrome via mTrPs of the Mm. scaleni (and pectoralis minor).

The diaphragm cannot be directly reached. Treatment can be performed via the paravertebral mTrPs of segments C4 (associated with tense neck) and T7.

30.5 EXAMINATION FOR TRIGGER POINT IDENTIFICATION

EXAMINATION FINDINGS	SEARCH FOR mTrPs IN
(Passive) thoracic spine flexion limited or painful or (active) straightening up painful	Back extensors (see Section 30.6)
Limited lateral movement	Thoracic autochthonic back extensors and contralateral abdominal muscles
Pain in the anterior intercostal region	Mm. intercostales, M. pectoralis (Sections 30.7 and 30.8), M. serratus anterior (Section 30.11), abdominal muscles
Pain in the posterior intercostal region	M. intercostales, M. serratus anterior (Section 30.11), M. serratus posterior inferior (Section 30.12), M. obliquus externus abdominis (Section 31.7), M. latissimus dorsi (Section 28.10)
Pain on inspiration – distinguish depending on location	M. pectoralis minor (Section 30.8), M. scaleni (Section 27.11), M. serratus posterior superior and anterior (Sections 30.10 and 30.11), Mm. intercostales externi, Mm. levatores costarum
Pain on expiration	Abdominal muscles (especially M. rectus abdominis), M. intercostales interni and intimi, M. serratus posterior inferior (Section 30.12), M. retractor costae, M. transversus thoracis, M. subcostalis; also note M. quadratus lumborum (Section 32.7)

Besides the functional examination, it is essential to the diagnosis of mTrPs to perform a thorough deep palpation of the cervical spine and shoulder muscles, buttocks and abdominal and lumbar spine muscles (Figure 30.1).

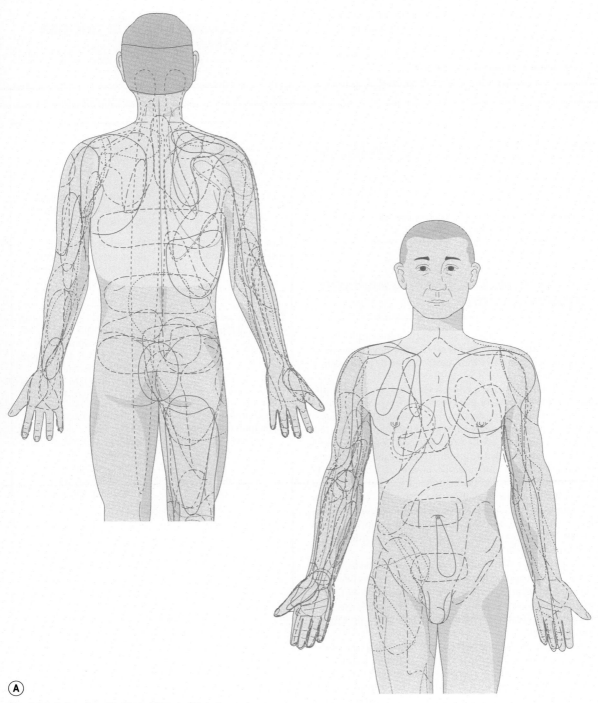

Ⓐ

Fig. 30.1 Pain referral pattern (a) and affected muscles

Continued

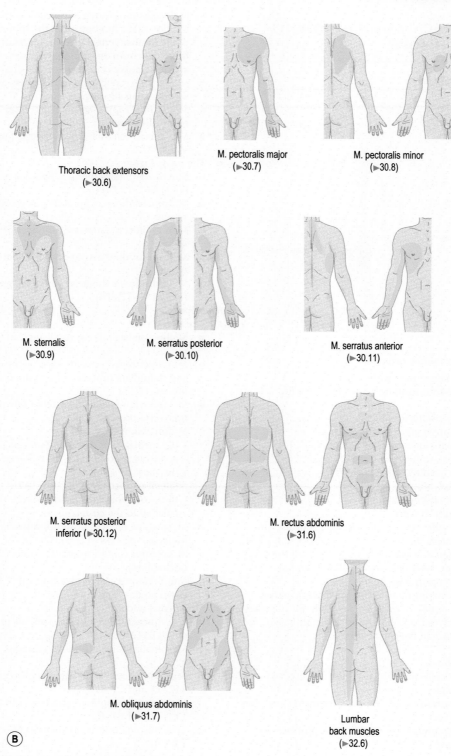

Thoracic back extensors
(▶30.6)

M. pectoralis major
(▶30.7)

M. pectoralis minor
(▶30.8)

M. sternalis
(▶30.9)

M. serratus posterior
(▶30.10)

M. serratus anterior
(▶30.11)

M. serratus posterior
inferior (▶30.12)

M. rectus abdominis
(▶31.6)

M. obliquus abdominis
(▶31.7)

Lumbar
back muscles
(▶32.6)

(B)

Fig. 30.1—cont'd (b) of the thoracic spine and thorax.

30.6 THORACIC AUTOCHTHONOUS BACK EXTENSORS

30.6.1 Anatomy

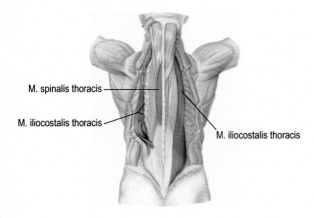

M. spinalis thoracis

M. iliocostalis thoracis

M. iliocostalis thoracis

The Mm. erector spinae comprise:

- superficial, lateral tract with:
  - muscle bands running vertically, in the thoracic area:
    – M. iliocostalis thoracis,
    – Mm. intertransversarii thoracis,
    – M. longissimus cervicis,
    – M. longissimus thoracis;
  - muscles running transversely:
    – Mm. splenii,
    – Mm. levatores costarum;
- deep medial tract with:
  - the vertically running muscles bands of the Mm. interspinales thoracis and the M. spinalis thoracis,
  - running in a diagonal superior direction the deep-lying Mm. rotatores, Mm. multifidii and M. semispinalis thoracis.

Innervation: posterior branches of the thoracic nerves (M. iliocostalis thoracis), posterior and anterior branches of the spinal nerves (Mm. intertransversarii thoracis), posterior branches of the spinal nerves.

Origin
- The lateral tract:
  - M. iliocostalis thoracis: 12th–7th ribs medial to the costal angle,
  - Mm. intertransversarii thoracis: transverse processes of T12–T10,
  - M. longissimus cervicis: transverse processes of T6–T1 and C7–C3,

- M. longissimus thoracis: together with the M. iliocostalis lumborum of the spinous process of the lumbar vertebrae, dorsal facet of the sacrum, frequently from the mamillary process of L2 and L1 and the transverse process of C12–T6,
  - M. splenius cervicis: spinous process of T3–C6, supraspinous ligament,
  - M. splenius capitis: spinous processes of C3–C7, nuchal ligament,
  - Mm. levatores costarum: transverse processes of T11–C7.
- The medial tract:
  - Mm. interspinales thoracis: spinous processes of (T12) T11–T2 (T1),
  - M. spinalis thoracis: spinous processes of (T4) T3–T1 and C7–C6,
  - Mm. rotatores: transverse processes of the thoracic spine,
  - Mm. multifidi: transverse processes of the thoracic spine,
  - M. semispinalis thoracis: transverse processes of (T12) T11–T7 (T6).

Insertion
- The lateral tract:
  - M. iliocostalis thoracis: costal angle of (rib 6) rib 7–rib 1,
  - Mm. intertransversarii thoracis: accessory process and mamillary process of L1 to the transverse process of T11,
  - M. longissimus cervicis: posterior tuberculum of the transverse process of C5–C2,
  - M. longissimus thoracis:
    – the medial part: mamillary process of L5, accessory process of L4–L1, tranverse processes of the thoracic spine,
    – lateral part: costal process of L4–L1, thoracolumbar fascia (deep layer), rib 12–rib 2 (medial to the costal angle);
  - M. splenius cervicis: posterior tubercle of the transverse process of (C3) C2–C1,
  - M. splenius capitis: mastoid process (superior nuchal line),
  - Mm. levatores costarum: rib 12–rib 1 lateral to the costal angle.
- The medial tract:
  - Mm. interspinales thoracis: spinous processes of (T1) T12–T3 (T2),
  - M. spinalis thoracis: spinous processes of (T10) T9–T2,
  - Mm. rotatores: root of spinous processes of L3–L1, T12–T1 and C7–C2,
  - Mm. multifidi: spinous processes of L5–L12, T12–T1 and C7–C2,
  - M. semispinalis thoracis: spinous processes of (T4) T3–C6.

Function

- Bending to one side, bilateral extension of the vertebral column:
  - M. erector spinae,
  - M. iliocostalis thoracis,
  - Mm. intertransversarii thoracis,
  - M. longissimus cervicis,
  - M. longissimus thoracis,
  - M. spinalis thoracis.
- Bending to one side and rotation of the cervical spine and head to the same side, bilateral extension of the cervical spine: M. splenius cervicis, M. splenius capitis.
- Segmental extension: M. interspinalis thoracis.
- One-sided rotation, bilateral extension: M. semispinalis thoracis.
- One-sided rotation and lateral flexion, bilateral extension: Mm. rotatores and multifidi.
- Raising the ribs, leaning to the side and rotation of the vertebral column: Mm. levatores costarum.

30.6.2 Patient symptoms

- Stabbing and/or dull, pressing pain in the area of the thoracic spine.
- Chest tightness.
- Pain when sitting down for long periods.
- Non-specific preliminary diagnosis: degenerative vertebral column syndrome, segmental functional disorder (blockage), 'lumbago', 'slipped disc'.

30.6.3 Trigger points

It is not often possible to attribute the mTrP precisely to an individual muscle because of the complex anatomical and functional situation.

30.6.4 Diagnosis

Questioning
- Acute or repetitive strain?
- Trauma?
- Cold, draughts?
- For chronic back pain and predominantly somatic disease careful psychological evaluation is required (work, relationships)

Inspection
- Protective posture.
- Postural problems and asymmetry.
- Scoliosis, torsion.

Physical examination
- Examine the patient sitting on a couch or in a supine position.

- Painful restriction of movement, especially during flexion and/or rotation.
- Segmental functional examination.
- Kibler fold (skin-rolling test).
- Firm palpation (pressure): delimitation of mTrPs in the M. rhomboideus by precise palpation.

Technical examination
- Only use imaging if there is a good reason to suspect findings (back pain guidelines).
- Possibly to rule out coronary heart disease.

30.6.5 Specific aspects

- Many 'non-specific' types of back pain are caused by mTrPs.
- Scoliosis, torsion and many degenerative changes do not usually explain the extent of the symptoms, so patients should not fixate on these structural aspects (can lead to iatrogenic chronification).

> 'For every patient plagued by pain with pathological findings in X-rays, MRI or CT, there is someone with the same pathological findings who does not have any pain.' Overlooking psychosocial factors is not a trifling offence, it is a 'professional error'.

- Individual multimodal treatment plan for chronic pain.
- If the patient is under great and chronic strain refer the patient to a specialised interdisciplinary treatment unit for a multimodal treatment plan.

30.6.6 Therapy

Instructions for manual trigger point therapy

- When sitting, the thoracic parts of the lateral tract (M. iliocostalis and M. longissimus) are more active than the lumbar parts, so look for mTrPs appropriate to problems when sitting.
- If spinous processes are tender, the mTrPs are usually deep in the medial tract (Mm. semispinales, multifidi, rotatores).
- With mTrPs in the muscles of the medial tract the referred pain area is usually small and in the local surroundings so local treatment is necessary for lumbar pain.
- Treatment of the deep parts is strenuous so use aids (trigger point sticks) to relieve the fingers.

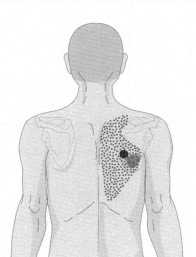

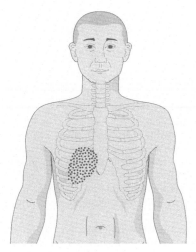

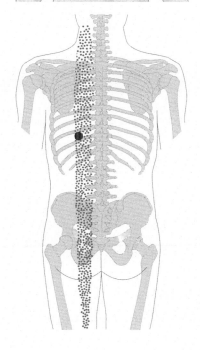

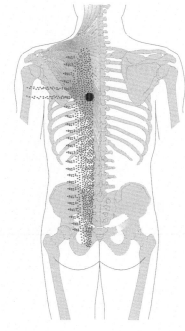

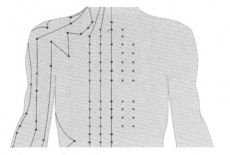

mTrP	LOCATION	RADIATION	MTRP→ ACUPUNCTURE POINT
1	M. iliocostalis thoracis (between the shoulder blade and the proc. spinosi, variable, but often in the area of BL 43 (T4)	Dorsally over all the muscles and ventrally	BL 13–BL 15, BL 42–BL 44
2	In the superficial lateral tract: multiple locations possible, predominantly close to the vertebral column approx. 4–5 finger widths next to the median line) in the M. longissimus cervicis thoracis and iliocostalis thoracis	Segmental, superiorly and inferiorly	Points on the inner and outer bladder meridian: BL 11–BL 21, BL 41–BL 50
3	In the deep medial part: multiple locations possible, close to the vertebral column (approx. 1–2 finger widths next to the median line) in the Mm. interspinalis and spinalis, Mm. rotatores, Mm. multifidi, Mm. semispinalis	Predominantly segmental	Extra-R 1 (Hua tuo jiaji) and inner bladder meridian (BL 11–BL 21)

Stretching

- It is not possible to stretch the individual muscles, only the whole tract.
- The patient sits on a chair and hunches their back like a cat.
- Allow the arms to hang down between the legs.
- The therapist's hands clasp the thoracic spine.
- Supporting the stretching with breathing techniques or postisometric relaxation techniques improves the success rate of the treatment.
- Stretching while seated with the legs fully extended is not ideal as it is predominantly the lumbar spine that is exercised.

Physical procedures

- Wraps and compresses, laser treatment, shock wave therapy, TENS.

Infiltration techniques/dry needling

- Treatment in prone position.
- If the patient is very tense, begin with contralateral superficial needling.
- In the thoracic area no deep filtration/needling lateral to the inner bladder meridian (**warning**: pneumothorax), tangential insertion here (photo, left).
- Depending on location and constitution long needles necessary (up to 8 cm), but maximum distance

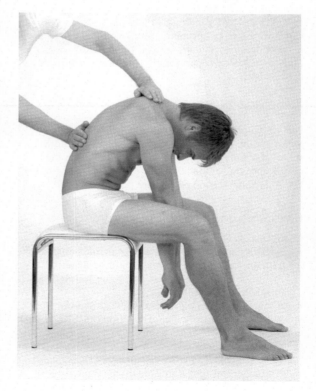

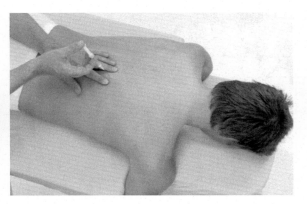

of 3 cm from the spinous process of the vertebral body (photo, right).
- Gentle segmental mobilisation following needling.
- Note respiratory excursions.

Classical Chinese acupuncture

Local and locoregional points (also contralateral): Extra-R 1 (Hua tuo jiaji), BL 11–BL 21, BL 41–BL 50, SI 6–SI 14 (choice depends on affected segments); Ashi points superficially in the segment (like a belt, Gleditsch's Very Point technique).
Distal points: BL 40, BL 58, BL 60, BL 62, SI 3, SI 6, GB 41, KI 3, Extra-AH 7 ('Yaotongdian'), SI 26.
Control points/symptomatic points: KI 3, KI 7, SP 6, heart and/or pericardial points, if the circle of function is affected, particularly if ventrally referred, tight feeling.

Microsystem acupuncture

Ear: vertebral column, sympathic ganglia, Shenmen, Jérôme point; points of the muscle zone of the thoracic spine representation (next to the anthelix fold in the direction of the antihelix).
YNSA: D zone; E zone of the base point.

Kiiko Matsumoto acupuncture

M. iliocostalis thoracis
- If the region around SP 3 is very painful on palpation, the distal points should be needled first; SP 5 and SP 9 (metal and water points) instead of SP 3.
- If there is a neurological cause: CV 12 and CV 10.
- With tenderness in the area of KI 2 (fire point), KI 7 (metal point) and KI 10 (water point) should be needled; the angle of the needle (especially at KI 7) should correlate with the release of pressure in the area KI 2.
- For tenderness in the area of GB 26 (Daimai): KI 7.

- For tenderness in the area of GB 25 (Mu point of the kidney): KI 7 and SP 9.
- For relief of pain in the area of the M. iliocostalis lumborum needling of points in the area of the navel (KI 16, CV 7, CV 9).
- If the patient is lying down, needling of a point 1 cm lateral to BL 40.

M. spinalis thoracis
- With tenderness in the area of the M. semispinalis thoracis at the level of T6–T9: PC 6 or (with tenderness at PC 8) PC 3 and PC 5.
- If the patient is standing BL 9 on both sides (diagonally or at a 45° angle).
- Hua tuo jiaji in the area of T10–T12 on both sides at an angle of 45° in the direction of the vertebral column.

M. semispinalis thoracis
- With tenderness at the level of T6–T9: PC 6 or (with tenderness at PC 8) PC 3 and PC 5,
- If the patient is standing: BL 59 on both sides (diagonally or at an angle of 45°),
- Hua tuo jiaji between T10 and T12, at an angle of 45° in the direction of the vertebral column,

Mm. intertransversarii thoracis
- If there are symptoms in the area between T1 and T3: Nagano's immune point 1 between LI 10 and LI 11.
- For symptoms in the area of T4: Hashimoto's eye point.
- For symptoms in the area of T7: BL 58 (insertion angle 15–45° with the flow of the meridian).
- For symptoms in the area of T9: ipsilateral (sometimes also both sides) BL 44 and/or BL 49 (insertion angle 115–45°, most painful site, with the flow of the meridian).
- For symptoms in the area of T12: SP 3 (insertion angle 45° with the flow of the meridian).

Psychosomatics/relaxation

- Psychosomatic aspects: anxiety, anxiety avoidance behaviour, work and/or social stress, bullying: a categorical denial of psychosomatic factors is often indicative.

- A tight feeling in the chest is often evidence of deep-seated anxiety and fear.
- Relaxation techniques can be individually selected depending on personal preferences. Give preference to techniques which also have physical benefits (Qigong, breathing therapy, Glaser psychotonics, etc.).
- Learning pain and stress management strategies.

30.6.7 Patient recommendations

Autostretching

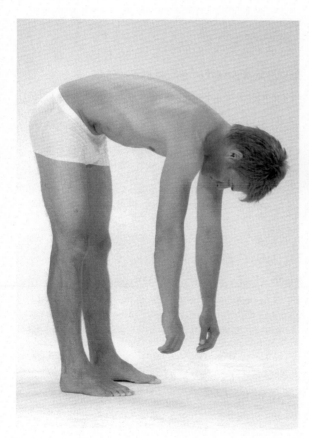

- Standing with legs straight.
- Bend upper body forwards, let arms hang down, lower head.
- Support with breathing and muscle relaxation technique.
- Depending on limitations to movement forwards and down or forwards to the side, gentle flexion to the side is also possible.

- Isolated stretching of individual muscle parts of the thoracic back extensors is almost impossible.

Additional measures

- Explanation and activation of the patient are key.
- Point out associations with psychosocial factors.
- Squeeze out mTrPs by lying on a tennis ball.
- Rhythm of daily life (interrupt long periods of sitting down, move about in between).
- Correct posture while sitting and standing.
- Orthopaedic correction only if body asymmetry is pronounced.
- Relaxed position while seated (support in the thoracolumbar transition).
- Ergonomics (work position, leisure activities).
- Functional training of the muscles (coordinative interplay of muscles and mobility training, build-up of strength is not the main thing); note: with standard back exercises there is a risk of acquiring a stereotypical behaviour pattern or strengthening the anxiety avoidance behaviour.
- Motivation of patient to take exercise.
- Design a home exercise programme as part of the physiotherapeutic treatment.

30.7 M. PECTORALIS MAJOR

30.7.1 Anatomy

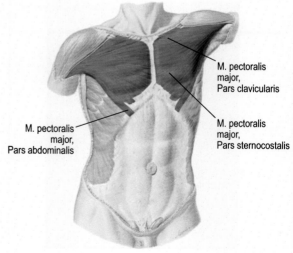

M. pectoralis major, Pars clavicularis

M. pectoralis major, Pars sternocostalis

M. pectoralis major, Pars abdominalis

Innervation: Nn. pectorales medialis and lateralis (plexus brachialis, pars infra-/supraclavicularis); the fibres converge to a broad tendon in the form of a flat pocket open at the top.

Origin

- Clavicular part: clavicle (sternal part).
- Pars sternocostalis: manubrium and corpus sterni, costal cartilage ribs 1–6.
- Pars abdominalis: rectus sheath (anterior layer).

Insertion: crest of the greater tubercle of the humerus.

Function

- Shoulder joint: adduction (particularly effective if the arms are lifted), medial rotation, clavicular part: anteversion.
- Pectoral girdle: lowering, anteversion.
- Thorax: lifting the sternum and widening the thorax (accessory muscles when breathing in deeply).

30.7.2 Patient symptoms

- Pain in the area of the thorax and the ulnar side of the upper extremities.
- Chest tightness.
- 'Heart pain'.
- Tension in the breast.
- Preliminary diagnosis: functional heart disease, tendinitis of the biceps tendon, intercostal neuralgia.

30.7.3 Trigger points

mTrP LOCATION		RADIATION	mTrP→ ACUPUNCTURE POINT
1	Clavicular part	Anterior shoulder, anterior chest (near the heart), upper arm, sometimes medial forearm	LU 1
2	Pars sternocostalis	Anterior chest (near heart), upper arm, forearm and as far as the ulnar fingers	ST 15

30.7.4 Diagnosis

Questioning

- Hyperabduction trauma?
- Lung disease with increased work on inspiration?

Inspection

- Shoulder protraction.
- Slumped sitting.

Physical examination

- Slight restriction especially on retroversion and/or elevation.
- Medial rotation against resistance can be painful.
- Weakness of the interscapular muscles.
- Examination in supine position with arms in various positions (range from abduction to elevation and lateral rotation) with concomitant muscle palpation.

Technical examination: if necessary, exclusion of cardiac or pulmonary disease.

30.7.5 Specific aspects

- The M. pectoralis is often secondarily affected with cardiac and pulmonary disease, e.g. prolonged pain following coronary infarction; however, it can also simulate relevant diseases.
- Longer existing shortening leads to strain of the M. trapezius (medial part) and the Mm. rhomboidei.
- Simons and Travell describe an arrhythmia mTrP in the M. pectoralis major below the fifth rib between the mamillary line and the sternum.

30.7.6 Therapy

Instructions for manual trigger point therapy

- Direct treatment of the mTrPs in the proximal fibre parts with pressure against the ribs (supine position with prestretching).
- Lateral fibres and distal fibre parts with pinch grip.
- Fascia separation technique to the anterior deltoid muscle.

Stretching

Patient in supine position:

- lateral scapular border on the edge of the bed, shoulder in abduction, retroversion, slight lateral rotation, unaffected arm in adduction and lateral rotation,
- keep hand next to patient at the appropriate origin:
  - clavicular part: clavicle (sternal part),
  - pars sternocostalis: manubrium and corpus sterni, costal cartilage ribs 1–6 (photo, top),
  - pars abdominalis: rectus sheath, (anterior layer), lower ribs;
- hand furthest from patient grasps forearm,

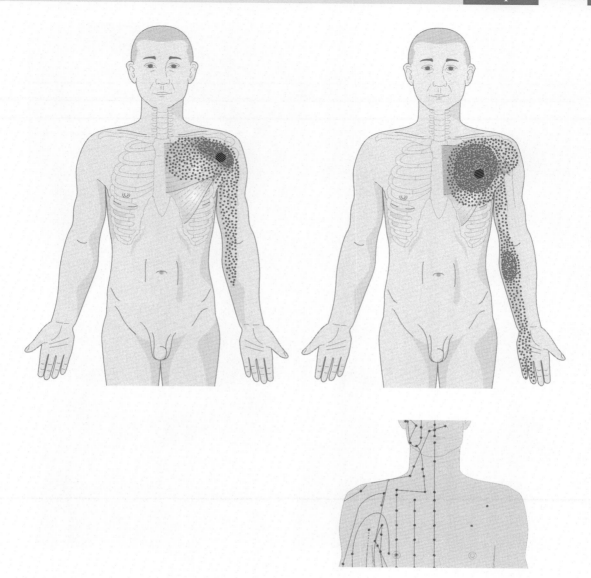

- stretch in the direction of lateral rotation and elevation depending on the affected muscle parts.

Stretching also possible while seated (photo, bottom):

- the therapist stands behind the patient,
- the holding position can be varied (e.g. for men and women).

Physical procedures

- Easily accessible for most procedures (note: pacemaker).

Infiltration techniques/dry needling

- Patient in supine position.
- Mobilise affected muscle parts in pinch grip.

- Infiltration/needling from anterior in direction of own finger.
- Treat medial parts strictly tangentially and vertically towards the ribs.

Classical Chinese acupuncture

Local and locoregional points (also contralateral): LU 1, ST 14, ST 15, ST 16, CV 18, KI 23, SP 9, PC 1, KI 22.

Distal points: ST 40 (meridian point, calms difficulty in breathing, calms the mind), ST 45 (meridian point, acute, generally calming).

Control points/symptomatic points: PC 6 (chest tightness, heart and/or pericardial points, if the circle of function is

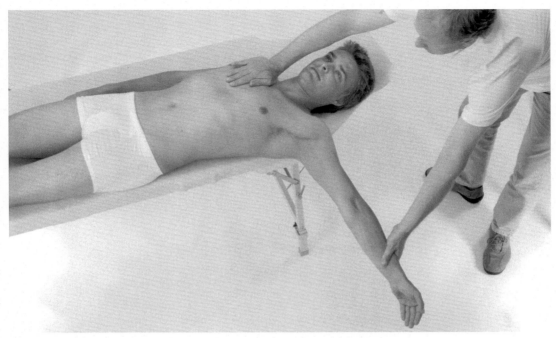

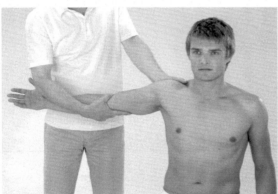

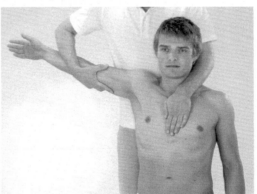

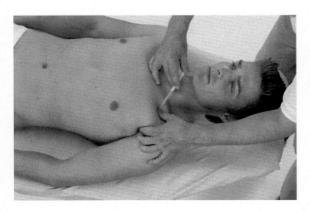

affected: tightness, psychosomatic disorders), LU 4 (widens the chest), CV 17.

Microsystem acupuncture

Ear: points of the muscle zone of the thoracic spine representation (next to the antihelix fold in the direction of the helix).
YNSA: E zone of the base point.

Kiiko Matsumoto acupuncture

- Symptoms in the area of the medial insertion: TH 9 and GB 40 (for slow or normal pulse) or TH and GB 41 (for fast pulse); PC 6 and SP 3 are other options.
- For symptoms in the sternal insertion area: PC 6 and SP 3.

- For symptoms in the lateral part of the muscle: LU 5 or LU 5 in combination with LU 8 ipsilaterally (particularly if palpation of LU 10 is painful); insertion angle 10–15°.
- For painful palpation of HT 8: HT 3 and HT 3 in combination with HT 5; insertion angle 10–15°.
- For painful palpation of PC 8: PC 3 and PC 5 instead of PC 6 to reduce pain at PC.

Psychosomatics/relaxation

- Anxiety in the sense of increased anxious tension or as expression of masked anxiety disease with right chest and external pressure.
- For anxious patients, the exclusion of cardiac or pulmonary disease can bring great relief and release therapeutic potential.

30.7.7 Recommendations for the patient

Autostretching

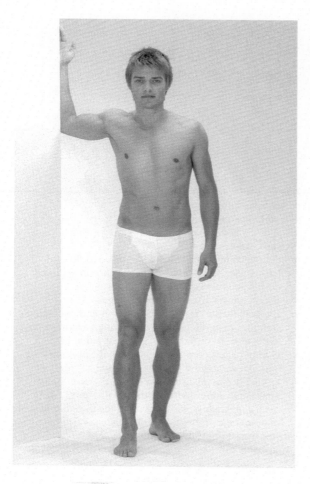

- A door frame is very suitable.
- Shoulder in 90° abduction.
- Flexion at the elbow.
- Elbow and hand are supported on the door frame.
- Stretch through rotation of the upper body to the opposite side.
- Vary level of abduction or elevation depending on the affected fibres to achieve optimum extension (trial and error).

Additional measures

- Regular stretching.
- Correct posture while sitting and standing (ergonomic check at workplace).
- Autotherapy is possible (directly with pressure against the ribs or with pinch grip).

30.8 M. PECTORALIS MINOR

30.8.1 Anatomy

Innervation: Nn. pectorales medialis and lateralis (plexus brachialis, pars infra-/supraclavicularis)
Origin: (2nd) 3rd–5th rib (close to the bone cartilage border).
Insertion: tip of the coracoid process of the scapula.
Function
- Pectoral girdle: lowering, anteversion.
- Thorax: lifting the upper ribs and widening the thorax (accessory muscles when breathing in deeply).

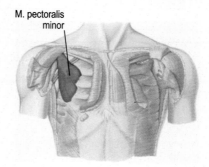

M. pectoralis minor

30.8.2 Patient symptoms

- Pain at the anterior shoulder and anterior upper chest area, sometimes worse on inspiration.
- Pain similar to precardiac and angina pectoris symptoms if the left side is affected.
- Possible preliminary diagnoses: radiculopathy C7/C8, thoracic outlet syndrome, tendinitis supraspinalis, epicondylopathy medialis (golfer's elbow).

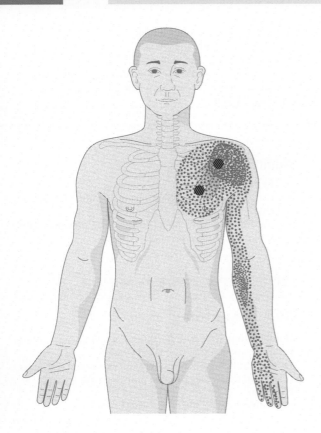

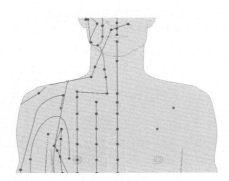

30.8.3 Trigger points

mTrP	LOCATION	RADIATION	mTrP↩ ACUPUNCTURE POINT
1	Close to origin at the 4th rib	Anterior chest, anterior shoulder	ST 15
2	Inferiorly from the coracoid process	Anterior chest, anterior shoulder, ulnar upper arm as far as the ulnar fingers	LU 1

30.8.4 Diagnosis

Questioning
- Fall on extended arm (pushing of the scapula in a dorsal direction)?
- Asthma?

- Use of walking aids?
- Posture when seated?
- Carrying a rucksack?

Inspection
- Shoulder protraction.
- Round shoulders.
- Women with large breasts who are wearing a bra.

Physical examination
- Retroversion limited with arm abducted 90°.
- Lifting the shoulders against resistance in supine position: weakness?
- Thoracoscapular articulation reduced.
- Hyperabduction test (lateral rotation and maximum elevation) as evidence of impingement syndrome: hypoaesthesia and disappearance of radial pulse.
- During palpation place the arm on the abdomen so that the M. pectoralis major is relaxed.
- Further differentiation of mTrPs in the Mm. pectoralis major and minor by the course of the fibres (taut band); pinch grip palpation using the thumb, index or middle finger deep in the axillary area is also possible.

Technical examination: with impingement syndrome use X-ray to rule out a neck rib or high 1first rib if a trial treatment does not produce any improvement.

30.8.5 Specific aspects

- Impingement syndrome with compression of the brachial plexus and the axillary artery; usually referred myofascial pain can be found in combination with neuropathic pain due to nerve compression or symptoms like a perfusion disorder.
- Frequently contraction caused by posture.
- Both pectoral muscles are often affected.
- With the M. trapezius pars ascendens the M. pectoralis minor forms an agonist/antagonist unit for lifting and lowering the shoulders, so this part of the M. trapezius should also be treated.

30.8.6 Specific treatment

Instructions for manual trigger point therapy

- Indirect treatment of mTrPs (from supine position) through the M. pectoralis major.
- Direct treatment of mTrPs below the M. pectoralis major (from supine position of lateral decubitus, shoulder protraction) with hand flat, fingertips under the axillary fold in the direction of the clavicle.
- With active depression of the scapula, palpation of the tense fibres of the M. pectoralis minor is easily possible.

Stretching

- Patient in the supine position.
- Scapula on the edge of the bed.
- Arm abducted 90°.
- Elbow flexed.
- Hand next to patient grasps the medial border of the scapula and pushes the scapula forwards.
- The hand away from the patient, lateral rotation of the arm which is abducted 90° and flexed at the elbow.

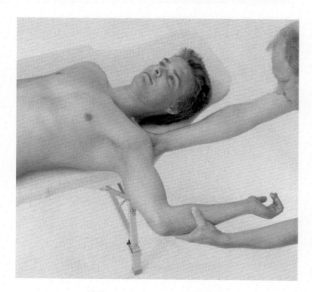

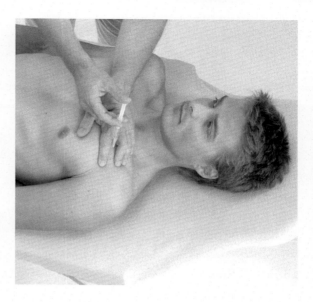

Physical procedures

- Most procedures can have a moderately deep effect.

Infiltration techniques/dry needling

- Patient in supine position.
- mTrP 1:
  - strong mobilisation of the muscle with index or middle finger in the deep axillary area as support,
  - angle of insertion tangentially into the muscle belly from medial to lateral and diagonally in a inferior direction (so that there is no danger of a pneumothorax).
- mTrP 2: mobilisation is not always possible here, so remain flat and tangential with angle of insertion 90° to the course of the ribs.

Classical Chinese acupuncture

Local and locoregional points (also contralateral): LU 1, LU 2, ST 15, KI 27, SI 14, SI 15, SP 20.
Distal points: LU 7, ST 38.
Control points/symptomatic points: for thoracic tightness: HT 5, HT 7, PC 6.

Microsystem acupuncture

Ear: points of the muscle zone of the thoracic spine representation (next to the antihelix fold in the direction of the helix).
YNSA: E zone of the base point.

Kiiko Matsumoto acupuncture

- HT 3 ipsilateral.
- For tenderness in the area of LU 10: LU 5 and LU 8.
- If LU 10 is not tender: LU 5.

Psychosomatics/relaxation

- Tight feeling, feeling of 'not wanting to be there' (see Ch. 12).
- Consider depression if the shoulders are lowered.
- Breathing therapy with widening.
- Self-assurance exercises: 'head back, chest out'.

30.8.7 Recommendations for the patient

Autostretching

- Patient stands at the table or at a window sill.
- Hand support at the back with arms extended.
- Stretch by lowering the body (e.g. bend knees).

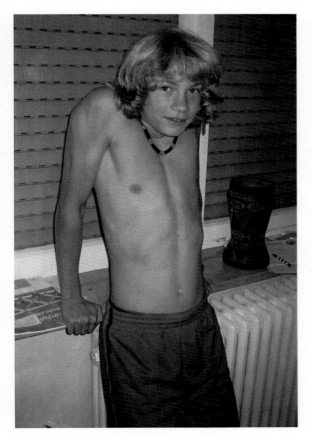

Additional measures

- Sit upright and lift shoulders (behind the head), lower the shoulders to correct posture (sitting, standing).
- Padding and weight distribution for bra wearers with large breasts.

30.9 M. STERNALIS

30.9.1 Anatomy

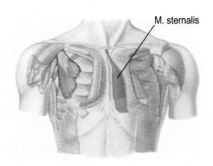

M. sternalis

The anatomy and course of the muscle can vary!

Innervation: branches of the pectoral nerves (brachial plexus, supraclavicular part) or intercostal nerves (thoracic nerves) (inconstant muscle about 5%).
Origin: sternal margin (on the fascia pectoralis).
Insertion: radiates into the fascia.
Function: contraction of the skin of the chest, tightens the fascia.

30.9.2 Patient symptoms

- Not dependent on motion, deep-seated sternal pain.
- This muscle rarely entertains retrosternal pain or causes symptoms similar to angina pectoris.

30.9.3 Trigger points

	mTrP LOCATION	RADIATION	mTrP→ ACUPUNCTURE POINT
1	Superficial sternal area, 2–3 finger widths next to the midline	Retrosternal, occasional anterior shoulder, ulnar upper arm	KI 24

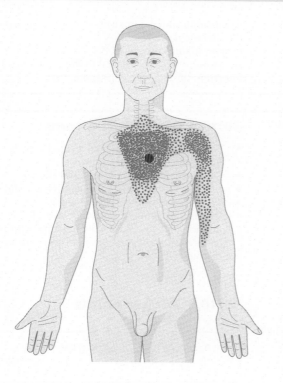

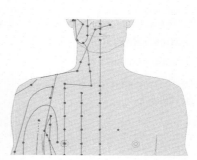

30.9.4 Diagnosis

Questioning: pain not dependent on motion.
Inspection: no information.
Physical examination: palpation.
Technical examination: exclusion of coronary heart disease.

30.9.5 Specific aspects

- Only present in very few people (2–15% depending on examination).
- mTrPs are frequently in common with the M. pectoralis.
- In rare cases the cause of pain is similar to angina pectoris (deceitful because it is not dependent on motion).
- May often be observed as concomitant finding in patient with heart disease, but treat in any case.

30.9.6 Therapy

Instructions for manual trigger point therapy

- Trigger point resolution by pressure.

Stretching

- Stretching not possible, only automassage.

Physical procedures

- Moist heat, laser.

Infiltration techniques/dry needling

- Identification with flat palpation, hold the mTrP firmly with two fingers.
- Insert needle tangentially and push slowly forward.
- mTrPs are superficial.

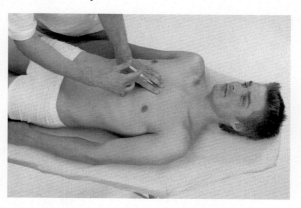

Classical Chinese acupuncture

Local and locoregional points (also contralateral): KI 23, KI 24, KI 25, CV 17, CV 18, CV 19.
Distal points: HT 3, KI 10, BL 13, BL 15.
Control points/symptomatic points: GV 20, if anxiety symptoms KI 3, BL 23.

415

Microsystem acupuncture

Ear: points of the muscle zone of the thoracic spine representation (next to the antihelix fold in the direction of the helix).
YNSA: E zone of the base point.

Kiiko Matsumoto acupuncture

- With tenderness over the kidney meridian between KI 21 and KI 27: KI 7 (metal point) and KI 10 (water point); insertion angle 15–45° with the flow of the meridian; insertion angle for KI 10: 45–90° (with the flow of the meridian).
- For tenderness at KI 27: HT 7.
- For tenderness on both sides between KI 21 and KI 27: TH 9 together with GB 40 or PC 6 (to harmonise sympathic and parasympathetic nervous system).

Psychosomatics/relaxation

- Possibly resolution of anxiety.

30.9.7 Recommendations for the patient

- Autostretching of this muscle is not possible, although automassage can be carried out.

30.10 M. SERRATUS POSTERIOR SUPERIOR

30.10.1 Anatomy

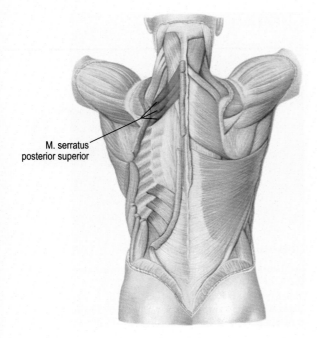

M. serratus posterior superior

Innervation: anterior branches of the cervical nerve (C6) to the thoracic nerve (T2).
Origin: spinous process of C6, C7 and T1, T2.
Insertion: rib 2–rib 5 (lateral to the costal angle).
Function: lifting ribs 2–5 (inspiration).

30.10.2 Patient symptoms

- Severe, deep seated, dorsal shoulder pain, which is frequently resistant to treatment.
- Pain at the dorsal upper arm and elbow.
- Feeling of numbness in the ulnar part of the hand.
- Symptoms dependent on breathing.
- Possible preliminary diagnoses: radiculopathy C8, thoracic outlet syndrome, neuropathic pain syndrome of uncertain cause, perfusion disorders, chronic bursitis olecrani.

30.10.3 Trigger points

mTrP	LOCATION	RADIATION	mTrP→ ACUPUNCTURE POINT
1	Medial border of the scapula or below the scapula, always in the upper half of the scapula, variable at the level of T3 or T4	Local, deep-seated pain in the upper part of the scapula	BL 42, BL 43

30.10.4 Diagnosis

Questioning
- Working at a desk which is too high?
- Chronic lung disease.

Inspection: slight excursion of breath especially during inspiration.

Physical examination
- Carry out deep breathing.
- Pressure on the scapula makes it worse.
- Palpation with the patient seated and upper body leaning forward with arms adducted in order to reach optimum abduction of the scapula.
- Palpation difficult because palpation must be through the trapezius and the rhomboid muscles.
- It is crucial that the known pain is caused or made worse by pressure.

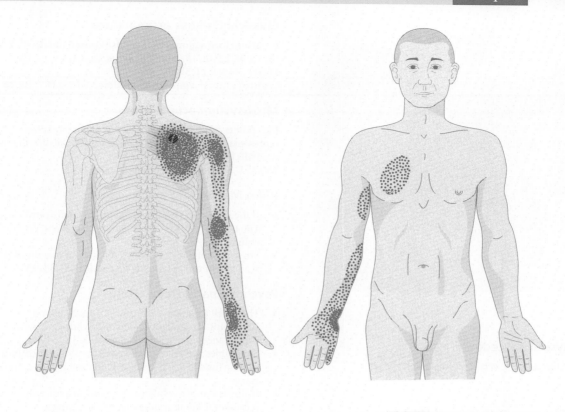

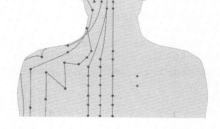

30.10.5 Specific aspects

- mTrPs in the M. serratus posterior superior have a very strong tendency to spread.
- A common concomitant finding is a segmental functional disorder (blocking) in the area T1–T3.
- Examine the M. scalenii at the same time, as these may also be affected but can also show the relevant pain pattern.

30.10.6 Therapy

Instructions for manual trigger point therapy

- Only indirect treatment possible through the fibres of the M. trapezius pars transversa and Mm. rhomboidei.

- mTrP often lie in the area of the muscle which is normally covered by the scapula: initial ventralisation of the scapula required.

Stretching

- The patient sits on a chair.
- Extend the arms to hang down between the legs.
- One of the therapist's hands lies on the spinous processes C6–T2.
- The other hand lies on the chest medial to the ventralised scapula.
- Inspiration.
- For stretching the hand is placed on the spinous process of the vertebral body and the other hand stretches the muscle inferiorly and laterally along the course of the ribs while breathing out slowly.

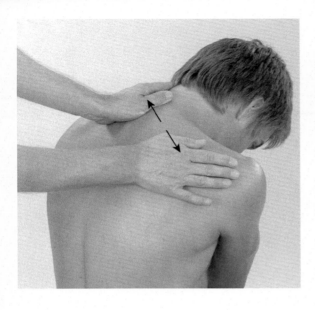

Physical procedures

- Needs to be very deep-reaching.

Infiltration techniques/dry needling

- Risk of pneumothorax if carried out incorrectly.
- Isolate mTrP on a rib.
- Insertion flat and tangentially and directed at a rib.
- Note the direction of the muscle twitch reaction: if a horizontal twitch is observed, it is more likely that an mTrP in the trapezius has been found.

Classical Chinese acupuncture

Local and locoregional points (also contralateral): BL 41–BL 43, BL 12–BL 15, Hua tuo points, Ex-R 1, CV 12, CV 13.
Distal points: BL 58, BL 57.
Control points/symptomatic points: LU 5, LU 7, BL 13.

Microsystem acupuncture

Ear: points of the muscle zone of the thoracic spine representation (next to the antihelix fold in the direction of the helix).
YNSA: E zone of the base point.

Kiiko Matsumoto acupuncture

- If the patient is standing: Hua tuo jiaji between T1 and T5, at an angle of 45° in the direction of the vertebral column.
- For symptoms in the area of the medial margin of the scapula (in the area of BL 42 and BL 45): BL 25.

Psychosomatics/relaxation

- The mTrP frequently corresponds to BL 43, an important acupuncture point with wide-ranging significance ('the inside of the inside').
- Sometimes the mTrP can be an expression of a disorder of lung function in the sense of an extended functional image.
- If this is the case, wide-ranging measures may be required: these may go so far as life changes.

30.10.7 Recommendations for the patient

Autostretching

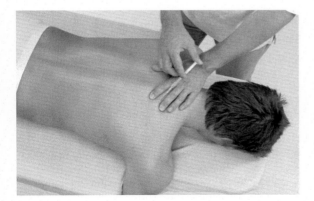

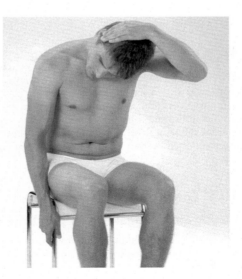

- Isolated autostretching is difficult.
- In the position shown, the M. serratus posterior superior is partially stretched at the same time.

Additional measures

- Self-treatment (with a tennis ball).
- Improvement in coordination between chest and abdominal breathing.
- Breathing therapy.

30.11 M. SERRATUS ANTERIOR

30.11.1 Anatomy

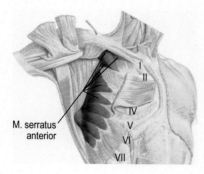

I
II
IV
V
VI
VII

M. serratus anterior

Innervation: thoracic nerve (plexus brachialis, pars supraclavicularis).

Origin

- Pars superior: 1st–2nd ribs (moderately converging).
- Medial part: 2nd–4th ribs (divergent).
- Inferior part: 5th–(8th) 9th ribs (strongly converging); dovetailed with the original processes of the M. obliquus abdominis externus.

Insertion

- Pars superior: superior angle of the scapula.
- Medial part: medial border of the scapula.
- Inferior part: inferior angle of the scapula.

Function

- Pectoral girdle: all parts: abduction of the scapula; together with the rhomboids pressing the scapula to the thorax (wing of scapula if one of the antagonists is missing); superior part: lifting; medial part: lowering; inferior part: lowering, lateral rotation (for elevation of the arm over the horizontal).
- Thorax: if the scapula is fixed lifting of the ribs (inspiration).

30.11.2 Patient symptoms

- Thoracic pain on the affected side.
- Lateral decubitus on the affected side painful.

- Pain on inspiration.
- Possible preliminary diagnoses: intercostal neuralgia, thoracic pain of uncertain cause.

30.11.3 Trigger points

mTrP	LOCATION	RADIATION	mTrP↔ ACUPUNCTURE POINT
1	Frequently central at the level of the nipple but also variable throughout the muscle	Lateral thorax, medial forearm as far as the 4th and 5th digits lower cervical spine	SP 21

30.11.4 Diagnosis

Questioning

- Lateral recumbent position unpleasant?
- Stabbing pains in the side during sport?
- Fall on arm with twisting of the scapula, e.g. while skiing?
- Lifting of heavy objects?
- Excessive press-ups?

Inspection

- Round shoulders as a result of rotation and abduction of the scapula with severe protrusion of the spina scapulae.
- Monitor the scapulohumeral articulation when flexing and adducting the arm compared to the other side.
- Slight excursion of breath.
- Wing of scapula as evidence of damage to the innervating thoracic nerve.

Physical examination

- Stretching test: both elbows are flexed (upper arm at the side) and taken back – deep inspiration – pain on the affected side.
- Lateral position with retroverted shoulder and flexed elbow (elbow up and to the back), then bring elbow down to the bed: limited movement when the sides are compared.
- Lying back against the wall while standing – observe the scapula – the affected side is slightly more raised from the thorax.

30.11.5 Specific aspects

- Sometimes cause of therapy-resistant cervical spine symptoms (lower cervical spine).

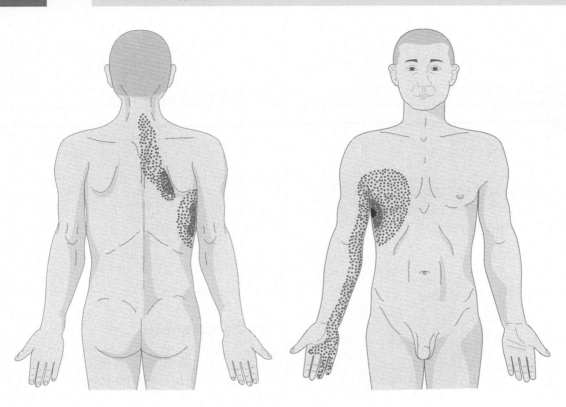

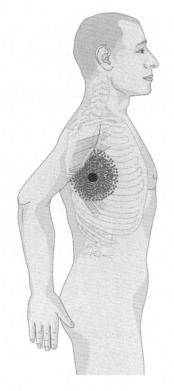

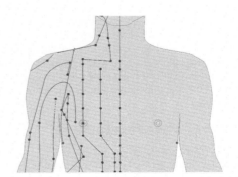

- Reciprocal influence of mTrPs in the serratus and subscapularis muscle.
- Likely to be caused by twisting movement.

30.11.6 Therapy

Instructions for manual trigger point therapy

- If the scapula is in maximum retraction (patient on their side) other parts of the muscle become accessible for direct palpation and treatment.
- Cranial fibres (to ribs 1–3) frequently have mTrPs.
- Indirect treatment of the fibre parts in the area of the medial border of the scapula through the M. trapezius pars transversa and Mm. rhomboidei. Access from the medial margin of scapula (patient in lateral decubitus or prone position).
- Mobilisation of the scapulothoracic articular space, lifting of the medial margin of the shoulder blade and the inferior angle of scapula.

Stretching

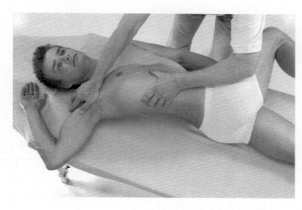

- Patient lying on the side not affected.
- Upper body dorsally rotated.
- Abduction and retroversion in the shoulder.
- Stretching through pressure on the upper arm in a dorsal direction and concomitant inspiration.
- Focus on breathing.

Physical procedures

- Laser, ultrasound, hydrotherapy and thermotherapy.

Infiltration techniques/dry needling

- Patient in lateral decubitus position.
- Depending on the position of the mTrP place the patient on their non-affected side with upper body slightly rotated to the back, arm in adduction and anteversion.

- Flat infiltration in pinch grip diagonally to the course of the ribs.
- **Warning:** pneumothorax with vertical injection or needling.

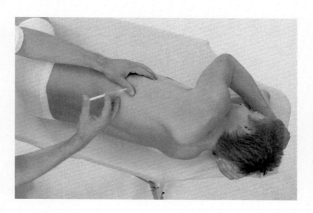

Classical Chinese acupuncture

Local and locoregional points (also contralateral): SP 17, SP 21, GB 22.
Distal points: HT 5, SP 1, GB 31, Ex-AH 3.
Control points/symptomatic points: HT 1 (thoracic tightness), PC 6, GB 34.

Microsystem acupuncture

Ear: points of the muscle zone of the thoracic spine representation (next to the antihelix fold in the direction of the helix).
YNSA: E zone of the base point.

Kiiko Matsumoto acupuncture

- With tenderness at SP 21: SP 5 and SP 9 ipsilaterally (metal and water points).
- GB 1 ipsilaterally (angle of insertion 15–45° in direction GB 2) and GB 34 (diagonal needling).

Psychosomatics/relaxation

- Similar to the subscapularis muscle (the approach for needling is also similar): narrowing the anterior chest (heart) space, protective posture.
- Inner tension.
- Relaxation exercises focusing on breathing.

30.11.7 Recommendations for the patient

Autostretching

- The patient sits on a chair.
- Hold the scapula in place with one hand on seat or backrest.
- Breathe in deeply.

421

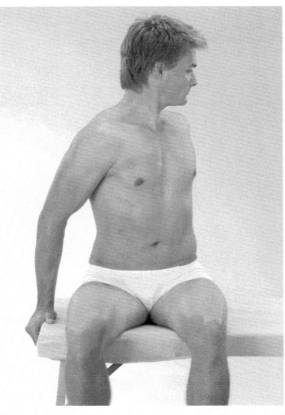

30.12 M. SERRATUS POSTERIOR INFERIOR

30.12.1 Anatomy

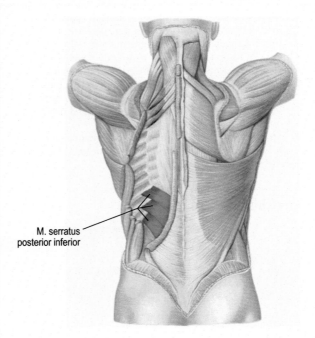

M. serratus posterior inferior

Innervation: anterior branches from the thoracic nerve (T11) to the lumbar nerve (L2).
Origin: spinous process of T11, T12 and L1, L2.
Insertion: 9th–12th rib (inferior margin).
Function: lowering ribs 9–12 (breathing out); as antagonist to traction effect of diaphragm, also active during forced inspiration.

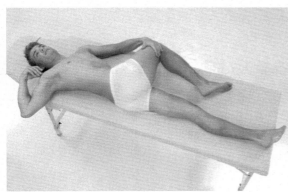

- Then rotation with concomitant slow expiration.
- Alternative: stretching in lateral decubitus, then rotation of the upper body dorsally (photo, bottom).

Additional measures

- Breathing therapy (e.g. Middendorf breathwork).
- 'Deep breaths'.

30.12.2 Patient symptoms

- Deep thoracic back pain, located paravertebrally lower thoracic spine as far as the thoracolumbar transition.
- Thoracic pain on rotation.
- Pain on breathing out.
- Possible preliminary diagnoses: renal disease without definite correlation, radiculopathy T9–T12, degenerative lumbar spine syndrome.

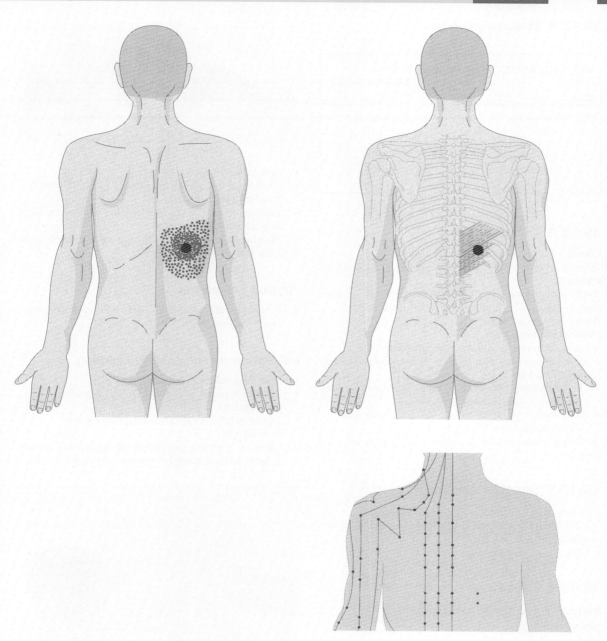

30.12.3 Trigger points

mTrP	LOCATION	RADIATION	mTrP↔ ACUPUNCTURE POINT
1	3–4 finger widths paravertebrally to the spinous processes T8–T12	Predominantly local	BL 47, BL 48

30.12.4 Diagnosis

Questioning: acute strain of trunk through carrying an object over a long distance with concomitant rotation?
Inspection: evidence of scoliosis? Protective posture with slightly twisted vertebral column (slight rotation and flexion on affected side)
Physical examination
- Pain on rotation of trunk (contralaterally).
- The pain recedes with rotation and flexion movement on affected side.
- Examination of the whole thoracic spine and lumbar spine required to rule out other causes.
- Palpation through M. erector spinae occasionally difficult (course of fibres).
Technical examination: possibly to rule out renal disease.

30.12.5 Specific aspects

- Frequently concomitant segmental functional disorder (blockade) in the area of the thoracolumbar transition.
- Focus on breathing out.

30.12.6 Therapy

Instructions on manual trigger point therapy

- Treatment through strong pressure with the patient lying on their side (positioning as for stretching).
- First treat mTrPs of the Mm. quadratus lumborum, latissimus dorsi, iliocostalis and longissimus.

Stretching

- Comfortable lateral decubitus supported with soft rolls.

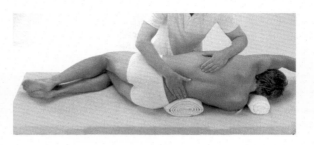

- Arm in elevation.
- Fixation of the spinous processes of T11–L2 with the hand furthest from the head.
- Traction on ribs 9–11 with the hand close to the head in a craniolateral direction.
- Breathe out during stretching and extend the arm to the floor ('make it long').

Physical procedures

- Particularly thermotherapy, drawing-out procedures (e.g. cupping), laser, TENS.

Infiltration techniques/dry needling

- **Warning:** risk of pneumothorax.
- Treatment possible in prone or lateral position (side not affected).
- Isolate mTrP on a rib (two-finger protection technique).
- Cautious approach to mTrP in the direction of the ribs (ribs 9–12 depending on the position of the mTrP).

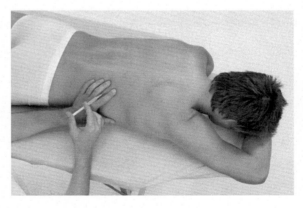

Classical Chinese acupuncture

Local and locoregional points (also contralateral): BL 47, BL 48, BL 49, BL 50, BL 18, BL 19, BL 20, BL 21, Hua tuo points, GB 25.
Distal points: BL 58 or BL 40 depending on sensitivity and reactibility.

Control points/symptomatic points: GB 34 with renal disease (kidney Qi weakness or similar) according to TCM.

Microsystem acupuncture

Ear: points of the muscle zone of the thoracic spine representation (next to the antihelix fold in the direction of the helix).
YNSA: E zone of the base point.

Kiiko Matsumoto acupuncture

- If the patient is standing: Hua tuo jiaji between T12 and L2, at an angle of 45°.
- With tenderness in the area of L2–L3 needling of a point approximately 1 cm lateral to BL 40, ipsilaterally, angle of insertion 15–45° along the course of the bladder meridian.

Psychosomatics/relaxation

- As for all back pain.

30.12.7 Recommendations for the patient

Autostretching

- Stable lateral decubitus position (affected side on top, upper leg in hip and knee flexion).
- Extension by rotation of the upper body in a dorsal direction while breathing out.

- Maintain position and stretch further by breathing out and in.
- In contrast to the M. serratus posterior superior (see Section 30.10), which is stretched in a similar manner, the arm on the affected side can here be laid down.

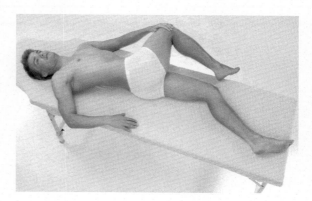

Additional measures

- Lumbar support when seated.
- Self-treatment with a tennis ball.
- Partner massage with cupping.
- Attempt orthopaedic correction with pronounced body asymmetry (inserts, heel wedges if leg difference >1 cm).
- Change mattress (harder mattress usually required so the back does not 'sag').

Chapter | 31 |

Abdomen

Dominik Irnich

31.1 FUNCTIONAL ASSOCIATIONS

The abdominal muscles and the visceral organs are closely connected functionally and segmentally with the lumbar spine (Ch. 32), the pelvis and the thorax, and they tension the anterior lower trunk area in a star shape. mTrPs of the abdominal muscles can be caused by visceral diseases and also by segmental disorders of the lumbar spine and attempts at compensation by more distant structures. Changes here affect the whole body, not just along the anterior muscle chains of the trunk but also along the whole vertebral column and right out to the extremities and even visceral function (see below).

Cutivisceral reflexes were described by Head and McKenzie back in 1900. A pathology of the internal organs can lead to dermal hyperalgesic zones in the area of the anterior wall of the trunk (head zones). They can usually be detected with the aid of a detailed sensory examination. Various authors also describe maximum zones of increased sensitivity in these skin areas.

Head used these skin regions therapeutically with the application of an irritant such as a mustard plaster. Chinese acupuncture also describes acupuncture points where perfusing and spasmolytic effects are attributed when they are irritated.

Analogously, musculoskeletal reflexes must also be assumed, which becomes routine if the abdominal muscles are carefully examined as well as internal diseases considered. mTrPs are regularly found in the straight and transverse abdominal muscles. However, simple segmental allocation is difficult as the viscerotome and myotome do not correspond to the extent of the dermatome and the innervation of the viscera is largely via the autonomic nervous system. Nevertheless, mTrPs are regularly found with visceral diseases and experience shows that differentiated trigger point treatment often leads to long-term improvement in visceral symptoms.

> Simons and Travell, as well as other authors, even assume that untreated mTrPs in the abdominal muscles can lead to functional disorders of the internal organs. There is no doubt that mTrPs can simulate visceral symptoms.

31.2 PSYCHOSOMATIC ASSOCIATIONS

The abdomen often represents the interaction of emotions and intuition with understanding and thought. Today, we know that the so-called emotional intelligence is an essential prerequisite for 'correct' decisions. This is shown in linguistic use: 'making a decision based on gut feeling'. Even in Chinese medicine, logic is attributed to the spleen; that is, the abdomen.

Brain research substantiates the influence of understanding *through* emotion, which is definitely more pronounced than the possibility of the understanding influencing the emotions. This conflict can be expressed as visceral symptoms: 'decisions give you a stomach ache'.

A one-sided and exclusively somatic understanding of disease would deny that trusting absolutely in reasoning and forcibly suppressing subjective and emotional truth does not lead to serious visceral functional disorders.

http://dx.doi.org/10.1016/B978-0-7020-4312-3.00031-3

It seems plausible that the abdominal muscles may be agents and carriers of this conflict.

A concomitant autonomic reaction is very common in the treatment of mTrPs, and not just in the abdominal space; it is as if there is an emotional component to the cause as well as physical tension. This is audible in the sounds of peristalsis, which are described in psychodynamics (a method of physical therapy) as 'psychoperistalsis'.

In TCM heartburn is said to occur as a symptom of anger or brooding and worry ('anger in the belly', 'worry causing a hole in the belly').

A well-relaxed abdomen indicates that a person has a stable core: 'Hara' as centre of strength below the navel in Eastern medicine (see Section 22.3, Ch. 32).

31.3 SYMPTOMS

The referral pattern for mTrPs in the abdominal muscles is usually locoregional, sometimes with referred pain as far as the lumbar spine/iliac crest or lower thoracic region. Pain can also occur in the inguinal or genital areas as far as the proximal medial side of the thigh.

A series of visceral symptoms can also be associated with abdominal mTrPs: nausea, heartburn, feelings of pressure or fullness, cramp-like symptoms and tight chest, as well as symptoms similar to angina or dysmenorrhoea.

With all abdominal symptoms, a trial treatment of locoregional mTrPs together with the relevant segmental paravertebral points can be helpful and therefore makes sense. Symptoms which can be attributed to postoperative adhesions can also be improved through the treatment of abdominal mTrPs.

31.4 DIAGNOSTIC AND THERAPEUTIC CONSIDERATIONS

Pronounced lumbar lordosis is usually associated with weakened abdominal muscles. The treatment of mTrPs can be sensible, as can correction of posture and training to build up the muscles.

Chronic symptoms in the pelvic area can occur as a result of strong traction of the abdominal muscles which may often be asymmetrical and are usually associated with muscular mTrPs (Pontari and Ruggieri 2008; Slocumb 1984). The occurrence of mTrPs is often associated with changes in the structure of the abdomen (e.g. space-occupying lesion, hernia, following surgery affecting the muscles or the symmetry). It often seems that mTrPs store the pain after an operation.

Treatment of mTrPs can also be considered for pain in the abdominal area during respiration or to improve respiratory volume for athletes.

The following tip comes from treatment of sternosymphysal strain with its wide-reaching effects on the whole locomotor system.

> Tenderness of the tuberculum pubicum (transition of the upper margin of the pubic bone to the inguinal ligament) as the inferior insertion of the transverse abdominal muscles is a good indicator of a tension disorder. As an example, infiltration and treatment of the relevant mTrPs may bring rapid relief for back pain.

31.5 EXAMINATION FOR mTrP IDENTIFICATION

mTrPs can be found by palpation in this area; this is best done by passive stretching. The patient lies in the supine position and is asked to breathe in deeply into the abdomen and hold their breath (Figure 31.1).

EXAMINATION FINDINGS	TRIGGER POINT SEARCH IN
Pain when straightening the upper body from the supine position	M. rectus abdominis (Section 31.6) Consider the M. pyramidalis (Section 31.8) for pain in the area of the symphysis
Pain when straightening the upper body from the supine position with pain at the end of expiration	Diaphragm: physiotherapy with loosening of the diaphragm
Pain with rotation of the upper body from the supine position (see Section 31.7)	• Pain on active side • Contraction pain: M. obliquus abdominis externus • Stretching pain: M. obliquus abdominis internus • Pain on stretched side • Contraction pain: M. obliquus abdominis internus • Stretching pain: M. obliquus abdominis externus

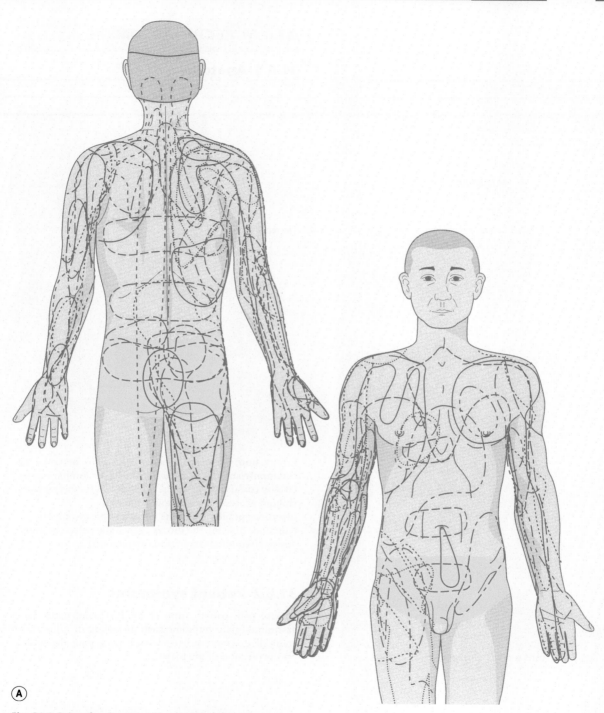

(A)

Fig. 31.1 Pain referral pattern (a) and affected muscles

Continued

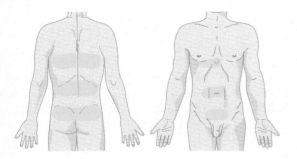

M. rectus abdominis
(▶31.6)

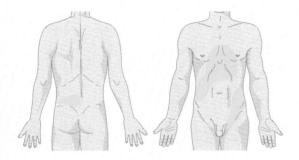

M. obliquus abdominis
(▶31.7)

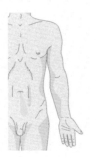

M. pyramidalis
(▶31.8)

(B)

Fig. 31.1—cont'd (b) in the abdomen

31.6 M. RECTUS ABDOMINIS

31.6.1 Anatomy

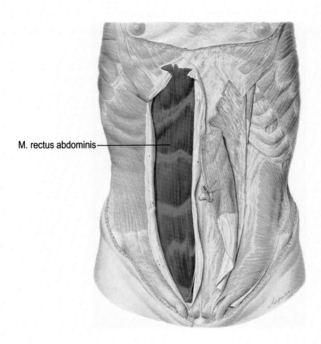

M. rectus abdominis

Innervation: intercostal nerves (thoracic nerves); less commonly anterior branches of the upper lumbar nerves.
Origin: costal cartilage of the 5th–7th ribs (lateral surface), xiphoid process, costoxiphoid ligament.
Insertion: pubic crest of the coccyx, pubic symphysis.
Function: drawing the thorax against the pelvis, bearing down, abdominal respiration (exspiration).

31.6.2 Patient symptoms

Diverse pain pattern from abdominal pain, particularly gastrointestinal symptoms such as feeling of fullness, to cramp-like symptoms, to classical back pain depending on the position of the mTrP.

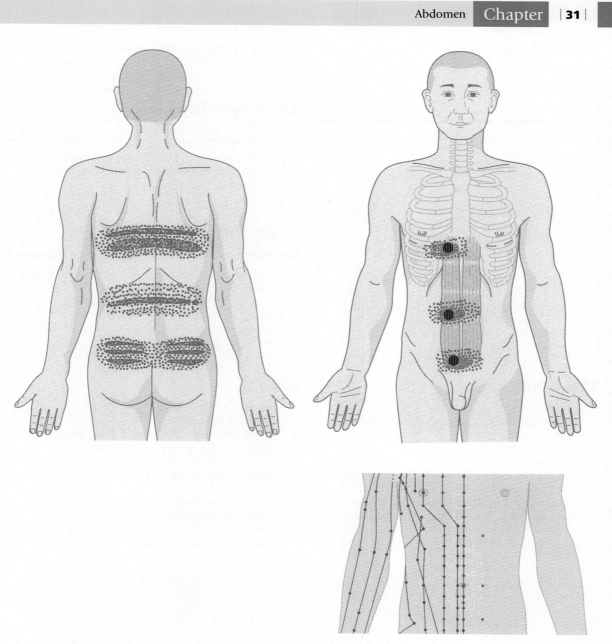

31.6.3 Trigger points

mTrP	LOCATION	RADIATION	mTrP↔ ACUPUNCTURE POINT
1	At the level of the upper abdomen	Thoracic spine on both sides; deep projection into the stomach	ST 19, ST 20
2	Periumbilical	Middle abdomen thoracic spine/ lumbar spine (area of the thoracolumbar transition)	ST 25, KI 16
3	Between the symphysis and the navel	Lower abdomen lumbar spine	KI 13, ST 28

31.6.4 Diagnosis

Questioning
- Abdominal muscle training or other biomechanical strain?
- Gastrointestinal disease or symptoms?
- Abdominal operation?

Inspection: observation of abdominal breath excursion.

Physical examination
- Palpation while standing, seated or lying down.
- Allow abdominal muscles to relax (lift head, shoulders and legs: if this provides relief it is more likely a visceral disorder).

Technical examination: examination of the visceral organs depending on the findings.

31.6.5 Specific aspects

- Often occur after abdominal muscle training or other strain of the abdominal muscles.
- Symptoms caused by mTrPs in the M. rectus abdominis are a classical expression of somatovisceral and viscerosomatic interplay.

31.6.6 Therapy

Instructions on manual trigger point therapy

- Gently pretense the muscles (counter traction with other hand) or use an underlay.
- Include in the treatment the insertion site at the sternum and neighbouring costal arch.
- Include treatment at the insertion site at the pubic bone.

Stretching

- Patient in supine position.
- Lengthwise stretching:
- support in the area of lumbar lordosis, which already reaches a stretch of the M. rectus abdominis,
- with maximum inspiration the thorax is pushed in a superior direction and the pelvis in a nferior direction with the two hands.
- Transverse stretching:
- patient in supine position without underlay,
- place thumbs or fists of both hands next to the rectus sheath and stretch laterally.

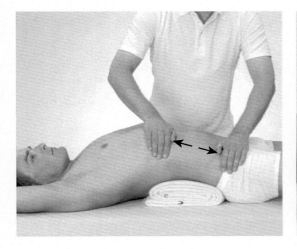

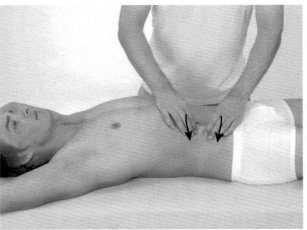

Physical procedures

- Thermotherapy, wraps, compresses, laser.

Infiltration techniques/dry needling

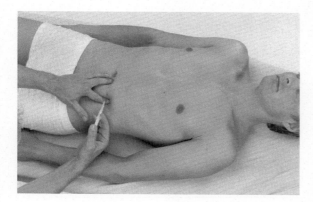

- Lateral infiltration with fixed mTrPs.
- Two-finger protection technique.
- Tangential insertion.

Classical Chinese acupuncture

Local and locoregional points (also contralateral): ST 19–ST 28, KI 13–KI 21, CV 4, CV 14, LR 12, LR 14.
Distal points: ST 36, KI 9, SP 3, points of the bladder meridian in the affected segments.
Control points/symptomatic points: depending on the symptoms according to TCM, e.g. PC 6 for fullness, GB 24, GB 25 for abdominal cramps, SP 8 for lower abdominal symptoms, GB 41 for belt-shaped pain below the navel, LR 5 for inguinal or genital pain.

Microsystem acupuncture

Ear: segment-related thoracic spine or lumbar spine representation.

Kiiko Matsumoto acupuncture

- With the patient in the prone position also BL 17, BL 20 and BL 21 (needling angle 15 to 45° downwards with the flow of the meridian).
- Hua tuo jiaji in the area from T10, T11 and T12, needling at an angle of 45° in the direction of the vertebral column.

Psychosomatics/relaxation

- Too many demands or stress from other people in close contact: feeling small, digestive disorders.
- Exercises for opening the abdomen.

31.6.7 Recommendations for the patient

Autostretching

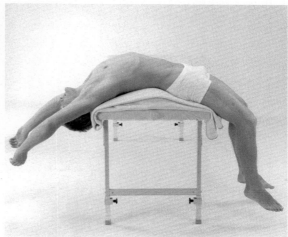

- Autostretching is illustrated for young mobile people who have strains caused by abdominal training.
- It is sensible to provide support in the area of lumbar lordosis.
- For older or less mobile patients, it is usually sufficient to lean against the edge of the bed with a pillow under the vertebral column and the upper arms elevated.
- Deep inspiration during autostretching.

Additional measures

- Correct posture while sitting and standing.
- Avoid perpetuating and causative factors (inadequate forms of abdominal muscle training, sitting incorrectly, etc.).
- Ergonomics (work position, leisure activities).
- Functional training (coordination, not strength) of the muscles, e.g. practise pelvic rocking or abdominal breathing.

433

31.7 M. OBLIQUUS ABDOMINIS (EXTERNUS AND INTERNUS)

31.7.1 Anatomy

Innervation: inferior intercostal nerves (thoracic nerves); iliohypogastricus nerve; ilioinguinal nerve (lumbar plexus).
Origin
- M. obliquus abdominis externus: 5th–12th rib (lateral surface, interlinked with the spinous processes of origin of the M. serratus anterior).
- M. obliquus abdominis internus: thoracolumbar fascia (superficial layer), intermediate line of the iliac crest, inguinal ligament (lateral two-thirds).

Insertion:

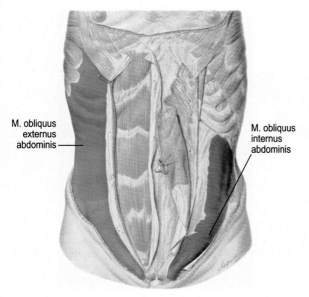

M. obliquus externus abdominis

M. obliquus internus abdominis

- M. obliquus abdominis externus: external labium of the iliac crest, inguinal ligament, tuberculum pubicum, pubic crest, linea alba (involved in construction of the anterior layer of the rectus sheath).
- M. obliquus abdominis internus: costal cartilage of the (9th) 10th–12th rib (lower margin), linea alba (above the arcuate line involved in the construction of the anterior and posterior layers of the rectus sheath under which all tendon fibres run into the anterior layer). In men the lowest fibres split off to form the M. cremaster and run into the spermatic cord.

Function:
- M. obliquus abdominis externus: one-sided action: rotation of the thorax to the opposite side, lateral flexion of the vertebral column; action on both sides.

Drawing the thorax against the pelvis, bearing down, abdominal respiration (expiration).
- M. obliquus abdominis internus: one-sided action: rotation of the thorax to the same side, lateral flexion of the vertebral column; action on both sides. Drawing the thorax against the pelvis, bearing down, abdominal respiration (expiration). The cremaster muscle draws the testicle upwards with the tunica testis.

31.7.2 Patient symptoms

- Pain in the upper abdomen (can also depend on respiration) or abdomen.
- Visceral symptoms in the upper abdomen (e.g. heartburn, feeling of fullness) or in the abdomen (cramp-like or spastic symptoms).
- Inguinal pain.
- Back pain (from thoracolumbar to lumbosacral area).

31.7.3 Trigger points

mTrP	LOCATION	RADIATION	mTrP→ ACUPUNCTURE POINT
1	Upper part of M. obliquus externus	Epigastric, thoracolumbar vertebral column	SP 14, BL 52
2	Lower part of M. obliquus externus or M. obliquus internus	Abdomen, pelvis, inguinal area, lumbar spine	GB 25, GB 26, LR 13

31.7.4 Diagnosis

Questioning
- Lifting heavy object with rotated trunk while holding one's breath?
- Birth?
- Abdominal muscle training?
- Abdominal operation?

Inspection: observation of abdominal breath excursion.
Physical examination: examination with the patient seated with slight ipsilateral rotation of the upper parts.
Technical examination: examination of the visceral organs depending on the findings.

31.7.5 Specific aspects

- mTrPs often lie surprisingly laterally and dorsally in the area between the 12th rib and the iliac crest.

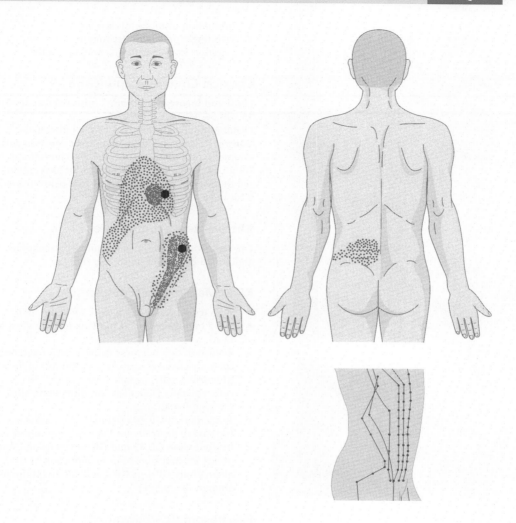

- It is not often possible to attribute mTrPs precisely to one of the transverse abdominal muscles.
- Simons and Travell describe an 'eructation point' immediately below the costal angle of the 12th rib which is associated with belching or even vomiting.

31.7.6 Therapy

Instructions for manual trigger point therapy

- Gently pretense the muscles (counter traction with other hand).
- Treatment in seated position for lateral parts.
- Treatment in supine position for anterior and inferior parts.

Stretching

- Lengthwise stretching:
- push towards iliac crest,
- traction on the contralateral costal arch (above) with deep inspiration.
- Transverse stretching M. obliquus externus:
- supine position,
- patient's arms elevated,
- place under lumbar spine,
- push in laterocaudal direction (middle).
- Transverse stretching M. obliquus internus:
- push in laterocranial direction (below).

Physical procedures

- Thermotherapy, wraps, compresses, laser.

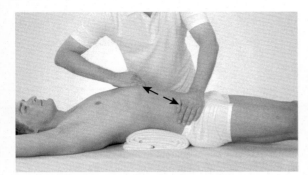

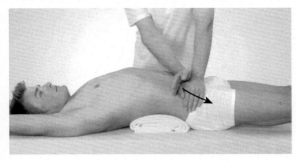

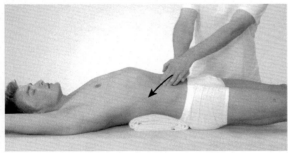

Infiltration techniques/dry needling

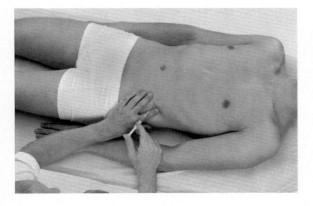

- Infiltration from lateral direction.
- Two-finger protection technique.
- Injection from lateral direction, tangential.

Classical Chinese acupuncture

Local and locoregional points (also contralateral): GB 25, GB 26, LR 13, SP 14, BL 52.
Distal points: depending on affected meridian.
Control points/symptomatic points: depending on the symptoms according to TCM, e.g. PC 6 for fullness, GB 24, GB 25 for abdominal cramps, SP 8 for lower abdominal symptoms, GB 41 for belt-shaped pain below the navel, LR 5 for inguinal or genital pain.

Microsystem acupuncture

Ear: segment-related thoracic spine representation, abdominal projection point, e.g. zero.

Kiiko Matsumoto acupuncture

- With tenderness at SP 2: SP 3, SP 5 and SP 9.
- ST 12 on both sides, needle diagonally in the direction LI 15.
- Reduction of tenderness at the superior anterior iliac spine also reduces tenderness in the area of the muscle: KI 9 ipsilaterally, in some cases also ST 30 contralaterally (superficial needling in the direction of the symphysis).
- Tenderness at GB 26 (Dai mai): KI 7 ipsilaterally (upwards); generally for the treatment of this muscle.
- In some cases GB 43 and GB 44 (metal and water point) are best suited for the reduction of tenderness; alternatively GB 1 or GB 2 and GB 28 (at the superior anterior iliac spine).

Psychosomatics/relaxation

- Too many demands or stress from other people in close contact.
- Feeling small, digestive disorders.
- Exercises for opening the abdomen.

31.7.7 Recommendations for the patient

Autostretching

- Autostretching is illustrated for young mobile people who have strains caused by abdominal training.
- It is sensible to provide support in the area of lumbar lordosis.
- Autostretching using gravity (allow arm to fall over and behind the head) and breathing excursions with deep expiration and inspiration.
- Alternative:

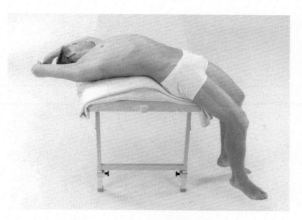

- lateral decubitus position with knees bent,
- then rotate the upper body contralaterally (dorsally) and stretch,
- extend abducted arm and allow to fall downwards: use gravity.
- Complex stretching while seated under upper body rotation.

Additional measures

- Correct posture while sitting and standing.
- Avoid perpetuating and causative factors (inadequate forms of abdominal muscle training, sitting incorrectly, etc.).
- Ergonomics (work position, leisure activities).
- Functional training (coordination, not strength) of the muscles, e.g. practise pelvic rocking or abdominal breathing.

31.8 M. PYRAMIDALIS

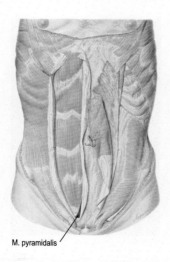

M. pyramidalis

31.8.1 Anatomy

Innervation: inferior intercostal nerves (thoracic nerves) (inconsistent muscle).
Origin: pubic crest of the coccyx, pubic symphysis (anterior to the M. rectus abdominis)
Insertion: linea alba.
Function: tensing the linea alba.

31.8.2 Patient symptoms

- Dull pressing pain above the symphysis.
- Lower abdominal pain.

31.8.3 Trigger points

mTrP	LOCATION	RADIATION	mTrP↔ ACUPUNCTURE POINT
1	Above the symphysis	Local, pubic bone: lower abdomen	KI 12, KI 13

31.8.4 Diagnosis

Questioning: abdominal muscle training? Trauma, e.g. operation?
Inspection: normal.
Physical examination: palpation only.
Technical examination: examination of the pelvic organs depending on the findings.

31.8.5 Specific aspects

- mTrPs often lie an surprising distance in a dorsal direction.
- The muscle is not regularly available.
- Occasionally involved with painful menstruation as well.
- Frequently together with mTrPs in the M. rectus abdominis.

31.8.6 Therapy

Instructions for manual trigger point therapy

- Cannot be distinguished by palpation from the M. rectus abdominis.
- Is also automatically treated with the treatment of the most inferior parts of the M. rectus abdominis and its insertion site at the pubic bone.

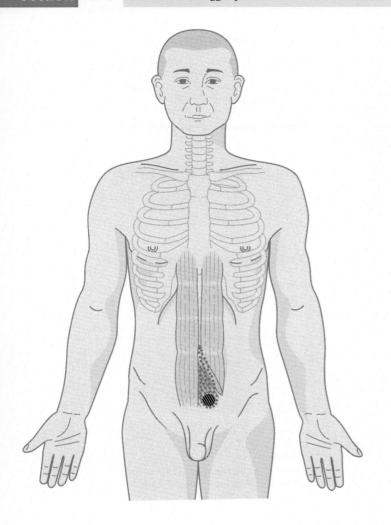

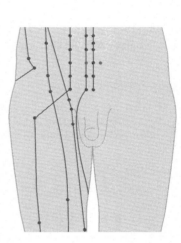

Stretching

With maximum inspiration the thorax is pushed in a superior direction and the pelvis in a inferior direction (see M. rectus abdominis, Section 31.6).

Physical procedures

- Thermotherapy, wraps, compresses, laser.

Infiltration techniques/dry needling

- Two-finger protection technique.
- Palpate the symphysis to delineate.

Classical Chinese acupuncture

Local and locoregional points (also contralateral): KI 12, KI 13, CV 2, CV 3.

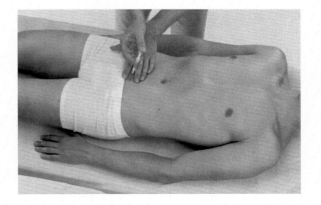

Distal points: KI 10, SP 8.
Control points/symptomatic points: segmental needling: Shu points BL 31, BL 32, BL 33, BL 34; KI 5 and/or KI 6 for menstrual symptoms.

Microsystem acupuncture

Ear: segment-related thoracic spine representation.

Kiiko Matsumoto acupuncture

- If there is a neurological cause: CV 12 and CV 10.
- For tenderness at ST 30 (border of pubic bone): ST 13 ipsilaterally and/or contralaterally; needling upwards in the direction of the shoulder, insertion angle 10°; if this point is not effective a point on the other superior anterior iliac spine should be found and needled (particularly in the area of the insertion of the inguinal ligament at GB 27 for the reduction of tenderness at ST 30).
- Tenderness in the muscle: CV 21, angle of insertion 10–15°; Hua tuo jiaji at the level T11 or T12.

Psychosomatics/relaxation

- For lower abdominal pain and if in association with other muscles in the area (M. rectus abdominis) consider disorders of sexual function.

31.8.7 Recommendations for the patient

Autostretching

- As for M. rectus abdominis (Section 31.6).
- Deep inspiration during autostretching.
- Isolated autostretching of this muscle is not possible, although automassage can be carried out.

Additional measures

- Avoid perpetuating and causative factors (inadequate forms of abdominal muscle training, sitting incorrectly, etc.).
- Functional training (coordination, not strength) of the muscles, e.g. practise pelvic rocking or abdominal breathing.

Chapter | **32** |

Lumbar spine, pelvis and hip region (pelvic girdle)

Dominik Irnich

32.1 FUNCTIONAL ASSOCIATIONS

The pelvis and its position play a key role in the whole lo-comotor system as a non-static, mobile base for the verte-bral column. Disorders have an effect not just along the vertebral column but also as far as the atlanto-occipital joint region, the muscles of mastication and the extremi-ties. The significance which has always been conferred on the base is indicated in the name of the bone which repre-sents the dorsal centre between the two halves of the pelvis: the sacrum ('sacred bone').

Summarising the lower part of the trunk as the lumbar, pelvic and hip region originates from manual medicine. It developed from experience of the many functional associations of the relevant joint connections. Besides the locomotor segments of the lumbar spine, the iliosacral joint – with its blockades and malpositions and related pelvic problems – plays a large role.

> mTrPs of the lumbar paravertebral muscles radiate and affect not only the buttocks, and as far as the ankle (segmental functional associations); pain in the lower lumbar spine and iliosacral area can also result in mTrPs of the buttocks, thigh and lower leg muscles.

In trigger point therapy we look for changes in muscles that run over the iliosacral joint or may affect its position, as for all joint disorders, which is in contrast to manual medicine.

We take note of associations between agonists and antag-onists in the lower trunk and lumbar, pelvic and hip region. The antagonists for the back muscles can be found in the abdominal muscles and the hip flexor, the M. iliopsoas (Section 32.8). The coordinated working of these muscles is more important than a simple antagonistic conflict. The overall tone of the trunk muscles is important for the state of tension of the upper and lower abdominal space. This is essential for maintaining upright posture and muffling blunt trauma. The special significance of the lower abdomen in all powerful physical actions as well as calm centring is shown in the terms 'Hara' or 'Dantian': the power centre in the middle below the navel. This is not just static: a relaxed abdomen is important for all move-ments (Qigong, Tai chi, etc.)

32.2 PSYCHOSOMATIC ASSOCIATIONS

We must basically assume that chronic back pain, resulting in restrictions to quality of life, in the majority of cases oc-curs under the influence of psychosocial stress factors. The lumbar, pelvic and hip region, as the base of the vertebral column, also say a great deal about the condition of a per-son in their world.

- A hyperlordotic lumbar spine with flexion position of the pelvis in the hip joints, when the patient seems 'in a rush', often correlates with tense muscles of the buttocks ('drawing in the tail') and an anxious insecure attitude to life (trying to escape) with lack of security in the sense of not having enough 'guts'.

http://dx.doi.org/10.1016/B978-0-7020-4312-3.00032-5

- However, a forward posture can be an expression of alert interest. The back is relaxed and the eyes gleam with curiosity.
- A body posture with a relaxed almost kyphotic lumbar spine, with the pelvis extended into the hip joints, correlates with someone who is well-balanced, confident and composed.

Back pain often represents the tip of the iceberg (iceberg model). If the biomechanics are out of order and there are mTrPs, there is often chronic stress not only in the tense muscles but also in the whole person. External posture in the form of lordosis or a stiff back often corresponds to an inner posture of anxiety or endurance. Behaviour may therefore be withdrawn, both somatically and mentally (i.e. psychologically or spiritually). Support from behind or an awareness of support is missing.

From the somatopsychological experience of acupuncture this can lead to a correlation with 'inherited' energy. By this we understand a relationship to our forefathers who keep the back clear or provide support imparting a safe background for physical and spiritual stability. If the family history is suggestive, systemic therapy can be helpful.

32.3 SYMPTOMS

With myofascial disorders of the lumbar spine region the symptoms can be locoregional but can also radiate to the abdomen and/or the legs, as well as sometimes in a superior direction to the thoracic spine. This can be explained by neurophysiological/segmental associations and the functional anatomy:

- painful tension of the lumbar spine and buttocks muscles (pain quality often dull and oppressive),
- limited mobility ('stiff back'), different on each side, e.g. of the M. quadratus lumborum, also with asymmetrical posture and even functional pelvic obliquity (tilted pelvis) and a lateral shift of the upper body in relation to the pelvis,
- sensitivity to cold, definite improvement with warmth,
- pain in bed in the morning which is relieved with movement,
- pain and symptoms radiating from the lumbar spine:
  - to the dorsal or lateral buttocks/hip region,
  - into the leg, depending on the level of the segment dorsally, laterally or even ventrally, also beyond the knee (in 1936 Kellgren showed, in an investigation of healthy students, that by injecting hypertonic saline solution irritation of the paravertebral lumbar spine muscles could be reproduced and can lead to pain referred as far as the ankle),
  - to the abdomen and lower body including the inguinal area; mTrPs of the paravertebral muscles at the level of the sacrum can also radiate to the urogenital system and even cause irritable bladder symptoms with the urge to urinate. Gastrointestinal

symptoms can also be caused via mTrPs of the paravertebral muscles of the lumbar spine associated with the segment (see also Ch. 31).

mTrPs of the buttocks muscles can radiate to the lower lumbar spine and the sacrum ('iliosacral joint'). Their referral area also runs distally as far as the ankles. At the front, referral is as far as the inguinal area which is also functionally closely associated (for precise differentiation of vertebral column syndrome see Sections 14.1.4 and 14.2).

32.4 DIAGNOSTIC AND THERAPEUTIC CONSIDERATIONS (FIGURE 32.1)

The standing posture is diagnostically very interesting and depends on a number of factors. Shortening of the M. quadriceps femoris (Section 33.9) and the ischiocrural muscles (Section 33.10) leads to reduced mobility of the pelvis in the hip joints. This can lead to a general stiffness and strain on the lumbosacral transition. If the M. iliopsoas (Section 32.8) is also shortened, the pelvis is even more fixed. If the hip flexors are more strongly shortened with flexion of the pelvis in the hip joints and resulting hyperlordosis of the lumbar spine, the whole lumbar spine–pelvis–hip region can become permanently deformed and strained. Besides tension in the buttocks region, it is also typical for the patient to demonstrate a gait with a short step length. Hyperlordosis of the lumbar spine can also be caused, however, by hardening and shortening of the paravertebral lumbar muscles including the M. quadratus lumborum.

Like tension in the buttocks, this all results in an abnormal, strained standing posture. It correlates functionally, especially with hardening of the lumbar muscles, with hardening of the calf muscles. The reverse also applies and is therapeutically useful in both directions; tense leg muscles often relax after treatment of the paravertebral muscles, particularly with dry needling in the relevant segment. The lumbar muscles can become looser after successful treatment of mTrPs in the calves and ischiocrural muscles.

The quality of the arch of the foot also affects all the postural muscles (especially the paravertebral ones). Flattening of the arch, as in flat or spread feet in particular, leads to the leg axis turning inwards when standing or walking. This leads to a change in the tension and length of the muscles of the buttocks and affects mobility. This can lead to symptoms in the lumbar, pelvic and hip region. When bending the knees, this disorder is seen in the form of premature touching of the knee joints and lifting the heels. As a differential diagnosis, especially in women with a narrow pelvis, consider antetorsion syndrome due to hip dysplasia.

It is easy to examine a patient's stability. Just ask the patient to stand still. The therapist grasps the area of the iliosacral joints from behind and pushes the patient forward. If the patient is able to remain standing and resist the pressure, this indicates good function of the interplay

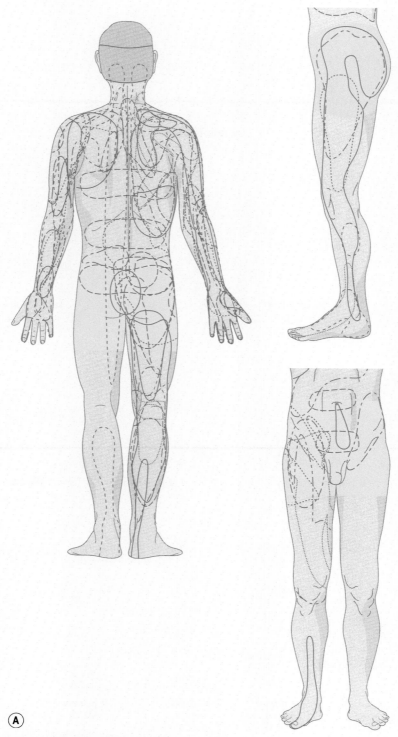

Fig. 32.1 Pain referral pattern (a) and affected muscles

Continued

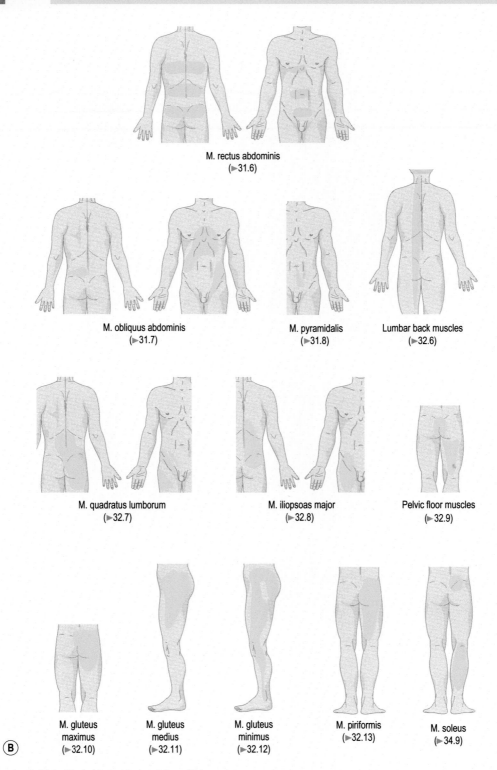

M. rectus abdominis
(►31.6)

M. obliquus abdominis
(►31.7)

M. pyramidalis
(►31.8)

Lumbar back muscles
(►32.6)

M. quadratus lumborum
(►32.7)

M. iliopsoas major
(►32.8)

Pelvic floor muscles
(►32.9)

M. gluteus
maximus
(►32.10)

M. gluteus
medius
(►32.11)

M. gluteus
minimus
(►32.12)

M. piriformis
(►32.13)

M. soleus
(►34.9)

B

Fig. 32.1—cont'd (b) in the lumbar spine, pelvis and hip region.

between legs and the lumbar–pelvic–hip region. There are two typical reactions if there are any disorders:

- a soft labile back that gives way in the sense of hyperlordosis of the lumbar spine and then falling or walking forwards,
- a hard, guarding back where the patient leans back stiffly against the therapist and goes onto their toes. This latter pattern leads to general strain on the lumbar spine, particularly the intervertebral discs and facet joints.

It is sensible to consider abdominal breathing during inspection when the patient is in the seated, standing and supine positions. A drawn-in, hard abdomen with reduced mobility on inspiration correlates with back, abdomen and lower body symptoms (see below) and is a good indication for trigger point treatment if more gentle methods including breathing therapy are insufficiently successful.

32.5 EXAMINATION FOR TRIGGER POINT IDENTIFICATION

Besides the functional examination, it is essential to the diagnosis of mTrPs to carry out thorough deep palpation of the lumbar–pelvic–hip region including the buttocks, abdominal and hip flexor muscles.

32.6 LUMBAR AUTOCHTHONOUS BACK MUSCLES

32.6.1 Anatomy

M. erector spinae

- Superficial, lateral tract with
  - straight muscle bands:
    – M. iliocostalis lumborum,
    – M. longissimus,
    – Mm. intertransversarii laterales and mediales lumborum (deeper-lying);
  - transverse muscles: *M. splenii (only cervicothoracic).*
- Deep medial tract with
  - straight muscle bands:
    – M. interspinalis lumborum,
    – M. spinalis thoracis (lumbar part);
  - transverse muscles: running superiorly, deep-lying:
    – Mm. rotatores,
    – Mm. multifidi.

EXAMINATION FINDINGS	TRIGGER POINT SEARCH IN (SEQUENCE DEPENDING ON SIGNIFICANCE)
Lumbar spine flexion limited or painful	Back extensors (see Section 32.6)
Straightening up is painful	Back extensors (see Section 32.6)
Limited lateral movement	Autochthonic lumbar back extensors incl. M. quadratus lumborum (Section 32.7) (contralateral), M. obliquus externus and internus
Standing flexion test	Back extensors ipsilaterally and/or ischiocrural muscles (Section 33.10) contralaterally
Anterior ilium	Back extensors (Section 32.6) ipsilaterally and/or M. iliopsoas (Section 32.8) ipsilaterally, M. rectus femoris, M. sartorius ipsilaterally
Posterior ilium	Ischiocrural muscles (Section 33.10) ipsilaterally
Limited rotation	Mm. rotatores (Section 32.6) (deep part of the lumbar autochthonous back extensors) ipsilaterally
Segmental function disorder (p.a. stress)	Relevant segmental paravertebral muscles
Pain on active hip flexion	M. rectus femoris, M. iliopsoas (Section 32.8) (from 90° single hip flexor!), M. tensor fasciae latae (Section 33.7), M. sartorius, M. gluteus medius and minimus (anterior part in each case) (Sections 32.11 and 32.12), M. pectineus (Section 33.8), M. adductor longus (Section 33.8)
Pain in the buttocks when running and at rest with increased lateral hip rotation	M. gluteus maximus and medius (dorsal part) (Sections 32.10 and 32.11), M. piriformis (Section 32.13), M. gemelli (Section 32.13), M. rectus femoris, M. obturatorius externus (Section 33.8), M. adductor brevis (Section 33.8), M. pectineus (Section 33.8), M. quadriceps femoris (Section 33.9), M. adductor longus and magnus (Section 33.8), M. biceps femoris (caput longum) (Section 33.10), M. sartorius

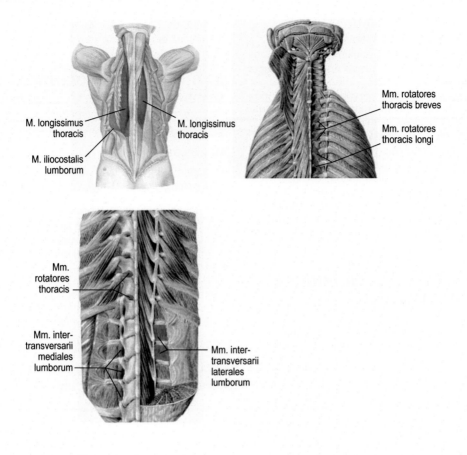

M. longissimus thoracis

M. longissimus thoracis

M. iliocostalis lumborum

Mm. rotatores thoracis breves

Mm. rotatores thoracis longi

Mm. rotatores thoracis

Mm. inter-transversarii mediales lumborum

Mm. inter-transversarii laterales lumborum

Innervation: dorsal branches of the spinal nerves.
Origin

- The lateral tract
  - M. iliocostalis lumborum together with M. longissimus thoracis from spinous processes of lumbar spine, posterior facet of sacrum, iliac crest (posterior third), fascia thoracolumbalis.
  - M. longissimus thoracis: together with the M. iliocostalis lumborum of the spinous processes of the lumbar spine, dorsal facet of the sacrum, frequently from the mamillary process of L2 and L1 and the transverse process of T12–T6.
  - Mm. intertransversarii laterales and mediales lumborum: iliac tuberosity, costal and accessory process of L6–L1, transverse process of T12.
- The medial tract
  - M. interspinalis lumborum: spinous processes of L5–L1.
  - M. spinalis thoracis: spinous process of (L3) L2, L1 and T12–T10 (closely associated with the M. longissimus thoracis).
  - Mm. rotatores: mamillary process of lumbar spine, transverse process of the thoracic spine (the long

rotator muscles each miss out a vertebra, the short rotators run to the next highest vertebra).
  - Mm. multifidi: posterior facet of the sacrum, posterior sacroiliac ligament, iliac crest (posterior part), mamillary process of the lumbar spine, transverse process of the thoracic spine (the muscle fibres miss out vertebrae 2–4).

Insertion

- The lateral tract
  - M. iliocostalis lumborum: 5th–12th rib (at the costal angle).
  - M. longissimus thoracis: the medial tract: mamillary process of L5, accessory process of L4–L1, transverse processes of the thoracic spine: lateral part: costal process of L4–L1, thoracolumbar fascia (deep layer), rib 12–rib 2 (medial to the costal angle).
  - Mm. intertransversarii laterales and mediales lumborum: costal process of L5, transverse process of T1, mamillary process of L4–L2.
- The medial tract
  - M. interspinalis lumborum: median sacral crest (upper margin), spinous process of L5–L2.

- M. spinalis thoracis: spinous processes of (T10) T9–T2 (closely associated with the multifidi muscles).
- Mm. rotatores: root of spinous processes of L3–L1 and T12–T1.
- Mm. multifidi: spinous processes of L5–L1 and T12–T1.

Function

- M. erector spinae: bending to one side, bilateral extension of the vertebral column.
- M. iliocostalis lumborum: bending to one side, bilateral extension.
- M. longissimus thoracis: bending to one side, bilateral extension.
- Mm. intertransversarii laterales and mediales lumborum: bending to one side, bilateral extension.
- M. interspinalis lumborum: segmental extension.
- M. spinalis thoracis: bending to one side, bilateral extension of the vertebral column.
- M. rotatores und multifidi: one-sided rotation and lateral flexion, bilateral extension.

32.6.2 Patient symptoms

- Dull, pressing, lumbar pain on one or both sides.
- Referral possible in a superior, inferior, gluteal or anterior direction or into the thigh.
- Painful restriction of movement (especially during extension and/or rotation).
- Non-specific preliminary diagnosis: degenerative vertebral column syndrome, blockage, lumbago, 'slipped disc', sciatica.

32.6.3 Trigger points

- mTrPs can be found throughout the lumbar back muscles.
- It is not often possible to attribute the mTrPs precisely to an individual muscle because of the complex anatomical and functional situation.
- Common predilectional sites are the classical acupuncture points in this area.
- If several mTrPs are active, the referral pattern can be complex, especially in combination with mTrPs in the M. quadratus lumborum (Section 32.7) and the gluteal muscles (see Sections 32.10–32.12).

	mTrP LOCATION	RADIATION	mTrP→ ACUPUNCTURE POINT
1	Multiple locations in the longissimus and iliocostalis lumborum muscles in the superficial lateral part (approx. 4–5 finger widths next to the median line)	Segmental, superiorly and inferiorly, gluteal region, thigh	Points on the inner and outer bladder meridian BL 22–BL 26, BL 51–BL 52, Ex-R 4, Ex-R 6
2	Multiple locations in the deep medial part (approx. 1–2 finger widths next to the median line) in the Mm. interspinalis and spinalis, Mm. rotatores, Mm. multifidi, Mm. semispinalis	Predominantly segmental, i.e. horizontal (occasionally posterior, lateral even anterior)	Extra-R 2 (Hua tuo jiaji) and inner bladder meridian (BL 22–BL 26)

32.6.4 Diagnosis

Questioning

- Acute or repetitive strain?
- Trauma? Cold, draughts?
- For chronic back pain and predominantly somatic disease careful psychological evaluation (work, relationships, sexuality).

Inspection

- Protective posture.
- Postural problems and asymmetry.
- Scoliosis or other deformity.

Physical examination

- Full examination of the vertebral column necessary (see Section 13.6 and Ch. 32).
- Examination standing, sitting, in supine position and lateral decubitus position.
- Painful restriction of movement.
- Flexion up to 45°: indicates M. erector spinae (main weight-bearing at flexion up to 45°).
- Rotation pain: indicates deep-seated M. rotatores and M. multifidi.
- Pain on extension: indicates M. interspinalis lumborum (segmental extension) and M. erector spinae.
- Leaning to the side with pain on the affected side: indicates M. iliocostalis lumborum.
- Segmental functional examination (mobility).
- Note co-reaction of segment, e.g. hyperaesthesia to mechanical and/or thermal stimuli, segmental connective tissue reaction (Kibler fold).
- The affected dermatome lies inferiorly to the motion segment.
- Palpation in prone position (possibly pillow under the abdomen to raise the lumbar lordosis): Proceed systematically from superior to inferior:

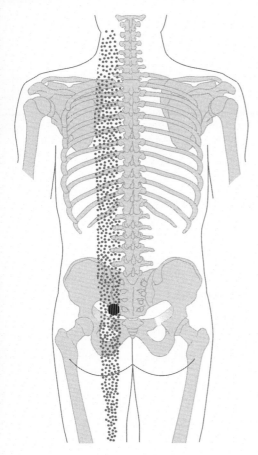

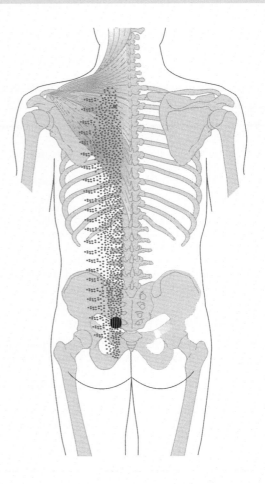

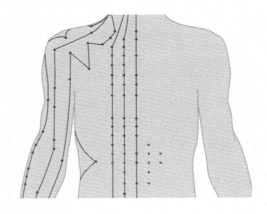

1. begin at the lateral margin of the M. erector spinae,
2. then at the level of the M. erector spinae,
3. medial margin of the M. erector spinae,
4. between the spinous process and the medial margin of the M. erector spinae.

- Firm pressure for palpation for mTrPs in the deep muscles.
- If radiculopathy is suspected differentiated neurological examination, otherwise basic neurological examination.

Technical examination

- Note the guidelines for back pain diagnosis, i.e. no extensive tests with acute back pain, if fever, weight loss, bladder or rectal disorder, or progressive neurological disorders can be excluded (and there is no history of fractures or tumours).
- Radiological tests for long-term back pain with no response to therapy, depending on the findings.

32.6.5 Specific aspects

- Many 'non-specific' back pains are caused by mTrPs.
- With almost all patient there are mTrPs independently of the primary cause of the back pain.
- Chronic back pain is a biopsychosocial event.
- Explanation and activation of the patient are key.
- Long-term effects have only been shown for multimodal treatment plans. These include explanation and information, physiotherapy, behavioural therapy, medical training and gaining competence in own responsibility for handling the disease by learning and improving with relaxation, body awareness, dealing with stress, and social competence. Unresolved workplace problems and continuous examinations and reports can themselves lead to a lack of success with these plans.
- If the patient is under great and chronic strain referral to specialised interdisciplinary treatment unit
- Many patients with fibromyalgia, chronic fatigue syndrome and somatoform pain disorders also suffer from back pain, often myofascially caused.

32.6.6 Therapy

Instructions for manual trigger point therapy

- When sitting, the thoracic parts of the lateral tract (M. iliocostalis and M. longissimus) are more active than the lumbar parts so look for mTrPs appropriate to problems when sitting.
- If spinous processes are tender, the mTrPs are usually deep in the medial tract (Mm. semispinales, multifidi, rotatores).

- With mTrPs in the muscles of the medial tract the referred pain area is usually small and in the local surroundings so local treatment is necessary for lumbar pain.
- Treatment of the deep parts is strenuous so use aids (trigger point sticks) to relieve the fingers.

Stretching

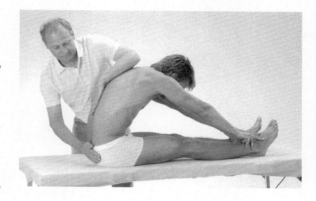

- The patient sits on the couch.
- Upper body leaning forwards with arms extended.
- The therapist supports the flexion in the area of the lumbar spine with pressure and traction so that the arm close to the head nestles against the thoracic spine.
- The hand away from the head tries to fix the sacrum.
- Realistically, this exercise only leads to slight extension but its use helps with improving the doctor–patient relationship.

Physical procedures

- All physical procedures are suitable; note the depth of penetration in each case; make use of segmental reflex effects.

Infiltration/dry needling

- Treatment is usually in the prone position as the anatomy is somewhat changed in the lateral decubitus position.
- Hand tensioning technique for the deep muscles, vertical insertion.
- Pinch grip for the superficial muscles, diagonal insertion.
- Place the and flat during the injection (broad area of activation of Aβ-fibres via mechanoreceptors so less needle pain).

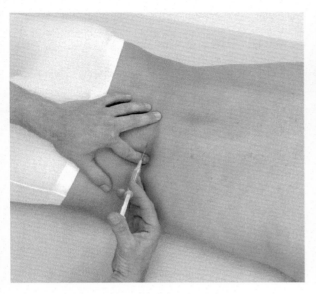
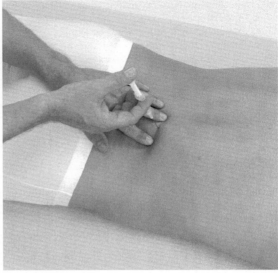

- If the patient is very tense, begin with contralateral superficial needling or use contralateral spot technique.
- Depending on location and constitution long needles required (up to 8 cm).
- During treatment of the superficial M. erector spinae the local muscle reaction is often visible and tangible.
- Mm. rotatores (only L1–L3):
  - vertical insertion 1.5 finger widths next to the spinous process (T12–L2),
  - deepen slowly,
  - overcome first resistance (especially with acupuncture needles (thoracolumbar fascia),
  - on contact with the transverse process guide needle inferiorly and alter to medial.
- Mm. multifidi (L1–L5):
  - vertical insertion 1.5 finger widths next to the spinous process (T12–L5),
  - deepen slowly,
  - overcome first resistance (especially with acupuncture needles) (thoracolumbar fascia),
  - on contact with the transverse process withdraw needle and change needle direction to medial,
  - gentle segmental mobilisation following needling.

Classical Chinese acupuncture

Local and locoregional points (also contralateral): BL 22–BL 26, BL 51–BL 52, Ex-R 4, Ex-R 6 (lateral tract), Ex-R 2 (Hua tuo jiaji), BL 22–BL 26 (medial tract), Ex-R 5, GV 3, GV 4, GV 5, Ashi points superficially in the segment (belt-shaped, Gleditsch Very Point technique).

Distal points
- SI 3 (with acute symptoms, strong manual stimulation or electrostimulation), SI 6, NP 67 ('dislocation point', 3 cun distal LI 11, at the margin of the M. extensor

digitorum longus), König/Wancura experience point; Ex-AH 7 (Yao tong dian): lumbago point, BL 40 (especially for acute symptoms, strong manual stimulation or electrostimulation), BL 40, BL 58 on both sides, local), BL 60, BL 62, CV 26 (especially for acute symptoms, strong manual stimulation or electrostimulation), CV 4, CV 6: anterior stabilisation, KI 2 (especially for acute symptoms, strong manual stimulation or electrostimulation): acute point.
- Moxa plan for acute strain: 3 moxa cylinders (cones) CV 6 and BL 23, 7 moxa cylinders (cones) CV 4, BL 29, CV 2.

Control points/symptomatic points: for chronic back pain the symptoms should be distinguished in accordance with TCM, for moisture (especially heaviness and feeling of swelling) SP 6, SP 9, for sensitivity to cold: KI 3, GV 4, moxibustion, GB 34 (tendon masterpoint), GB 25 (kidney alarm point).

Microsystem acupuncture

Ear: vertebral column, sympathic ganglia, Shenmen, Jérôme point; lumbar spine representation on the antihelix or directly next to it in the direction of the helix.
YNSA: D zone in the temporal area (Y zone), D1–D5 points preauricular.
NPS-O (Siener): point area at the lateral malleolus.
Mouth: intraoral at the canine tooth, lower jaw or extraoral analogue point.

Kiiko Matsumoto acupuncture

- If there is a neurological cause: CV 12 and CV 10.
- For tenderness at KI 2 (fire point): KI 7 (metal point) and KI 10 (water point), angle of insertion (especially at KI 7) depending on tenderness at KI 2.

- Tenderness at GB 25 (Dai mai): KI 7 (for reduction of tenderness and symptoms of the M. iliocostalis).
- For tenderness in the area of the navel: GB 25 (Mu point of the kidney) and KI 7 and SP 9.
- For tension in the area of the navel: KI 16, CV 7 and CV 9.
- For tenderness in the area of the M. iliocostalis: point 1 cm laterally from BL 40.

M. iliocostalis lumborum

- If there is a neurological cause: CV 12 and CV 10.
- For tenderness at KI 2 (fire point): KI 7 (metal point) and KI 10 (water point), insertion angle depending on tenderness at KI 2.
- Tenderness at GB 26 (Dai mai): KI 7.
- Tenderpoints in the area of the navel (KI 16, CV 7, CV 9).
- For tenderness in the area of the muscle: needle point 1 cm laterally from BL 40.

Mm. intertransversarii laterales and mediales lumborum

- Tenderness at GB 26 (Dai mai): KI 7 ipsilaterally (with the flow of the meridian).

Mm. interspinales lumborum

- Tenderness at GB 26 (Dai mai): KI 7 ipsilaterally (with the flow of the meridian).
- Tenderness in the area of the Huato Jiaji at the level L2–L3: BL 40 ipsilaterally, insertion angle 15–45°.

M. interspinalis thoracis

- Tenderness in the area of the Huato Jiaji at the level T7: BL 58 ipsilaterally, insertion angle 15–45° (with the flow of the meridian).

Mm. rotatores

- Tenderness at GB 26 (Dai mai): KI 7 ipsilaterally (with the flow of the meridian).

Psychosomatics/relaxation

- Psychosomatic aspects: anxiety, anxiety avoidance behaviour, work and/or social stress, bullying, problems with sexuality with lumbar symptoms: a categorical denial of psychosomatic factors is often indicative.
- Learning pain and stress management strategies.
- Relaxation techniques can be individually selected depending on personal preferences. Give preference to techniques which also have physical benefits (Qigong, breathing therapy, yoga, Glaser psychotonics).
- Yoga and Qigong include exercises to keep the vertebral column upright and at the same time impart calm and composure (see Ch. 24).

32.6.7 Recommendations for the patient

Autostretching

The following stretching exercises should be individually selected depending on the overall mobility of the patient or used in combination. They are more effective than passive extension.

- First exercise (left): sitting with legs crossed with the upper body flexed slightly forward. Traction can be increased by placing the closed hands over the feet.
- Second exercise (right): in the supine position flex the thigh on the affected side and draw to the body with both hands so that the head and knee are flexed, lift the hips and roll to the back (rocking movement); the exercise can then be carried out depending on development with just flexion of the leg of the affected side.
- Third exercise (bottom): the patient kneels, buttocks on heels (**warning:** knee joint problems), and flexes the back until the head lies between the knees.

Additional measures

- Point out associations with psychosocial factors.
- Squeeze out mTrPs by lying on a tennis ball (pressure massage).
- Partner massage with cupping.
- Rhythm of daily life (interrupt long periods of sitting down, move about in between).
- Changes in the environment to adjust to the back should only be made if there are actual structural changes in the vertebral column (very rare). If too much value is placed on these measures this can lead to chronification.
- Work out a home exercise programme as part of the physiotherapeutic treatment. Functional training of the muscles (coordinative interaction of the muscles, anterior stabilisation and mobility training, build-up of strength is not the focus).
- **Warning:** with standard back training there is a risk of acquiring stereotypical behaviour patterns or strengthening the anxiety avoidance behaviour.
- Lifting heavy objects in a manner suitable for the back, but deconditioning – incorrect movement – pain.
- Orthopaedic correction with pronounced body asymmetry (inserts, heel wedges if leg difference is >1 cm).
- Instruct relatives on handling partner's pain.

32.7 M. QUADRATUS LUMBORUM

32.7.1 Anatomy

Innervation: Rr. musculares (plexus lumbalis); N. intercostalis (N. thoracicus (T12)).

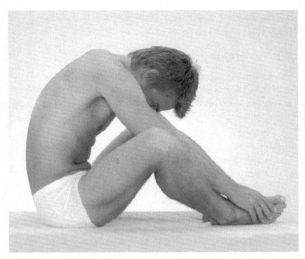
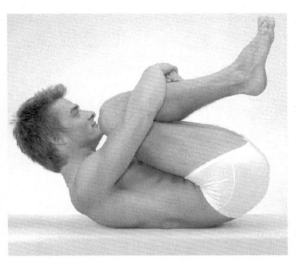
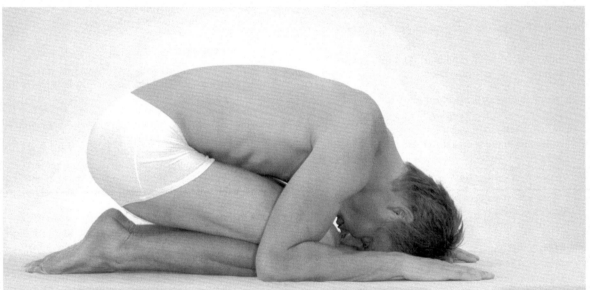

Origin: labium internum of the crista iliaca (posterior third), Lig. iliolumbale.
Insertion: 12th rib (medial area), costal process of L4–L1.
Function: lateral flexion of the vertebral column, lowering of the ribs (expiration), lifts the hips.

32.7.2 Patient symptoms

- Classic lumbar back pain with high pain intensity, limited mobility, pain referral into the gluteal and/or hip region and intolerable pain.
- Dull, oppressive, myofascial pain, but often also stabbing pain on movement.

- Possible preliminary diagnoses: degenerative lumbar spine syndrome, radiculopathy (especially with involvement of the gluteal muscles), iliosacral joint dysfunction, coxarthrosis, bursitis trochanterica, nephropathy.

32.7.3 Trigger points
32.7.4 Diagnosis

Questioning
- Lifting heavy objects in rotated position?
- Trauma, e.g. fall.

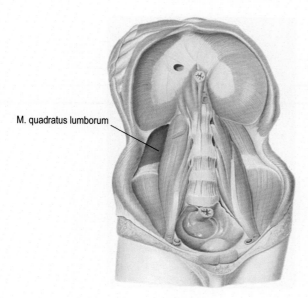

M. quadratus lumborum

mTrP LOCATION	RADIATION	mTrP→ ACUPUNCTURE POINT
1 In the upper medial part of the muscle 2–3 finger widths below the medial area of the 12th rib, predominantly in the fibres which run vertically	Paravertebral lumbar, dermatome L1–L3, hips laterally	BL 51, BL 52
2 In the middle and lower part of the muscle, predominantly in the diagonally running fibres	Paravertebral, lumbar, gluteal, hips, lateral thigh	BL 23, BL 24, Ex-R 6 Ex-R 7

- Mother with child (frequent carrying, heavy child?).
- Tight-fisted?

Inspection
- Lumbar scoliosis?
- Ask the patient to turn from side to side while lying down: high pain intensity.

Physical examination
- Full examination of the vertebral column necessary (see Section 13.6 and Ch. 32).

- Examination of the pelvic tilt while standing and when seated (palpation of the iliac crest and the SIPS (spina iliaca post. sup.) comparing the sides): if there is a deviation in both positions, shortening of the M. quadratus lumborum is a possible cause (the affected side is higher).
- Contralateral lateral inclination, flexion of the vertebral column, and occasionally ipsilateral lateral inclination may be painfully limited.
- The extent of the lateral inclination can be estimated if the arms and hands are placed on the side of the leg during lateral flexion: mark the tip of the middle finger in each case at the end of the movement and compare the sides.
- Examination for difference in leg length.
- Palpation while seated and in lateral extension position (see below). The flat hand presses medially to laterally around the M. erector spinae (between the ribs and the iliac crest), at the lateral border try to surround the muscles and exercise pressure in an anteromedial direction with the fingers: mTrPs can often not be directly palpated, but appropriate pressure regularly causes the known pain if mTrPs are present.
- If the pain is superiorly referred, there may be mTrPs in the M. latissimus dorsi.
- Frequently segmental functional disorder/ hypomobility (T11–L4).
- Kibler fold positive at T11/T12, with deeper paravertebral tenderness at the level of L2–L4.
- Examination for satellite trigger points in the gluteal muscles.

Technical examination
- Laboratory tests, with ultrasound if nephropathy is the suspected medical diagnosis.
- Radiological measurement for evidence of difference in leg length.

32.7.5 Specific aspects

- Muscular basis of the posterior abdominal wall.
- Complex course of fibres so various referral patterns have been described.
- For chronic lumbar back pain, mTrPs in the M. quadratus lumborum are very often an important pain causing and maintaining factor.
- Include the transverse abdominal muscles in the treatment plan.

32.7.6 Therapy

Instructions for manual trigger point therapy

- Iliocostal fibres are easily palpable and treatable at the insertion site at the iliac crest.
- In the treatment of the M. quadratus lumborum parts of the transverse abdominal muscles, the

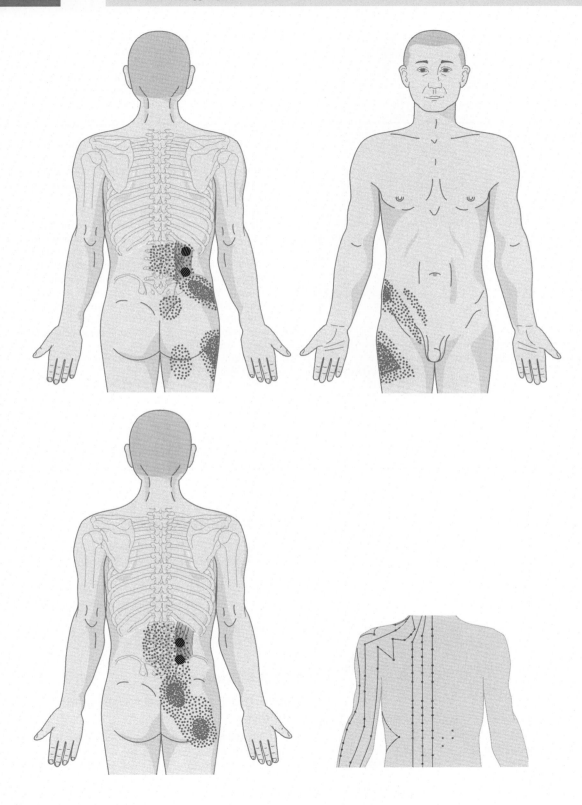

M. longissimus, M. latissimus dorsi and M. serratus posterior inferior are treated at the same time.

- Important with low back pain: it is worth taking your time and being very thorough with treatment.
- Frequently primary mTrPs.

Stretching

Lengthwise stretching: with this form of lengthwise stretching, muscles such as the M. obliquus abdomini and the M. tensor fasciae latae are also stretched; these are frequently affected in the sense of muscle function chains.

- Patient lying on the unaffected side.
- Lateral flexion of the trunk by lying on a firm pillow shaped to fit between the ribs and the iliac crest.
- The upper arm is elevated to its maximum (placed over the other side of the head).
- The upper leg is extended and the lower leg flexed at the hip and knee.
- The therapist stands behind the patient, the hand close to the head lies on the lateral thorax (over ribs 7–11), the hand away from the head on the iliac crest.

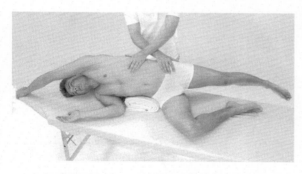

- Extension by superior and gentle anterior traction on the thorax and inferior and slightly dorsal traction on the iliac crest.

Transverse stretching

- Position as for lengthwise stretching.
- The therapist stands in front of the patient.
- The hand away from the head lies on the side and back of the iliac crest, the hand by the head lies with the ball of the thumb or the fist on the muscle from the side (deep between the ribs and the iliac crest, as inferiorly as possible).
- Extension by traction on the iliac crest in an anterior direction and pressure in a medial direction.

Lengthwise extension is frequently more effective here and is sufficient.

Physical procedures

- TENS, segmental counter-irritation, cupping (blood-cupping, cupping without bloodletting), cupping head massage.

Infiltration techniques/dry needling

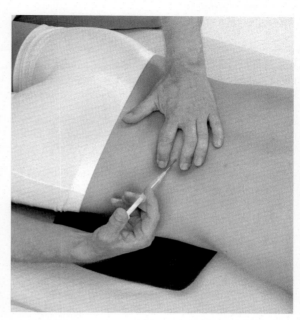

The M. quadratus lumborum is a flat muscle so advance slowly after a depth of 3 cm and pay attention to information from the patient!

- Patient in prone position.
- Dry needling is advantageous as the risk of complications is less and location is better when using an atraumatic needle point.
- Needle length 5–8 cm (depending on patient's build).
- Proceed from a lateral direction:
  - the flat, non-treating hand presses medially to laterally around the M. erector spinae (between the ribs and the iliac crest), at the lateral border try to surround the muscles and exercise pressure in an anteromedial direction with the fingers: with typical pain provocation the mTrPs are released by spreading the index and middle finger but maintaining medial pressure,
  - push the needle forward slowly; once contact is made with a transverse process the maximum required depth has been achieved, so withdraw the needle to the subcutaneous area, change direction and push forward again,
  - injection/dry needling from a lateral direction through the M. latissimus dorsi,
  - no deep injection superior to the spinous process of L2; **warning:** risk of pneumothorax,
  - **warning:** kidneys, inject as dorsally as possible.

- Proceed from a dorsal direction:
  - this is the choice when the lateral procedure is unsuccessful,
  - 2–4 finger widths next to the spinous process.

Classical Chinese acupuncture

Local and locoregional points (also contralateral): BL 23, BL 24, BL 52, Ex-R 6 (Yao yi), Ex-R 7 (Yao yan): important and often effective points in the area of origin of the muscle; segmental needling using Very Point (frequently points which are sensitive as far as the lateral trunk); GV 3, GV 4, BL 54.

Distal points

- SI 3 (especially with acute symptoms, strong manual stimulation or electrostimulation), SI 6, NP 67 (for acute symptoms, strong manual stimulation or electrostimulation), ('dislocation point', 3 cun distal LI 11, at the margin of the M. extensor digitorum longus), König/Wancura experience point; Ex-AH 7 (Yao tong dian): lumbago point, BL 40 (especially for acute symptoms, strong manual stimulation or electrostimulation), BL 58, BL 60, BL 62, CV 26 (especially for acute symptoms, strong manual stimulation or electrostimulation), CV 4, CV 6: anterior stabilisation, KI 2 (especially for acute symptoms, strong manual stimulation or electrostimulation): acute point.
- Moxa plan for acute strain: 3 moxa cylinders (cones) CV 6 and BL 23, 7 moxa cylinders (cones) CV 4, BL 29, CV 2.

Control points/symptomatic points: for chronic back pain the symptoms should be differentiated using TCM. For moisture (especially feeling of heaviness or swelling) SP 6, SP 9, for sensitivity to cold: KI 3, GV 4, moxibustion, GB 34 (tendon masterpoint), GB 25 (kidney alarm point).

Microsystem acupuncture

Ear: lumbar spine representation on the anthelix or directly next to it in the direction of the helix.
YNSA: D zone in the temporal area (Y zone), D1–D5 points preauricular.
NPS-O (Siener): point area at the lateral malleolus.
Mouth: intraoral at the canine tooth, lower jaw or extraoral analogue point.

Kiiko Matsumoto acupuncture

- With painful palpation in the area of SP 3 (general muscle-relaxing point) before needling of the point, needling of distal points.
- Alternative: SP 5 (metal point) and SP 9 (water point).

Psychosomatics/relaxation techniques

- For chronic back pain, long-term review of the psychoemotional and social factors indispensable (see Section 32.2).
- 'Strengthen your back', 'keep your back clear', i.e. search for potential support in specific life situations.
- Relaxation techniques must be individually chosen together with the patient.
- Qigong, yoga for physical strength (e.g. straightening the pelvis in the sense of anterior stabilisation) while simultaneously addressing mental and spiritual aspects.

32.7.7 Recommendations for the patient

Autostretching

Patient lying on the side not affected (see above).

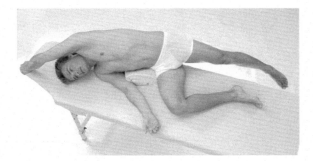

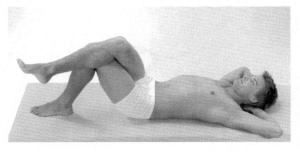

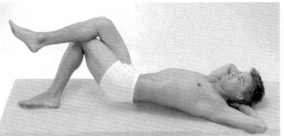

- Lateral flexion of the trunk by lying on a firm pillow shaped to fit between the ribs and the iliac crest.
- The upper arm is elevated to its maximum (placed over the other side of the head).
- The upper leg is extended and the lower leg flexed at the hip and knee.
- Stretching is performed by gravity extending the leg (allow it to hang over).

Gentle stretching can be carried out in the supine position (centre and below).

- Patient in supine position.
- Hands under back of head.
- The leg on the affected side is placed over the other leg.
- Press the knee on the affected side to the bed so that the hips go with it or are lifted.

Additional measures

- Lift heavy weights correctly to protect the back.
- Making up for true difference in leg length. The patient should feel relief and improvement. If the locomotor system has compensated well for decades for the difference (especially in elderly people), levelling out can lead to deterioration and can be a disadvantage: trial for 4 weeks.
- Change to a soft mattress or place a 2 cm-thick wooden board lengthwise under the mattress.
- Alternately lift left and right hips lying in the supine position in bed.
- Do not sit on loose change.
- For acute symptoms relief through:
  - avoidance of combined flexion and rotation movement in everyday life, e.g. sitting down or getting up,
  - avoid bending down,
  - sleep on one side with a pillow between the legs (avoid pelvic tilt at the same time as flexion),
  - knee roll for those who sleep on their back.
- **Warning:** for chronic back pain, take great care about acquired pathological behaviour patterns or continuous deviant patterns: mental anxiety can be made worse, the patient feels 'disabled' more than often necessary, the symptoms become the focus of everyday life as a result of complicated postural and motion correction.
- Self-treatment (with a tennis ball).
- Rhythm of daily life (interrupt long periods of sitting down, move about in between).
- Relaxed position while seated (support in the thoracolumbar transition).
- Orthopaedic correction with pronounced body asymmetry (inserts, heel wedges if leg difference is >1 cm).

32.8 M. ILIOPSOAS MAJOR

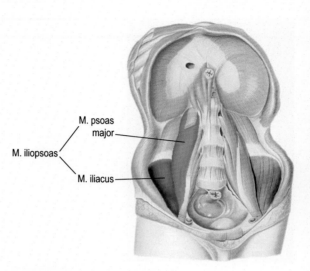

M. psoas major

M. iliopsoas

M. iliacus

32.8.1 Anatomy

Innervation: rotator muscles (lumbar plexus).
Origin
- M. iliacus: iliac fossa, inferior anterior iliac spine, anterior capsule of the hip joint.
- M. psoas major: superficial layer: lateral surface of the body from T12 to L4, intervertebral discs, deep layer: costal process from L1 to L4.

Insertion: trochanter minor and bordering area of the medial labium of the linea aspera.
Function
- Lumbar spine: lateral flexion, extension (hyperlordosis).
- Hip joint: flexion, medial rotation (lateral rotation with concomitant contraction of the Mm. glutei).

32.8.2 Patient symptoms

- Classical lumbago and sciatica with predominantly vertical pain pattern.
- Pain worse when standing with the vertebral column upright.
- Pain worse when standing up from a seated position.
- Lumbosacral pain when getting up after sitting down for a long time (M. iliacus).
- Back pain at night in supine or prone position (M. iliacus).
- Possible preliminary diagnoses: degenerative lumbar spine syndrome, spondylitis ankylosis, meralgia paraesthetica, 'failed back surgery syndrome', coxarthrosis, periarthropathia coxae, inguinal hernia, 'chronic appendicitis'.

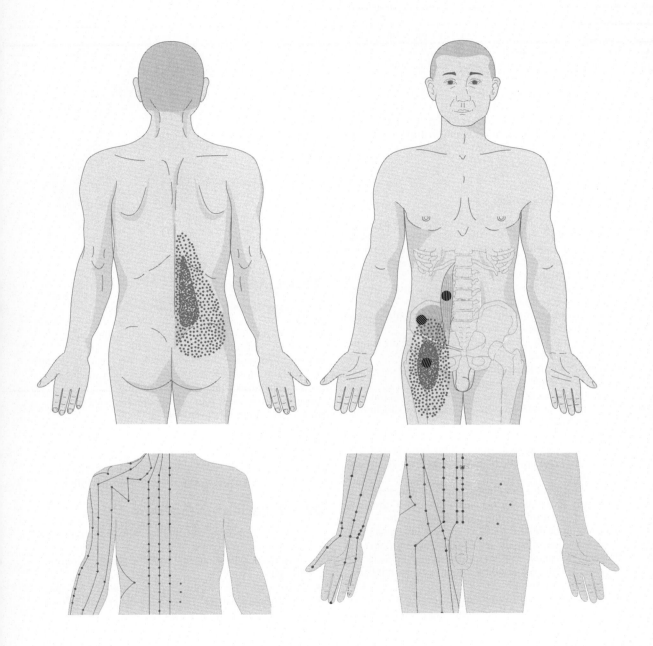

32.8.3 Trigger points

mTrP	LOCATION	RADIATION	mTrP→ ACUPUNCTURE POINT
1	In the psoas major and minor at the level of L1–L4 paravertebrally	Paravertebrally from the thoracolumbar transition to the sacrum, sometimes to the opposite side as well	BL 23, BL 24, BL 25, Ex-R 2 Hua tuo jiaji (L1–L4)
2	In the iliacus at the medial wall of the iliac fossa	Paravertebral and lumbosacral, hips including the inguinal area, dorsal, anterior and lateral thigh, rarely lower leg and foot	SP 14, Ex-BB 1, Ex-BB Ti tuo (3.5 cun lateral to KI 13)
3	In the iliopsoas below the inguinal ligament (middle area)	As mTrP 1 and mTrP 2, lesser pelvis	LR 11, SP 12

mTrP 1 and mTrP 2 require a certain amount of time as it is a slow careful procedure to avoid reflex tensioning of the abdominal wall muscles and the abdominal organs, needing relatively deep strong pressure with the palpation finger while avoiding a guarding or tickling reaction, so the non-palpating hand is place contralaterally flat with light pressure.

- mTrP 1: palpation finger lateral to the M. rectus abdominis at the level of the navel, slow medial pressure against the transverse processes of the lumbar spine, usually a distinction can be made between pain caused by compression of the bowel (slight, diffuse pain) and pain caused by pressure on the psoas (strong pain, localised, causes the known pain symptoms after pressing for a long time), difficulties in patients who are obese or have a very muscular abdominal wall, same procedure superiorly and inferiorly to the navel.
- mTrP 2: therapist sits on the affected side, and places the palmar surface and thumb on the gluteus minimus, index, middle and ring fingers carry out flexion with all finger joints and follow the iliac crest to the iliac fossa, palpation along the iliac fossa and palpate deeply, increase pressure from medial to lateral when reach sensitive or hardened site (try compression of the muscle against the iliac fossa).
- mTrP 3: between the inguinal ligament and the trochanter minor, one or two finger widths lateral to the middle of the thigh (seen from the anterior), to be sure the muscle is located, ask the patient to flex the hips slightly.
- Frequently associated hypomobility of the iliosacral joint.

Technical examination: ultrasound; CT if aortic aneurysm is suspected.

32.8.4 Diagnosis

Questioning
- Excessive, non-optimum abdominal muscle training, e.g. sit-ups up to 90° hip flexion.
- Football (shooting at goal), rowing? Dancing? Cross-country skiing? Hurdling?
- Condition following hip operation?

Inspection
- When standing, the affected leg has as little weight on it as possible and is slightly flexed.
- Hyperlordosis of the lumbar spine.

Physical examination
- Look for shortening in associated with extension.
- Relief of lumbosacral pain when the hips are flexed.
- Painfully limited extension of the vertebral column with lateral flexion to the ipsilateral side (iliacus), painfully limited extension of the vertebral column with lateral flexion to the contralateral side (psoas).
- No pain when coughing or breathing (more likely the Mm. quadratus lumborum).
- Palpation in supine position with relaxed abdominal wall, possibly slight elevation of the upper body.

32.8.5 Specific aspects

- For chronic lumbosacral back pain, the iliopsoas is very often an important factor for causing and maintaining pain (biopsychosocial event).
- The most affected muscle for walking, running and jumping.
- Frequently involved in 'adductor problems' in footballers (inguinal pain).
- Concomitant pain with coxarthrosis.
- Psoas compression with aortic aneurysm.
- Possibly visceral pain projection (especially the intestine).
- Impingement syndrome:
  - N. cutaneus femoralis in the M. iliacus,
  - N. femoralis, N. genitofemoralis, N. ilioinguinalis, N. iliohypogastricus in the M. psoas.

32.8.6 Therapy

Instructions for manual trigger point therapy

- Treatment of the M. iliacus:
  - patient sits or lies on their side or back,
  - mTrPs in the M. iliacus are often far away in a cranio-dorsal direction (on the medial side of the ilium).
- Treatment of the M. psoas:
  - the patient lies on their back,
  - use the fingers to slowly palpate deeply (from the lateral margin of the M. rectus abdominis),
  - by drawing up the leg (flexion in the hip joint) and stretching (extension in the hip joint) the tension and release of the psoas can definitely be perceived (note: abdominal aorta and/or urethra).
- mTrPs are often at the site where the psoas and iliacus come together.
- Also check and if necessary treat the insertion site at the trochanter minor.
- Frequently primary mTrPs.
- One of the key muscles in low back pain.

Stretching

- Transverse stretching of the iliacus muscle (top left):
  - patient lies on the back with the hips slightly flexed,
  - ulnar aide of the therapist's hand on the iliac fossa, possibly supported by other hand,
  - pressure down and medially ('stretching out').
- Stretching of the iliopsoas in lateral decubitus (top right):
  - patient lying on the side not affected,
  - hand by the head holds the pelvis in place,
  - hand away from head grasps the whole leg and guides it to his own body and stretches by means of hyperextension in the hips.
- Lengthwise stretching of the iliopsoas (below):
  - patient on their back with buttocks at the edge of the bed,
  - even out lumbar spine lordosis with pillows,
  - the patient holds the leg not affected with both hands at the knee so that it is fully flexed at the hip and knee,
  - the therapist stands at the medial side of the affected leg and grasps the thigh just above the knee (below left) with the hand near the head,
  - the hand away from the head grasps the lower leg above the ankle,
  - stretching by extension in the knee joint and subsequent hyperextension in the hip joint so that the hips are slightly rotated medially (below right).

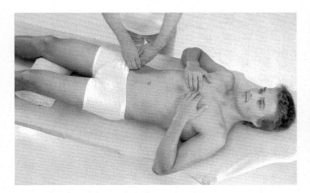
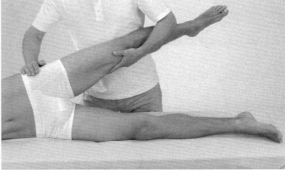
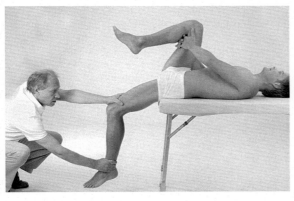
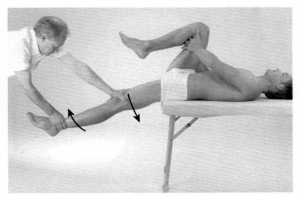

Physical procedures

- mTrP 1: segmental-reflex e.g. with TENS or (moist) heat pack on the abdomen along the course of the muscle.
- mTrP 2: laser, ultrasound.
- mTrP 3: all procedures possible.

Infiltration/dry needling

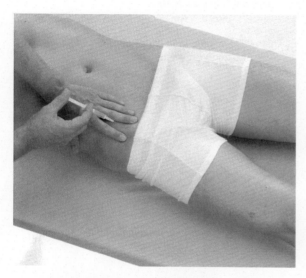

For mTrP 1 and mTrP 2 dry needling only with prior needling of distal points and not until specific manual treatment has been unsuccessful with intensive concomitant home exercise programme.

mTrP 1
- Prerequisite: specific experience in infiltration techniques near the vertebral column, normal blood clotting (note: NSAIDs).
- Needle length at least 8 cm.
- Treatment only from dorsal direction and dry needling only with slow pushing forward of the needle.
- Palpation in prone position with pillow under the abdomen to raise the lumbar lordosis.
- Insertion three finger widths lateral to the spinous process (L1–L4 possible).
- With paraesthesia withdraw needle as far as the subcutis and change the needle direction slightly in a inferior direction.
- With bone contact (transverse process) change the needle direction slightly in a superior direction.
- Stimulation of the mTrP if the known symptoms can be caused.
- There is usually a pronounced 'post-treatment muscle soreness' (explain to the patient).
- CT-controlled treatment may be indicated for specific cases with great stain caused by pain and resistance to treatment. A LA injection is also possible in such cases.

mTrP 2
- Dry needling is preferable to infiltration as there is less danger of nerve irritation or injury.
- In the supine position, possibly with the hip joint slightly flexed.
- The therapist should be seated to make sure the needle can be introduced safely.
- Procedure as for palpation: once the point is located it is released by spreading the index and middle fingers while keeping the pressure the same.
- Insertion between the two fingers.
- Push the needle slowly forward at the medial side of the ilium (not directly at the periosteum) until the mTrP is reached.

mTrP 3
- In the supine position, thigh slightly abducted and flexed.
- Hand span technique.
- Location of the femoral artery.
- Vertical insertion of at least one finger width next to the femoral artery (anatomy from medial to lateral: V. femoralis, A. femoralis, N. femoralis).

Classical Chinese acupuncture

Local and locoregional points (also contralateral): BL 22–BL 26, Hua tuo jiaji, BL 51 and BL 52, segmental needling using the Very Point technique (sensitive points often as far as the lateral trunk) at the level of T11–L2, depending on sensitivity, no needling of SP 14, Ex-BB 1, Ex-BB Ti Tuo for M. iliacus (bowel injury), Ashi points especially on the thigh.

Distal points
- SI 3 (for acute symptoms, strong manual stimulation or electrostimulation): meridian point (Yang–Yang axis), switch point CV with paravertebral lumbar pain; SI 6; GB 41 (for acute symptoms, strong manual stimulation or electrostimulation): belt-shaped pain (switch point Dai mai), Ex-AH 7 (Yao tong dian): lumbago point, NP 67 (for acute symptoms, strong manual stimulation or electrostimulation) ('dislocation point', 3 cun distal to LI 11, at the margin of the M. extensor digitorum longus), König/Wancura experience point, LU 3: M. iliopsoas (from Perschke), BL 62: M. iliacus (from Perschke), BL 40 (for acute symptoms, strong manual stimulation or electrostimulation); BL 60 and BL 62 for paravertebral lumbar pain; CV 26; CV 4, CV 6: anterior stabilisation, GB 31 for lateral (hip) pain, GB 37 for lateral (hip) pain, GB 39 for lateral (hip) pain, KI 2 (especially for acute symptoms, strong manual stimulation or electrostimulation): acute point.
- Moxa plan for acute strain: 3 moxa cylinders (cones) CV 6 and BL 23, 7 moxa cylinders (cones) CV 4, BL 29, CV 2.

Control points/symptomatic points: for chronic back pain the symptoms should be distinguished in accordance with TCM, for moisture (especially heaviness and feeling of swelling) SP 6, SP 9, for sensitivity to cold: KI 3, GV 4, moxibustion, GB 34 (tendon masterpoint), GB 25 (kidney alarm point).

Microsystem acupuncture

Ear: lumbar spine representation on the antihelix or directly next to it in the direction of the helix.
YNSA: D zone in the temporal area (Y zone), D1–D5 points preauricular.
NPS-O (Siener): point area at the lateral malleolus.
Mouth: intraoral at the canine tooth, lower jaw or extraoral analogue point.

Kiiko Matsumoto acupuncture

- If there is a neurological cause: CV 12 and CV 10.

Psychosomatics/relaxation

- For chronic back pain, long-term review of the psychoemotional and social factors indispensable (see Section 32.2).
- 'Strengthen your back', 'keep your back clear', i.e. search for potential support in specific life situations.
- For abnormal anxiety symptoms psychiatric investigation.
- Relaxation techniques must be individually chosen together with the patient.
- Qigong and yoga for physical strength (e.g. straightening the pelvis in the sense of anterior stabilisation) while simultaneously addressing mental and spiritual aspects.
- Body awareness.
- Psychosomatic aspects: sexuality (strain, demands, lack of emotionality), emotional cold, psychoemotional, social and/or work-related stress.

32.8.7 Recommendations for the patient

Autostretching

- Supine position.
- Possibly support the lumbar spine to avoid strain on the vertebral column.
- Buttocks on the edge of the bed.

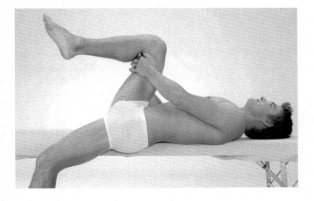

- Leg that is not affected should be flexed at the knee and hip.
- Both hands surround the lower thigh and draw the thigh to the body.
- Traction as a result of gravity in the affected leg.

Additional measures

- Mobilisation of the iliosacral joint.
- Adapt training for athletes.
- If the symptoms are obstinate try exercises in a warm bath.
- Instruction for functional abdominal muscle training (to avoid strain on the iliopsoas).

32.9 PELVIC FLOOR MUSCLES

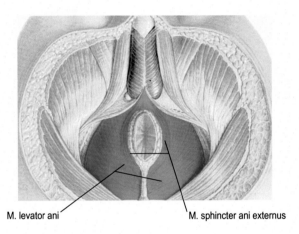

M. levator ani   M. sphincter ani externus

32.9.1 Anatomy

Innervation
- M. coccygeus: direct branches from the sacral plexus.
- M. levator ani: direct branches from the sacral plexus.
- M sphincter ani externus: pudendal nerve.

Origin
- M. coccygeus: spina ischiadica.
- M. levator ani (M. pubococcygeus, M. levator prostatae, M. pubovaginalis, M. puborectalis, M. iliococcygeus): tendinous arch of the levator ani muscle (= arch-shaped strengthening of the obturator fascia from the pubic symphysis to the ischial spine), bridging the M. obturatorius internus.
- M sphincter ani externus: subcutaneous part: fibres in front of and behind the anus to the corium; superficial part. From the centre of the perineum to the anococcygeum ligament; deep part: ring-shaped a few centimetres above the latter around the anal canal.

Insertion

- M. coccygeus: lateral surface of the lower sacrum and coccyx.
- M. levator ani: radiates into the M. sphincter ani externus, runs to the sacrum and coccyx.
- M sphincter ani externus: subcutaneous part: fibres in front of and behind the anus to the corium; superficial part: from the centre of the perineum to the anococcygeum ligament; deep part: ring-shaped a few centimetres above the latter around the anal canal.

Function

- M. coccygeus: strengthens the pelvic floor.
- M. levator ani: tenses the pelvic floor, crucial sphincter muscle for the anus ('puborectal loop'), the free medial margin forms the gateway for the entry of the urogenital organs, acts as a carrier belt for the pelvic floor.

- M sphincter ani externus: lateral, transversely striated (voluntarily innervated) sphincter muscle for the anus.'

32.9.2 Patient symptoms

- Pain when sitting down (especially the M. levator ani).
- Pain in the sacrum, coccyx, rectum (especially the M. levator ani).
- Rather diffuse pain in the anal and/or genital region.
- Stabbing pain on defecation.
- Dyspareunia.
- Possible preliminary diagnoses: coccygodynia, proctalgia fugax, haemorrhoids, iliosacral joint blockade, levator ani syndrome, chronic abacterial prostatitis, facet joint arthrosis L4 and L5.

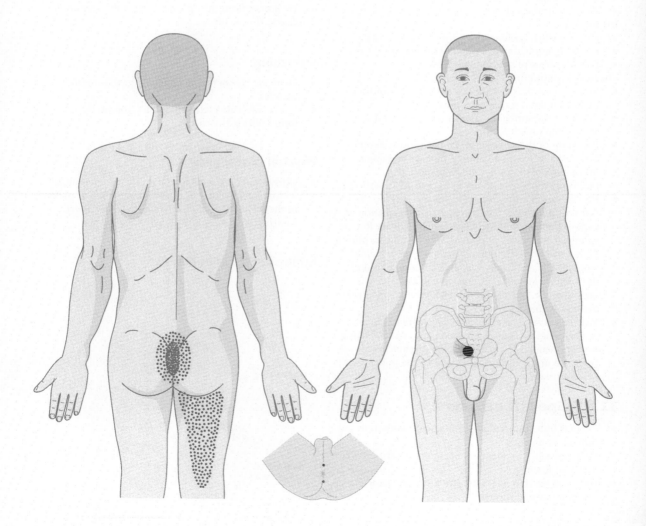

32.9.3 Trigger points

mTrP	LOCATION	RADIATION	mTrP→ ACUPUNCTURE POINT
1	In the posterior half of the pelvic floor: M. levator ani, M. ischiococcygeus, M. sphincter internus	Coccyx, anus, 'inner' inguinal area, medial thigh	GV 1
2	In the posterior half of the pelvic floor: M. levator ani, M. bulbospongiosus, M. ischiocavernosus, M. transversus perinei	Genital region, posterior thigh	CV 1

32.9.4 Diagnosis

Questioning
- Perineal tear? (with second- and third-degree perineal tear the muscles are not affected).
- Previous urological operation?

Inspection
- Stiffness when walking, often legs slightly spread apart.
- Cautious sitting down, sitting on the edge of the chair.
- Hyperlordosis of the lumbar spine.

Physical examination
- Respect the privacy of the patient (e.g. do not keep them waiting in an exposed position).
- Begin by examining the gluteal muscles and the abdominal muscles.
- Palpation of the external pelvic floor in the supine position and maximally flexed hips and knees or lithotomy position: M. ischiocavernosus, M. bulbospongiosus, M. transversus peronei superficialis.
- Rectal examination: using a lubricant, Jendratschek move or breathing manoeuvre, circular palpation at various depths with alternating hand, palpate the M. sphincter ani (tonus), dorsal M. levator ani pars pubica (allow the pelvic floor to contract slightly), contact with the Lig. anococcygeum and Os coccygeus and dorsolateral M. ischiococcygeus with Lig. sacrotuberale, counter pressure with thumb or finger of the other hand if possible.
- Vaginal examination in lithotomy position: M. bulbospongiosus (cautious pinch grip, test by asking for contraction of the introitus), M. ischiocavernosus (pressure in the distal vagina against the pubic bone), M. levator ani.

32.9.5 Specific aspects

- There is little knowledge of the referral pattern of the individual muscles.
- High resistance to treatment for internal haemorrhoids and anal fissures.
- Increased tension of the M. gluteus maximus if the M. levator ani is affected.

32.9.6 Therapy

Instructions for manual trigger point therapy

- Treatment from the outside or from the rectum or vagina is possible.

Stretching

- There are no stretching exercises for the specific muscles.
- It is possible to stretch the M. levator ani by immobilising the coccyx.

Physical procedures

- Ultrasound (2 W/cm² for 10 min) from the outside with a finger in the rectum or vagina as counter pressure to the ultrasound head; stretching using an anal stretcher.

Infiltration/dry needling

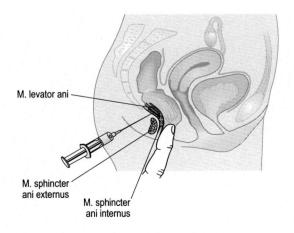

M. levator ani

M. sphincter ani externus

M. sphincter ani internus

- Infiltration is preferable.
- Infiltration of the M. sphincter ani, M. levator ani, M. ischiocavernosus, M. bulbospongiosus in men and M. ischiococcygeus is possible.
- Superficial anaesthesia (LA ointment, LA spray).
- Location of the mTrP from the rectum or vagina.
- Push the needle forward in the direction of the finger until the taut band or mTrP is reached.
- Therapeutic alternative: blockade of the pudendal nerve with low-concentration LA followed by trigger point massage.

Classical Chinese acupuncture

Local and locoregional points (also contralateral): CV 1, CV 2, CV 3, GV 1, GV 2, Ex-R 9 (Yao qi):median line, 2 cun superior to the tip of the coccyx.
Distal points: ST 4: correspondence anal–oral, GV 20: meridian point, GV 26: meridian point, CV 24: meridian point, BL 27–BL 31: segmental needling S1–S4.
Control points/symptomatic points: LI 4 (analgesia), LR 2 (2nd Shu point, effect on the lesser pelvis and genital area), LR 3 (muscle tension), LR 5 (Luo point, effect on gynaecological disorders and genital area), KI 10 (effect on sexuality disorders), SP 6 (effect on sexuality disorders, especially men), SP 8 (effect on cramp-like pain in the lesser pelvis).

Microsystem acupuncture

Ear: lumbar spine representation on the antihelix or directly next to it in the direction of the helix.
YNSA: D zone in the temporal area (Y zone), D1–D5 points preauricular.
NPS-O (Siener): point area at the lateral malleolus.
Mouth: intraoral at the canine tooth, lower jaw or extraoral analogue point.

Kiiko Matsumoto acupuncture

- For pressure pain in the area of KI 2 (fire point): KI 7 (metal point) and KI 10 (water point), needling angle (particularly with KI 7) should correlate with the relief of pain in the area of KI 2.

Psychosomatics/relaxation

- Psychosomatic aspects: sexuality (opening, dedication, emotional cold), letting go, compulsion.
- Careful study of sexual problems; possibly couples therapy.
- Exercises to improve body awareness.
- Letting go symptoms.
- For suspected compulsion arrange for specialist investigation.

32.9.7 Recommendations for the patient

- Watch out for upright posture when seated.
- Self-massage.
- 'Progressive muscle relaxation' in the pelvic area.
- Pelvic floor exercises.
- Pelvic floor training (e.g. with vaginal balls).

32.10 M. GLUTEUS MAXIMUS

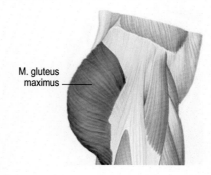

M. gluteus maximus

32.10.1 Anatomy

Innervation: N. gluteus inferior (plexus sacralis).
Origin: facies glutea of the ala ossis ilium (dorsal to the linea glutea posterior), facies posterior of the os sacrum, fascia thoracolumbalis, Lig. sacrotuberale.
Insertion
- Superior part: tibia below the lateral condyle (over the iliotibial tract). Between the trochanter major and tractus iliotibialis lies the bursa trochanterica musculi glutei maximi.
- Inferior part: tuberositas glutea, septum intermusculare femoris laterale.

Function
- Hip joint superior part: extension, lateral rotation, abduction.
- Hip joint inferior part: extension, lateral rotation, adduction.
- Knee joint (over the iliotibial tract): extension.

32.10.2 Patient symptoms

- Pain when walking on rising ground.
- Sharp or burning pain when sitting.
- Possible preliminary diagnoses: lumbago, periarthropathia coxae, iliosacral joint blockade, coccygodynia, chronic bursitis trochanterica, failed back surgery.

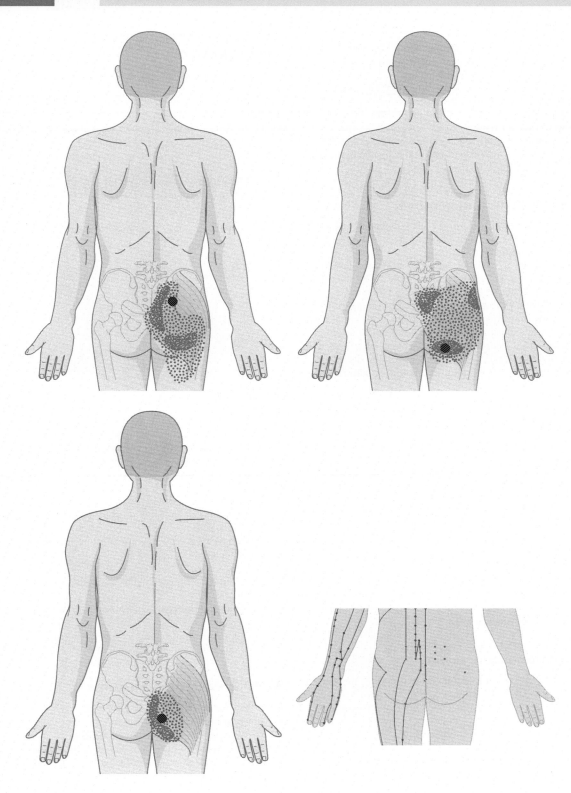

32.10.3 Trigger points

mTrP	LOCATION	RADIATION	mTrP→ ACUPUNCTURE POIN
1	In the medial part of the muscle, lateral sacrum, at the level of the sacral foramina II–IV	Predominantly in the area of the muscle, sacral hiatus	Lateral to BL 28–BL 30, BL 53, BL 54
2	In the medial part of the muscle	Hip region	GB 30
3	At the inferior end, in the fold of the buttocks	Sacral hiatus 1 in the dorsal thigh (upper third)	BL 36

32.10.4 Diagnosis

Questioning
- Intramuscular injection?
- Fall, trauma? Previous hip operation?
- Regular swimming training (especially freestyle)?
- Back training?
- Sitting on a lot of loose change, e.g. on a long car journey.

Inspection
- Gait with the leg laterally rotated and abducted so that the affected leg only bears weight briefly (limp).
- Restless when seated.

Physical examination
- Pain when lifting an object from the ground with vertebral column extended and knees flexed (lifting an object protecting the back).
- Pain provocation by bending forward while seated on a chair.
- Length test in supine position: flex the knee in the direction of the opposite shoulder so that the hips are medially rotated.
- Simple palpation in lateral decubitus with slightly flexed hips (affected side uppermost) with pillow between the legs, initially vertically to the course of the fibres in order to identify the muscle band, then pinch grip.
- mTrP 2 lie superficially (mTrPs can also lie underneath in the M. gluteus medius or in the M. piriformis): use pinch grip palpation to delimit.

- Examination of the iliosacral joint (iliosacral joint hypomobility is frequently associated with mTrPs in the M. gluteus maximus).

Technical examination
- If the pain is resistant to therapy use ultrasound to exclude bursitis subtrochanterica.
- X-ray: exclusion of iliosacral joint arthrosis.

32.10.5 Specific aspects

- Location of the mTrPs is simple but delimitation in the M. gluteus medius is occasionally difficult.
- For patients who have had back training, lifting to protect the back can lead to strain of the gluteal muscles.
- Frequently associated with coxarthrosis (protective posture).

32.10.6 Therapy

Instructions for manual trigger point therapy
- Mobilisation of the iliosacral joint.
- Many mTrPs immediately close to the insertion line along the lateral sacral margin as far as the coccyx.
- Fascia separation technique to the quadratus femoris muscle.
- Also treat the fascia lata (three-quarters of all muscle fibres of the gluteus maximus radiate into the iliotibial tract).

Massage
- Functional massage in the prone position with knee joint flexed 90°.
- Therapist stands on the side to be stretched.
- The hand close to the foot grasps the flexed leg at the ankle.
- The thumb of the hand near the head is placed on the mTrP and the sacrum held in place with the fingers of the same hand to suppress any further movement in the pelvis.
- While the mTrP is massaged the leg is dynamically moved at the ankle by the hand by the foot in the direction of medial rotation of the hips.

Stretching
- Patient lying on the side not affected.
- The leg underneath is in hip extension.
- The affected leg is in hip flexion and adduction.
- Stretching along the course of the fibres.
- Alternative in prone position (see massage): the therapist holds the pelvis in place with pressure on the superior anterior iliac spine with concomitant flexion in the hip joint.
- Choose the technique that allows the patient to feel optimum stretching.

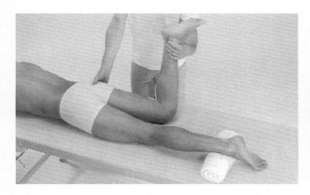

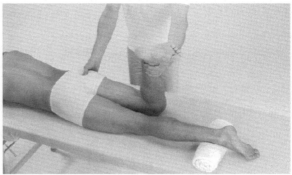

Physical procedures

- All physical procedures are possible.

Infiltration techniques/dry needling

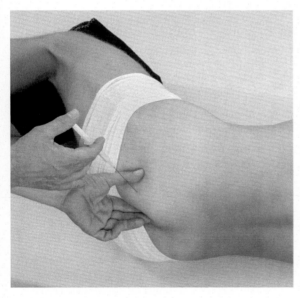

- Treatment in lateral decubitus position on the unaffected side with a pillow between the legs and moderately flexed hip joint and flexed knee joint (90°).
- Pinch grip is usually possible.
- Needle length 5 cm.
- With mTrP 1 superficial paraesthesia can be caused by irritation of the Nn. clunium medii.
- mTrP 2 can be superficial (2–4 cm).
- **Note:** N. ischiadicus (withdraw immediately if paraesthesia is caused).

Classical Chinese acupuncture

Local and locoregional points (also contralateral): BL 28, BL 32; BL 29, BL 33; BL 30, BL 34; BL 54, BL 35, BL 36, Ex-R 8 (Shi qi zhui), Ex-R 9 (Yao qi), GB 30, Ashi points.

Distal points: Ex-AH 7 (Yao tong dian): lumbago point, BL 40: meridian point (He point), BL 55: meridian point, muscle function chain, BL 60: meridian point, BL 62: meridian point, ST 25–ST 28: anterior abdominal muscles, SP 14, Ex-BB 1, Ex-BB Ti Tuo, LR 11, SP 12: hip flexors (antagonists), GB 39: meridian point.
Control points/symptomatic points: for moisture (especially feeling of heaviness or swelling) SP 6, SP 9, for sensitivity to cold: KI 3, GV 4, moxibustion, GB 34 (tendon masterpoint).

Microsystem acupuncture

Ear: hips, Jérôme point; lumbar spine representation on the antihelix or directly next to it in the direction of the helix.
YNSA: D zone in the temporal area (Y zone), D1–D5 points preauricular.
NPS-O (Siener): point area at the lateral malleolus.
Mouth: intraoral at the canine tooth, lower jaw or extraoral analogue point.

Kiiko Matsumoto acupuncture

- For tenderness in the area of GB 26 (Daimai): KI 7.

Psychosomatics/relaxation

- 'Straighten up', 'watch your posture'.
- Head pushed forward and hanging down with rounded back in the sense of an insufficient body posture as expression of depression (allowing the head and vertebral column to hang down).
- Qigong and yoga place particular value on an upright spine.

32.10.7 Recommendations for the patient

Autostretching

- Supine position.

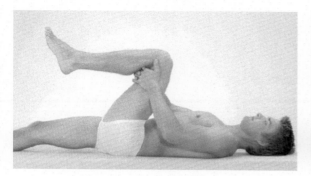
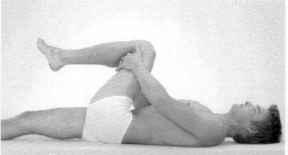

- Surround the thigh on the affected side with both hands with the hip and knee joints flexed.
- Traction first upwards then in the direction of the opposite shoulder.
- Or exercise while seated (note: lumbar spine).

Additional measures

- Mobilisation of the iliosacral joint.
- Regular autostretching with postisometric relaxation (see above).
- Squeeze out mTrP by lying on a tennis ball.
- Swimming on back or side.

32.11 M. GLUTEUS MEDIUS

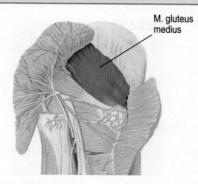

M. gluteus medius

32.11.1 Anatomy

Innervation: N. gluteus superior (plexus sacralis).
Origin: facies glutea of the ala ossis ilium (between lineae gluteae anterior and posterior).
Insertion: trochanter major (tip and lateral margin).
Function

- Hip joint anterior part: abduction, flexion, medial rotation.
- Hip joint posterior part: abduction, extension, lateral rotation.

32.11.2 Patient symptoms

- Classical lumbago and/or hip pain.
- Pain when walking, sitting and lying on side (sleeping on affected side).
- Possible preliminary diagnoses: lumbago, coxarthrosis, periarthropathia coxae, iliosacral joint blockade, chronic bursitis trochanterica.

32.11.3 Trigger points

mTrP	LOCATION	RADIATION	mTrP↔ ACUPUNCTURE POINT
1	In the upper part of the muscle close to the origin below the iliac crest	Whole lumbar spine, rarely in the lateral thigh	BL 53
2	In the upper part of the muscle close to the insertion, above the trochanter major and 2–4 finger widths in the direction of the vertebral column	Lumbar spine, sacrum, lateral and anterior thigh	–

32.11.4 Diagnosis

Questioning

- Intramuscular injection?
- Fall, trauma?
- Previous hip operation?
- Long-term weight-bearing on one side (work, sport)?

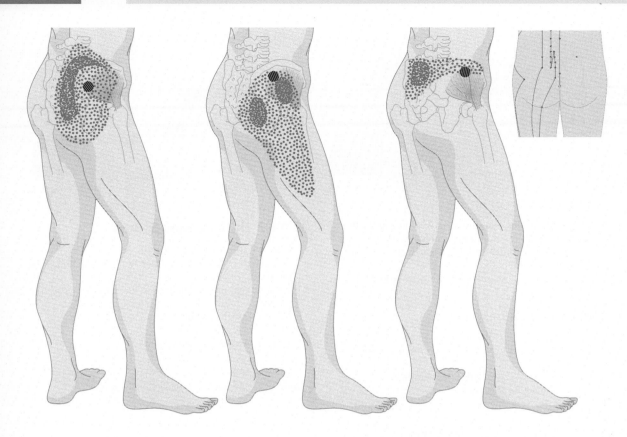

- Sitting on a lot of loose change, e.g. on a long car journey

Inspection: gait with laterally rotated and abducted leg (limp).

Physical examination

- Hips: pain on adduction and abduction against resistance.
- Length test in lateral decubitus (on non-affected side) for the more horizontally running fibres. Upper part of affected leg with slightly flexed hips and slightly flexed knee joint (backwards) over the couch, adducted at the hip (anteromedial traction) see also Autostretching, below.
- Length test in lateral decubitus (on non-affected side) for the lateral, more vertically running fibres: upper part of affected leg with hips and knee joint stretched (forwards) over the couch, adducted at the hip (traction forward and down).
- Palpation in lateral decubitus position (affected side up) with pillow between the legs.

Technical examination

- Resistance to therapy.
- Ultrasound: exclusion of bursitis subtrochanterica.
- X-ray: exclusion of iliosacral joint arthrosis.

32.11.5 Specific aspects

- Location of the mTrPs is simple, but demarcation of the individual muscles is occasionally difficult.
- Frequently associated with coxarthrosis (protective posture)

32.11.6 Therapy

Instructions for manual trigger point therapy

- Treatment of the parts covered by the M. gluteus maximus is strenuous so use aids (trigger point sticks) to relieve the fingers.

Stretching

- Begin in lateral decubitus position.
- Leg on affected side bent.
- Then turn the upper body to the affected side, shoulders/thoracic spine remain in supine position as far as possible.
- Place the affected leg over the unaffected leg.

470

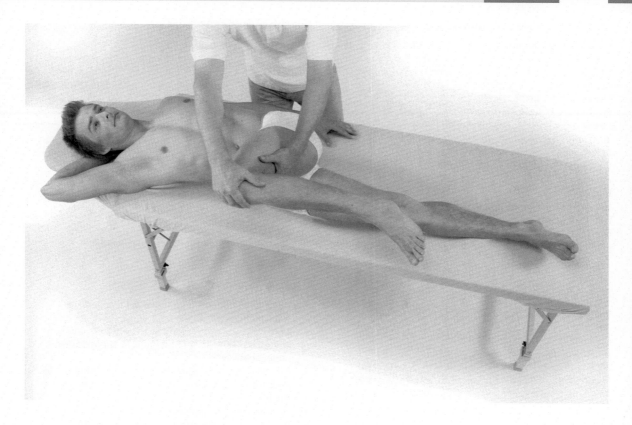

- Stretch by pressure on the knee of the affected leg towards the floor.
- Together with the patient find the optimum position leading to extension of the affected muscle parts.

Physical procedures

- All physical procedures are possible, for mTrP 2 penetration depth ≥6 cm.

Infiltration techniques/dry needling

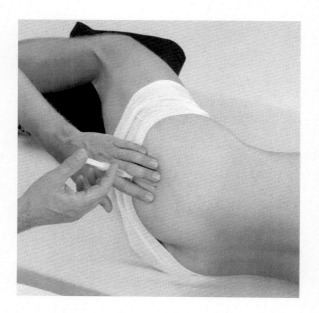

- Treatment with the patient lying on the unaffected side.
- Pillow between the legs.
- Hip joint moderately flexed and knee flexion (90°).
- Needle length: mTrP 1: 5 cm; mTrP 2: 5–7 cm.
- mTrP 1: pinch grip.
- mTrP 2: finger protection technique for deeper muscle parts below the M. gluteus maximus.
- **Note:** N. ischiadicus (withdraw immediately if paraesthesia is caused).

Classical Chinese acupuncture

Local and locoregional points (also contralateral): level of sacral foramen 2: BL 28, BL 32, BL 53; level of sacral foramen 3: BL 29, BL 33; level of sacral foramen 4: BL 30, BL 34, BL 54.

Other points: BL 35, BL 36, Ex-R 8 (Shi Qi Zhui), Ex-R 9 (Yao Qi), GB 30, Ashi points.

Distal points: Ex-AH 7 (Yao tong dian): lumbago point, BL 40 (He point) for lumbago, BL 55, muscle function chain, BL 60, BL 62 (for lumbago), GB 31 for lateral pain, GB 39 for lateral pain, ST 25 to ST 28: anterior abdominal muscles, SP 14, Ex-BB 1, Ex-BB Ti Tuo, LR 11, SP 12: hip flexors (antagonists).

Control points/symptomatic points: for moisture (especially feeling of heaviness or swelling) SP 6, SP 9, for sensitivity to cold: KI 3, GV 4, moxibustion, GB 34 (tendon masterpoint), LR 3 (Yuan point):psychological balance, spasmolytic.

Microsystem acupuncture

Ear: hips, Jérôme point; lumbar spine representation on the anthelix or directly next to it in the direction of the helix.

YNSA: D zone in the temporal area (Y zone), D1–D5 points preauricular.

NPS-O (Siener): point area at the lateral malleolus.

Mouth: intraoral at the canine tooth, lower jaw or extraoral analogue point.

Kiiko Matsumoto acupuncture

- Tenderness in the area of the navel: GB 25 (Mu point of the kidney) and KI 7 and SP 9.

Psychosomatics/relaxation

- Predominantly pain located on the side.
- For anger, rage (especially suppressed), aggression, aggression inhibition verbalisation and exercises to reduce tension. Pure relaxation alone can often make things worse, so try physical burn-out beforehand (sports therapy, exercise therapy).
- Psychosomatic aspects: pain in the area of the hips can occasionally have something to do with anger, rage (especially suppressed), aggression, aggression inhibition.
- Predominantly pain located on the back.
- See lumbar autochthonous back muscles (see Section 32.6).

32.11.7 Recommendations for the patient

Autostretching

- Begin with patient lying on the unaffected side.
- Leg on affected side bent.
- Then turn the upper body to the affected side, shoulders/thoracic spine remain in supine position as far as possible.
- Affected leg with slightly flexed hips and slightly flexed knee joint (backwards) over the couch, adducted at the hip.
- Use of gravity for stretching.
- Possibly reinforce with light pressure on the lateral knee joint.
- The careful trying out of the individual optimum extension position is crucial

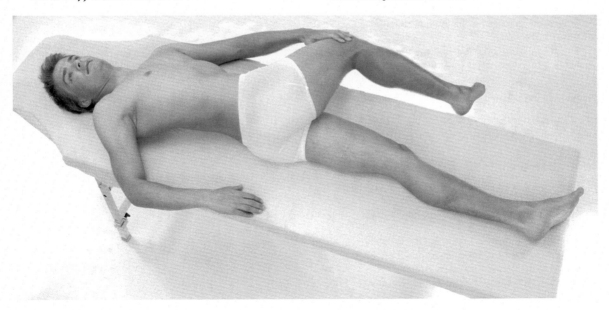

Additional measures

- Autostretching with postisometric relaxation (see above).
- Squeeze out mTrPs by lying on a tennis ball.
- Pillow between the legs for those who sleep on their side.

32.12 M. GLUTEUS MINIMUS

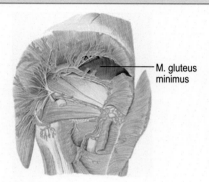

M. gluteus minimus

32.12.1 Anatomy

Innervation: N. gluteus superior (plexus sacralis).
Origin: facies glutea of the ala ossis ilium (between lineae gluteae anterior and posterior).
Insertion: trochanter major (tip and lateral margin).
Function: hip joint:
- anterior part: abduction, flexion, medial rotation,
- dorsal part: abduction, extension, lateral rotation.

32.12.2 Patient symptoms

- Hip pain, deep-seated lumbago.
- Pain when standing up after sitting for a long time or lying on the affected side is characteristic.
- Pain when crossing the legs.
- Possible preliminary diagnoses: lumbago, periarthropathia coxae, coxarthrosis, sciatica, chronic bursitis subtrochanterica, radiculopathy (L5 or S1).

32.12.3 Trigger points

mTrP	LOCATION	RADIATION	mTrP→ ACUPUNCTURE POINT
1	Between the anterior gluteal line	Gluteal, local, dorsal and lateral thigh	–
2	Between the iliac crest and the trochanter major	Gluteal, lateral thigh over the lower leg to the external malleolus	GB 29

(row 2 continued) and muscle, one hand width below the iliac crest

32.12.4 Diagnosis

Questioning
- Intramuscular injection?
- Fall, trauma?
- Condition following hip operation?
- Strain from standing for too long?
Inspection: protective limp.
Physical examination
- Examination of the hips and lower lumbar spine.
- Pain during hip adduction.
- mTrPs are accessible only with pressure palpation, so must be long enough (at least 10 s of pressure and ask the patient whether it causes the typical pain).
- mTrPs in the M. gluteus minimus frequently occur together with functional disorder in the iliosacral joint.

32.12.5 Specific aspects

- Location of the mTrPs is simple but demarcation of the individual gluteal muscles is difficult where they overlap.
- Frequently associated with coxarthrosis (protective posture).

32.12.6 Therapy

Instructions for manual trigger point therapy
- Treatment of the parts covered by the Mm. gluteus maximus and medius (anteriorly from the M. tensor fasciae latae) is strenuous so use aids (trigger point sticks) to relieve the fingers.
- In the area where the M. gluteus medius covers the M. gluteus minimus the two muscles cannot be distinguished by palpation.

Stretching
- Lateral decubitus position.
- Extension and adduction of the thigh on the affected side by gravity.
- Slight hip flexion and medial rotation as well as adduction.
- The therapist gently guides the stretching movements as gravity is too powerful.
- Fibres of the M. gluteus medius and the M. tensor fasciae lata are usually stretched at the same time.

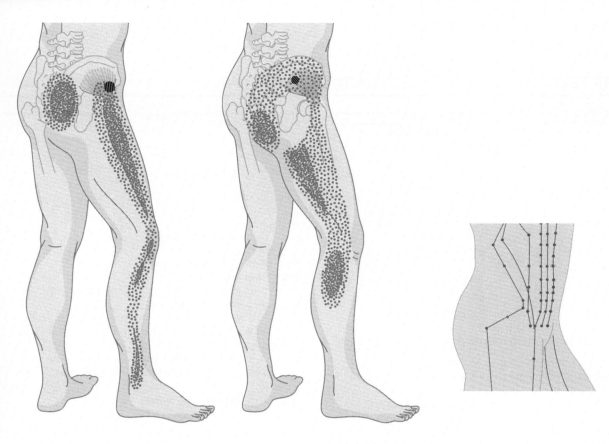

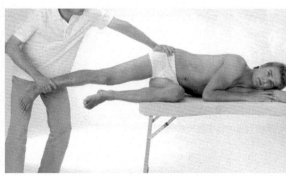

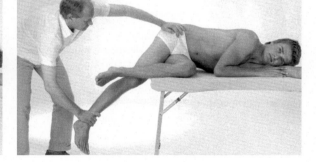

Physical procedures

- All physical procedures possible, for mTrP 2 use a penetration depth ≥6 cm.

Infiltration techniques/dry needling

- Perform treatment with the patient lying on the unaffected side.
- Moderately flexed hip joint.

- Pillow between the legs.
- Needle length: mTrP 1: 5 cm; mTrP 2: 6–8 cm.
- Finger protection technique.
- **Note:** N. ischiadicus (withdraw immediately if paraesthesia is caused).

Classical Chinese acupuncture

Local and locoregional points (also contralateral): BL 28, BL 32, BL 53 (sacral foramen 2); BL 29, BL 33 (sacral foramen

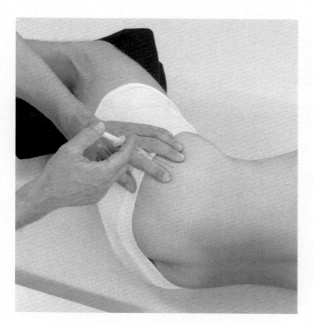

3); BL 30, BL 34, BL 54 (foramen sacrale 4); other points: GB 30, lower point of the hip (over trochanter major).

Distal points: BL 40 for lumbago, BL 58 for dorsal pain; GB 31–GB 33 for lateral pain; LR 10, LR 11, SP 12 adductors (antagonists).

Control points/symptomatic points: GB 34 (tendons masterpoint); LR 3 (Yuan point): psychological balance, spasmolytic.

Microsystem acupuncture

Ear: hips, Jérôme point; lumbar spine representation on the anthelix or directly next to it.

YNSA: D zone in the temporal area (Y zone), D1–D5 points preauricular.

NPS-O (Siener): point area at the lateral malleolus.

Mouth: intraoral at the canine tooth, lower jaw or extraoral analogue point.

Kiiko Matsumoto acupuncture

• Tenderness in the area of the navel: KI 16, CV 7, CV 9.

Psychosomatics/relaxation

• For anger, rage (especially suppressed), aggression, aggression inhibition verbalisation and exercises to reduce tension. Pure relaxation alone can often make things worse, so initially try physical burn-out (sports therapy, exercise therapy).

• Pain in the area of the hips can occasionally have something to do with anger, rage (especially suppressed), aggression or aggression inhibition.

32.12.7 Recommendations for the patient

Autostretching

• Patient on the unaffected side on the lower edge of the bed.

• The healthy leg is bent and lies with the outside still fully on the bed.

• The affected leg is stretched behind the foot using gravity while it swings freely out over the edge of the bed.

• Tension/relaxation by lifting the leg against gravity.

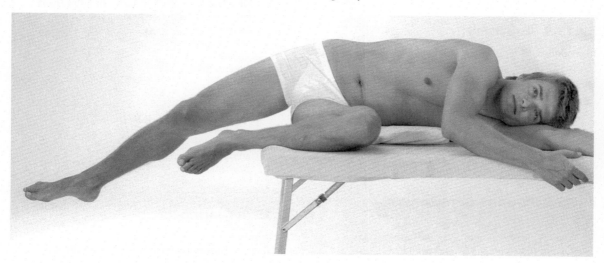

- Find optimum stretching position by rotation of the hips (medial versus lateral rotation; the hip rotators are also stretched with lateral rotation).
- The M. tensor fasciae lata is usually stretched at the same time.

Additional measures

- Autostretching with postisometric relaxation (see above).
- Squeeze out mTrPs by lying on a tennis ball.
- Pillow between the legs for those who sleep on their side.

32.13 M. PIRIFORMIS

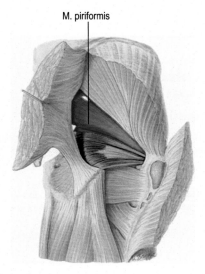

M. piriformis

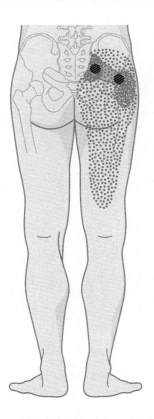

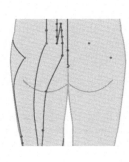

32.13.3 Trigger points

mTrP	LOCATION	RADIATION	mTrP→ ACUPUNCTURE POINT
1	On a line between the sacral hiatus and the greater trochanter, close to the vertebral column	Iliosacral area, dorsal thigh	BL 54 Ex Huan Zhong
2	On a line between the sacral hiatus and the greater trochanter, close to the hip	Hips, dorsal thigh	GB 30

32.13.1 Anatomy

Innervation: N. ischiadicus and/or N. musculi piriformis (plexus sacralis).
Origin
- Pelvic facet of the sacrum (laterally and between the pelvic sacral foramina of S3 and S4).
- Greater sciatic notch (close to the sacrum).
Insertion: trochanter major (medial surface of the tip).
Function: hip joint: adduction, extension, lateral rotation.

32.13.2 Patient symptoms

- Lumbosciatic pain of varying degrees.
- Possible preliminary diagnoses: lumbago, sciatica, iliosacral joint blockade, coccygodynia.

32.13.4 Diagnosis

Questioning
- Long car journey (especially if right leg affected)?

- Acute strain?
- Trauma with leg medially rotated?

Inspection

- Restless when sitting.
- Lateral rotation of the affected leg in relaxed supine position.

Physical examination

- Painful medial rotation of the hips.
- Palpation with patient lying on the unaffected side with hip joint on the affected side flexed.
- Indirect palpation through gluteal muscles: pain referred with strong pressure.
- Iliosacral joint hypomobility often involved.
- Careful neurological examination for paraesthesia, dysaesthesia or other neurological symptoms.

Technical examination

- X-ray: if the pain is resistant to therapy to exclude iliosacral joint arthrosis.
- Neurophysiological examination if there are neurological symptoms.

32.13.5 Specific aspects

- Mixed symptoms possible: symptoms caused by nerve entrapment (N. ischiadicus, N. gluteus superior) and direct referral pattern.
- Piriformis syndrome caused by joint dysfunction, nerve entrapment and mTrPs in the piriformis muscle.
- Occurs with tension after long car journeys (right leg, accelerator pedal).
- The other lateral hip rotators are also often affected (Mm. gemellus superior and inferior, Mm. obturatorius externus and internus, M. quadratus femoris).
- Agonist of the M. gluteus maximus.
- Iliosacral joint hypomobility and position of the sacrum also often involved.

32.13.6 Therapy

Instructions for manual trigger point therapy

- Palpation and treatment (patient in prone or lateral position) through the M. gluteus maximus, completely covering all the deep lateral rotators.
- M. piriformis: division of the connecting line between the superior posterior iliac spine and the greater trochanter; at the first divisional point from a proximal direction inwards the piriformis enters the sciatic foramen: palpation.
- Rectal/vaginal treatment of the area of origin of the piriformis (anterior side of the sacrum) possible.
- The gemelli and internal obturators are difficult to distinguish.

- M. quadratus femoris (between the ischial tuberosity and the intertrochanteric crest) frequently with mTrPs (with coxarthrosis).

Stretching

- Patient lying on the unaffected side.
- The affected leg is flexed at the hips at 90° and pressed down over the underlying leg over the bed (additional light pressure on the knee joint).
- Make sure that the patient remains on the side of the pelvis (see therapist's right hand in the photo).

Physical procedures

- Deep effect required (minimum 8 cm).

Infiltration techniques/dry needling

- Patient lying on the unaffected side.
- Hip joint on the affected side slightly flexed.
- Long needles required (up to 10 cm if the patient is of sturdy build).
- The mTrP is held in place using a two-finger technique.
- The other lateral hip rotators are treated in the same session (Mm. gemellus superior and inferior, Mm. obturatorius externus and internus, M. quadratus femoris).
- **Note:** N. ischiadicus (withdraw immediately if paraesthesia is caused).

Classical Chinese acupuncture

Local and locoregional points (also contralateral): BL 54, GB 30, Ex Huan Zhong (in the middle of the association GB 30 and GV 2), GV 2; BL 29, BL 33 (at the level of sacral foramen I); BL 30, BL 34, BL 54 (at the level of sacral foramen 4); lower point of the hip (over trochanter major).
Distal points: BL 40: meridian point (He point) for lumbago, BL 58: meridian point for dorsal pain, GB 31: meridian point for lateral pain, GB 32, GB 33, GB 39: meridian points for lateral pain, BL 22, BL 23, BL 24, BL 25, BL 26, BL 51, BL 52, Hua tuo jiaji, BL 51, BL 52: local points of the M. iliopsoas (antagonist), deep needling.
Control points/symptomatic points: GB 41 (Dai mai switch point) with belt-shaped pain, GB 34 (tendons masterpoint), LR 3 (Yuan point): psychological balance, spasmolytic.

Microsystem acupuncture

Ear: lumbar spine representation on the antihelix or directly next to it in the direction of the helix.
YNSA: D zone in the temporal area (Y zone), D1–D5 points preauricular.
NPS-O (Siener): point area at the lateral malleolus.

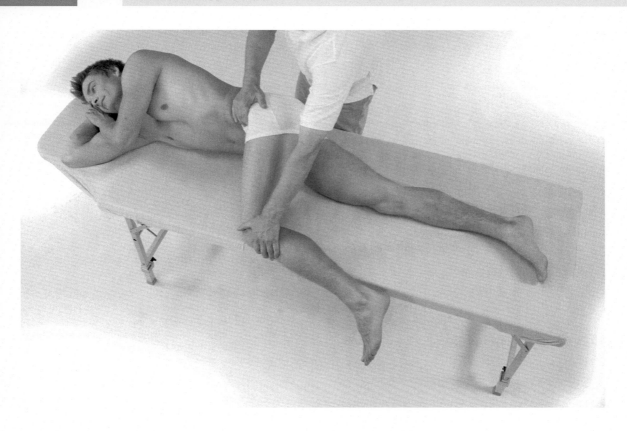

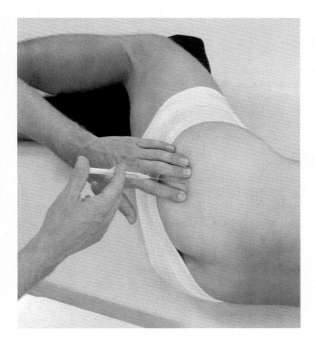

Mouth: intraoral at the canine tooth, lower jaw or extraoral analogue point.

Kiiko Matsumoto acupuncture

- If the patient is lying down, needling of a point 1 cm lateral to BL 40.

Psychosomatics/relaxation

- Relaxation training for stressed drivers ('meditation pause').

32.13.7 Recommendations for the patient

Autostretching

- Patient in supine position.
- Leg on the affected side flexed at the hip and knee joints.
- Place the foot flat next to the knee of the unaffected side.
- The hand on the affected side is placed on the superior anterior iliac spine and presses the pelvis onto the bed.
- The hand on the unaffected side surrounds the knee joint and presses it down until tension can be felt.

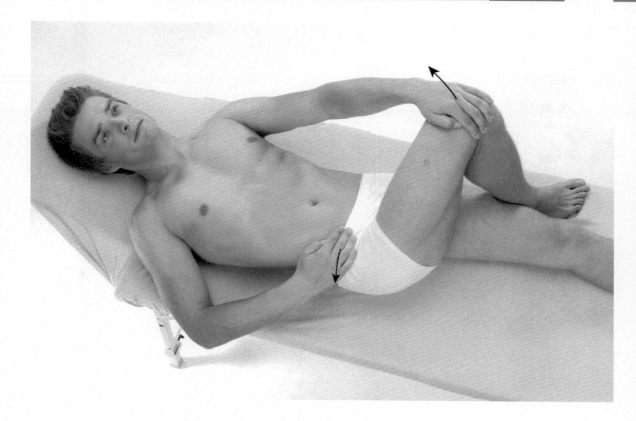

Additional measures

- Iliosacral joint mobilisation.
- Pillow between the legs for those who sleep on their side.

- Autotreatment with a tennis ball (for pins and needles exercise pressure on the sciatic nerve: push the ball away).
- Pause and stretch for long-distance drivers.

Chapter 33

Hips, thighs and knees

Dominik Irnich

The associations between the hip joint and lumbar spine with the pelvis are described in Ch. 32. The hip joint is discussed here with the relevant muscles – the hip flexors and extensors, rotators and abductors and adductors – as well as the knee joint with the relevant muscles and functions.

33.1 FUNCTIONAL ASSOCIATIONS

33.1.1 Hips

The hip joint is a ball-and-socket joint and enables movement between the lower extremity and the trunk. While standing and walking the body weight rests on the hip joint of the supporting leg; the free leg is moved.

Both hip joints must be balanced by distal asymmetry. Deformities such as hip dysplasia with coxa antetorta disturb the equilibrium of the knees and feet and even strain the vertebral column, leading to limping.

The hip joint is moved by a number of muscle groups, as follows.

- The lateral rotators regularly play an important part in any symptoms. They control the powerful and fast medial rotation of the thigh at the start of the standing phase, when walking or running. The short lateral rotators, particularly the piriformis muscles (see Section 32.13), can also irritate these as they are anatomically very close to the sciatic nerve (entrapment). Insufficient attention is often paid to the psoas muscle (see Section 32.8), which is of great significance as a hip flexor together with the iliacus muscle, particularly after 90°. The psoas also influences the position of the iliosacral joint because of its origin at the lumbar spine, and also with asymmetrical traction in the form of pelvic manipulation.

- Clinically at least as important are the effects of bilateral shortening of the hip flexors (Mm. iliopsoas (see Section 32.8) and rectus femoris) with increased flexion of the pelvic in the hip joints and consequent increased lumbar spine lordosis with strain on the dorsal structures. It is not just with coxarthrosis that this leads to a gait with small steps.

- The gluteus maximus (see Section 32.10) is a key muscle for standing upright and for pushing off. The gluteus medius (see Section 32.11) is a stabiliser for standing on one leg.

33.1.2 Knee

With this joint the emphasis is more on the dynamic stabilising and control function of the muscles, in addition to knee extension and forward locomotion. The contribution of the quadriceps to forward motion is relatively more important in running rather than walking, where the calf and buttocks muscles play a bigger role. The quadriceps also play a particular role in controlling the patella.

The function of the vastus medialis muscle is correction of medial traction on the patella, which arises as a result of an imbalance between the lateral line further down the femoral shaft and the straight thigh muscles (Mm. rectus femoris and vastus intermedius, further strengthened by the vastus lateralis) compared to the weight axis.

The significance of control of the patella is indicated by the fact that most cases of gonarthrosis begin in the retropatellar compartment. Too much traction from the hardened, shortened vastus medialis, especially when combined with weakness of the lateral traction belt of the thigh (by the iliotibial tract tensed by the tensor fasciae latae and the gluteus maximus), can influence the occurrence of medially pronounced gonarthrosis. If the vastus medialis is

http://dx.doi.org/10.1016/B978-0-7020-4312-3.00033-7

hardened, it can no longer control the patella properly with the vastus lateralis, which contributes to retropatellar problems and can lead to general strain and to deformity of the knee. In footballers functional shortening of the rectus femoris occurs mainly in the shooting leg with the formation of mTrPs.

The knee flexor also represents an anatomically and functionally interesting zone: because of the hard bony anterior and lateral limitation, extension is only possibly in a posterior direction. A joint effusion here can form a Baker cyst. With taut bands in the regional muscles, the pressure on the vessels and nerves that run through the area can be tangibly increased; this is particularly pronounced in flexion.

33.2 PSYCHOSOMATIC ASPECTS

33.2.1 Hip joint

Symptoms in the lateral area (i.e. in the area of the gluteus minimus; see Section 32.12) and the iliotibial tract, and rotation symptoms can correlate with mental tension and withheld rage.

The case of a patient who attended with pain of uncertain cause radiating from the left lateral hip to the lateral malleolus (for acupuncturists: gallbladder meridian) and for whom the symptoms could clearly be reproduced by mTrPs of the gluteus minimus was impressive. When the topic of rage was approached, she breathed in deeply and said that her daughter was trying to have her declared mentally incompetent so that she could get her inheritance earlier!

Heterotopic ossification in juveniles in the area of the iliotibial tract without external trauma during the parents' divorce battle also fits in here.

Tension disorders and mTrPs in the dorsal buttocks often correlate with a 'clenching the buttocks' – control as a result of anxiety, often associated with the double meaning of insecurity.

With the inguinal flexors and adductors (in the Yin area) it may be about vulnerability and protecting oneself, especially the genital area. With shortening of the iliopsoas, being mentally 'driven' often plays a part as well and may go so far as nervous exhaustion or burn-out syndrome. Acupuncturists know this by the term 'kidney Yin emptiness'. With the adductors it may also be about suppressed anxiety (caused by a sense of being hurt) and then, after resolution, in the positive sense about 'power'.

33.2.2 Knee joint

The knee joint is associated with being on 'bended knee' – or avoiding doing so – a conflict with authority, although it is also an expression of weakness or control of emotions. We go 'weak at the knees' when excited or especially

anxious. A key muscle here is the M. vastus medialis. It is not just important for the prevention and treatment of medial knee problems or arthritis, it is also essential for full or hyperextension. Fully extended knees are part of a military bearing or childish defiance. In our experience mTrPs of this muscle and the other parts of the M. quadriceps femoris can activate feelings of weakness (which, as a result of self-acceptance, in the end leads to true strength, which needs no strengthening). The knee is also involved in a secure stance, as is the whole lower extremity (see Ch. 32).

33.3 SYMPTOMS

Hips: typical of 'periarthropathic pain' so the pain of mTrPs tends to be of a dull, dragging character with symptoms which come on gradually and are improved with warmth. However, stabbing pain caused by strain can also have a myofascial cause.

Knee joint: myofascial pain and functional disorders can cause or imitate many symptoms. Examination and treatment of mTrPs could prevent many knee arthroscopies, which may not produce any findings and may be unsuccessful.

mTrPs in the M. vastus medialis can 'imitate' damage to the medial ligament and the medial meniscus, although without impingement (for more, see Section 33.5).

33.4 DIAGNOSTIC AND THERAPEUTIC CONSIDERATIONS

33.4.1 Hips

It is barely possible to distinguish myofascial periarthropathy from coxarthrosis or the history of the pain. Although an X-ray will show the extent of narrowing of the joint space and any reactive/degenerative changes, it cannot show what part it has played in the current symptoms. This is only possible by clinical examination and attempted mTrP therapy.

The significance of mTrPs in hip pain can be seen in the long-known fact that there are people who suffer from severe pain with little radiological evidence of changes; and vice versa, it is not uncommon for people with pronounced coxarthrosis in X-rays to suffer relatively few symptoms.

An X-ray of the pelvis can occasionally show visible productive fibrosis as calcified muscle insertions, and indication of too much tension in the muscles.

Besides releasing hardening and improving mobility, we must not forget that restricted motion primarily caused by the muscles can also have a protective function, for example if there is impingement of the hip joint by slight hip dysplasia (i.e. the neck of the femur touching the acetabular rim if the shape is distorted). More precise investigation using CT or MRI would be sensible here.

Otherwise, it is always sensible to at least carry out a trial treatment, no matter what part the myofascial disorder plays in the symptoms. This also applies before and after a hip replacement. Even when the joint is thankfully back in order again, we must not forget that the muscles are often still in disarray and the deviant movements, protective postures and pain are still stored in the mTrPs.

After the operation there is often weakness of the abductors with Trendelenburg gait or Duchenne gait pattern; we should not just consider the changed biomechanics caused by the steeper neck of the femur as a result of the hip replacement, providing an unfamiliar lever for the abductors, we should also treat the abductors and adductors. It is often not possible to exercise the abductors until they have been released, and shortened adductors can contribute to weakness of the abductors through reciprocal innervation.

33.4.2 Knee

Besides a consideration of stance and tension of the lower leg (see Ch. 34) the shape of the muscle is also meaningful. With knee problems it is usually the vastus medialis which atrophies first. Treatment of the taut bands can provide rapid improvement as the muscle is released and more easily exercised. Functionally, the stabilisation capability of the muscle is of interest when standing on one leg and when running.

33.5 EXAMINATION FOR mTrP IDENTIFICATION

33.5.1 Examination for mTrP identification in the hip joint

During passive/assistive examination, ask the patient where it 'pulls' every time there is limited or painful movement, then palpate this area!

LIMITED FUNCTION OR MOVEMENT	SEARCH FOR mTrP IN
Flexion with extended knee	Ischiocrural muscles[1]
Flexion with knee bent as well	Mm. gluteus maximus (see Section 32.10), medius (see Section 32.11) and to some extent also minimus (see Section 32.12), M. adductor magnus (see Section 33.8), M. quadratus femoris
Extension[2]	M. rectus femoris, M. psoas (see Section 32.8), M. iliacus, M. tensor fasciae latae (see Section 33.7), M. sartorius, M. pectineus, M. adductor longus (see Section 33.8)
Medial rotation	M. gluteus maximus and medius (dorsal part) (Sections 32.10, 32.10), M. piriformis (Section 32.13), M. gemelli (Section 32.13), M. rectus femoris, M. obturatorius externus (Section 33.8), M. adductor brevis (Section 33.8), M. pectineus (Section 33.8), M. quadratus femoris, M. adductor longus and magnus (Section 33.8), M. biceps femoris (caput longum) (Section 33.10), M. sartorius
Lateral rotation[3]	Mm. gluteus minimus (Section 32.12) and medius (Section 32.11), M. tensor fasciae latae (Section 33.7), Mm. semimembranosus and semitendinosus (Section 33.10), sometimes also adductors
Abduction	All adductors, M. semimembranosus (Section 33.10), M. iliopsoas (Section 32.8), M. biceps femoris (caput longum) and M. semitendinosus (Section 33.10), M. quadratus femoris, M. obturatorius externus (Section 33.8))
Adduction	Mm. gluteus medius (Section 32.11) and minimus (Section 32.12), M. tensor fasciae latae (Section 33.7), M. rectus femoris, M. piriformis (Section 32.13), M. sartorius
Flexion > 120° with medial rotation and adduction	M. piriformis (Section 32.13)

[1]The influence of the ischiocrural muscles (Mm. biceps femoris caput longum, semitendinosus and semimembranosus) on limited hip flexion can be easily delimited. As this is a two-joint muscle which also runs over the knee joint, try flexion first with the leg extended as for the Lasègue test and then with the knee bent.
[2]In the prone position or with the Thomas grip: maximally flex the knee and hip on the opposite side and then observe whether the knee on the side being examined is drawn upwards.
[3]Can also be examined in the prone position for good comparison of the sides.

A simple clinical sign: a stance or gait with increased lateral rotation of one or both feet indicates shortening of the lateral rotators of the hip, particularly the M. gluteus maximus and medius (dorsal part) and the M. piriformis.

33.5.2 Examination for mTrP identification in the knee joint

Palpation plays a bigger part here than examination of function.

LIMITED FUNCTION OR MOVEMENT	SEARCH FOR mTrPs IN
Medial	M. vastus medialis, M. adductor magnus and M. gracilis (Section 33.8)
Retropatellar, 'in the knee' or insertion of the patellar tendon: tibial tuberosity	Whole M. quadriceps (Section 33.9); besides the M. rectus femoris the deep M. vastus intermedius is particularly important and is frequently overlooked
Lateral/lateroventral	M. vastus lateralis, tractus iliotibialis (insertion at the tuberculum gerdii) with M. tensor fasciae latae (Section 33.7)
Lateral proximal lower leg	Mm. peroneus longus and brevis (Section 34.7)
Back of the knee (central or lateral)	M. gastrocnemius (Section 34.8), M. popliteus (Section 33.11), M. biceps femoris (Section 33.10) (insertion at the head of the fibula) and M. plantaris (Section 34.9)

33.6 FUNCTIONAL EXAMINATIONS

Shortening of the M. quadriceps femoris (Section 33.9) is very common, and examination must distinguish between the two-jointed rectus femoris, which can also flex in the hip joint, and the vastus muscles, which can only extend the knee joint (Figure 33.1).

RESTRICTED MOVEMENT	SEARCH FOR mTrPs IN
Knee flexion only with concomitant hip extension	M. rectus femoris
Knee flexion: also with hip flexion	Mm. vastus intermedius, medialis and lateralis, M. tensor fasciae latae (Section 33.7)

Extension	Mm. semimembranosus, semitendinosus and biceps femoris (Section 33.10), M. gracilis (Section 33.8), M. sartorius, Mm. gastrocnemii (Section 34.8), M. plantaris (Section 34.9)
Medial rotation	M. biceps femoris (Section 33.10), M. gastrocnemius (caput laterale) (34.8), M. tensor fasciae latae (Section 33.7)
Lateral rotation	Mm. semimembranosus, semitendinosus (Section 33.10), M. popliteus (33.11), M. sartorius, M. gastrocnemius (caput mediale) (34.8), M. gracilis (Section 33.8), M. plantaris (34.9)

33.7 M. TENSOR FASCIAE LATAE

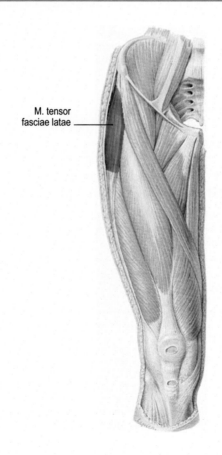

M. tensor fasciae latae

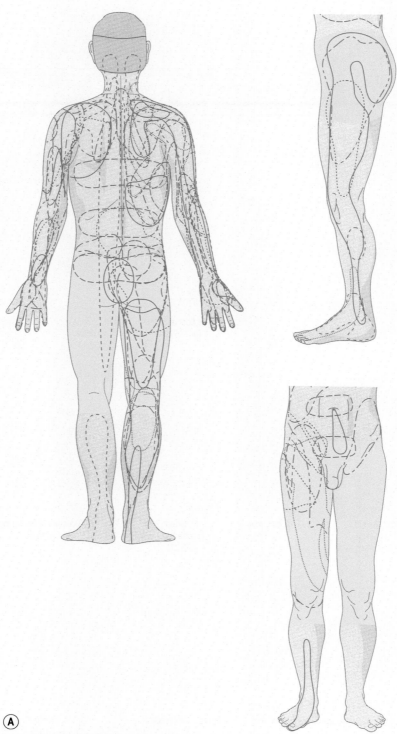

Ⓐ

Fig. 33.1 Pain referral pattern (a) and affected muscles

Continued

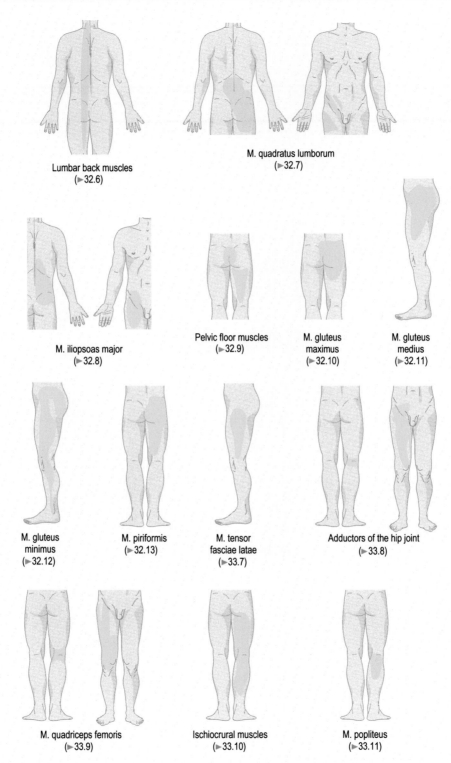

Lumbar back muscles
(▶32.6)

M. quadratus lumborum
(▶32.7)

M. iliopsoas major
(▶32.8)

Pelvic floor muscles
(▶32.9)

M. gluteus
maximus
(▶32.10)

M. gluteus
medius
(▶32.11)

M. gluteus
minimus
(▶32.12)

M. piriformis
(▶32.13)

M. tensor
fasciae latae
(▶33.7)

Adductors of the hip joint
(▶33.8)

B

M. quadriceps femoris
(▶33.9)

Ischiocrural muscles
(▶33.10)

M. popliteus
(▶33.11)

Fig. 33.1—cont'd (b) of the hip, thigh and knee.

33.7.1 Anatomy

Innervation: N. gluteus superior.
Origin: superior anterior iliac spine.
Insertion: lateral end of the tibia (over the iliotibial tract below the lateral condyle).
Function
- Hip joint: abduction, flexion, medial rotation.
- Knee joint: stabilisation in the extension position.

33.7.2 Patient symptoms

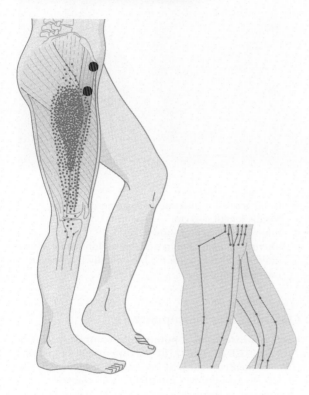

- Pain when walking, in the hips, at the lateral thigh and lower leg.
- 'Deep-seated' hip pain.
- Pain when lying on the affected side.
- Possible preliminary diagnoses: coxarthrosis, bursitis trochanterica, radiculopathy (L3, L4, L5), meralgia paraesthetica.

33.7.3 Trigger points

mTrP	LOCATION	RADIATION	mTrP↔ ACUPUNCTURE POINT
1	Two finger widths below the superior anterior iliac spine	Greater trochanter, gluteal region, lateral thigh	GB 29 (one finger width ventral)
2	1.5 hand widths below the superior anterior iliac spine	Lateral hips, lateral thigh, lateral tibial condyle, lateral thigh to lateral malleolus	–

33.7.4 Diagnosis

Questioning
- Long car journey?
- Long walk leaning to the side?
- Previous hip operation?

Inspection
- Slightly flexed hips when standing (upper body leaning forward).
- In slim people a strained M. tensor fasciae lata may be visibly prominent.

Physical examination
- Painfully limited hip extension and adduction.
- Test for shortening in the supine position with the buttocks at the lower edge of the bed. Hip joint and knee joint flexion on the unaffected side, both hands draw the thigh to the body (maximum flexion on the unaffected side): test extension (such as iliopsoas) and adduction on the free leg.
- Testing abduction capability with the patient lying on the unaffected side.
- Difference in leg length is possible in examination in the supine position.
- Palpation with the patient lying on the back and the unaffected side: strong pressure may be needed, as the muscle can be strong and deep.

Technical examination: X-ray the hips if coxarthrosis is suspected.

33.7.5 Specific aspects

- Associated mTrPs can often be found in the M. gluteus minimus.
- Frequently associated with coxarthrosis (protective posture).

33.7.6 Therapy

Instructions for manual trigger point therapy

- Treatment of mTrPs in the area of the posterolateral fibres: patient in lateral decubitus position.
- Treatment of mTrPs in the area of the anteromedial fibres: patient in supine position.
- Fascia separation technique to M. sartorius.

Stretching

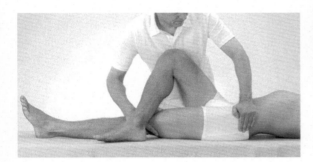

- Patient in supine position.
- Place the unaffected leg over the affected leg.
- With the hand nearest the foot, the therapist grasps the thigh of the affected leg and pulls in the direction of adduction.
- The hand closer to the head holds the hips in place.

Alternative:

- Patient lying on the unaffected side.
- The therapist stands behind the patient.
- The leg underneath is flexed 90° at the hip and knee joint.
- The upper leg is extended and slightly rotated laterally.
- The therapist's hand nearest the head grasps the pelvis and holds it in position from a dorsal direction.
- The hand away from the head grasps the knee joint from below (laterally).
- Stretching by extension and adduction of the hips (traction in direction of own abdomen).

Physical procedures

- All physical procedures are possible.

Infiltration techniques/dry needling

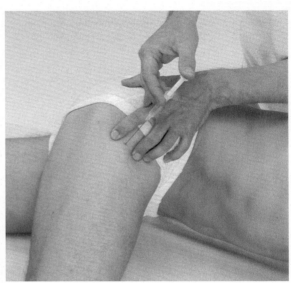

- Good access for injection and dry needling.
- Needle length 4–6 cm.
- Injection in position shown
- Alternative: treatment in supine position with a pillow under the knees to flex the hips slightly (muscles in relaxed position).

Classical Chinese acupuncture

Local and locoregional points (also contralateral): GB 29, GB 30, GB 31, GB 32, BL 54, lower point of the hip (over trochanter major), ST 34, Ex-BF 1 (point pair), GB 27, GB 28, Ashi points (important, as no classical acupuncture in the muscle area of the M. tensor fasciae lata).

Distal points: GB 32, GB 37; GB 39, LR 10, 11, SP 12: adductors (antagonists), BL 23–BL 25: segmental effects (sensitive, dermatome), BL 25–BL 27 segmental effects (motor function).

Control points/symptomatic points: GB 34 (meridian point and tendons masterpoint); LR 3 (Yuan point): psychological balance, spasmolytic.

Microsystem acupuncture

Ear: hip representation.
YNSA: D zone/points preauricular, D1–D5.
NPS-O (Siener): point area at the medial malleolus.

Kiiko Matsumoto acupuncture

- For painful palpation of the insertion of the inguinal ligament at the superior anterior iliac spine: KI 9.
- Tenderness in the lower area of the fascia: LR 8 and GB 34.
- Tenderness in the medial area of the inguinal ligament: ST 13 on both sides.
- In some cases the points GB 43 and GB 44 have relieved tenderness in this muscle.
- If the metal and water points of the gallbladder meridian do not have any effect, GB 1 or GB 2 and GB 28 (on the superior anterior iliac spine) relieve tenderness.

Psychosomatic aspects/relaxation

- Avoidance of relaxation techniques with one-sided weight-bearing, e.g. lotus position in yoga.
- Treat the lateral axis.

33.7.7 Recommendations for the patient

Autostretching

- Patient on the unaffected side on the lower edge of the bed.
- Pillow under the lumbar spine.
- Flex the lower leg at the hip and knee, stretch the upper leg and extend at the hip.
- Rotate the upper leg laterally and allow to fall (adduction).
- Autostretching similarly to M. gluteus minimus.

Additional measures

- Self-treatment with a tennis ball.
- Sufficient breaks on long car journeys.
- Avoid one-sided posture with flexed hip or frequent changes of position.

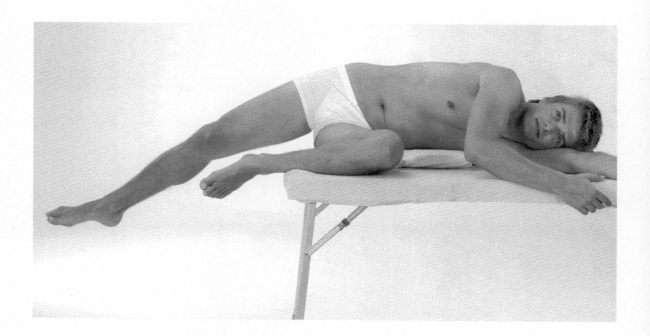

33.8 HIP JOINT ADDUCTORS

33.8.1 Anatomy

The medial group of the muscles of the thigh is also described as an adductor group because of its main function:

- M. gracilis,
- M. pectineus,
- M. adductor brevis,
- M. adductor longus,
- M. adductor magnus,
- M. adductor minimus (represents a proximal incomplete split from the M. adductor magnus),
- M. obturatorius externus.

Innervation
- N. obturatorius (plexus lumbalis): M. gracilis, M. pectineus, M. adductor magnus, M. adductor brevis, M. adductor longus, M. obturatorius externus.
- N. femoralis (plexus lumbalis): M. pectineus.
- N. ischiadicus (tibial part: plexus sacralis): M. adductor magnus.

Origin
- M. gracilis: inferior branch pubic bone (medial edge, along the symphysis).
- M. pectineus: pectors of the pubic bone.
- M. adductor brevis: inferior branch of the pubic bone (closer to the obturator foramen than M. adductor longus).
- M. adductor longus: pubic bone (below the pubic crest to the symphysis).
- M. adductor magnus: inferior branch of the pubic bone, branch and tuberosity of the ischial bone (medial margin).
- M. obturatorius externus: circumference of obturator foramen (lateral surface), obturator membrane.

Insertion
- M. gracilis: proximal end of tibia (medial to the tibial tuberosity).
- M. pectineus: linea pectinea of the femur.
- M. adductor brevis: labium mediale of the linea aspera (proximal third).
- M. adductor longus: labium mediale of the linea aspera (middle third).
- M. adductor magnus: medial labium of the linea aspera (proximal two-thirds), tuberosity, tuberculum adductorium (hiatus adductorius between both insertions).

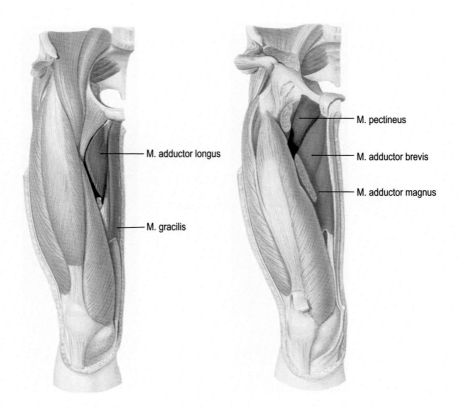

M. adductor longus

M. gracilis

M. pectineus

M. adductor brevis

M. adductor magnus

- M. obturatorius externus: sinewy in the trochanteric fossa.

Function
- Hip joint:
  - adduction, flexion, lateral rotation: M. gracilis, M. pectineus, M. adductor brevis, M. obturatorius externus,
  - adduction, flexion, lateral rotation, most anterior fibres medial rotation: M. adductor longus,
  - adduction, lateral rotation, flexion (anterior part), extension (posterior part): M. adductor magnus.
- Knee joint (flexion, medial rotation): M. gracilis.

33.8.2 Patient symptoms

- Inguinal pain.
- Medial knee pain.
- Rarely pelvic pain.

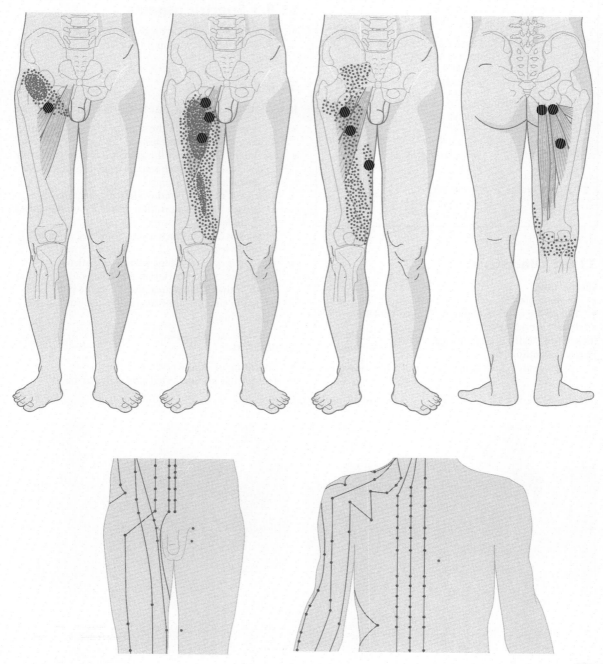

33.8.3 Trigger points

mTrP	LOCATION	RADIATION	mTrP→ ACUPUNCTURE POINT
1	M. pectineus	Inguinal area	SP 12, SP 13
2	M. adductor brevis	Inguinal area, anterior and medial thigh	SP 12, SP 13
3	M. adductor longus	Inguinal area, anterior and medial thigh, medial knee	LR 10, LR 11
4	M. adductor magnus	Inguinal area, anterior and medial thigh, referral to pelvis, medial knee	LR 11, SP 11
5	M. gracilis	Medial thigh, medial knee and knee flexor	LR 9

33.8.4 Diagnosis

Questioning
- Football player?
- Fall on ice or when skiing with overextension?
- Inguinal operation?

Inspection: 'as if walking on eggs'

Physical examination
- mTrPs easily palpable or symptoms easily caused by pressure.

- Adduction against resistance painful, especially with flexed hips.
- Tenderness between the sartorius and adductor longus muscles in the Patrick test (see Stretching, below).
- Delimitation of coxarthrosis using medial rotation (painful only if arthritis is present).

Technical examination: if necessary perform a hip X-ray.

33.8.5 Specific aspects

- mTrPs in the adductor brevis are the most common cause of inguinal pain in footballers.

33.8.6 Therapy

Instructions for manual trigger point therapy

- Treatment of mTrPs in the adductor longus: patient in supine position, Patrick test.
- Treatment of mTrPs in the adductor brevis: patient in supine position, Patrick test, treatment through the pectineus/adductor longus.
- Treatment of mTrPs in the adductor magnus:
  - patient in supine position, lower leg on therapist's shoulder,
  - patient lies on affected side, lower leg extended, upper leg bent.
- Treatment of mTrP in the pectineus: patient in supine position, Patrick test, palpation of the femoral artery in the inguinal area, medial to the pulse palpation site the pectineus runs to the pubic bone superior branch.

Stretching

- Stretching in supine position.
- Hold pelvis on unaffected side with one hand.

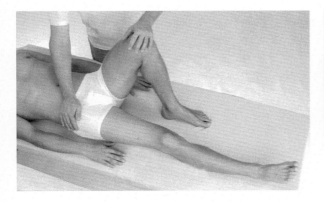 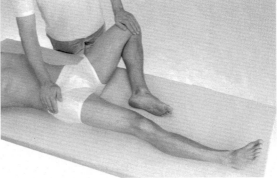

- With the other hand stretch with pressure on the flexed knee in the direction of hip joint abduction.

Physical procedures

- Combine all physical and thermal applications, especially for (top) athletes.

Infiltration techniques/dry needling

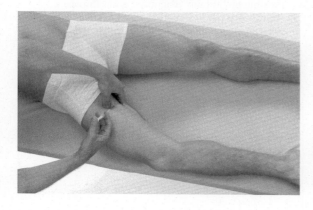

- Affected leg abducted and slightly flexed at the knee joint.
- Muscles in pinch grip.
- Before infiltration into the adductors always delimit the femoral artery and vein and the femoral nerve.

Classical Chinese acupuncture

Local and locoregional points (also contralateral): LR 9, LR 10, LR 11, SP 10, SP 11, SP 12; lower point of the hip (approx. hand width distal to the trochanter major along the course of the tractus iliotibialis); GB 27, GB 28. Antagonists: Mm. gluteus minimus and medius tensor fasciae.
Distal points: GB 34, ST 34, SP 5; LR 3 can immediately improvement abduction capacity: test; BL 25–BL 27: segmental effects; LU 1.
Control points/symptomatic points: GB 34 (meridian point and tendons masterpoint); LR 3 (Yuan point): psychological balance, spasmolytic.

Microsystem acupuncture

Ear: hip representation.
YNSA: D zone/points preauricular, D1–D5.
NPS-O (Siener): point area at the medial malleolus.

Kiiko Matsumoto acupuncture

M. pectineus:
- tenderness in the medial area of the inguinal ligament: ST 13 on both sides,
- in some cases needling of GB 43 and GB 44 (metal and water point) or possibly GB 1 and GB 2 as well as GB 28 may help (superior anterior iliac spine).
M. obturatorius externus:
- ipsilateral to LR 3 or LR 4 together with GB 40 or GB 41 and BL 60 and KI 3,
- ipsilateral to BL 66 and BL 67 (particularly for tenderness in the area of BL 60).

Psychosomatic aspects/relaxation

- Pressure to perform among athletes? Person plagued with stress? Protection of the lower body/genital region.

33.8.7 Recommendations for the patient
Autostretching

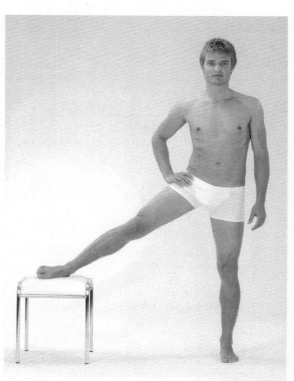

- Spread the affected leg and place the medial edge of the foot on a chair.
- Stretch by leaning to the affected side and apply pressure with the hand on the hip on the affected side.

Additional measures

- Instruction for regular stretching and treatment (stretching and strengthening the antagonists).

33.9 M. QUADRICEPS FEMORIS

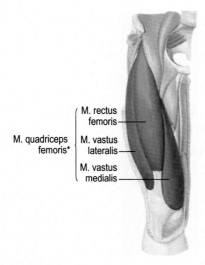

M. quadriceps femoris*
- M. rectus femoris
- M. vastus lateralis
- M. vastus medialis

33.9.1 Anatomy

- M. rectus femoris: two joints.
- Mm. vasti medialis, lateralis and intermedius: single joint.

Innervation: N. femoralis (plexus lumbalis).

Origin

- M. rectus femoris, caput rectum: inferior anterior iliac spine.
- M. rectus femoris, caput reflexum: cranial margin of acetabulum.
- M. vastus medialis: medial lip of the linea aspera of the femur (lower two-thirds).
- M. vastus lateralis: greater trochanter (distal circumference), lateral lip of the linea aspera.
- M. vastus intermedius: anterior facet of the femur (upper two-thirds).
- M. articularis genus: anterior facet of the femur (distal quarter).

Insertion: patella (proximal and lateral margins), tibial tuberosity (over patellar ligament), proximal end of tibia (area lateral to the tibial tuberosity over patellar retinaculum).

Function

- Hip joint (only M. rectus femoris): flexion.
- Knee joint: extension.

33.9.2 Patient symptoms

- Pain in the thigh and knee, occasionally accompanied by hip pain.
- Pain when walking.
- Weakness in the knee joint, e.g. when going up stairs.
- Weakness in the hips when carrying heavy objects.
- Possible preliminary diagnoses: gonarthrosis, coxarthrosis, chondropathia patellae, chronic bursitis suprapatellaris, meralgia paraesthetica.

33.9.3 Trigger points

mTrP	LOCATION	RADIATION	mTrP→ ACUPUNCTURE POINT
1	M. rectus femoris, frequently close to the origin but also along the course	Anterior knee and distal thigh	SP 11, ST 31, ST 32, ST 33
2	M. vastus medialis	Medial knee, distal medial thigh	SP 10
3	M. vastus lateralis, 3–4 predilection sites	Lateral knee, back of knee, thigh laterally to hips	ST 34, GB 31, GB 32
4	M. vastus intermedius:	Medial and anterior knee, thigh, hip	ST 31, SP 11

33.9.4 Diagnosis

Questioning

- Strain when riding a bike, skiing or climbing a hill?
- Previous knee joint injury or immobilisation of affected extremity?
- Previous hip operation?

Inspection: flat foot, genu valgus, stiff gait because of incomplete flexion or extension of the knee joint, lateral patellar dislocation.

Physical examination

- Differentiated examination of the knee with known provocation test to exclude internal knee or joint damage, hypomobility of the patella.

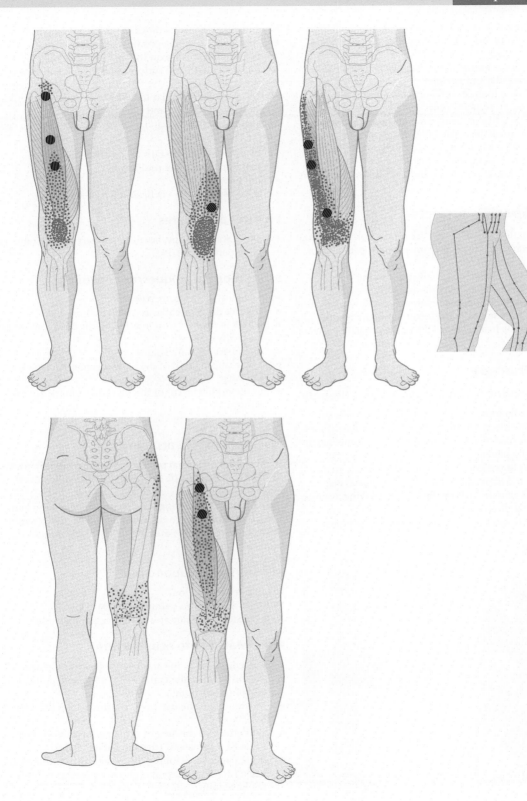

- Shortening of parts of the quadriceps, subpatellar pain when pushing the patella likely indicator of patellar chondropathy.
- There is often a muscular imbalance between the Mm. vastus medialis and lateralis.
- Knee flexion limited with concomitant hip joint extension: M. rectus femoris.
- Knee flexion limited with concomitant flexed hip: M. vastus medialis or lateralis or intermedius.
- Careful palpation of the whole thigh, mTrPs in the intermedius usually not palpable.

Technical examination: depending on findings exclusion of relevant arthritis.

33.9.5 Specific aspects

- mTrPs in the quadriceps are an almost normal finding with coxarthrosis and gonarthrosis with pain and/or limited function.
- A shortened quadriceps predisposes to the development of patellar chondropathy.
- mTrPs can often be permanently cured only when mTrP-induced tension of the ischiocrural muscles is treated.
- There can be ligamentary TrPs in the medial or lateral ligament.

33.9.6 Therapy

Instructions for manual trigger point therapy

- M. rectus femoris: mTrPs occasionally immediately next to the insertion site (inferior anterior iliac spine).
- M. vastus medialis: relevant mTrPs often immediately next to the patella.
- M. vastus intermedius: can only be indirectly treated through the M. rectus femoris/M. vastus lateralis.
- M. vastus lateralis: mTrPs often lie an amazing distance in a dorsal direction.
- Use aids (trigger point sticks) to relieve the fingers.

Stretching

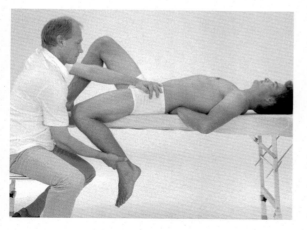

M. rectus femoris, sometimes M. vastus intermedius:
- stretching in supine position on edge of bed,
- the fixing hand lies on the iliac spine,
- the stretching hand surrounds the ankle and flexes the knee.

M. vastus medialis similar to adductors: patient in supine position, hip abducted and flexed and stretching via knee joint flexion with hand on ankle and pushing the heal towards the buttocks.

Mm. vasti medialis, lateralis and intermedius:
- stretching in supine position,
- hip flexed,
- therapist stretches via flexion in the knee joint.

Physical procedures

- Shock wave therapy, laser therapy, wraps and poultices for superficial mTrPs.

Infiltration techniques/dry needling

- Many mTrP are easily palpable.
- Delimit the femoral artery, vein and nerve.
- mTrPs in the M. vastus intermedius lie deep (below the M. rectus femoris).
- The injection is illustrated:
- in the upper mTrP of the M. rectus femoris (photo, top left),
- in the middle mTrP of the M. rectus femoris (photo, bottom left),
- in the M. vastus medialis (photo, top right).

Classical Chinese acupuncture

Local and locoregional points (also contralateral): ST 31, ST 32, ST 33, ST 34, GB 31, GB 32, SP 10, SP 11; Ex-BF 1, Ex-BF 2, Ex-BF 3.
Distal points: depending on affected meridian and axis.
Control points/symptomatic points: GB 34, LR 3 (tension reduction for M. vastus medialis), KI 3/BL 62 for stance problems.

Microsystem acupuncture

Ear: hip representation.
YNSA: D zone/points preauricular, D1–D5.
NPS-O (Siener): point area at the medial malleolus.

Kiiko Matsumoto acupuncture

- For tenderness in the area of the M. vastus medialis: ST 44 and ST 45 ipsilateral and GB 43 (metal point) and GB 44 (water point).
- In addition, if there is a neurological cause: KG 12 and KG 10.
- Tenderness in the area of the superior anterior iliac spine KI 9 ipsilateral (needling at an angle).
- If the patient is standing: BL 20 and BL 21, insertion angle 15–45°; these points also improve the mobility of the knee joint.

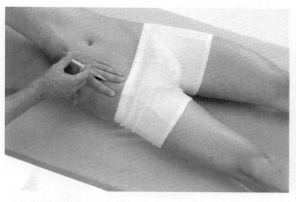
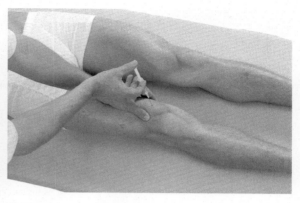
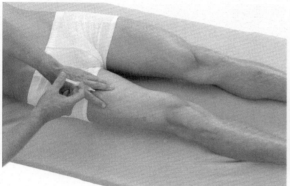
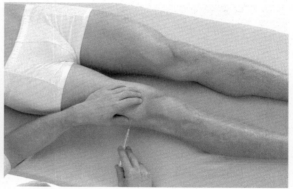

Psychosomatic aspects/relaxation

- Stability/steadfastness, Qigong: 'standing like a pine tree'.

33.9.7 Recommendations for the patient

Autostretching

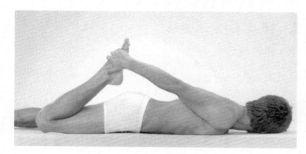

- In the prone position traction on the back of the foot in the direction of knee joint flexion.
- Standing with hyperextended hip and flexed knee joint.
- Stretching hand on the back of the foot or the ankle and traction in the direction of knee joint flexion.

Additional measures

- Avoid strengthening exercises (lack of muscle strength is rarely a problem).
- Practise standing on one leg, at first on level ground then on sloping or uneven ground for dynamic stabilisation.
- Automassage with golf ball.
- Correction of foot deformities.

33.10 ISCHIOCRURAL MUSCLES

33.10.1 Anatomy

The ischiocrural muscles are composed of the dorsal muscles of the thigh:

- M. biceps femoris,
- M. semitendinosus,
- M. semimembranosus.

Innervation

- N. ischiadicus, tibial part (plexus sacralis): M. biceps femoris, caput longum; M. semitendinosus, M. semimembranosus.
- N. ischiadicus, fibular part (plexus sacralis): M. biceps femoris, caput breve

497

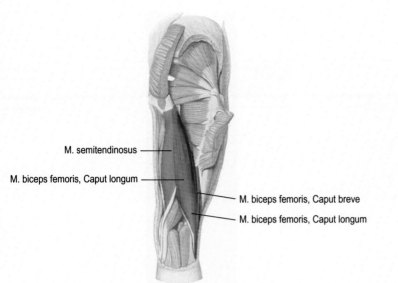

M. semitendinosus

M. biceps femoris, Caput longum

M. biceps femoris, Caput breve

M. biceps femoris, Caput longum

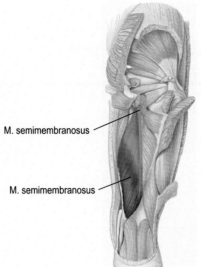

M. semimembranosus

M. semimembranosus

Origin
- M. biceps femoris:
  - long head: ischial tuberosity together with M. semitendinosus,
  - short head: middle third of the lateral lip of the linea aspera.
- M. semitendinosus: ischial tuberosity together with the long head of the bicipitis femoris muscles.
- M. semimembranosus: tuber ischiadicum.

Insertion
- M. biceps femoris: fibular head (separates the fibular collateral ligament), radiates into the crural fascia.
- M. semitendinosus; medial surface of the tibial tuberosity.
- M. semimembranosus: proximal end of the tibia below the medial condyle, posterior capsule of the knee joint, oblique popliteal ligament, fascia of the M. popliteus.

Function
- Knee joint:
  - flexion, medial rotation: M. semitendinosus, M. semimembranosus,
  - flexion, lateral rotation: M. biceps femoris.

- Hip joint:
  - extension, adduction, medial rotation: M. semitendinosus, M. semimembranosus,
  - extension, adduction, lateral rotation: M. biceps femoris.

33.10.2 Patient symptoms

- Gluteal pain and at the dorsal thigh when walking.
- Pain at the back of the knee.
- Pain when standing up from a seated position.
- Possible diagnoses: sciatica, radiculopathy, iliosacral joint blockade, chronic knee pain.

33.10.3 Trigger points

33.10.4 Diagnosis

Questioning
- Long run? Short-term strain, e.g. after sport?
- Car accident (abrupt strain)?

Inspection: standing up from seated position painful.

mTrP	LOCATION	RADIATION	mTrP→ ACUPUNCTURE POINT
1	M. biceps femoris	Dorsal thigh, back of knee	BL 37, BL 38
2	M. semitendinosus, M. semimembranosus	Buttocks, dorsal thigh, back of knee	LR 9

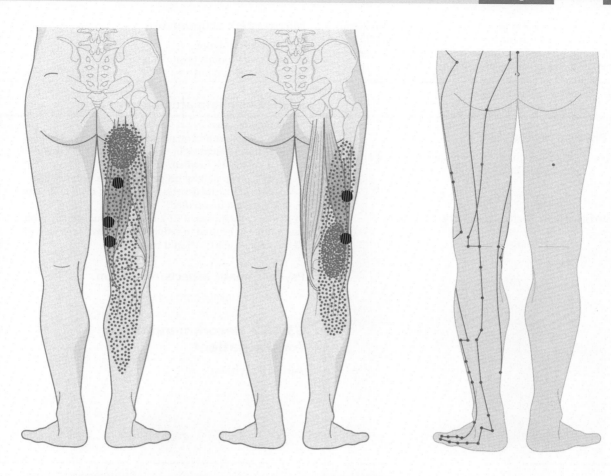

Physical examination: hip flexion and knee joint extension painful, particularly lifting the extended leg leads to dorsal pain in the area of the muscles (delimitation to true Lasègue).

33.10.5 Specific aspects

- Dysfunction of the ischiocrural muscles leads to strain of the quadriceps.
- Insertion tendinosis at the ischial tuberosity due to chronic strain.

33.10.6 Therapy

Instructions for manual trigger point therapy

- M. semitendinosus: muscle fibres (and mTrPs) are predominantly in the proximal half of the thigh.
- M. semimembranosus: muscle fibres (and mTrPs) are predominantly in the distal half of the thigh.
- M. biceps caput breve: access medially and laterally to the tendon of the M. biceps caput longum deep in the distal half of the dorsal femur.
- Use aids (trigger point sticks) to relieve the fingers.

Stretching

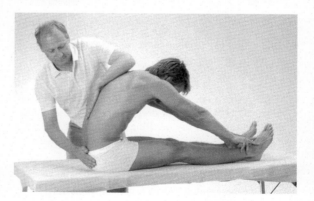

- This position stretches the lumbar autochthonous back muscles (see Section 32.6) and the ischiocrural muscles at the same time.

- A second possibility for stretching is to left the extended leg and flex at the hip while lying down until the appropriate traction can be felt (as for Lasègue).
- Depending on the muscle parts affected, the hips should be medially rotated (= lowering of the extended leg in a lateral direction).

Physical procedures

- Laser treatment, shock wave therapy, wraps and compresses, TENS.

Infiltration techniques/dry needling

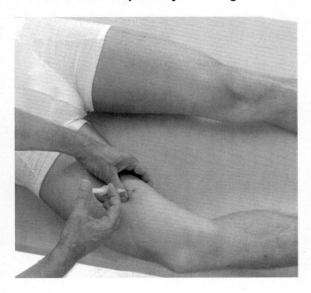

- Infiltration easy using two-finger protection technique or pinch grip.
- M. semimembranosus and M. semitendinosus can be to some extent easily mobilised.
- There are frequently several mTrPs close to each other.
- **Note:** N. ischiadicus: for deep mTrPs push the needle forward carefully, dry needling is better here.

Classical Chinese acupuncture

Local and locoregional points (also contralateral): LR 8, LR 9, BL 36, BL 37, BL 38, BL 39, BL 40.
Distal points: BL 63, BL 64, BL 65, SI 6, treat points for M. quadriceps at the same time (Section 33.9). Other bladder points in the M. erector spinae.
Control points/symptomatic points: GB 34, KI 3 for pain at night.

Microsystem acupuncture

Ear: hip representation.
YNSA: D zone/points preauricular, D1–D5.
NPS-O (Siener): point area at the medial malleolus.

Kiiko Matsumoto acupuncture

M. semitendinosus:
- if KI 2 is not painful on palpation this point can be used to reduce tenderness in the area of KI 10; otherwise KI 7 should be needled,
- if LR 2 is not painful on palpation this point can be used to reduce tenderness in the area of LR 8; otherwise LR 4 should be needled.

M. semimembranosus: if KI 2 is not painful on palpation this point can be used to reduce tenderness in the area of KI 10; otherwise KI 7 should be needled.

Psychosomatic aspects/relaxation

- The performance aspect is important.

33.10.7 Recommendations for the patient

Autostretching

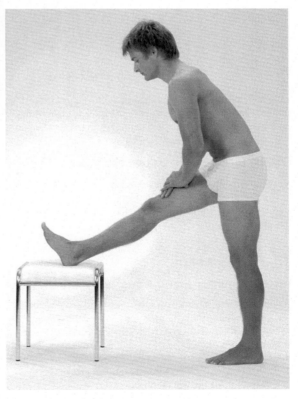

- Stretching while standing with the foot on a stool or chair.
- Stretch further by flexing the hip.
- Frequent regular stretching can be very successful.
- Avoid compression of the muscles when sitting, for example by using cushions.
- Make sure the saddle is at the correct height when riding a bicycle.
- Self-treatment with a tennis ball.

33.11 M. POPLITEUS

33.11.1 Anatomy

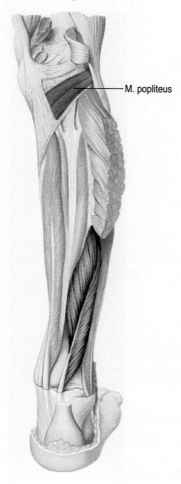

— M. popliteus

Innervation: tibial nerve (sciatic nerve).
Origin: lateral condyle of the femur.
Insertion: posterior facet of the tibia above the linea musculi solei.
Function: knee joint: flexion, medial rotation.

33.11.2 Patient symptoms

- Pain at the back of the knee, especially when squatting or running on sloping paths.
- Possible preliminary diagnoses: popliteus tendinitis, Baker cyst.

33.11.3 Trigger points

mTrP	LOCATION	RADIA-TION	mTrP→ ACUPUNCTURE POINT
1	Dispersed in the muscle	Back of knee, dorsal upper thigh	BL 55

33.11.4 Diagnosis

Questioning
- Rotation trauma in extension position of the knee, e.g. slipping or twisting?
- Strain when going downhill?

Physical examination
- Passive lateral rotation inhibited while seated and 90° flexed knee joint.
- Palpation just below the knee joint fold between the tendons of the M. biceps femoris and M. gastrocnemius.
- Tenderness over tendon and belly of muscle.

Technical examination: exclusion of knee joint pathology.

33.11.5 Specific aspects

- It is not unusual for chronic knee pain to be caused after an operation on athletes, especially footballers.

33.11.6 Therapy

Instructions for manual trigger point therapy
- Patient in prone position, knee flexed:
- treatment at the insertion site at proximal third of the tibia (dorsal side),
- treatment medial to the pulse palpation site at the back of the knee.
- The popliteus muscle can be felt over guided medial/lateral rotation of the knee joint, it is extended with passive lateral rotation at the end of the range of motion.

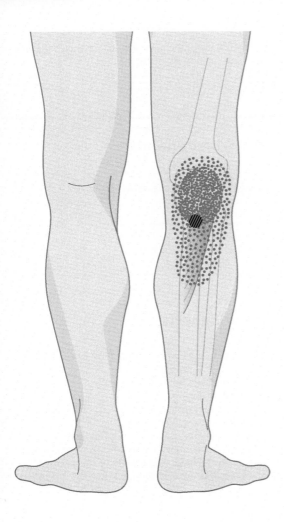

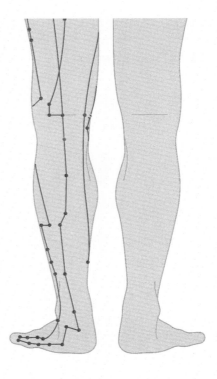

Stretching

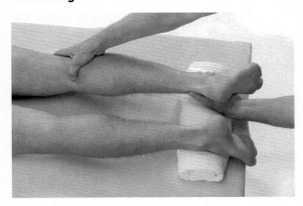

- Patient in prone position, feet supported by pillow.
- One of the therapist's hands supports the knee.
- The other hand grasps the ankle, foot slightly pronated.
- Stretch by traction and lateral rotation of the ankle.

Physical procedures

- Laser therapy, heat treatment.

Infiltration techniques/dry needling

- Patient in prone position, feet supported by pillow.
- Injection with two-finger protection technique.
- **Note:** popliteal artery and vein, tibial nerve and fibular nerve, therefore good delineation of the mTrPs and cautious infiltration.
- Dry needling less traumatic.

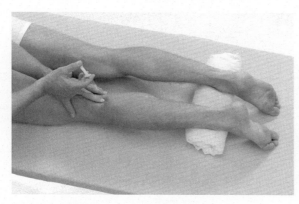

Classical Chinese acupuncture

Local and locoregional points (also contralateral): BL 39, BL 40, BL 55, BL 56.
Distal points: BL 62, KI 3.
Control points/symptomatic points: only if there are additional symptoms after differentiation.

Microsystem acupuncture

Ear: hip representation.
YNSA: D zone/points preauricular, D1–D5.
NPS-O (Siener): point area at the medial malleolus.

Kiiko Matsumoto acupuncture

- SP 9 can be used as the locoregional point, insertion angle 10–45° along the course of the spleen meridian.
- BL 20 and BL 21 (Shu points of spleen and stomach) ipsilaterally: insertion angle 15–90° (depending on easing of tenderness).

3.11.7 Recommendations for the patient

Autostretching

- Autostretching only partly possible.
- Patient in prone position.
- Feet supported and hanging over end of bed.
- Stretching by lateral rotation/supination.
- Multiple repetitions are necessary (1–20 times lateral rotation for 20 s).

Additional measures

- Shoes without inserts.

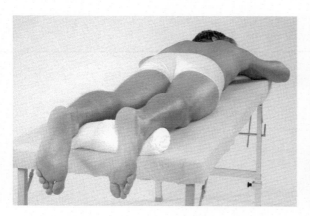

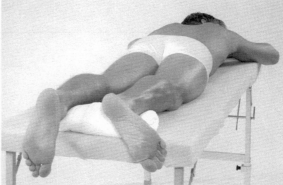

Chapter | 34 |

Lower leg and foot

Dominik Irnich

34.1 FUNCTIONAL ASSOCIATIONS

The foot and lower leg represent the base of the body. About half of all adults have significant changes in the fore-foot or arch of the foot. Functional or structural disorders at this level demand compensation mechanisms from the structures constructed therefrom, and sometimes these demands are too great. This usually has effects on the whole locomotor system.

The foot has a complex structure and does not just provide a secure stance; it also transfers the power of movement to the ground. The muscles of the foot and lower leg have to adjust to differently shaped and structured ground and at the same time dynamically stabilise the ankle to avoid injuries to the ligaments. The functioning of the sensorimotor system is a prerequisite, as we have to be 'good on our feet' to be aware of the ground.

Besides the standard anatomy of foot deformities (see below), Larsen's spiral dynamics view (1998) is also interesting. This sees the whole arch of the foot (and the whole body) as being dynamically stabilised in a three-dimensional screw system. This is vividly compared to a cloth where the two ends are 'wrung out' against each other so it curves up with the ends removed from each other in an S-shape, finishing in a spiral. The characteristically healthy foot has no problem moving and also forms a shock absorber. Hallux valgus is (even) a consequence of a disorder of this spiral screw shape and the dynamic stabilisation of the whole foot. It can be immediately improved by reconstruction of the arch of the foot by the therapist's hand. For this to hold under strain by the patient's own muscles, intensive 'foot training' is needed with improvement in perception, coordination training of individual muscle function and strengthening of the muscles.

These positive experiences are often disputed, but, even so, the muscles can play a relevant role in maintenance and even correction of the arch of the foot, so it is possible to at least relieve the symptoms with treatment of mTrPs and to relieve and strengthen strained compensation mechanisms.

34.2 PSYCHOSOMATIC ASPECTS

A functional disorder in the area of the foot may express lack of stability; difficultt with or lack of feeling 'rooted' or 'grounded'. This is similar to the relationship of the dorsal system of acupuncture:

- the kidney meridian has its first point on the sole of the foot (deep-rootedness and lack of familiarity),
- the bladder meridian runs over the calf to the lateral border of the foot (security, creating space).

Disorders of the calf muscles with possible insecure stance do not just correlate with local symptoms but also with what is often extremely treatment-resistant pain of the foot muscles or even a calcaneal spur. The latter can prevent running away (from something).

The mythology of the Achilles tendon is interesting when associated with hardening of the calf muscles and the whole postural system. Achilles was the hero who was almost entirely protected from injury when his mother dipped him into the River Styx by holding on to his heel. This could be used as an analogy for armour against pain following traumatic early childhood experiences.

http://dx.doi.org/10.1016/B978-0-7020-4312-3.00034-9

34.3 SYMPTOMS

Local symptoms can be caused by mTrP as well:

- achillodynia: M. triceps surae,
- night cramps in the calf: M. triceps surae,
- calcaneal spur: M. quadratus plantae, M. triceps surae,
- symptoms of polyarthritis: M. interossei,
- numbness and pain in the area between the first and second metatarsals: entrapment of the deep fibular nerve by the fibularis longus muscle below the head of the fibula,
- many other foot symptoms.

In principle, any symptoms of the locomotor apparatus can also be caused by pathology in the area of the foot/lower leg, which is why examination is always sensible. For example, pelvic obliquity can result from a functional difference in leg length if the foot is misaligned; this may not be compensated due to prior damage to the lumbar, thoracic or cervical spine and can cause headaches. A series of mTrPs may also be found in the weight-bearing muscles (along the muscle function chains), which can in their turn cause their own vicious circle.

Lumbar spine or buttock pain can also be caused by mTrPs in the M. triceps surae.

34.4 DIAGNOSTIC AND THERAPEUTIC CONSIDERATIONS

The most common malposition of the foot is pes transverso planus (spread foot), where the transverse arch of the forefoot drops. This spreads the toes out in a fan shape and shifts weight-bearing into the middle of the forefoot on the second and third metatarsals. This often also spreads the foot as well as causing pain. mTrPs are usually found in muscles which tighten the arch of the foot: Mm. peroneus longus (Section 34.7), tibialis anterior (Section 34.6) and short muscles of the sole of the foot (M. adductor hallucis (Section 34.11), Mm interossei).

Pes planus (flat foot/fallen arches) is usually the result of spread foot, because if the transverse arch of the foot drops it is virtually inevitable that the lengthwise arch also drops. 'Flat foot' is when the medial lengthwise arch is flat on the ground. Appropriate mTrPs are usually found in the Mm. flexor hallucis longus, digitorum longus (Section 34.12), tibialis posterior (Section 34.10) and the short muscles of the sole of the foot.

Pes valgus is usually associated with pes planus. If the longitudinal arch of the foot in particular has dropped severely, the foot pronates, which can put great stress on the ankle and the tendons and ligaments. Active mTrPs are mostly found in the stressed muscles which support the ankle and try to compensate (Mm. gastrocnemius (Section 34.8), soleus (Section 34.9), tibialis posterior (Section 34.10) and anterior

(Section 34.6), flexor digitorum longus (Section 34.12) and flexor hallucis longus (Section 34.12)). However, latent mTrPs in the pronators which often fix the malposition by shortening should also be treated for optimum success of treatment (Mm. peroneus longus, brevis and tertius, extensor digitorum longus, extensor hallucis longus).

For talipes cavus (hollow foot), which can be either hereditary or acquired, large parts of the arch of the foot do not lie on the floor. The consequence is a concentration of the supported body weight on the toes and heel. With hollow foot, the foot is relatively immobile at the ankle as a result of shortening of the pronators (Mm. peroneus longus, brevis and tertius (Section 34.7), extensor digitorum longus (Section 34.11), extensor hallucis longus (Section 34.11)) with relevant latent mTrPs. Hollow foot is, in general, also susceptible to injury resulting from lack of stability caused by the lack of control in the middle of the foot.

The most common disease of the forefoot is hallux valgus. This can be caused by relevant predisposition or by badly fitting shoes: approximately three-quarters of all those affected are women. Women's shoes are often pointed and frequently have high heels as well, so the toes are 'pressed' into shape with almost the whole body weight, causing strain and eventually damage on the transverse arch.

Hallux rigidus is when the unnatural position of the joint has degenerated until it has developed into severe arthritis in the metatarsophalangeal joint of the big toe. Direct mTrPs for the relief of symptoms are usually found in the M. extensor hallucis longus, adductor hallucis (Section 34.11) and the lateral head of the M. flexor hallucis brevis (Section 34.12); they can also occur in the M. peroneus longus (Section 34.7) as a result of incorrect motion of the foot.

> If the arch of the foot suddenly collapses, consider rupture of the M. tibialis posterior; consider lateral X-ray of the foot with and without weight-bearing.

Dudley J. Morton described structural variations in the skeleton of the foot in 1935 (the Morton anomaly; from *The Human Foot*): it is characterised by hypermobility of the first metatarsal with a weak longitudinal plantar ligament and a relatively short first metatarsal (second toe longer than the big toe, which occurs in approximately 40% of the population; Harris, Beath 1949). Although not directly painful, these anomalies can involve functional changes. The hypermobility of the first metatarsal strains the Mm. tibialis posterior (Section 34.10) and flexor digitorum longus (Section 34.12), and a big toe which is too short usually causes pronation and strain of the M. peroneus longus (Section 34.7).

Although treatment of the active and latent mTrPs provides only marginal correction of the malposition, it does relieve the symptoms, improve the mechanisms of compensation and reduce or prevent spreading of the symptoms in a superior direction. The interplay with appropriate correction by, for example, inserts and strengthening of the foot muscles (going barefoot or trying spiral dynamics) can often reconstruct satisfactory functionality.

For pain on active movement or isometric testing, the classification may be reversed, such as with painful plantar flexion (e.g. walking on the toes): look in the Mm. gastrocnemius, soleus, etc.

TREATMENT TIP

The whole arch of the foot can also be improved by the application of kinesiotape for traction from the medial back of the foot proximal to the big toe diagonally over the sole of the foot to the lateral heel under/behind the lateral malleolus. It also helps to train proprioception and activates the appropriate muscles.

Disorders may also not just spread in a superior direction from the foot or lower leg. Disorders in a more superior position may also cause malposition or strain on the feet. One example is increased medial rotation of the legs due to coxa antetorta as a result of hip dysplasia.

As with all regions, it is not just the muscles with active mTrPs (pain on tension) stressed by compensation which should be treated to strengthen their power and coordination and capacity for stabilisation. Of course, the antagonists that may sustain latent mTrPs through shortening must also be sought and treated.

34.6 M. TIBIALIS ANTERIOR

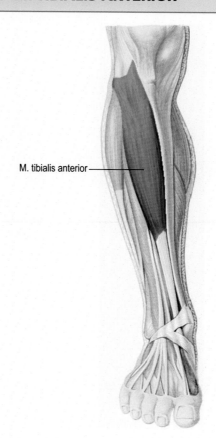

M. tibialis anterior

34.5 EXAMINATION FOR mTrP IDENTIFICATION

Clinical examination with careful palpation of the locoregional muscles is crucial for finding mTrPs, at least in the foot and the whole of the lower leg (Figure 34.1).

LIMITED MOVEMENT	SEARCH FOR mTrPs IN
Upper ankle joint	
Plantar flexion	M. tibialis anterior (Section 34.6), Mm. extensor digitorum longus, extensor hallucis longus (Section 34.11), M. peroneus tertius (Section 34.7)
Dorsal extension	M. gastrocnemius (Section 34.8), M. soleus (Section 34.9), Mm. flexor hallucis longus and flexor digitorum longus (Section 34.12), M. tibialis posterior (Section 34.10), M. peroneus longus and brevis (Section 34.7)
Lower ankle joint	
Supination	Mm. peroneus longus, brevis and tertius (Section 34.7), Mm. extensor digitorum longus and extensor hallucis longus (Section 34.11) and, depending on position, M. tibialis anterior (Section 34.6)
Pronation	M. gastrocnemius (Section 34.8), M. soleus (Section 34.9), M. tibialis posterior (Section 34.10) and anterior (34.6), Mm. flexor digitorum longus and flexor hallucis longus (Section 34.12)

34.6.1 Anatomy

Innervation: N. fibularis profundus (sciatic nerve).
Origin: proximal end of the tibia (below the lateral condyle), lateral facet of the tibia (upper two thirds), interosseous membrane, deep fascia of leg.
Insertion: base of the first metatarsal (medial border), medial cuneiform bone (plantar surface).

507

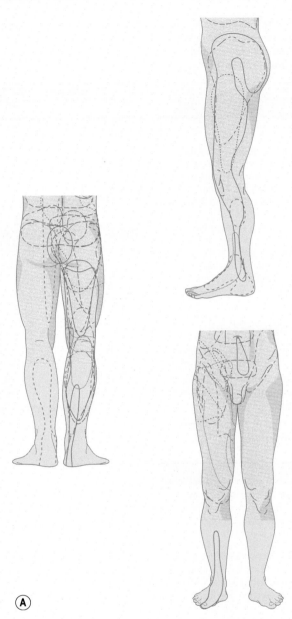

Ⓐ

Fig. 34.1 Pain referral pattern (a) and affected muscles

Continued

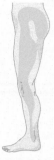
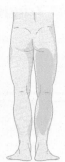
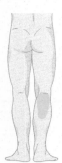
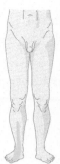

M. gluteus
minimus
(▶32.12)

Hamstrings
(▶33.10)

M. popliteus
(▶33.11)

M. tibialis
anterior
(▶34.6)

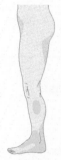
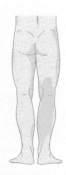
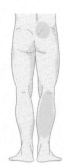

Mm. peronei
(▶34.7)

M. gastrocnemius
(▶34.8)

M. soleus
(▶34.9)

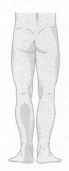
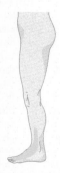
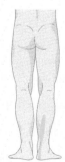

M. tibialis posterior
(▶34.10)

Mm. extensor
hallucis longus
(▶34.11)

Mm. flexor
digitorum
(▶34.12)

Fig. 34.1—cont'd (b) of the lower leg and foot.

Function
- Ankle: dorsal flexion.
- Ankle: supination.

34.6.2 Patient symptoms

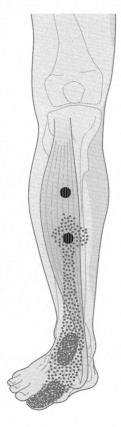

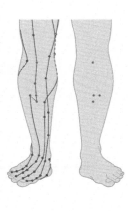

- Dragging pain when running or jogging, shortly after starting (during rolling of the foot over the heel).
- Pain cannot be very well located on the back of the foot or the medial malleolus.
- Light pain directly at the tibia at the upper third of the lower leg.
- Balance slightly insecure (tendency to fall backwards).
- With chronic symptoms there is additional lateral knee joint pain.
- Persistent symptoms following trauma (e.g. fracture at head of tibia).
- Possible preliminary diagnoses: ankle arthritis, chronic radiculopathy L5, recurrent blockade of the head of the fibula, tibial border syndrome.

34.6.3 Trigger points

mTrP	LOCATION	RADIATION	mTrP ↔ ACUPUNCTURE POINT
1	At the transition from the upper third to the lower two-thirds of the muscle, approximately two finger widths lateral to the tibial border	Forming a line in a inferior direction, also over the tibial border, ankle and back of foot (anteromedial) first and second toe, rarely superior	ST 36
2	Between the middle and lower third of the muscle	Local circular, anterior ankle	ST 38, ST 39, ST 40

34.6.4 Diagnosis

Questioning
- Jogger?
- Worn-out shoes?
- High-heeled shoes or pumps?
- Walking for long periods on downward sloping ground (mountain walking)?
- Sprinter?
- Slightly one-sided gait insecurity?
- Frequent car journeys with steep accelerator pedal?

Inspection: observe the patient walking barefoot (walking on toes?).

Physical examination
- Supine position with knee roll.
- Palpation of the tibial border laterally in the direction of the fibres.
- On identification of a hardened bundle of fibres palpation from superior to inferior along the fibre bundle until the maximum pain point is found.
- Snapping palpation here often causes dorsal flexion and inversion of the foot.
- At the same time examine the M. peroneus longus (antagonist), M. extensor digitorum longus (agonist in the ankle) and the head of the fibula (origin M. peroneus longus).
- Paraesthesia, severe tenderness and strong, passive extension pain indicate an anterior compartment syndrome.

Technical examination: measurement of intramuscular pressure if compartment syndrome is suspected.

34.6.5 Specific aspects

- According to TCM there are functional associations with the epigastrium and abdomen.
- Very ambitious people who go running or walking tend to have mTrPs in the M. tibialis anterior. Leisure runners run the risk of the development of anterior compartment syndrome if they do not roll over the heel (those who run on their toes or the balls of their feet).
- Sprinters are particularly disposed to tibial mTrPs (strengthen balance training).
- Anterior compartment syndrome should not be overlooked.

34.6.6 Therapy

Instructions for manual trigger point therapy

- Easy access to treatment (as superficial).
- Fascia separation technique between fascia of anterior tibial muscle and periosteum of the tibia.
- Frequently 'forward-back' problem, then treat mTrPs in the tensed and shortened calf muscles.

Stretching

- Patient in supine position.
- Roll or pillow below the knee (15–30° flexion of the knee).
- Foot hangs freely over the edge of the bed.
- The therapist stands laterally and grasps the tibia just above the ankle with one hand.
- The other hand grasps the mid-foot.
- Dorsal flexion (plantar flexion) of the foot and pronation (aversion and abduction).
- Postisometric relaxation is sensible.
- Transverse lateral stretching with the balls of both thumbs.

Physical procedures

- Electrotherapy, shock waves, laser treatment, TENS.

Infiltration techniques/dry needling

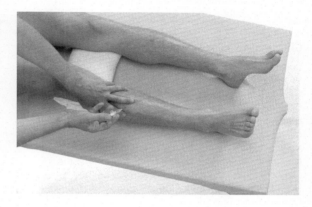

- Supine position, roll or pillow below the knee (15–30° flexion of the knee).
- Foot in normal neutral position.
- Needle length 2–4 cm.
- The same procedure for mTrPs 1 and 2.
- Fast, powerful insertion through the relatively strong fascia.
- Hold the mTrP with the second and third finger placed superiorly and inferiorly to the mTrP on the affected band.
- Vertical needle insertion.
- As large mTrPs or several small mTrPs may lie in the immediate vicinity, the needle may be withdrawn to the subcutis following injection of a small amount of LA and probed in a new direction. In this case use a longer-acting LA to be able to identify mTrPs together with the patient.
- Injection depth 2–4 cm.
- Smooth from proximal to distal after treatment.

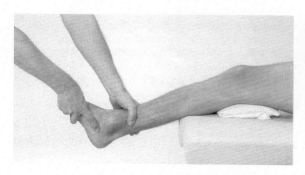

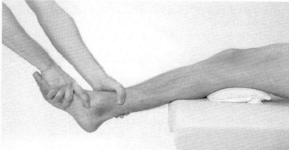

- **Warning:** anterior compartment syndrome so do not use invasive techniques that have a tendency to cause bleeding.
- **Warning:** anterior tibial artery with very deep injection/needling (>4 cm).
- Irritation at the level of L4–S1 paravertebrally can relieve acute pain (dermatome).

Classical Chinese acupuncture

Local and locoregional points (also contralateral): ST 36, ST 37, ST 38, ST 39, ST 40 (in the M. tibialis), GB 34 (below and in front of the head of the fibula), GB 37, GB 38 (antagonist treatment, M. peroneus longus), GB 36 traditionally also psychosomatic disorders, GB 39 (antagonist treatment, tendon of the M. peroneus longus), SP 5 and LR 4 (medial to the tendon of the M. tibialis anterior): muscle tension can occasionally be influenced as well, Ex-BF 7 (M. tibialis anterior), Ex-BF 6 (M. peroneus longus). Consider moxibustion as well (especially local stomach points).

Distal points: SP 3: source point for concomitant digestive disorders, symptoms of gastroenteritis, SP 4: Luo point (balances stomach meridian), anatomical relationship to tendon of the anterior tibialis muscle, LI 10: corresponding point on the forearm (Yang–Yang axis), BL 25: segmental effects (sensitive, dermatome), BL 26–BL 28: segmental effects (motor function).

Control points/symptomatic points: LR 3 (effect on muscle tension); SP 21 (large Luo vessel of the spleen).

Microsystem acupuncture

- **Ear:** point detection of the triangular fossa.
- **YNSA:** D zone.
- **NPS-O:** point detection in the area around the lateral/medial malleolus.

Kiiko Matsumoto acupuncture

- Tenderness along the stomach Qi line (M. tibialis anterior): CV 12, transverse needling. BL 11 ipsilateral vertical to the course of the fibres along the meridian.

Psychosomatic aspects/relaxation

- Information for ambitious athletes/leisure runners (cognitive approach).
- Recommend walking consciously in a relaxed manner (full foot-roll action) on level ground.
- Psychosomatic aspects: lack of grounding, too much pride (e.g. no rest or recuperation phases in sport).

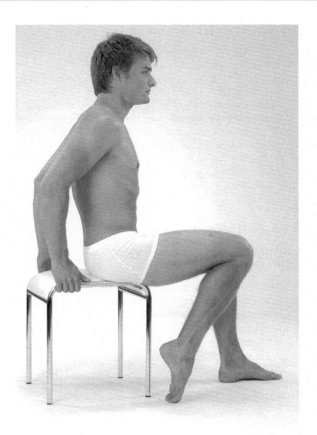

34.6.7 Recommendations for the patient

Autostretching

- The patient sits on a chair.
- Flexes the knee on the affected side and guides foot backwards.
- Presses the toes or back of the foot to the ground.

Alternatively:

- patient sits on a chair with legs crossed,
- using both hands, stretch the foot in plantar flexion and pronation,
- vary positions slightly until optimum stretch is felt,
- runners should pay attention to their running technique: rolling the foot over the heel,
- compensate for drop foot with inserts,
- if the accelerator pedal is too high, heighten the insert to avoid permanent dorsal flexion,
- when asleep keep the ankle in the neutral position with a foot support,
- use heel cushion as a shock absorber,
- strengthening (walking on heels),
- regular autostretching (sitting on heels),
- standing on one leg: practise balancing.

34.7 MM. PERONEI (FIBULARES) LONGUS AND BREVIS

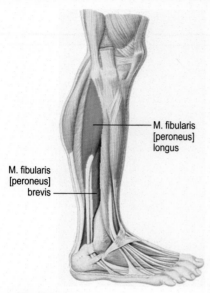

M. fibularis [peroneus] longus

M. fibularis [peroneus] brevis

34.7.1 Anatomy

Innervation: N. fibularis profundus (sciatic nerve).
Origin
- M. peroneus longus: head of fibula, lateral facet and posterior border of fibula (proximal two-thirds), intermuscular septum of anterior and posterior crus, deep fascia of leg.
- Peroneus brevis: lateral facet and posterior border of fibula (distal half), intermuscular septum of anterior and posterior crus.

Insertion
- M. peroneus longus tuberosities of first and second metatarsals, intermediate cuneiform bone (plantar surface).
- Peroneus brevis: tuberosity of fifth metatarsal, tendons to little toe.

Function
- Ankle: plantar flexion.
- Ankle: pronation.
- Secure transverse arch in mid-foot.

34.7.2 Patient symptoms

- Pain at the lateral lower leg and foot.
- Feeling of unstable ankle.
- Paraesthesia on compression of the common peroneal nerve.
- Frequent ankle sprains (supination trauma).
- Possible preliminary diagnoses: arthritis of the ankle joint, radiculopathy S1 (especially if accompanied by entrapment syndrome of the common peroneus

nerve), recurrent blockades of the head of the fibula, Baker cyst (without more serious symptoms in the knee area, but in the upper part of the lower leg).

34.7.3 Trigger points

> Radiation of mTrPs of the peroneus muscles corresponds to the gallbladder meridian of TCM!

mTrP LOCATION	RADIATION	mTrP ↔ ACUPUNCTURE POINT
1	In the peroneus longus two to three finger widths below the head of the fibula, frequently related mTrPs	Inferiorly in the lateral lower leg, into the lateral ankle and the posterior lateral part of the foot (not Achilles tendon)	GB 34GB 36
2	Peroneus brevis	Inferiorly in the lateral ankle and partly on the lateral back of the foot	GB 38

34.7.4 Diagnosis

Questioning
- Sprained ankle? Multiple supination trauma?
- Long-term immobilisation after ankle trauma?
- Types of sport where you have to hold your body up on the toes (running, throwing, boxing)?
- Long car journeys (steep accelerator pedal)?

Inspection
- Calluses.
- Worn-out soles on the shoes.
- Excessive pronation when walking.

Physical examination
- Supine position with knee roll.
- Palpation with the thumb, the hand grasps the tibia, the other fingers serve as resistance to the medial side of the lower leg.
- Narrow muscle so strands are difficult to delineate with transverse palpation.
- Paraesthesia, diffuse, severe tenderness and strong, passive extension pain indicate an anterior compartment syndrome.

Technical examination: measurement of intramuscular pressure if compartment syndrome is suspected.

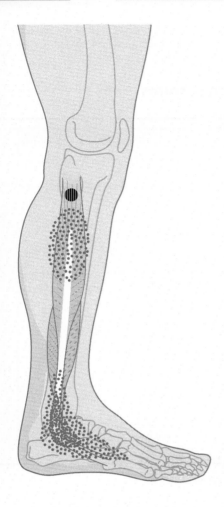
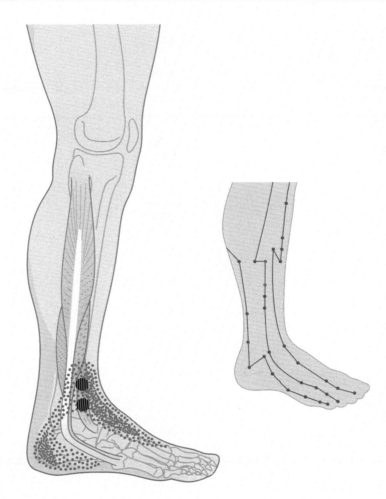

34.7.5 Specific aspects

- The Mm. peronei act as antagonists to the M. tibialis anterior during various sporting activities (throwing, jumping) so both muscles are frequently affected when strained.
- There are often satellite trigger points in the M. peroneus longus when there are mTrPs in the M. gluteus minimus or M. tensor fasciae lata.
- As with the M. tibialis anterior athletes are often affected (over-ambitious leisure athletes, unbalanced training with professional athletes).
- Lateral anterior compartment syndrome should not be overlooked.
- Identifier muscle S1.

34.7.6 Therapy

Instructions for manual trigger point therapy

- Easy access and treatment.

- Combination of mobilisation of the head of the fibula and the tarsal bones is desirable.

Stretching

- Patient in prone position.
- Roll or pillow below the ankle (15–30° flexion of the knee).
- Foot hangs freely over the edge of the bed.
- The therapist grasps the distal fibula to hold it in place and simultaneously feel the muscle tension.
- The other hand grasps the mid-foot.
- The foot is dorsally extended and placed in supine position.
- Postisometric relaxation is sensible.

Physical procedures

- Easily accessible for all physical procedures with penetration depth 2–6 cm, e.g. electrotherapy, shock waves, laser.

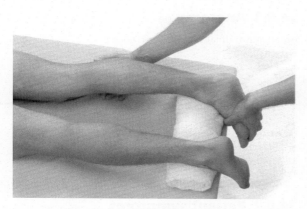

Infiltration techniques/dry needling

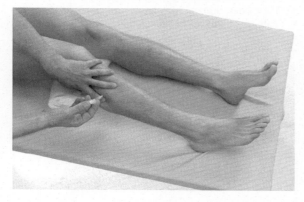

- Very dilute LA (e.g. lidocaine 0.25%, ropivacaine 0.2%) to avoid nerve block.
- Patient on side not to be treated or in supine position, knee slightly flexed, with the lower leg to be treated lying flat (long or several cushions from the knee to the ankle).
- Foot in normal neutral position.
- Needle length 2–4 cm, a 2 cm needle is often sufficient for mTrP 2.
- Palpation of the head of the fibula.
- Possible location of the common peroneus nerve behind the head of the fibula.
- Hold the mTrP with the second and third finger placed superiorly and inferiorly to the mTrP on the affected band.
- Vertical needle insertion.
- Smooth from proximal to distal after treatment.
- Irritation at the level of L4–S2 paravertebrally can relieve acute pain (dermatome).
- **Warning:** lateral anterior compartment syndrome so do not use invasive techniques that have a tendency to cause bleeding.

Classical Chinese acupuncture

Local and locoregional points (also contralateral): GB 34, GB 36, GB 37, GB 38, GB 39, Ex-BF 6 (2 cun distal to GB 34), BL 60, BL 61, BL 62, BL 63 (always close to the tendon of the Mm. peronei, BL 64, Ex-BF 9 (tip of the lateral malleolus, for muscle cramps).

Distal points: GB 29: meridian or muscle function chain (M. tensor fasciae lata), GB 31: meridian or muscle function chain, GB 32: meridian or muscle function chain, TH 5: mTrP 2, corresponding point on the forearm (Yang–Yang axis), TH 9 and the Ashi points situated distally from it on the TH meridian: mTrP 1, corresponding points on the forearm (Yang–Yang axis), neuralgia-type pain, Ashi points in the M. gluteus minimus: muscle function chain, BL 26, BL 27: segmental effects (sensitive, dermatome), BL 26–BL 29: segmental effects (motor function).

Control points/symptomatic points: LR 3 (muscle tension, only foot point in the supply area of the deep peroneus nerve), SP 6 (crossing of the 3 Yin) for motion disorder of the lower extremity, SP 9 for swelling/feeling of swelling.

Microsystem acupuncture

Ear: point detection of the triangular fossa.
YNSA: D zone.
NPS-O: point detection in the area around the lateral/medial malleolus.

Kiiko Matsumoto acupuncture

- Generally muscle-relaxing points such as SP 3 ipsilaterally and ST 22 on the right, Hua tuo jiaji between T10 and T12.

Psychosomatic aspects/relaxation

- Information for ambitious athletes/leisure runners (cognitive approach).
- Walking in a conscious and relaxed manner.

34.7.7 Recommendations for the patient

Autostretching

- The patient sits on a chair or a couch.
- Single-legged tailor position.
- The foot is dorsally extended and placed in supine position.
- Postisometric relaxation is sensible.

Additional measures

- Shoe with good foot bed (stabilising lateral side).
- Avoid knee stockings/socks with tight band.
- For convalescence and prevention: skipping, trampolining (in measured amounts) followed by (auto)stretching.
- Exercises on a wobble board (using a spotter).
- Standing on one leg: practise balancing – dynamic stabilisation.

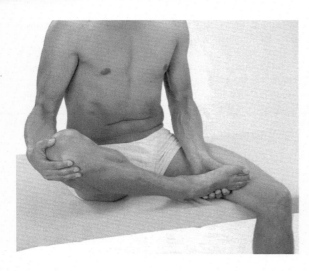

34.8 M. GASTROCNEMIUS

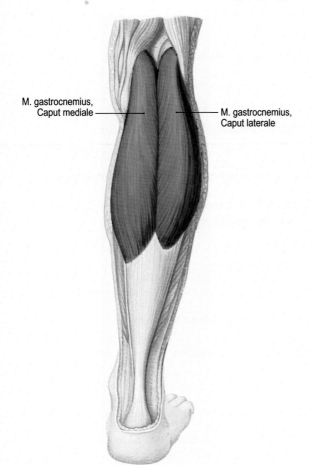

M. gastrocnemius, Caput mediale

M. gastrocnemius, Caput laterale

34.8.1 Anatomy

Innervation: tibial nerve (sciatic nerve).
Origin
- Medial head: popliteal facet of the femur (proximal to the medial condyle).
- Lateral head: popliteal facet of the femur (proximal to the lateral condyle).

Insertion: calcaneal tuberosity over Achilles tendon.
Function
- Knee joint: flexion.
- Ankle: plantar flexion.
- Ankle: supination.

34.8.2 Patient symptoms

- Cramp-like pain, frequently at night.
- Pain when riding a bicycle.
- Pain at the back of the knee on exertion (e.g. climbing).
- Pain on the Achilles tendon.
- Possible preliminary diagnoses: sciatica, chronically pulled calf muscle, suspected thrombosis, thrombophlebitis, Baker cyst, knee joint arthritis, radiculopathy S1 (S2), peripheral arterial occlusive disease (PAOD), achillodynia.

34.8.3 Trigger points

	mTrP LOCATION	RADIATION	mTrP ↔ ACUPUNCTURE POINT
1	M. gastrocnemius, caput mediale, upper to middle parts	Dorsal lower leg, Achilles tendon, sole of foot, medial knee joint	SP 8
2	M. gastrocnemius, caput laterale, upper to middle parts	Dorsal lower leg, back of knee	BL 58
3	Between the medial and lateral heads of the M. gastrocnemius (occasionally also tendinous trigger points)	Dorsal lower leg (along bladder meridian)	BL 55, BL 56, BL 57

34.8.4 Diagnosis

Questioning
- Long mountain tour or strenuous cycling (saddle too low?) especially in cold and/or wet weather.

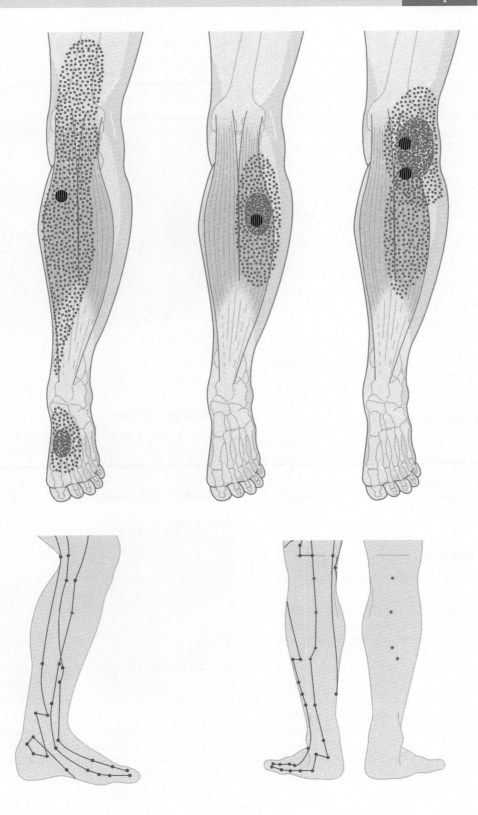

- Trauma to the lower leg, ankle?
- Ankle fracture?
- Walking plaster?

Inspection
- Flat-footed, stiff-legged gait.
- Limited knee joint extension with heel on the floor.
- Achilles tendon thickening with symptoms for a long time.

Physical examination
- Patient in prone position with a role or firm narrow cushion under the ankle so that the ankle is in neutral position.
- If the muscle is too tense in this position, ask the patient to kneel.
- Initially use crosswise palpation to locate the bands of muscle.
- Then palpate with pinch grip or pressure along the muscle band.
- Look for associated mTrPs in the soleus and the ischiocrural muscles.
- Palpate the popliteal fossa.
- Lasègue sign negative.
- Achilles tendon reflex not weakened.

Technical examination
- Nerve conduction speed is radiculopathy suspected.
- Doppler ultrasound, phlebography is thrombosis, thrombophlebitis suspected.
- Angiographic examination if PAOD suspected.

34.8.5 Specific aspects

- Remaining in an unphysiological seated position for too long (e.g. chair too low at workplace) predisposes to development.
- Many related mTrPs in the muscle.
- There are frequently associated mTrPs in the soleus, the ischiocrural muscles and the gluteus maximus and medius.

34.8.6 Therapy

Instructions for manual trigger point therapy

- Easy access and treatment.
- Use aids (trigger point sticks) to relieve the fingers.
- Fascia stretching technique prestretch the muscles (patient takes a step forward) and works the muscle fascia by pressing down on the ankle.

Stretching

- Patient in supine position.
- Leg extended, foot hangs freely over the edge of the bed.
- The therapist stands to the side and grasps the ankle to hold it in place.
- The other hand grasps the heel so the forearm lies on the ball of the foot.

- Stretch the muscle with dorsal flexion.
- Postisometric relaxation with prestretching in dorsal extension.
- Transverse stretching in prone position with belly of muscle between both thumbs and fingers (with both hands).

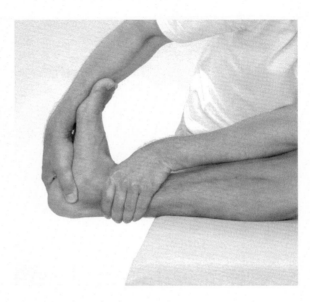

Physical procedures

- Easily accessible for all physical procedures with penetration depth 2–6 cm, for example electrotherapy, shock waves, laser, TENS.

Infiltration techniques/dry needling

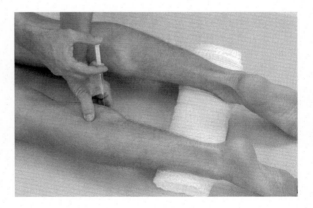

If there are several related mTrPs in the muscle, dry needling is frequently more effective with low pain needling if the relevant distal points and microsystem points are needled before the local treatment.

- mTrP 1
  - Patient in prone position.
  - Place a roll or firm narrow cushion under the ankle so that it is in the neutral position.
- mTrP 2
  - Patient lying on the unaffected side.
  - Knee slightly flexed, with the lower leg to be treated lying flat (long or several cushions from the knee to the ankle).
  - Foot in normal neutral position.
  - Vertical needle insertion.
- mTrP 3
  - If there are mTrPs at the medial border of the lateral head or at the lateral margin of the medial head, use the same procedure for mTrP 1.
  - If there are tendinous mTrPs between both heads of the muscle: Superficial needling without insertion into the tendon.
  - Smooth out from proximal to distal after treatment.
  - Irritation at the level of S1–S2 paravertebrally can relieve acute pain (dermatome).

Classical Chinese acupuncture

Local and locoregional points (also contralateral): BL 40, BL 55, BL 56, BL 57, BL 58, BL 59, BL 60, BL 61, KI 3, KI 5, KI 6, KI 7, SP 7, SP 8 (with dorsal needling mTrPs in the medial head can be reached), four short needles (superficial) medial and lateral to the Achilles tendon.
Distal points: SI 3 (for tenderness): meridian (Yang–Yang axis), SI 6 (for tenderness): meridian (Yang–Yang axis), BL 10 (for tenderness): meridian point, BL 32, BL 33: segmental effects (sensitive, dermatome S1, S2), BL 25, BL 26, BL 31, BL 32: segmental effects (sciatic nerve, motor function).
Control points/symptomatic points: for concomitant paratendinitis of the Achilles tendon SP 6, SP 9.

Microsystem acupuncture

Ear: point detection of the triangular fossa.
YNSA: D zone.
NPS-O: point detection in the area around the lateral/medial malleolus.

Kiiko Matsumoto acupuncture

- Important point for reduction of tenderness: BL 25 (superior posterior iliac spine).
- Muscle can be pinched with thumb and index finger at three sites from proximal to distal. Important: find correct insertion angle (and correct insertion depth).
- Use longer needles for overweight patients.

Psychosomatic aspects/relaxation

- Straightening up (strengthening self-awareness).
- Psychosomatic aspects: stooped gait with depression, lack of support (weakened dorsal postural axis).

34.8.7 Recommendations for the patient

Autostretching

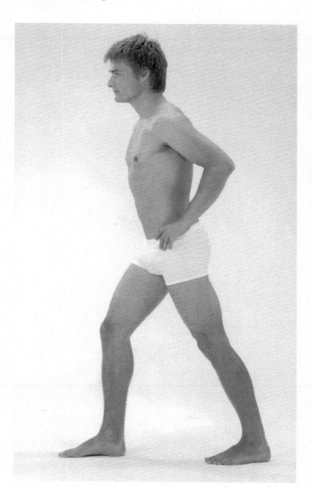

Auto-stretching while standing:

- step forward and stand with both feet firmly placed (floor contact with the whole of the sole of the foot),
- possibly use the contralateral hand for support on a wall,
- both feet pointing forward, upper body straight,
- with the weight on the front leg bend the knee of the front leg to exercise traction on the gastrocnemius.

Autostretching while seated:

- sit on the floor with the back against a wall,
- hold a towel round the soles of the feet with both hands and pull towards body (alternate tension and relaxation).

Additional measures

- Sit on heels and clasp a tennis ball between the thighs and lower legs to work the calf muscles with small movements.
- Make sure the work chair is at the correct height.
- Make sure the bicycle saddle is at the correct height.
- Do not wear long socks with cuffs that are too tight.
- Keep calves warm.
- Do not wear high-heeled shoes.

34.9 M. SOLEUS

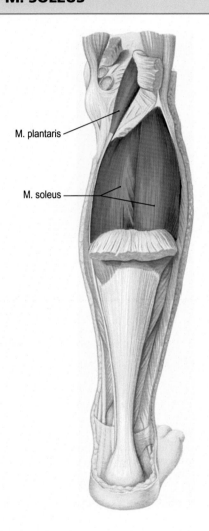

M. plantaris

M. soleus

34.9.1 Anatomy

Innervation: tibial nerve (sciatic nerve).
Origin: fibular head, posterior facet and posterior border of the fibula (proximal third), posterior facet of the tibia (at

and below the soleus muscle line), tendinous arch of the soleus muscle.
Insertion: calcaneal tuberosity over Achilles tendon.
Function
- Knee joint: flexion.
- Ankle: plantar flexion.
- Ankle: supination.

34.9.2 Patient symptoms

- Severe pain in the heel.
- Pain in the calf (rarely cramp).
- Pain on the Achilles tendon (as for calcaneal spur).
- Limited dorsal flexion.
- Slight feeling of instability at the knee when walking.
- Possible preliminary diagnoses: achillodynia, thrombophlebitis, calcaneal spur, Baker cyst, radiculopathy S1.

34.9.3 Trigger points

	mTrP LOCATION	RADIATION	mTrP → ACUPUNCTURE POINT
1	Deep mTrPs in the upper third of the muscle below the lateral head of the gastrocnemius	Distally along the calf, partly along the Achilles tendon	–
2	Deep mTrPs in the lower third of the muscle below the lateral head of the gastrocnemius	Lower calf and Achilles tendon radiating into the ipsilateral iliosacral joint and lumbar area	BL 58
3	In the distal part of the muscle, dorsomedial	Lower calf and Achilles tendon	LR 6, SP 7, (KI 9)

Diagnosis

Questioning
- Almost a fall (slipped)?
- Excessive jogging on sloping ground?
- PAOD (there are frequently concomitant mTrPs here).
Inspection: ask a patient to pick up an object from the floor with an upright stance (dorsal extension of the

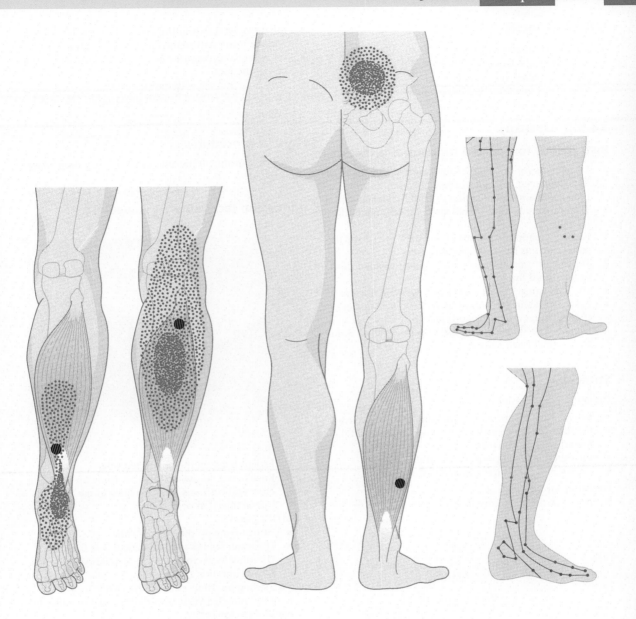

ankle and concomitant knee flexion difficult or painful?).

Physical examination

- Palpation:
  - mTrP 1: on knees on a soft chair or bed with the ankle in neutral position (foot hangs over the edge of the bed), flat palpation,
  - mTrPs 2 and 3: lying on affected side, the knee is flexed 90°, with the lower leg to be palpated lying flat (long or several cushions from the knee to the ankle), pinch grip.

- Test dorsal flexion in the ankle in prone position with knee flexed 90°.
- Achilles tendon reflex can be slightly weakened.

Technical examination

- Doppler ultrasound.
- Phlebography if thrombosis or thrombophlebitis suspected.
- Radiological investigation if true leg-length difference is suspected.
- Neurophysiological and/or radiological investigation if Achilles tendon reflex is limited (S1).

34.9.4 Specific aspects

- Frequently associated with tibialis anterior syndrome.
- mTrPs in the soleus described by Simons and Travell as 'growing pains' in children.
- The soleus functions as a 'vein pump'.

34.9.5 Therapy

Instructions for manual trigger point therapy

- Distal parts (not covered by the gastrocnemius) can be directly treated (patient in prone position: finger pressure in anterior direction or with hands on waist).
- Treat proximal parts through the gastrocnemius and/or laterally.
- Fascia separation technique between the soleus and the gastrocnemius from a lateral direction.
- Thoroughly treat the insertion region (proximal third of the dorsal fibula).
- Use aids (trigger point sticks) to relieve the fingers.
- Fascial stretching technique: prestretch the muscles (patient takes a step forward) and work the muscle fascia by pressing down on the ankle; work from distal to proximal (vein valves).

Stretching

Patient in prone position:

- flex affected leg 90° at the knee and extend upwards,
- the therapist uses one hand to grasp the heel and the forearm lies on the toes,
- the other hand supports the leg at the ankle,
- extension by pressure in dorsal flexion.

Patient in supine position:

- staged positioning knee flexed 70–90°,

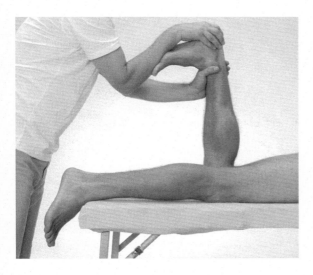

- the therapist stands to the side and grasps the ankle and the lower part of the tibia with the left hand,
- the other hand grasps the heel so the forearm lies on the ball of the foot,
- stretch the muscle with dorsal flexion,
- postisometric relaxation with prestretching in dorsal extension.

Physical procedures

- Physical treatment procedures with a very deep effect for mTrP 1.

Infiltration techniques/dry needling

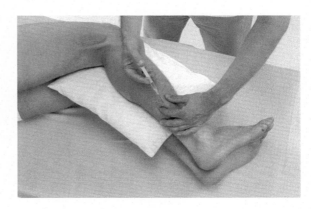

- mTrP 1
  - Patient lying on the unaffected side.
  - Knee flexed 90°, with the lower leg lying flat (long or several cushions from the knee to the ankle).
  - Lateral injection or needling.
- mTrPs 2 and 3
  - Patient lying on the affected side.
  - The lower leg lies with the lateral side flat.
  - The other leg is crossed over and is flexed at the hip.
  - Medial injection or needling.
- Fast, strong insertion as the fascia coat is tough.
- If a local muscle twitch reaction is caused it is like an Achilles tendon reflex.

Classical Chinese acupuncture

Local and locoregional points (also contralateral): BL 39, BL 40, BL 57, BL 58 (TrP 2 often rather superior), BL 60, BL 61, LR 6, SP 7 (a deep-seated mTrP can often be directly needled via these points if the needle is in the correct direction), LR 5, KI 9, KI 3, KI 5, 4 short needles (superficial) medial and lateral to the Achilles tendon.
Distal points: SI 3 (for tenderness), meridian (Yang–Yang axis), SI 6 (for tenderness), meridian (Yang–Yang axis), BL

10 (for tenderness), meridian point, BL 32, BL 33, segmental effects (sensitive, dermatome S1, S2), BL 25, BL 26, BL 31, BL 32, segmental effects (sciatic nerve, motor function).
Control points/symptomatic points: for concomitant paratendinitis of the Achilles tendon SP 6, SP 9.

Microsystem acupuncture

Ear: points on the toe representation.

Kiiko Matsumoto acupuncture

- As for M. gastrocnemius (Section 34.8).

34.9.6 Recommendations for the patient

Autostretching

- Affected leg flexed at 90°, with the foot placed behind the body axis at the same time (heel supported).
- The unaffected leg is placed parallel (feet parallel) in front of the body axis.
- For extension push body focus forwards.

Additional measures

- At night keep the foot in the neutral position with foot support.
- Stretch before and after sporting activity.
- Avoid long-term restriction of perfusion in the soleus. There is a risk of this if, e.g., the lower leg is placed on a stool (muscle compression).
- If it is necessary to go upstairs avoid dorsal flexion of the ankle (gastrocnemius).
- Sit on heels and clasp a tennis ball between the thighs and lower legs to work the calf muscles with slow movements (move weight sideways).

34.10 M. TIBIALIS POSTERIOR

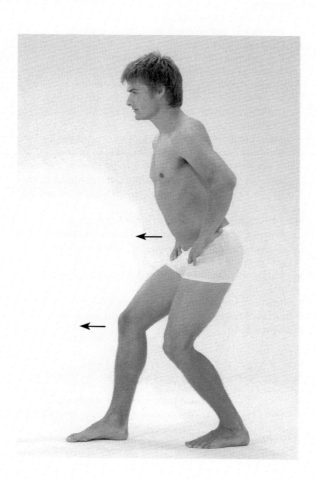

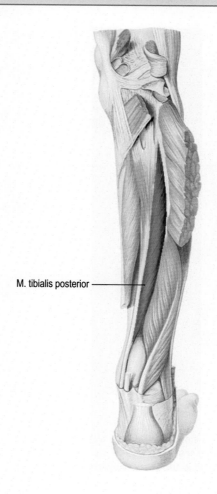

M. tibialis posterior

34.10.1 Anatomy

Innervation: tibial nerve (sciatic nerve).
Origin: interosseous membrane, posterior facet of tibia and fibula (proximal half bordering on interosseous membrane).
Insertion: navicular bone tuberosity, cuneiform bones I–III (plantar surface), base of metatarsals II–IV.
Function
- Ankle: plantar flexion.
- Ankle: supination.

34.10.2 Patient symptoms

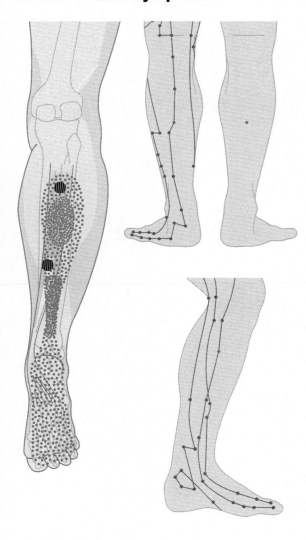

- Pain when running or walking, especially in the Achilles tendon.
- Possible preliminary diagnoses: achillodynia.

34.10.3 Trigger points

mTrP	LOCATION	RADIATION	mTrP → ACUPUNCTURE POINT
1	In the upper part of the muscle	Dorsal calf, Achilles tendon and back of foot	BL 57
2	In the lower part of the muscle	Achilles tendon and back of foot	SP 8

34.10.4 Diagnosis

Questioning
- Lot of running on uneven ground?
- Excessive jogging?
- Ankle pronation trauma?

Inspection
- Foot turned outwards when standing.
- Flat-footed gait (everted and abducted foot).

Physical examination
- Pressure palpation with one or two fingers with patient in the prone position with a roll or firm narrow cushion under the ankle so that the ankle is in the neutral position. Then try to work the fingers deep between the heads of the gastrocnemius and press firmly.
- Lateral palpation (from medial) in prone position with 90° flexed knee joint and ankle in neutral position. The therapist stands to one side and exercises pressure with the fingers on the posterior border of the tibia between the soleus and the flexor digitorum longus.
- Direct trigger palpation is usually difficult to impossible, although the pain symptoms can often be triggered with lengthy pressure ($\geq$10 s) on the sensitive site over the muscle.
- Lifting the heel from standing on one leg is weak or painful.

Technical examination: measurement of intramuscular pressure if deep compartment syndrome is suspected.

34.10.5 Specific aspects

- Treatment-resistant symptoms as for achillodynia.
- Deep (posterior) compartment syndrome should not be overlooked.
- Infiltration using cannulas should not be performed.

34.10.6 Treatment

Instructions for manual trigger point therapy

- Only indirect treatment through the gastrocnemius and soleus is possible.
- Mobilisation of the interosseous membrane between tibia and fibula (region of origin of the tibialis posterior) by mobilisation of the fibula.

Stretching

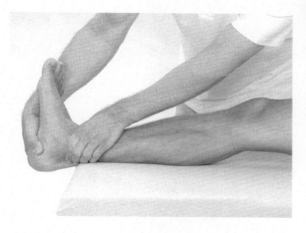

Isolated stretching of the tibialis posterior is difficult. If muscle shortening is pronounced the following procedure can be tried:

- patient in supine position, leg extended, foot hangs freely over the edge of the bed,
- the therapist stands to the side and grasps the tibia/ankle with the hand nearest the head,
- the hand furthest from the head grasps the heel (calcaneal tuberosity) with the lower forearm on the lateral side of the foot,
- pressure in the direction of dorsal flexion and pronation (eversion) so that the direction is varied slightly until the patient feels traction deep in the lower leg,
- traction can possibly be improved by passive extension of the toes,
- postisometric relaxation,
- stretching as for soleus, also use a wedge at the lateral margin of the foot.

Physical procedures

- Hardly any possibilities as the muscle is very deep-seated and is surrounded by vessels and nerve; an attempt with ultrasound may be possible.

Infiltration techniques/dry needling

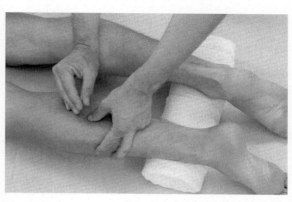

Infiltration cannot be recommended because of the anatomical situation; mTrP acupuncture can be chosen as an alternative as this can be performed in a less traumatic manner. A prerequisite is normal blood clotting.

- mTrP 1
  - Choose position and access that are appropriate to the result of palpation (medially at the posterior margin of the tibia or dorsally). That is, choose the access where the typical pain referral was most caused.
  - We recommend disinfection, then search for the mTrP with a sterile finger/thumb as described in the examination. Skin penetration immediately next to the palpation finger (or thumb) exercising pressure, so that parts of the overlying muscles are already displaced. Needle in the direction below the palpation finger, stretching a little with finger pressure.
  - If paraesthesia is caused, withdraw the needle and gently change direction.
  - Lateral anterior access and along the edge of the tibia is possible through the interosseous membrane (one finger width medial from ST 36).
- mTrP 2
  - The patient lies on the affected side, the lower leg lies flat on the lateral side, the other leg is crossed over and flexed at the hip.
  - Inferiorly lying mTrP can be reached from the medial posterior edge of the tibia (spleen meridian frequently SP 8).

Classical Chinese acupuncture

Local and locoregional points (also contralateral):
BL 57, ST 36, ST 37, ST 38 (deep needling), SP 7, SP 8, LR 5, LR 6, GB 35, GB 36, GB 37, GB 38, GB 39, KI 3, KI 5.

Distal points: SI 3 (for tenderness): meridian (Yang–Yang axis), SI 6 (for tenderness): meridian (Yang–Yang axis), BL 10 (for tenderness): meridian point, BL 32, BL 33: segmental effects (sensitive, dermatome S1, S2), BL 25, BL 26, BL 31, BL 32: segmental effects (sciatic nerve, motor function).

Control points/symptomatic points: SP 9 for swelling/feeling of swelling, GB 34 (masterpoint of the muscles and tendons).

Microsystem acupuncture

Ear: points on the toe represented.

Kiiko Matsumoto acupuncture

- With painful palpation of SP 2: SP 5 and SP 9 ipsilaterally.
- With inversion of the foot KI 6, BL 60 and ST 41; tapping of Yin Qiao and Yang Qiao to correct theinversion and prevent the occurrence of mTrP.

Psychosomatic aspects/relaxation

- If midlife crisis is suspected, motivation to 'age-appropriate' exercise.
- Psychosomatic aspects: excessive jogger (midlife crisis)?

34.10.7 Recommendations for the patient

Autostretching

- Autostretching of the posterior tibial muscle is not possible.

Additional measures

- Sit on heels and clasp a tennis ball between the thighs and lower legs to work the calf muscles with small, slow movements (move weight sideways).
- Running or jogging on smooth ground.
- Shoes with optimum sole and uppers (lateral stabilisation).

34.11 MM. EXTENSOR HALLUCIS LONGUS AND EXTENSOR DIGITORUM LONGUS

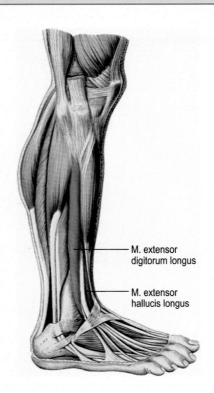

M. extensor digitorum longus

M. extensor hallucis longus

34.11.1 Anatomy

Innervation: N. fibularis profundus (sciatic nerve).
Origin
- M. extensor hallucis longus: medial facet of fibula (distal two-thirds), interosseous membrane, deep fascia of leg.
- M. extensor digitorum longus: proximal end of tibia (below the lateral condyle), anterior border of fibula, deep interosseous membrane, deep anterior intermuscular septum, deep fascia of leg.

Insertion
- M. extensor hallucis longus: base of the distal phalanx of the big toe, proximal phalanx.
- M. extensor digitorum longus: dorsal aponeuroses of the four lateral toes.

Function

- Ankle: dorsal flexion.
- Ankle:
  - pronation (M. extensor digitorum longus),
  - supination (M. extensor hallucis longus).
- Toe joints: extension (M. extensor digitorum longus).
- Joints of the big toe: extension (M. extensor hallucis longus).

34.11.2 Patient symptoms

- Anterior foot and toe pain.
- Occasionally anterior calf cramp.
- Pain when jumping (athletes, e.g. long jump).
- Possible preliminary diagnoses: ankle arthritis, synovitis of the metatarsophalangeal joints, radiculopathy L5 (mTrP 3), radiculopathy S1 (mTrP 2).

34.11.3 Trigger points

mTrP	LOCALISATION	RADIATION	mTrP ↔ ACUPUNCTURE POINT
1	In the upper part of the M. extensor digitorum longus	Along the muscle anterolateral lower leg and back of foot, tibia	–
2	In the upper part of the M. extensor digitorum longus	Lateral lower leg, lateral back of foot and little toe	GB 36
3	In the M. extensor digitorum hallucis longus	Over the back of the foot to the big toe	GB 37

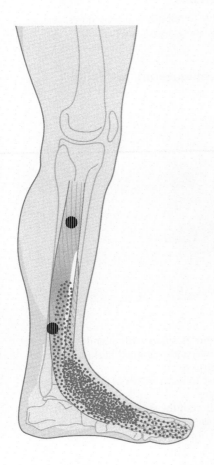

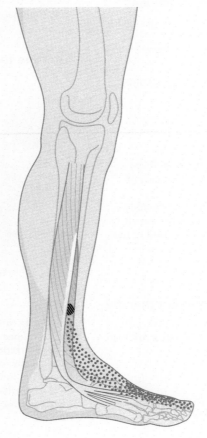

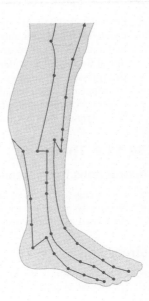

34.11.4 Diagnosis

Questioning
- Strain when running?
- Routinely wearing high-heeled shoes?
- History of trauma, e.g. fibula fracture?

Inspection: sinking of the forefoot when walking?

Physical examination
- Compare heel walking on both sides.
- Test the function of each individual toe (dorsal flexion against resistance).
- Palpation of the muscle belly lateral to the tibial muscle in supine position with slightly flexed knee (pillow, knee roll) with thumb or index finger.
- mTrPs in the M. extensor digitorum longus are easily palpable, mTrPs in the M. extensor hallucis longus only indirectly. However, the M. extensor hallucis longus can be distinguished with isolated dorsal flexion of the big toe.
- Sensory examination in the supply area of the fibular nerve (lateral lower leg and back of foot).

> The skin region between metatarsals I and II and digits I and II is supplied by the deep fibular nerve (LR 3 area).

Technical examination: nerve conduction speed if fibular nerve compression syndrome is suspected.

34.11.5 Specific aspects

- Secondary mTrPs can often be found in the synergists (M. tibialis anterior, fibularis muscles) and antagonists (M. gastrocnemius, M. soleus) of dorsal flexion in the ankle.
- Compression of the deep fibular nerve is possible.
- M. extensor hallucis longus is the identifier muscle L5.
- Often concomitant hypomobility of the head of the fibula (gentle mobilisation).

34.11.6 Therapy

Instructions for manual trigger point therapy

- Easy access to treatment (as mTrPs are superficial).
- Frequently 'forward-back' problem, then treat mTrPs in the tensed and shortened calf muscles.

Stretching

- Patient in supine position with slightly flexed knee (pillow, knee roll) and supported heel.

- The therapist grasps the forefoot with one hand and the other holds the leg below the knee joint.
- Increase dorsal extension with gentle pressure (pull down slightly, little pressure from above).

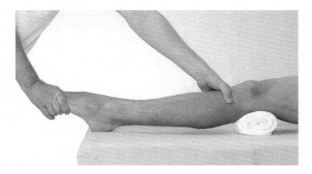

Physical procedures

- Easily accessible for all physical procedures, such as electrotherapy, shock waves, laser, TENS.

Infiltration techniques/dry needling

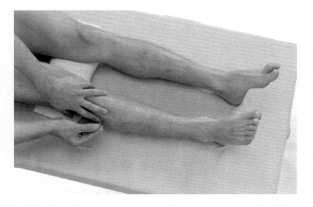

- Patient in supine position with slightly flexed knee (pillow, knee roll) and supported heel (ankle in neutral position).
- It is usually easy to reach mTrPs in the M. extensor digitorum longus.
- To avoid irritation of the superficial fibular nerve insert as close as possible to the margin of the tibialis muscle.

- Treatment of mTrPs in the M. extensor hallucis longus should be performed using dry needling (approximately 5–8 cm-long needle; **warning:** A. tibialis anterior, N. fibularis profundus), pay attention to blood clotting.

Classical Chinese acupuncture

Local and locoregional points (also contralateral): GB 34, GB 36, GB 37, GB 38, GB 39, GB 40, ST 41, LR 4, SP 5 (points at the transition from the back of the foot to the ankle), GB 41 (M. extensor digiti minimi), Dig. I: SP 2, SP 3, LR 2, LR 3, Dig. II: LR 2, LR 3, ST 43, ST 44, Dig. III: ST 43, ST 44, choose relevant Ashi points between Dig. III and IV, Dig. IV: Ashi points between Dig. III and IV, GB 42, GB 43, Dig. V: GB 42, GB 43, BL 65, BL 66, Bafeng (Ex-BF 10).
Distal points: TH 5 (for tenderness): meridian (Yang–Yang axis), TH 3 (for tenderness): meridian (Yang–Yang axis), Ba Xie: corresponding wrist points, BL 26, BL 31: segmental effects (sensitively, dermatome L5, S1), BL 25, BL 26, BL 31, BL 32: segmental effects (N. fibularis communis, motor function).
Control points/symptomatic points: SP 6 (crossing of the 3 Yin) motion disorder of the lower extremity, SP 9 for swelling/feeling of swelling.

Microsystem acupuncture

Ear: points on the toe represented.

Kiiko Matsumoto acupuncture

- If there is a neurological cause: CV 12 and CV 10.
- One or two points on the stomach Qi line, anterior and lateral side of the tibia between ST 36 and ST 41 between bones and muscles; needling angle 10–15° along the course of the stomach meridian.
- Generally relaxing points SP 3 (ipsilateral) and ST 22 (on the right, 'sphincter of Oddi point'), needled in exact location and exact angle.

Psychosomatic aspects/relaxation

- Information for ambitious athletes/leisure runners (cognitive approach).
- Recommend walking consciously in a relaxed manner (full foot-rolling action) on level ground.
- Psychosomatic aspects: lack of grounding, too much pride (e.g. no rest or recuperation phases in sport).

34.11.7 Recommendations for the patient

Autostretching

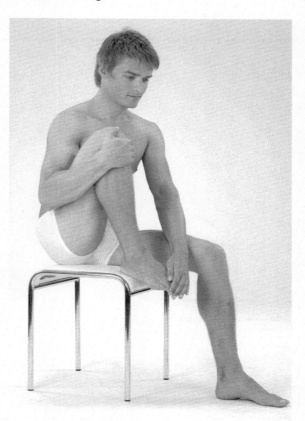

- The patient sits on a stool.
- Hip and knee joint flexed on affected side.
- Heel placed on the edge.
- Plantar flexion of ankle and toes.
- Further plantar extension with gentle pressure (pull down slightly, little pressure from above).

Additional measures

- Balancing objects (e.g. pen) while seated with dorsally flexed toes.
- Grasping objects such as a pen from the floor with the toes (antagonist training).
- If the accelerator pedal is too high, heighten the insert to avoid permanent dorsal flexion.
- When asleep keep the ankle in the neutral position with a foot support.

- Heel walking alternating with autostretching for strengthening.
- Regular autostretching (sitting on heels).
- Use heel cushion as shock absorber.
- Standing on one leg: practise balancing.

34.12 MM. FLEXOR DIGITORUM LONGUS AND FLEXOR HALLUCIS LONGUS

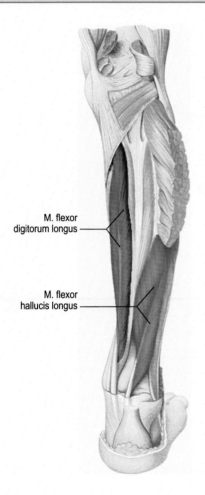

M. flexor digitorum longus

M. flexor hallucis longus

34.12.1 Anatomy

Innervation: tibial nerve (sciatic nerve).
Origin
- M. flexor digitorum longus: posterior facet of tibia (distal to the line of the soleus muscle), tendon arcade between tibia and fibula (proximal to the crural chiasm).

- M. flexor hallucis longus: posterior facet of fibula (distal two-thirds), interosseous membrane, intermuscular septum of posterior crus.

Insertion
- M. flexor digitorum longus: distal phalanx of second to fifth toes.
- M. flexor hallucis longus: distal phalanx of big toe.

Function
- Ankle: plantar flexion.
- Ankle: supination.
- Toe joints: flexion (M. flexor digitorum longus).
- Big toe joints: flexion (M. flexor hallucis longus).

34.12.2 Patient symptoms

- Pain in the forefoot and big toe.
- Possible preliminary diagnoses: ankle arthritis, synovitis of the metatarsophalangeal joints, radiculopathy L5 (mTrP 1), radiculopathy S1 (mTrP 2).

34.12.3 Trigger points

mTrP	LOCALISATION	RADIATION	mTrP ↔ ACUPUNCTURE POINT
1	Upper part of the M. flexor digitorum longus	Medial lower leg, medial malleolus, sole of foot	SP 8
2	M. flexor hallucis longus	Lateral lower leg over sole of foot to big toe	BL 59

34.12.4 Diagnosis

Questioning
- Sole inserts because of foot pain?
- Running or jogging on uneven ground?
- Walking for long periods barefoot on soft ground?

Inspection
- Foot deformity, high arch of foot.
- Muscular imbalance in foot when walking.
- Loss of balance when standing on toes.

Physical examination: pain on flexion of toes with plantar flexion of foot.
- mTrP 1
  - Patient lying on affected side, the knee is flexed 90°, with the lower leg to be palpated lying flat (long or several cushions from the knee to the ankle).
  - Palpation between the edge of the tibia and the soleus, possibly pinch grip.
- mTrP 2
  - Patient in prone position.
  - Finger palpation anterior to the Achilles tendon.

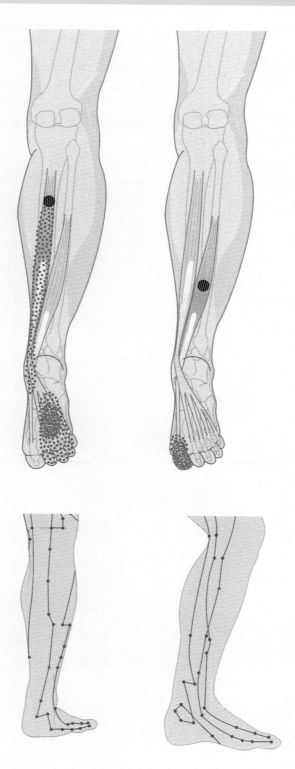

34.12.5 Specific aspects

- Frequent sports injury.
- Delimitation of mTrPs of the interossei.
- Development of hammer or claw toe deformity described.

34.12.6 Therapy

Instructions for manual trigger point therapy

- Treatment of the M. flexor digitorum longus: medially from the back of the tibia, in the distal half of the lower leg.
- Treatment of the M. flexor hallucis longus: laterally on the back of the fibula, at the distal two-thirds and in the area of the bordering interosseous membrane.

Stretching

- Patient in prone position with knee joint flexed 90°.
- Lateral rotation of the foot.
- Dorsal extension of the toes.
- Stretching via dorsal extension of the ankle (good lever).
- Stretching of M. flexor digitorum longus: as for soleus, initially also with wedge or similar to extend toes II–IV.

- Extension of M. flexor hallucis longus: as for soleus, initially also with wedge or similar to extend big toe.

Physical procedures

- Easily accessible for all physical procedures such as electrotherapy, shock waves, laser, TENS.

Infiltration techniques/dry needling

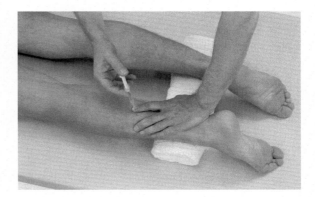

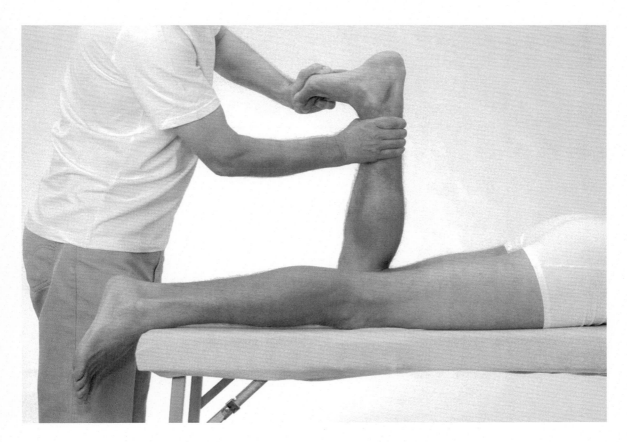

- Positioning as for palpation.
- Support pillow below distal shinbone.
- Two-finger protection technique.
- Usually problem-free injection or needling, but do not insert needle very deep (2–4 cm).

Classical Chinese acupuncture

Local and locoregional points (also contralateral):
BL 58, BL 59, BL 60, SP 7, SP 8, KI 3, KI 5, KI 8, KI 9, SP 2, SP 3, SP 4.
The following points should be needled deep than for the M. extensor digitorum (but not into the tendons!):
Dig. I: SP 2, SP 3, LR 2, LR 3; Dig. II: LR 2, LR 3, ST 43, ST 44; Dig. III: ST 43, ST 44, choose relevant Ashi points between Dig. III and IV; Dig. IV: Ashi points between Dig. III and IV, GB 42, GB 43; Dig. V: GB 42, GB 43, BL 65, BL 66, Bafeng (Ex-BF 10).
Distal points: relevant axis points (Yang–Yang axis) depending on pain referral, BL 32, BL 33: segmental effects (sensitive, dermatome S1, S2), BL 25, BL 26, BL 31, BL 32: segmental effects (sciatic nerve, motor function).

Microsystem acupuncture

Ear: points on the toe represented.

Kiiko Matsumoto acupuncture

M. flexor hallucis longus:
- if there is a neurological cause: CV 12 and CV 10,
- for tenderness in the area of KI 2 (fire point), needling of KI 7 (metal point) and KI 10 (water point), needling angle (particularly with KI 7) should correlate with the relief of pain in the area of KI 12,
- in some cases, if other muscles in the lower extremity are affected, needling of LU 8 (in the direction of LU 9),
- tension in the area of Hua tuo jiaji between T10 and T12: needling of these points at an angle of 45° in the direction of the vertebral column; if these points are palpable, needling of SP 3; after that needling Hua tuo jiaji to treat the pain,
- the combination of three points ('I-Hi-Kon') is effective, each 1 cm lateral to BL 40, BL 59 and BL 60; needling of points lateral to BL 40 and BL 59 at an angle of 15° with the flow of the

meridian; needling of BL 60 at an angle of 15–45° against the flow of the meridian.
M. flexor digitorum longus:
- for neurological cause CV 12 and CV 10,
- for tenderness in the area of ST 41 (fire point), ST 45 (metal point) and ST 44 (water point),
- for cold toes seven or eight direct moxa in the area of needle insertion.

34.12.7 Recommendations for the patient

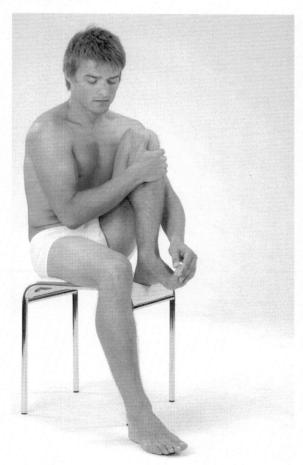

Autostretching

- The patient sits on a stool.
- Hip and knee flexed on the affected side, heel supported on the edge.
- Dorsal extension of ankle and toes.
- Stretch over further dorsal extension with gentle pressure (pull gently upwards).

Additional measures

- Grasping objects such as a pen from the floor with the toes.
- Balancing objects (e.g. pen) while seated with dorsally flexed toes (antagonist training).
- Do not wear shoes which limit the mobility of the big toe.

- Adapt running training when jogging.
- Autotreatment: sit on heels and clasp a tennis ball between the thighs and lower legs to work the calf muscles with small, slow movements (move weight sideways).

Bibliography

Aaron LA, Buchwald D. Chronic diffuse musculoskeletal pain, fibromyalgia and co-morbid unexplained clinical conditions, Best Pract. Res. Clin. Rheumatol (2003) 563–574.

Abele J. Schröpfkopfbehandlung. Theorie und Praxis, 6. Aufl, Haug, Stuttgart, 1999.

Acupuncture: NIH consensus development panel on acupuncture, J. Am. Med. Assoc. 280 (17) (1998) 1518–1524.

Acupuncture: Review and analysis of reports on controlled clinical trials, WHO, Geneva, 2002.

Adler R, Hemmler W. Praxis und Theorie der Anamnese, Gustav Fischer, Stuttgart, New York, 1986.

Allgemeine ärztliche Berufspflichten der ärztlichen Berufsordnung § 2 (abzurufen bei den Ärztekammern).

Almeida-Lopes L, et al. Comparison of the low level laser therapy effects on cultured human gingival fibroblasts proliferation using different irradiance and same fluence, Lasers Surg. Med. 29 (2001) 179–184.

Amberger R. Schulungsmaterial von Medi-ABC.

Andersen JH, Gaardboe O. Prevalence of persistent neck and upper limb pain in a historical cohort of sewing machine operators, Am. J. Ind. Med. 24 (1993) 677–687.

Appenzeller O. Reflex vasomotor function: Clinical and experimental studies in migraine, Res. Clin. Stud. Headache 6 (1978) 160–166.

Arndt R, Schulz H. Biologisches Grundgesetz, in: Großer Brockhaus, 2. Aufl, Brockhaus, Wiesbaden, 1953.

Auberger A, Biermann E. Schmerzausstrahlung und schmerzinduzierte Phänomene, in: Praktische Schmerztherapie, Thieme, Stuttgart, 1988.

Auroy J, et al. Major complications of regional anesthesia in France: The SOS regional anesthesia hotline service, Anesthesiology 97 (2002) 1274–1280.

AWMF-Leitlinie Behandlung akuter perioperativer und posttraumatischer Schmerzen AWMF Nr. 041/001 (21.05.2007).

Azevedo LH, et al. Influence of different power densities of LILT on cultured human fibroblast growth: a pilot study, Lasers Med. Sci. 21 (2006) 86–89.

Back pain. A systematic review within the framework of the Cochrane Collaboration Back Review Group, Spine 24 (1999) 1113–1123.

Bäcker M, Dobos GJ. Psychophysiologische Wirkmechanismen von Akupunktur in der Behandlung von Schmerzen, Dt Ztschr f Akup 49 (2006).

Bäcker M, Hammes M. Akupunktur in der Schmerztherapie, Urban & Fischer, München, 2004.

Bäcker M, et al. Akupunktur in der Schmerztherapie. Hypothesen zu adaptiven Prozessen, Forsch. Kompl. Med 11 (2004) 335–345.

Bäcker M, et al. Acupuncture: quo vadis? Dtsch. Med. Wochenschr. 131 (2006) 506–511.

Baldry P. Akupunktur, Triggerpunkte und muskuloskeletale Schmerzen, MLV, Uelzen, 1997.

Baling M. Der Arzt, sein Patient und die Krankheit, Klett, Stuttgart, 1957.

Banzer W, et al. Short-time effects of laser needle stimulation on the peripheral microcirculation assessed by laser Doppler spectroscopy and near-infrared spectroscopy, Photomed. Laser Surg. 24 (2006) 575–580.

Banzer W, Hübscher M, Schikora D. Laser-needle therapy for spontaneous osteonecrosis of the knee, Photomed. Laser Surg. 26 (4) (2008) 301–306.

Barker PJ, Briggs CA. Attachments of the posterior layer of lumbar fascia, Spine 24 (1999) 1757–1764.

Barker PJ, et al. Effects of tensioning the lumbar fasciae on segmental stiffness during flexion and extension: Young Investigator Award winner, Spine 15 (2006) 397–405.

Basmajian J. Muscles alive: Their function revealed with electromyography, Williams & Wilkins, Baltimore, 1978.

Basmajian J, Nyberg R. Rational Manual Therapies, Williams & Wilkins, Baltimore, 1993.

Bauer J. Warum ich fühle, was du fühlst. Intuitive Kommunikation und das Geheimnis der Spiegelzellen, 9. Aufl, Heyne, München, 2006.

Baxter GD. Therapeutic lasers: theory and practice, Churchill Livingstone, Edinburgh, 1994.

BDY - Berufsverband der Yogalehrenden in Deutschlan (Hrsg.), 'Der Weg des Yoga, Via Nova, Petersberg, 2007.

Bednar DA, et al. Observations on the pathomorphology of the thoracolumbar fascia in chronic mechanical back pain. A microscopic study, Spine 20 (1995) 1161–1164.

Bendtsen L, et al. Qualitatively altered nociception in chronic myofascial pain, Pain 65 (1996) 259–264.

Berghoff C, et al. Diagnostik bei Myalgien – Bundeseinheitliche Konsensuspapiere, Nervenheilkunde (2005) 703.

Berman BM, Swyers JP. Complementary medicine treatments for fibromyalgia syndrome, Baillières Best Pract. Res. Clin. Rheumatol (1999) 487–492.

Bernstein DA, Borkovec TD. Entspannungstraining. Handbuch der progressiven Muskelentspannung nach Jacobson, Pfeiffer, München, 1975.

Birch S, Jamison RN. Controlled trial of Japanese acupuncture for chronic myofascial neck pain: assessment of specific and nonspecific effects of treatment, Clin. J. Pain. 14 (1998) 248–255.

Bircher-Benner M. Ordnungsgesetze des Lebens, Bircher-Benner Verlag, Bad Homburg, 1999.

Bjordal JM, et al. Photoradiation in acute pain: a systematic review of possible mechanisms of action and clinical effects in randomized placebo-controlled trials, Photomed. Laser Surg. 24 (2006) 158–168.

Bjordal JM, et al. Short-term efficacy of physical interventions in osteoarthritic knee pain. A systematic review and meta-analysis of randomised placebo-controlled trials, BMC Musculoskelet. Disord (2007) 8–51.

Böcker W, et al. Pathologie, Urban & Schwarzenberg, München, 1997.

Bölts J. Qigong. Heilung mit Energie. Eine alte chinesische Gesundheitsmethode, Herder, Freiburg, 1994.

Bossy J. Die Mikrosysteme der Akupunktur, VGM, Essen, 1993.

Bouche K, et al. Comparison of postural control in unilateral stance between healthy controls and lumbar discectomy patients with and without pain, Eur. Spine J. 15 (2006) 423–432.

Braddom RL, et al. Physical Medicine & Rehabilitation, second ed., Saunders, Philadelphia, 2000.

Braun WL, et al. Regional anesthesia and local anesthetic-in-use systemic toxicity: seizure frequency and accompanying cardiovascular changes, Anesth. Analg. 8 (1995) 221–228.

Brenke R, Polonius D. Hydro- und Thermotherapie, in: Melchart D, et al. (Hrsg.), Naturheilverfahren, Schattauer, Stuttgart, New York, 2002, pp. 294–331.

Brosseau L, et al. Low level laser therapy for osteoarthritis and rheumatoid arthritis: a metaanalysis, J. Rheumatol. 27 (2000) 1961–1969.

Brückle W, et al. Gewebe-pO$_2$-Messung in der verspannten. Rückenmuskulatur (M. erector spinae), Z. Rheumatol. 49 (1990) 208–216.

Brumagne S, et al. Proprioceptive weighting changes in persons with low back pain and elderly persons during upright standing, Neurosci. Lett. 366 (2004) 63–66.

Brune K, et al. Schmerz, 1. Aufl, Springer, Berlin, Heidelberg. New York, 2001.

Bruns T, Praun N. Biofeedback, Vandenhoeck & Ruprecht, Göttingen, 2002.

Burdon RH. Superoxide and hydrogen peroxide in relation to mammalian cell proliferation, Free Radic. Biol. Med. 18 (1995) 775–794.

Buytendijk FJJ. Das Menschliche der menschlichen Bewegung, Nervenarzt 28 (1) (1957) S. 1 7, *28 Jahrgang 1. Heft.

Cantu RI, Grodin AJ. Myofascial Manipulation – Theory and Clinical Application, Aspen, 1992.

Carano A, Siciliani G. Effects of continuous and intermittent forces on human fibroblasts in vitro, J. Orthod. 18 (1996) 19–26.

Carlsson C. Acupuncture for chronic low back pain: a randomized placebo-controlled study, Clin. J. Pain. 17 (2001) 296–305.

Ceccherelli F. Comparison between superficial and deep acupuncture in the treatment of the shoulder's myofascial pain: a randomized and controlled study, Acupunct. Electrother. Res. 26 (2001) 229–238.

Ceccherelli F, et al. Comparison of superficial and deep acupuncture in the treatment of lumbar myofascial pain, Clin. J. Pain. 18 (2002) 149–153.

Ceylan Y, et al. The effects of infrared laser and medical treatments on pain and serotonin degradation products in patients with myofascial pain syndrome. A controlled trial, Rheumatol. Int. 24 (2004) 260–263.

Chaitow L. Neuromuskuläre Techniken in der Manuellen Medizin und Osteopathie, Urban & Fischer, München, 2002.

Chaitow L. Positional Release-Techniken in der Manuellen Medizin und Osteopathie, Urban & Fischer, München, 2003.

Chang CW, et al. Evidence of neuroaxonal degeneration in myofascial pain syndrome, Eur. J. Pain. 12 (2008) 1026–1030.

Chen CS, Ingber DE. Tensegrity and mechanoregulation: from skeleton to cytoskeleton, Osteoarthritis Cartilage 7 (1999) 81–94.

Chen E. Cross-sectional anatomy of acupoints, Churchill Livingstone, Edinburgh, 1995.

Chen Q, et al. Identification and quantification of myofascial taut bands with magnetic resonance elastography, Arch. Phys. Med. Rehabil. 88 (2007) 1658–1661.

Xinnong Cheng. Chinese acupuncture and moxibustion, 1. Aufl, Foreign Languages Press, Beijing, 1987.

Cherkin DC, et al. Physician variation in diagnostic testing for low back pain. Who you see is what you get, Arthritis Rheum. 37 (1994) 15–22.

Childers MK. Use of Botulinum Toxin Type A in Pain Management, Academic Information System, 1999.

Cholewicki J, et al. Stabilizing function of the trunk flexor-extensor muscles around neutral posture, Spine 22 (1997) 2207–2212.

Chu J, Schwartz I. The muscle twitch in myofascial pain relief: effects of acupuncture and other needling methods, Electromyogr. Clin. Neurophysiol. 42 (2002) 307–311.

Classen M, et al. (Hrsg.), Innere Medizin. Elsevier, Urban & Fischer, München, 2006.

Clauw DJ, Crofford LJ. Chronic widespread pain and fibromyalgia: what we know, and what we need to know, Best Pract. Res. Clin. Rheumatol. (2003) 685–701.

Clemente CD. Anatomy: a regional atlas of the human body, second ed., Urban & Schwarzenberg, Baltimore, 1981.

Conradi S, Smolenski UC. Testgütekriterien manualmedizinischer Tests bei Low-back-pain-Patienten Eine Literaturrecherche, Manuelle Medizin 43 (2005) 227–234.

Colwell HA. An essay on the history of electrotheapy and diagnosis, Heinemann, London, 1922.

Cottingham JT, et al. Shifts in pelvic inclination angle and parasympathetic tone produced by Rolfing soft tissue manipulation, Phys. Ther. 68 (1988) 1364–1370.

Cotton AM. A review of the principles and use of lasers in lower limb problems, Int. J. Low Extrem. Wounds 3 (2004) 133–142.

Cummings TM, White AR. Needling therapies in the management of myofascial trigger point pain: a systematic review, Arch. Phys. Med. Rehabil. 82 (2001) 986–992.

Dalai Lama. Die Essenz der Meditation, Ansata, München, 2001.

Dale R. The micro-acupuncture systems, vol. I–III, Dialectic Publ, Surfside, 1980/1985.

Danneskiold-Samsoe B, et al. Myofascial pain and the role of myoglobin, Scand. J. Rheumatol. 15 (1986) 174–178.

Deadman P, et al. A manual of acupuncture, J Chin Med Publ, Hove, East Sussex (UK), 1998.

Dejung B. Triggerpunkt- und Bindegewebsbehandlung – neue Wege in Physiotherapie und Rehabilitationsmedizin, Physiotherapeut 6 (1988) 3–12.

Dejung B. Der informierte Arzt, Gazette Medicale: Muskuär bedingter Schmerz, Sonderdruck DIA/GM, 12, (1991).

Dejung B. Triggerpunkt-Therapie: Die Behandlung akuter und chronischer Schmerzen im Bewegungsapparat mit manueller Triggerpunkt-Therapie und Dry Needling, 2. korrigierte Aufl, Huber, Bern, 2006 (1. Aufl. 2003).

Deutsche Ärztegesellschaft für Akupunktur (DÄGfA), Stellungnahme, DÄGfA, www.daegfa.de.

DGSS, http://www.dgss.org.

Dicke E, et al. Bindegewebsmassage, 6. Aufl, Hippokrates, Stuttgart 1982.

Dilling H, et al. Internationale Klassifikation psychischer Störungen. ICD-10 Kapitel V (F), S. 41 184, Huber, Bern, Göttingen, Toronto, 1991.

Dommerholt J, Simons DG. Myofascial pain syndromes – trigger points, J. Musculosk. Pain 15 (2007).

Dörner K. Der gute Arzt: Lehrbuch der ärztlichen Grundhaltung, Schattauer, Stuttgart, New York, 2001.

Dorsher PT. Acupuncture points and trigger points: anatomic and clinical correlations, Med. Acupunct. 17 (2006) 20–23.

Douglas A, et al. Entspannungs-Training. Handbuch der, progressiven Muskelentspannungnach Jacobsen, Klett-Cotta, Stuttgart, 2002.

Dressler D. Botulinum-Toxin-Therapie, Thieme, Stuttgart 1995.

Drewes AM, Jennum P. Epidemiology of myofascial pain, low back pain, morning stiffness and sleep-related complaionts in the general population, J. Musculosk. Pain 3 (Suppl. 1) (1995) 68 (Abstract).

Dvorak J, Dvorak V, et al. Manuelle Medizin, Diagnostik, 4. Aufl, Thieme, Stuttgart, New York, 1991.

Dworkin SF, Le Resche L. Research diagnostic criteria for temporomandibular disorders: review, criteria, examinations and specifications, critique, J. Craniomandib. Disord. 6 (4) (1992) 301–355.

Edel H. Fibel der Elektrodiagnostik und Elektrotherapie, 5. Aufl, Müller & Steinicke, München, 1983.

Egle UT, et al. Psychoanalytisch orientierte Gruppentherapie mit psychogenen Schmerzpatienten. Ein Beitrag zur Behandlungsmethodik, Psychother. Psychosom. Med. Psychol. 42 (1992) 79–90.

Egle UT, Nickel R. Kindheitsbelastungsfaktoren bei Patienten mit Somatoformen Störungen, Z. Psychosom. Med. Psychoanal. 44 (1998) 21–36.

Egle UT, et al. Die somatoforme Schmerzstörung, Deutsches Ärzteblatt 97 (2000) 1469–1472.

Eliade M. Yoga, Insel Verlag, Frankfurt a. M., 2004.

Elliott FA. Lancet 1 (1944) 47.

Eriksson MBE. Hazard from transcutaneous nerve stimulation in patients with pacemakers, Lancet 1 (1975) 13–19.

Eriksson MBE, Sölund BH. Transcutane Nervenstimulierung für Schmerzlinderung, Verl f Med Fischer, Heidelberg, 1979.

Ernst E. The efficacy of Phytodolor for the treatment of musculoskeletal pain – a systematic review of randomized clinical trials, Nat. Med. J. (1999) 14–17.

Ernst E, et al. Acupuncture for back pain: meta-analysis of randomised controlled trials and an update with data from the most recent studies, Schmerz 16 (2002) 129–139.

Fachinformationen der Roten Liste Service GmbH, Frankfurt/Main.

Fassbender HG, Wagener K. Morphologie und Pathogenese des Weichteil-Rheumatismus, Z. Rheumaforsch. 32 (1975) 355–374.

Feng TY. Treatment of soft tissue injury with traditional Chinese Medicine and Western medicine, People's Medical Publishing House, Beijing, 1983.

Fernández-de-las-Peñas C, et al. Myofascial trigger points and sensitization: an updated pain model for tension-type headache, Cephalalgia 27 (2007a) 383–393.

Fernández-de-Las-Peñas C, et al. Myofascial trigger points, neck mobility, and forward head posture in episodic tension-type headache, Headache 47 (2007b) 662–672.

Fernández-de-Las-Peñas C, et al. The role of myofascial trigger points in musculoskeletal pain syndromes of the head and neck, Curr. Pain Headache Rep. 11 (5) (2007c) 365–372.

Fernández-de-Las-Peñas C, et al. Referred pain elicited by manual exploration of the lateral rectus muscle in chronic tension-type headache, Pain Med. 10 (1) (2009) 43.

Fikáčová H, et al. Effectiveness of low-level laser therapy in temporomandibular joint disorders: a placebo-controlled study, Photomed. Laser Surg. 25 (2007) 297–303.

FIMM. Reproducibility and Validity Studies of Diagnostic Procedures in Manual/Musculoskeletal Medicine for Low back pain patients, Scientific Committee FIMM, 2001.

Findley T, Schleip R (Eds.), Fascia Research – Basic Science and

Implications for Conventional and Complementary Health Care, Elsevier Urban & Fischer, München, 2007.

Finestone DH, et al. Physical and psychiatric impairment in patients with myofascial pain syndrome compared to patients with fibromyalgia, J. Musculosk. Pain 3 (Suppl. 1) (1995) 86 (Abstract).

Finkel T. Redox-dependent signal transduction, FEBS Lett. 476 (2000) 52–54.

Fishbain DA, et al. Male and female chronic pain patients categorized by DSM-III psychiatric diagnostic criteria, Pain 26 (2) (1986) 181–197.

Fisher AA. Pressure threshold meter: ist use for quantification of tender points, Arch. Phys. Med. Rehabil. 67 (1986) 836–838.

Fisher AA. Pressure threshold measurement for diagnosis of myofascial pain and evaluation of treatment results, Clin. J. Pain. 2 (1987) 207.

Fisher AA. Local injections in pain management, trigger point needling with infiltration and somatic blocks, Phys. Med. Rehabil. Clin. N. Am. 6 (1995) 851–870.

Fisher P, Ward A. Medicine in Europe: complementary medicine in Europe, BMJ 309 (1994) 107–111.

Fleischhauer M, et al. Leitfaden Physiotherapie in der Orthopädie und Traumatologie, Urban & Fischer, München, 2002.

Flitney FW, Megson IL. Nitric oxide and the mechanism of rat vascular smooth muscle photorelaxation, J. Physiol. 550 (2003) 819–828.

Focks C. Leitfaden Akupunktur, Elsevier, Urban & Fischer, 2004.

Focks C, Hillenbrand N. Leitfaden Chinesische Medizin, Elsevier, Urban & Fischer, München, 2006.

Forth W, et al. Allgemeine und spezielle Pharmakolgie und Toxikologie, 6. Aufl, BI-Wiss.-Verlag, 1992.

Fourie WJ. Fascia lata: Merely a thigh stocking, or a coordinator of complex thigh muscular activity, in: Franz M, Schepank H (Eds.), Mood disorders. Prevalence and course of unspecified functional disorders from the epidemiologic and psychosomatic viewpoint, Z Arztl Fortbild Qualitätssich, vol. 91, 1997, pp. 723–727.

Freisens U. Pain in Europe, in: Medienkonferenz der Schweizerischen Gesellschaft für Gesundheitpolitik, publiziert in Mundipharma-Bulletin, Bern, 4.11.2003.

Freiwald J, et al. Neuere Forschungsergebnisse und deren praktische Umsetzung, Manuelle Medizin 1 (1999) 3–10.

Frettlöh, et al. Validation of the German Mainz Pain Staging System in different pain syndromes, Schmerz 17 (2003) 240–251.

Fricton JR, et al. Myofascial pain syndrome of the head and neck: A review of clinical characteristics of 164 patients, Oral Surg. Oral Med. Oral Pathol. 60 (1985) 615–623.

Fricton JR, et al. Myofascial pain syndrome: Electromyographic changes associated with local twitch response, Arch. Phys. Med. Rehabil. 66 (1986) 314–317.

Fricton JR. Etiology and management of masticatory myofascial pain, J. Musculosk. Pain 7 (1999) 143–160.

Fröhlich D, Fröhlich R. Das Piriformissyndrom: eine häufige Differentialdiagnose des lumbglutäalen Schmerzes, Manuelle Medizin 33 (1995) 7–10.

Furlan AD, et al. Massage for low-back pain: a systematic review within the framework of the Cochrane Collaboration Back Review Group, Spine 127 (2002) 1896–1910.

Garavello-Freitas I, et al. Low-power laser irradiation improves histomorphometrical parameters and bone matrix organization during tibia wound healing in rats, J. Photochem. Photobiol. B 70 (2003) 81–89.

Gautschi R. Latent myofascial trigger points: their effects on muscle activation and movement efficiency. Latente myofasziale Triggerpunkte: Ihre Wirkungen auf Muskelaktivität und Bewegungseffizienz, Manuelle Therapie 11 (2007) 32–34.

Gautschi R. Myofasziale Triggerpunkt-Therapie, in: van den Berg Frans (Hrsg.), Angewandte Physiologie, Bd. 4: Schmerzen verstehen und beeinflussen, 2. erw. Aufl, Thieme, Stuttgart, 2008, pp. 310–366.

Geissler L. Arzt und Patient – Begegnung im Gespräch, 3. erw. Aufl, Peter Hoffmann/Pharma Verlag, Frankfurt, 1992.

Gerdesmeyer L, et al. Physikalisch-technische Grundlagen der extrakorporalen Stoßwellentherapie (ESWT), Orthopäde 31 (2002) 610–617.

Gerwin R, Gevirtz R. Chronic myofascial pain: Iron insufficiency and coldness as risk factors, J. Musculosk. Pain 3 (Suppl. 1) (1995) 120 (Abstract).

Gerwin R, et al. Ultrasound identification of the myofascial triggerpoint, Muscle Nerve 20 (1997a) 767–768.

Gerwin R, et al. Interrater reliability in myofascial trigger point examination, Pain 69 (1997b) 65–73.

Gerwin RD, et al. An expansion of Simons' integrated hypothesis of trigger point formation, Curr. Pain Headache Rep. 8 (2004) 468–475.

Gessler M. Stumpf- und Phantomschmerzen, in: Pothmann R (Hrsg.), TENS, 2. Aufl, Hippokrates, Stuttgart, 1996, pp. 47–52.

Glaser V. Eutonie – das Verhaltensmuster menschlichen Wohlbefindens – Lehr- und Übungsbuch für Psychotonik® Glaser, 4. Aufl, Haug, Heidelberg, 1993.

Gleditsch JM. Akupunktur in der Hals-Nasen Ohrenheilkunde, Hippokrates Verlag, Stuttgart, 1997.

Gleditsch JM. Reflexzonen und Somatotopien, 9. Aufl, Urban & Fischer, München, 2005.

Gleditsch JM. Oral acupuncture in the therapy of craniomandibular dysfunction syndrome, Wien. Klin. Wochenschr. 118 (2006) 36–42.

Gleditsch JM. Lehrbuch und Atlas der MikroAkuPunktSysteme (MAPS). Grundlagen und Praxis der somatotopischen Therapie, KVM Dr. Kolster & Co 2. Aufl, 2007.

Gmunder R, Kissling R. The Efficacy of homeopathy in the treatment of chronic low back pain compared to standardized physiotherapy, Z. Orthop. Ihre Grenzgeb. 140 (2002) 503–508.

Goepel R, et al. Transcutane Nervensti-mulation bei Migräne-Patienten, Fortschr. Med. 103 (1985) 865.

Goldenberg DL, et al. Management of fibromyalgia syndrome, JAMA 292 (2004) 2388–2395.

Gran JT. The epidemiology of chronic generalized musculoskeletal pain, Best Pract. Res. Clin. Rheumatol. (2003) 547–561.

Granges G, Littlejohn GO. A comparative study of clinical signs in fibromyalgia/fibrositis syndrome, healthy and exercising subjects, J. Rheumatol. 20 (1993) 344–351.

Graven-Nielsen T, et al. Painful and non-painful pressure sensations from human skeletal muscle, Exp. Brain Res. 159 (2004) 273–283.

Grossarth-Maticek R. Systemische Epidemiologie und präventive Verhaltensmedizin chronischer Erkrankungen. Strategien zur Aufrechterhaltungen der Gesundheit, De Gruyter, Berlin, New York, 1999.

Grossarth-Maticek R. Selbstregulation, Autonomie und Gesundheit. Krankheitsfaktoren und soziale Gesundheitsressourcen im sozio-psycho-biologischen System, De Gruyter, Berlin, New York, 2003.

Guorui J. Qigong Yangsheng. Chinesische Übungen zur Stärkung der Lebenskraft, Fischer, Frankfurt/Main, 1996.

Guorui J. Die fünfzehn Ausdrucksformen des Taiji-Qigong, Medizinisch Literarische Verlagsanstalt, Uelzen, 1997.

Guorui J. Qigong Yangsheng, Medizinisch Literarische Verlagsanstalt, Uelzen, 1998.

Gür A, et al. Effects of low power laser and low dose amitriptyline therapy on clinical symptoms and quality of life in fibromyalgia: a single-blind, placebo-controlled trial, Rheumatol. Int. 22 (2002a) 188–193.

Gür A, et al. Efficacy of low power laser therapy in fibromyalgia: a single-blind, placebo-controlled trial, Lasers Med. Sci. 17 (2002b) 57–61.

Gür A, et al. Efficacy of 904 nm gallium arsenide low level laser therapy in the management of chronic myofascial pain in the neck: a double-blind and randomize-controlled trial, Lasers Surg. Med. 35 (2004) 229–235.

Hackethal HJ. Gesundheit und Lebensfreude durch Kranich Qigong, Maudrich, Wien, 2000.

Hakgüder A, et al. Efficacy of low level laser therapy in myofascial pain syndrome: an algometric and thermographic evaluation, Lasers Surg. Med. 33 (2003) 339–343.

Haltenhof H, et al. Beurteilung und Verbreitung komplementärmedizinischer Verfahren, Gesundheitswesen 57 (1995) 192–195.

Hamm A. Progressive Muskelentspannung, in: Vaitl D, Petermann F (Hrsg.), Handbuch der Entspannungsverfahren. Bd. 1: Grundlagen und Methoden, Psychologie Verlags Union, Weinheim, 1993.

Han C. Leitfaden Tuina, 2. AuflUrban & Fischer, München, 2005.

Han JS. Acupuncture and endorphins, Neurosci. Lett. 361 (1–3) (2004) 258–261.

Han JS. Acupuncture: neuropeptide release produced by electrical stimulation of different frequencies, Trends Neurosci. 26 (1) (2003) 17–22.

Hanna T. Beweglich sein, ein Leben lang, Kösel, Stuttgart, 2003.

Harris RI, Beath T. The short first metatarsal; its incidence and clinical significance, J. Bone Joint Surg. 31A (3) (1949) 553–565.

Hatzenbühler M, et al. Repetitorium Schmerztherapie, 2. Aufl, Springer, Heidelberg, 2007.

Hausdorf J, et al. Molecular basis for pain mediating properties of extracorporeal shock waves, Schmerz 18 (2004) 492–497.

Hawkins D, et al. Low level laser therapy (LLLT) as an effective therapeutic modality for delayed wound healing, Ann. N. Y. Acad. Sci. 1056 (2005) 486–493.

Head H. S nsibilitätstorungen der Haut, Berlin(1898).

Hecker H, et al. Ohr- Schädel-, Mund-, Hand-Akupunktur, 3. Aufl, Hippokrates, Stuttgart 2002.

Heilpraktikergesetz. http://de.wikipedia.org/wiki/Heilpraktikergesetz.

Helms JM. Acupuncture energetics: A clinical approach for physicians, Medical Acupuncture Publishers, Berkeley, 1995.

Hesse J, et al. Acupuncture versus metoprolol in migraine prophylaxis: a randomized trial of trigger point inactivation, J. Intern. Med. 235 (1994) 451–456.

Heydenreich A, et al. Handbuch der transkutanen Nervenstimulation schwa-medico, 6. Aufl, A.M.I.-Verlag, Gießen, 1995.

Hides JA, et al. Multifidus muscle recovery is not automatic after resolution of acute first episodes of low back pain, Spine 21 (1996) 276–279.

Hildenbrand G. Qigong – chinesische Heilkunde in Aktion, Akupunktur 27 (1999) 76–85.

Hillman SK. Interactive functional anatomy [DVD-ROM], Primal Pictures, London, 2002.

Ho KY, Tan KH. Botulinum toxin A for myofascial trigger point injection: a qualitative systematic review, Eur. J. Pain 11 (2007) 519–527.

Hodges PW, Richardson CA. Inefficient stabilization of the lumbar spine associated with low back pain. A motor control evaluation of the transversus abdominis, Spine 21 (1996) 2640–5650.

Hofmann E. Progressive Muskelentspannung. Ein Trainingsprogramm, Hogrefe, Göttingen, 1998.

Hoheisel U, et al. Excitatory and modulatory effects of inflammatory cytokines and neurotrophins on mechanosensitive group IV muscle afferents in the rat, Pain 114 (2005) 168–176.

Hoheisel U, et al. Sensitization of rat dorsal horn neurons by NGF-induced subthreshold potentials and low-frequency activation. A study employing intracellular recordings in vivo, Brain Res. 12 (2007) 34–43.

Hong CZ. Pathophysiology of myofascial trigger point, J. Formos. Med. Assoc. 95 (1996) 93–104.

Hong C, et al. Interexaminer reliability of the palpation of trigger points in the trunk and lower limb muscles, Arch. Phys. Med. Rehabil. 81 (2000) 258–264.

Hong CZ. Myofascial trigger point pathophysiology and correlation with acupuncture points, Acupunct. Med. 18 (2000) 41–47.

Bibliography

Hong CZ, Torigoe Y. Electrophysiological characteristics of localized twitch responses in responsive taut bands of rabbit skeletal muscle, J. Musculosk. Pain 2 (1994) 17–43.

Hou DR, et al. Immediate effects of various therapeutic modalities on cervical myofascial pain and trigger-point sensitivity, Arch. Phys. Med. Rehabil. 83 (2003) 1406–1414.

Huang Di Nei Jing (Yellow Emperor's Inner Classic), 100–200 bc.

Hubbard DR, Berkoff GM. Myofascial trigger points show spontaneous needle EMG activity, Spine 18 (1993) 1803–1807.

Huijing PA, et al. Extramuscular myofascial force transmission also occurs between synergistic muscles and antagonistic muscles, J. Electromyogr. Kinesiol. 17 (2007) 708–724.

Ilbuldu E, et al. Comparison of laser, dry needling, and placebo laser treatments in myofascial pain syndrome, Photomed. Laser Surg. 22 (2004) 306–311.

Irnich D. Münchner naturheilkundliches Schmerzintensivprogramm – Ein 3 Stufen Konzept, Dt Zeitschr f Akup 46 (2003) 45–49.

Irnich D, Beyer A. Neurobiologische Grundlagen der Akupunkturanalgesie, Schmerz 16 (2002) 93–102.

Irnich D, et al. Randomised trial of acupuncture compared with conventional massage and 'sham' laser acupuncture for treatment of chronic neck pain, BMJ 322 (2001) 1574–1577.

Irnich D, et al. Immediate effects of acupuncture on pain and mobility in chronic neck pain: results of a randomised, double-blind, placebo-controlled crossover trial, Pain 99 (2002) 83–89.

Irnich D, et al. (Munich Outpatient Program in Complementary and Alternative Medicine for Chronic Pain (MOCAM) – one year follow up (2005), Abstracts 11, in: World Congress on Pain, IASP-Press, Sydney, Australia, p. 639.

Jäckel WH, et al. Epidemiologie rheumatischer Beschwerden in der Bundesrepublik Deutschland, Z. Rheumatol. 52 (1993) 281–288.

Jacobson E. Entspannung als Therapie. Progressive Relaxation in Theorie und Praxis, Pfeiffer, München, 1990.

Janda V. Manuelle Muskelfunktionsdiagnostik, Elsevier, München, 2000.

Jeanmonod D, et al. Low threshold calcium spike bursts in the human thalamus, Brain 119 (1996) 363–375.

Jenckner FL. Nervenblockaden auf pharmakologischem und auf elektrischem Weg, 3. Aufl, Springer, Wien, New York 1980.

Jensen R, et al. Muscle tenderness and pressure pain thresholds in headache. A population study, Pain 52 (1993) 193–199.

Jones L. Strain Counterstrain, Urban & Fischer, München, 2004.

Junghans H, Schmorl G. Die gesunde und kranke Wirbelsäule in Röntgenbild und Klinik: pathologisch-anatomische Untersuchungen, Archiv und Atlas der normalen und pathologischen Anatomie in typischen Röntgenbildern, Band 43 von Fortschritte auf dem Gebiete der Röntgenstrahlen: Ergänzungsbd (1951).

Kaergaard A, Andersen JH. Musculoskeletal disorders of the neck and prevalence, incidence, and prognosis shoulders in female sewing machine operators, Occup. Environ. Med. 57 (2000) 528–534.

Kane K, Taub A. A history of local analgesia, Pain 1 (1975) 125.

Karlsson JO, et al. Effects of ultraviolet radiation on the tension and the cyclic GMP level of bovine mesenteric arteries, Life Sci. 34 (1984) 1555–1563.

Karnath HO, et al. The perception of body orientation after neck-proprioceptive stimulation. Effects of time and of visual cueing, Exp. Brain Res, 143 (2002) 350–353.

Kasai S, et al. Effect of low-power laser irradiation on impulse conduction in anesthetized rabbits, J. Clin. Laser Med. Surg. 14 (1996) 107–109.

Keidel D (Hrsg.), Kurzgefasstes Lehrbuch der Physiologie (gebundene Ausgabe), Thieme, Stuttgart, 1994.

Khadra M, et al. Effect of laser therapy on attachment, proliferation and differentiation of human osteoblast-like cells cultured on titanium implant material, Biomaterials 26 (2005) 3503–3509.

Knappe V, et al. Principles of lasers and biophotonic effects, Photomed. Laser Surg. 22 (2004) 411–417.

Köhle K, Raspe HH. Das Gespräch während der ärztlichen Visite. Empirische Untersuchungen, Urban & Schwarzenberg, München, Wien, Baltimore, 1982.

Kolár P. The sensomotor nature of postural function. Its fundamental role in rehabilitation of the motor system, J. Orthop. Med 21 (1999) 40–45.

Kolár P. Facilitation of agonist-antagonist co-activation by reflex stimulation, in: Liebenson C (Ed.), Rehabilitation of the spine, Lippincott, Williams & Wilkins, Philadelphia, 2006, pp. 531–565.

Korr IM. Proprioceptors and somatic dysfunction, J. Am. Osteop. Assoc. 74 (1975) 638–650.

Krampen G. Autogenes Training, in: Steinebach C (Hrsg.), Heilpädagogik für chronisch kranke Kinder und Jugendliche, Lambertus, Freiburg i. Br, 1997.

Krampen G. Einführungskurse zum Autogenen Training: Ein Lehr- und Übungsbuch für die psychosoziale Praxis, 2. Aufl, Verlag für Angewandte Psychologie Hogrefe, Göttingen, 1998.

Kuan TS, et al. The spinal cord connections of the myofascial trigger spots, Eur. J. Pain 11 (2007) 624–634.

Langemark M, Olesen J. Pericranial tenderness in tension headache. A blind, controlled study, Cephalalgia 7 (1987) 249–255.

Langen D. Autogenes Training. Dreimal täglich zwei Minuten abschalten, loslassen, erholen, Gräfe & Unzer, München, 1999.

Langer H. Allgemeinerkrankungen durch Störfelder (Trigeminusbereich), E. Fischer, Heidelberg, 1977.

Langevin HM, et al. Connective tissue fibroblast response to acupuncture: dose-dependent effect of bidirectional needle rotation, J. Altern. Complement. Med. 13 (2007) 355–360.

Larbig W. Schmerz, Kohlhammer, Stuttgart, 1982.

Larsen R. Anästhesie, 8. Aufl, Elsevier, Urban & Fischer, München, 2006.

Lavelle ED, et al. Myofascial trigger points, Anesthesiol. Clin. 25 (2007) 841–851.

LeBoeuf M. Imagination, Inspiration, Innovation. Kreative Kräfte nutzen, mvg, München, 1991.

Leitlinie Fibromyalgiesyndrom, www. leitlinien.net, HTML der Langversion, http://www.uni-duesseldorf.de/AWMF/ll/041-004.htm.

Leuner H. Lehrbuch des Katathymen Bilderlebens, Huber, Bern, Stuttgart, Toronto, 1994.

Levin S. The tensegrity-truss as a model for spine mechanics: biotensegrity, J. Mech. Med. Biol. 2 (2002) 375–388.

Lewit K. The needle effect in the relief of myofascial pain, Pain 6 (1979) 83–90.

Lewit K. The functional approach, J. Orthop. Med. 10 (1993) 73–77.

Lewit K. X ray of trunk rotation, J. Manipulative Physiol. Ther. 28 (1997) 454–458.

Lewit K. Editorial. Relationship of structure and function in the motor system, J. Orthop. Med 23 (2001) 45–46.

Lewit K. Criteria for the most physiological manipulative techniques, J. Orthop. Med. 27 (2003a) 50–53.

Lewit K. Verkettungen in der muskuloskelettalen, Medizin Funktionskrankheiten des Bewegungssystems 11 (2003b) 159–168.

Lewit K. Managing common pain syndromes and finding the key link, in: Liebenson C (Ed.), Rehabilitation of the Spine, Lippincott, Williams & Wilkins, 2006a, pp. 776–797.

Lewit K. Manuelle Medizin bei Funktionsstörungen des Bewegungssystems, 8. Aufl, Elsevier, Urban & Fischer, München, 2006b.

Licht G, et al. Untersuchung Myofaszialer Triggerpunkte ist reliabel! Intertester-Reliabilität überprüft an insgesamt 304 Muskeln, Manuelle Medizin 45 (2007) 402–408.

Lie FT, Skopek H. Chinesische Heilmassage, Maudrich, Wien, 1992.

Liebermann JS, et al. Skeletal muscle: structure, chemistry, and function, in: Downey JA, et al. (Ed.),

The Physiological Basis of Rehabilitation Medicine, second ed., Butterworth-Heinemann, Boston, 1994.

Lin TY, et al. Cervicogenic headache, J. Musculosk. Pain 3 (Suppl. 1) (1995) 151 (Abstract).

Lindel K. Muskeldehnung. Grundlagen – Differenzialdiagnostik – Therapeutische Dehnungen – Eigendehnungen, Springer, Heidelberg, 2006.

Linke WA, Leake MC. Multiple sources of passive stress relaxation in muscle fibres, Phys. Med. Biol. 49 (2004) 3613–3627.

Litscher G, Schikora D (Eds.), Laserneedle-Acupuncture. Science and Practice, Pabst Science Publishers, Lengerich, 2005.

Litscher G, et al. Acupuncture using laser needles modulates brain function: first evidence from functional transcranial Doppler sonography and functional magnetic resonance imaging, Lasers Med. Sci. 19 (2004) 6–11.

Loeser JD, et al. Relief of pain by transcutaneous stimulation, J. Neurosurg. 42 (1975) 308.

Lubart R, et al. Low-energy laser irradiation promotes cellular redox activity, Photomed. Laser Surg. 23 (2005) 3–9.

Lubart R, et al. Photochemistry and photobiology of light absorption by living cells, Photomed. Laser Surg. 24 (2006) 179–185.

Lucas, et al. Latent myofascial triggerpoints: their effects on muscle activation and movement efficieny, J. Bodywork Movement Therapies 8 (2004) 160–164.

Mackenzie J. Symptoms and their interpretation, London, 1909.

Maegawa Y, et al. Effects of near-infrared low-level laser irradiation on microcirculation, Lasers Surg. Med. 27 (2000) 427–437.

Magni G, et al. Chronic musculoskeletal pain and depressive symptoms in the general population. An analysis of the 1st National Health and Nutrition Examination, Survey data, Pain 43 (1990) 299–307.

Maier M. Extrakorporale Stoßwellentherapie – von der experimentellen Untersuchung zur differenzierten Indikation, Z.

Orthop. Ihre Grenzgeb. 141 (2003) 254–256.

Maier M, et al. Substance P and prostaglandin E2 release after shock wave application to the rabbit femur, Clin. Orthop. Relat. Res. 406 (2003) 237–245.

Marcus Schiltenwolf in FAZ-net vom 08.06.2008.

Matsumoto K, Euler D. Kiiko Matsumoto's Clinical Strategies, vol. 1, Kiiko Matsumoto Inte rnational, Natick, 2001.

McCue D. The effects of stress on physicians and their medical practice, N. Engl. J. Med. 8 (1982) 458–463.

Meerwein F. Das ärztliche Gespräch, 3. Aufl, Huber, Bern, Stuttgart, Toronto, 1986.

Meisekothen L. Myofascial pain syndrome: a multidisciplinary approach, Nurse Pract. (1995) 20.

Melchart D, et al. Prospective investigation of adverse effects of acupuncture in 97 733 patients, Arch. Intern. Med. 164 (2004) 104–105.

Melnick J. Treatment of trigger mechanism in gastrointestinal disease, N. Y. State J. Med. 54 (1954) 1324–1330.

Melzack R. Myofascial trigger points – relation to acupuncture and mechanisms of pain, Pain 3 (1981) 1–9.

Melzack R, Wall PD. Pain mechanisms: a new theory, Science 150 (1965) 971–979.

Melzack R, et al. Triggerpoints and acupuncture points for pain: correlations and implications, Pain 3 (1977) 3–23.

Meng ACL. Die traditionelle chinesische Massage: Tuina-Therapie, Haug, Heidelberg, 1981.

Mense S. Nociception from skeletal muscle in relation to clinical muscle pain, Pain 54 (1993) 241–289.

Mense S. Pathophysiologic basis of muscle pain syndroms, Phys. Med. Rehabil. Clin. N. Am. 8 (1997) 23–53.

Mense S. Neurobiological basis of muscle pain, Schmerz 13 (1999) 3–17.

Mense S, Hoheisel U. Stickstoffmonoxid-Mangel im Rückenmark, Schmerz 15 (2001) 19–25.

Mense S. Funktionelle Neuroanatomie und Schmerzreize, Schmerz 18 (2004a) 225–237.

Mense S. Neurobiological basis for the use of botulinum toxin in pain therapy, J. Neurol. 251 (Suppl. 1) (2004b) I/1–I/7.

Mense S, et al. Muscle pain, understanding its nature, diagnosis, and treatment, Lippincott Williams & Wilkins, Philadelphia, 2001.

Mergner T, et al. Role of vestibular and neck inputs for the perception of object motion in space, Exp. Brain Res. 89 (1992) 655–668.

Middendorf I. Der erfahrbare Atem. Eine Atemlehre, 8. Aufl, Junfermann, Paderborn, 1995.

Mink ASF, et al. Manuelle Therapie der Extremitäten, Urban & Fischer, München, 2001.

Mitchell JH, Schmidt RF. Cardiovascular reflex control by afferent fibers from skeletal muscle receptors, in: Shepherd, JT, et al. (Ed.), Handbook of physiology. Sect.2, vol.III, part 2, American Physiological Society, Bethesda, MD, 1977, pp. 623–658.

Mochizuki-Oda N, et al. Effects of near-infra-red laser irradiation on adenosine triphosphate and adenosine diphosphate contents of rat brain tissue, Neurosci. Lett. 323 (2002) 207–210.

Molcho S. Körpersprache, Mosaik, München, 1983.

Morton DJ. The Human Foot, Columbia University Press, New York, 1935.

Myers TW. Anatomy Trains: Myofasziale Leitungsbahnen, Elsevier Urban & Fischer, München, 2005.

Netter FH. Atlas of Human Anatomy, Ciba-Geigy, 1989.

Neumann HD. Manuelle Medizin, Einführung in Theorie, Diagnostik und Therapie, 3. Aufl, Springer, Berlin, Heidelberg, New York, 1989.

Niboyet JEH. Cours de médicine manuelle chinoise – première année, Maisonneuve, 1978.

Nice D, et al. Intertester reliability of judgments of the presence of trigger points in patients with low back pain, Arch. Phys. Med. Rehabil. 73 (1992) 893–898.

Nielsen AJ. Spray and stretch for myofascial pain, Phys. Ther. 58 (1978) 567–569.

Niemz MH. Laser-Tissue Interaction. Fundamentals and Appications, Springer, Berlin, 2003.

Njoo K, van der Does E. The occurence and inter-rater reliability of myofascial trigger points in the quadratus lumborum and gluteus medius: a prospective study in non-specific low back pain patients and controls in general practice, Pain 58 (1994) 317–323.

Nogier P. From Auriculotherapy to Auriculomedicine, Maisonneuve, Moulins-les-Metz, 1983.

Norbu N. Yantra Yoga: Yoga der Bewegungen, Edition Tsaparang, Gleisdorf, 1988.

O'Connor J, Bensky D. Acupuncture: a comprehensive text, Eastland Press, Chicago, 1981.

Offenbächer M, Stucki G. Physical therapy in the treatment of fibromyalgia, Scand. J. Rheumatol. Suppl. (2000) 78–85.

Ogal H, Kolster C. Propädeutik der Neuen Schädelakupunktur nach Yamamoto (YNSA), Hippokrates, Stuttgart, 2004.

Olschewski A. Progressive Muskelentspannung, Hüthig, Stuttgart, 1996.

O'Malley PG, et al. Antidepressant therapy for unexplained symptoms and symptom syndromes, J. Fam. Pract 48 (1999) 980–990.

Ombregt L, et al. A System of Orthopaedic Medicine, WB Saunders, Philadelphia, 1999.

Ostwald W. Die Welt der vernachlässigten Dimensionen. Eine Einführung in die moderne Kolloidchemie mit besonderer Berücksichtigung ihrer Anwendung, Steinkopf, Dresden und Leipzig, 1915.

Ots T. Klinische diagnostisch-therapeutische Mitteilung: Sternales Druck- und Engegefühl xiong men, Dt Ztschr f Akup 44 (4) (2002) 286–288.

Pal, et al. Effect of low intensity laser interaction with human skin fibroblast cells using fiber optic nano-probes, J. Photochem. Photobiol. B 86 (3) (2007) 252–261.

Panjabi MM. The stabilizing system of the spine. Part I, Function, dysfunction, adaption and enhancement, J. Spinal Disord 5 (1992a) 383–390.

Panjabi MM. The stabilizing system of the spine. Part II, Neutral zone and instability hypothesis, J. Spinal Disord 5 (1992b) 390–397.

Paramhans Swami Maheshwarananda, Yoga im täglichen Leben – Das System, Ibera, Wien.

Passarella S, et al. Increase in the ADP/ATP exchange in rat liver mitochondria irradiated in vitro by helium-neon laser, Biochem. Biophys. Res. Commun. 156 (1988) 978–986.

Patañjali, Die Wurzeln des Yoga: Die klassischen Lehrsprüche des Patañjali – die Grundlage aller Yoga-Systeme, O.W. Barth, Frankfurt.

Patijn J. Studien zur Reproduzierbarkeit und Validität diagnostischer Verfahren in der Manuellen Medizin, Manuelle Medizin 40 (2002) 339–351.

Paulus W, Schöps P. Schmerzsyndrome des Kopf- und Halsbereichs. Klinik, Diagnostik, medikamentöse und physikalische Therapie, Wissenschaftliche Verlagsgesellschaft, Stuttgart, 1998.

Pedrosa Gil F, et al. Parental bonding and alexithymia in adults with fibromyalgia, Psychosomatics 49 (2008) 115–122.

Perschke O. Atlas der Manuellen Therapie und Akupunkturmassage, Hippokrates, Stuttgart, 2001.

Petermann F, Vaitl D (Hrsg.), Handbuch der Entspannungsverfahren. Bd. 2: Anwendungen, Psychologie Verlags Union, Weinheim, 1994.

Philipp CM, Berlien HP. Physikalisch-medizinische Grundlagen, Laryngorhinootolgie 82 (2003) 1–20.

Pipelzadeh MH, Naylor IL. The in vitro enhancement of rat myofibroblast contractility by alterations to the pH of the physiological solution, Eur. J. Pharmacol. 357 (1998) 257–259.

Pischinger A. Zellstrukturen und Kolloidchemie, Wien. Klin. Wochenschr. 5 (1938) 130.

Pischinger A. Das System der Grundregulation, 3. Aufl, Haug, Heidelberg, 1980.

Pomeranz B. Wissenschaftliche Grundlagen der Akupunktur, in: Stux G, et al. (Eds.), Akupunktur, Springer, Hamburg, 1999, pp. 5–55.

Pontari MA, Ruggieri MR. Mechanisms in prostatitis/chronic pelvic pain syndrome, J. Urol. 179 (2008) 61–67.

Pothmann R. Transcutane elektrische Nervenstimulation, in: Pothmann R (Hrsg.), Chronische Schmerzen im Kindesalter, Hippokrates, Stuttgart, 1988.

Pothmann R (Ed.), TENS, 3. Aufl, Hippokrates, Stuttgart, 2003, pp. 47–52.

Pothmann R, Göbel U. Schmerzdiag-nostik und -therapie in der Kinder-onkologie, Klin. Pädiat. 198 (1986) 479–483.

Prado LG, et al. Isoform diversity of giant proteins in relation to passive and active contractile properties of rabbit skeletal muscles, J. Gen. Physiol. 126 (2005) 461–480.

Preusser W. Die Gelosenmassage, Hippokrates, Stuttgart, 1957.

Preusser W. Gelopunktur, Hippokrates, Stuttgart, 1961.

Preusser W. Regulationstherapie. Über palpable Kolloidveränderungen im Bindegewebe (Gelosenbehandlung), Haug, Heidelberg, 1987.

Putz R, et al. (Hrsg.), Sobotta Atlas der Anatomie des Menschen, 22. Aufl, Elsevier Urban & Fischer, München, 2006.

Rasmussen BK, et al. Epidemiology of headache in a general population – A prevalence study, J. Clin. Epidemiol. 44 (1991) 1147–1157.

Rasmussen BK, et al. Impact of headache on sickness absence and utilisation of medical services: A Danish population study, J. Epidemiol. Community Health 46 (1992) 443–446.

Rehfisch HP, Basler HD. Entspannung und Imagination, in: Basler HD, et al. (Hrsg.), Psychologische Schmerztherapie. Grundlagen, Krankheitsbilder, Behandlung, Springer, Berlin, Heidelberg, New York, 1999.

Richardson CA, et al. Therapeutic Exercise for spinal Stabilization in Low Back Pain, 2. Aufl, Churchill Livingstone, Edinburgh, 2004.

Richtlinien für die Physiotherapeuten Gesetz über die Berufe in der Physiotherapie vom 26, Mai(1994).

Rief W, Bierbaumer N. Biofeedback-Therapie. Grundlagen, Indikation und praktisches Vorgehen, Schattauer, Stuttgart, 2000.

Rief W, Hiller W. Somatoforme Störungen: Körperliche Symptome ohne organische Ursache, Huber, Bern, Göttingen, Toronto, 1992.

Roche P, et al. Modification of Haemophiliac Haemorrhage Pain by Transcutaneous Electrical Nerve Stimulation, Pain 21 (1985) 43–48.

Rolf I. Rolfing, Harper, London, 1997a.

Rolf I. Rolfing: Strukturelle Integration. Wandel und Gleichgewicht der Körperstruktur, Irisiana, München, 1997b.

Rosted P. Practical recommendations for the use of acupuncture in the treatment of temporomandibular disorders based on the outcome of published controlled studies, Oral. Dis. 7 (2001).

Sakyong Mipham. Wie der weite Raum. Die Kraft der Meditation, dtv, München, 2005.

Sammer U. Entspannung erfolgreich vermitteln. Progressive Muskelentspannung und andere Verfahren, Klett-Cotta, Stuttgart, 1999.

Scarinci IC, et al. Altered pain perception and psychosocial features among women with gastrointestinal disorders and history of abuse: a preliminary model, Am. J. Med. 97 (1997) 108–118.

Schade H. Über den Rheumatismus, insbesondere den Muskelrheuma-tismus (Myogelosen), MMW 4 (1921a) 95.

Schade H. Von der Bedeutung der Kolloide im menschlichen Körper, MMW 5 (1921b) 144.

Scharf HP, et al. (Ed.), Orthopädie und Unfallchirurgie, Elsevier, Urban & Fischer, München, 2008.

Schepank H. Beeinträchtigungs-Schwere-Score (BSS), Beltz, Weinheim, 1995.

Scherer H. Das Gleichgewicht, Springer, Berlin, 1997.

Schiffman EL, et al. The prevalence and treatment needs of subjects with temporomandibular disorders, J. Am. Dent. Assoc. 120 (1990) 295.

Schiltenwolf M, Henningsen P. Deutscher Ärzteverlag, Köln, 2007.

Schiltenwolf M. Heidelberg, Quelle: FAZ-net vom 8.6.2008.

Schleip R. Faszien und Nervensystem, Osteopathische Medizin 4 (2003) 20–28.

Schleip R. Fascial plasticity – a new neurobiological explanation, J. Bodywork Movement Therapies 7 (2002) 11 197; 104–116.

Schleip R, et al. Fascia is able to contract in a smooth muscle-like manner and thereby influence musculoskeletal mechanics, in: Liepsch D (Ed.), Proceedings of the 5th World Congress of Biomechanics, München, 2006, pp. 51–54.

Schmerzfragebögen, http://www.drk-schmerz-zentrum.de/content/07_infos/7–5_schmerzfragebogen.htm.

Schmidt KL, et al. Lehrbuch der Physikalischen Medizin und Rehabilitation, 6. Aufl, Gustav Fischer, Stuttgart, 1995.

Schneider W, et al. Manuelle Medizin, Thieme, Stuttgart, 1986.

Schneider W, et al. (Hrsg.), Sozialmedizinische Begutachtung in Psychosomatik und Psychotherapie, Huber, Bern, Göttingen, Toronto, 2001.

Schnorpfeil F, Reuter W (Hrsg.), Neurologische Untersuchung, Elsevier, Urban & Fischer, München, 2006.

Schüller BK, Neugebauer EAM. Evidenz zur Laserakupunktur bei orthopädischen Erkrankungen. Ein systematisches Review, Schmerz 22 (2008) 9–15.

Schultz JH. Das autogene Training, Thieme, Stuttgart, 1991.

Schwind P. Faszien- und Membran-Manipulation, Elsevier, München, 2004.

Seem M. Akupunktur und myofasziale Lösung, Medizinisch Literarische Verlagsgesellschaft mbH, Uelzen, 1999.

Seemann H, Nilges P. Schmerzdoku-mentation, in: Zenz M, Jurna I (Hrsg.), Lehrbuch der Schmerzther-apie: Grundlagen, Theorie und Praxis für Aus- und Weiterbildung, Wis-senschaftliche Verlagsgesellschaft GmbH, Stuttgart, 2001.

Senn E, Rusch D. Elektrotherapie: Gebräuchliche Verfahren der physikalischen Therapie; Grundlagen, Wirkungsweisen, Stellenwert, Thieme, Stuttgart, 1990.

Senn E. Wirbelsäulensyndrome, in: Brandt J, et al. (Hrsg.), Therapie und Verlauf neurologischer

Erkrankungen, 2. Aufl, Kohlhammer, Stuttgart, Berlin, Köln, 1993.

Servan-Schreiber D. Die Neue Medizin der Emotionen, Goldmann, München, 2006.

Sessle BJ, et al. Convergence of cutaneous, tooth pulp, visceral, neck and muscle afferents onto nociceptive and non-nociceptive neurones in trigeminal subnucleus caudalis (medullary dorsal horn) and its implications for referred pain, Pain 27 (1986) 219–235.

Shah JP. Integrating dry needling with new concepts of myofascial pain, muscle physiologie, and sensitisation, in: Audette J, Bailey A (Eds.), Integrative Pain Medicine, Humana Press, Totowa, 2008, pp. 107–122.

Shah JP, et al. An in vivo microanalytical technique for measuring the local biochemical milieu of human skeletal muscle, J. Appl. Physiol. 99 (2005) 1977–1984.

Shah JP, et al. Biochemicals associated with pain and inflammation are elevated in sites near to and remote from active myofascial trigger points, Arch. Phys. Med. Rehabil. 89 (2008) 16–23.

Shi S, Klotz U. Clinical use and pharmacological properties of selective COX-2 inhibitors, Eur. J. Clin. Pharm. 64 (2008) 233–252.

Siddall PJ, Cousins MJ. Spine update; spinal pin mechanisms, Spine 22 (1997) 98–104.

Siedentopf CM, et al. Functional magnetic resonance imaging detects activation of the visual association cortex during laser acupuncture of the foot in humans, Neurosci. Lett. 327 (2002) 53–56.

Siedentopf CM, et al. Laser acupuncture induced specific cerebral cortical and subcortical activations in humans, Lasers Med. Sci. 20 (2005) 68–73.

Siener R. NPSO – Neue Punktuelle Schmerz- und Organtherapie, Henrich, Wiesbaden, 1996.

Simons DG. Clinical and etiological update of myofascial pain from triggerpoints, J. Musculosk. Pain 4 (1/2) (1996) 93–121.

Simons DG. Review of enigmatic mTrPs as a common cause of enigmatic musculoskeletal pain and dysfunction, J. Electromyogr. Kinesiol. 14 (2004) 95–107.

Simons DG. New views of myofascial trigger points: Etiology and diagnosis, Arch. Phys. Med. Rehabil. 89 (1) (2008) 157–159.

Simons DG, Dommerholt J. Mysofascial pain syndrome – trigger points, J. Musculosk. Pain 13 (2005) 53–64.

Simons DG, Dommerholt J. Myofascial pain syndrome – trigger points literature review, J. Muscoskel. Pain 1 (15) (2007) 70–71.

Simons DG, Mense S. Understanding and measurement of muscle tone related to clinical muscle pain, Pain 75 (1998) 1–17.

Simons DG, Mense S. Diagnose und Therapie myofaszialer Triggerpunkte, Schmerz 17 (2003) 419–424.

Simon DG, Travell J. Myofascial trigger points, a possible explanation, Pain 10 (1981) 106–109.

Simons DG, et al. Myofascial Pain and Dysfunction, 2. Aufl, Williams & Wilkins, Baltimore, 1999.

Simunovic Z (Ed.), Lasers in medicine and dentistry: basic science and up-to-date clinical application of low level laser therapy: LLLT, Vitagraf, Rijeka, 2000.

Singer KP, Giles LGF. Manual therapy considerations at the thoracolumbar junction: an anatomical and functional perspective, J. Manipulative Physiol. Ther. 13 (1990) 83–88.

Skládal J, et al. Posturální funkce bránice, (Die posturale Funktion des Zwerchfells) Cs fysiol 19 (1970) 279–280.

Skootsky SA, et al. Prevalence of myofascial pain in general internal medicine practice, West. J. Med. 151 (1989) 157–160.

Slocumb JC. Neurological factors in chronic pelvic pain: trigger points and the abdominal pelvic pain syndrome, Am. J. Obstet. Gynecol. 149 (1984) 536–543.

Smith J. Structural Bodywork: an Introduction for Students and Practitioners, Churchill Livingstone, Edinburgh, 2005.

Smith M, et al. Acupuncture Treatment of Drug and Alcohol Abuse: 8 Years Experience Emphasizing Tonification rather than Sedation, Substance Abuse Division, Lincoln Hospital, New York, 1982.

Sola AE, et al. Incidence of hypersensitive areas in posterior shoulder muscles, Am. J. Phys. Med. 34 (1955) 585.

Spezzano C. Karten der Erkenntnis auf dem Weg nach innen/Das Buch der Erkenntnis, 9. Aufl, Via Nova, Petersberg, 2004.

Sriram A, Sriram R. Yoga und Gefühle, Theseus, Stuttgart, 2004.

Stecco C, et al. Anatomy of the deep fascia of the upper limb. Second part: study of innervation, Morphologie 292 (2007) 38–43.

Stein A, et al. Low-level laser irradiation promotes proliferation and differentiation of human osteoblasts in vitro, Photomed. Laser Surg. 23 (2005) 161–166.

Stetter F. Was geschieht, ist gut. Entspannungsverfahren in der Psychotherapie, Psychotherapeut 43 (1998) 209–220.

Stör W. Abrechnung in der Akupunktur, Elsevier, Urban & Fischer, München, 2006.

Stör W, Irnich D. Acupuncture: basics, practice, and evidence, Schmerz 23 (4) (2009) 405–417.

Strupp M, et al. Perceptual and oculomotor effects of neck muscle vibration in vestibular neuritis. Ipsilateral somatosensory substitution of vestibular function, Brain 121 (1998) 677–685.

Sun SC (Ed.), Atlas of Therapeutic Motion for Treatment and Health, Foreign Languages Press, Beijing, 1989.

Sun SC (Ed.), Chinese Massage Therapy, Shandong Science and Technology Press, Jinan, 1990.

Swami Vishnudevananda. Das große illustrierte Yoga Buch, J. Kamphausen, Bielefeld, 2001.

Taguchi T, et al. Neuroanatomical pathway of nociception originating in a low back muscle (multifidus) in the rat, Neurosci. Lett. 427 (2007) 22–27.

Tilscher H, Eder M. Reflextherapie, 2. Aufl, Hippokrates, Stuttgart, 1989.

Tough EA, et al. Acupuncture and dry needling in the management of myofascial trigger point pain: A systematic review and meta-analysis of randomised controlled trials, Eur. J. Pain (2008).

Tough EA, et al. Variability of criteria used to diagnose myofascial trigger point pain syndrome - Evidence from a review of the literature, Clin. J. Pain 23 (2007) 278–286.

Tramèr MR, et al. Quantitative estimation of rare adverse events which follow a biological progression: a new model applied to chronic NSAID use, Pain 85 (2000) 169–182.

Travell JG. Myopain Seminars, curriculum. http://www.painpoints.com/seminars.

Travell JG, Rinzler SH. The myofascial genesis of pain, Postgrad. Med. 11 (1952) 425–434.

Travell JG, Simons DG. Myofascial Pain and Dysfunction, vol. 1, The Trigger Point Manual, Williams & Wilkins, Baltimore, 1983 (2nd ed 1992).

Travell JG, Simons DG. Handbuch der Muskeltriggerpunkte (Trigger Point Manual), 2. Aufl, Urban & Fischer, München, Jena, 2002.

Travell JG, Simons DG. Flipchart Triggerpunkte, Elsevier, Urban & Fischer, München, 2004.

Trökes A. Das große Yogabuch, Verlag Gräfe & Unzer, München, 2000.

Tsuchiya K, et al. Diode laser irradiation selectively diminishes slow component of axonal volleys to dorsal roots from the saphenous nerve in the rat, Neurosci. Lett. 161 (1993) 65–68.

Uexküll Tv (Hrsg.), Psychosomatische Medizin, 3. Aufl, Urban und Schwarzenberg, München, 1986.

Unschuld P. Huang Di Nei Jing Su Wen: Nature, Knowledge, Imagery in an Ancient Chinese Medical Text, University of California Press, Berkeley, Los Angeles, London, 2003.

Usichenko T, et al. Auricular acupuncture for pain relief after ambulatory knee surgery: a randomized trial, CMAJ 176 (2007) 179–183.

Vaitl D, Petermann F (Hrsg.), Handbuch der Entspannungsverfahren. Bd. 1: Grundlagen und Methoden, Psychologie Verlags Union, Weinheim, 1993 (2000).

van den Berg F. Angewandte Physiologie: Therapie, Training, Tests, Thieme, Stuttgart, 2001.

van Koulil S, et al. Cognitive-behavioural therapies and exercise programmes for patients with fibromyalgia: state of the art and future directions, Ann. Rheum. Dis. 66 (2007) 571–581.

van Wingerden BAM. Connective Tissue in Rehabilitation, Scipro, Vaduz, 1995.

Vojta V, Peters A. Das Voita Prinzip, Springer, Heidelberg, 1993.

Voll R. Topographische Lage der Messpunkte der Elektroakupunktur, ML, Uelzen, 1973–1976.

von Harder Y. Paint herapy – legal reference points and stumbling blocks, Schmerz 21 (2007) 62–66.

Wagner B. Chinesische Meditationsform. Qigong: Von Bär und Tiger lernen. Serie Entspannungstechniken. Folge 1: Die Lebensenergie bündeln, Fortschr. Med. 117 (1999) 55.

Wancura J. Segment-Anatomie. Der Schlüssel zu Akupunktur, Neuraltherapie und Manualtherapie, Elsevier, Urban & Fischer, München, 2009.

Weber M. Nadeln aus Licht – Vorstellung einer neuen Therapiemethode, Dt Ztschr f Akup 48 (2005) 24–32.

Weeks VD, Travell JG. How to give painless injections. AMA Scientific Exhibits, Grune & Stratton, New York, 1957.

Weinberg RS, Hunt VV. Effects of structural integration on state-trait anxiety, J. Clin. Psychol. 35 (1979) 19–322.

Werner G, et al. Physikalische und Rehabilitative Medizin (Checkliste), Thieme, Stuttgart, 1997.

White A. E-mail correspondence from editor of Acupuncture in Medicine 2007.

Whittaker P. Laser acupuncture: past, present, and future, Lasers Med. Sci. 19 (2004) 69–80.

Whittaker P. Laser acupuncture and analgesia: preliminary evidence for a transient and opioid-mediated effect, in: Hamblin MR, et al. (Eds.), Proceedings of SPIE – Volume 6140 Mechanisms for Low-Light Therapy, 2006.

Williams NH, et al. Randomized osteopathic manipulation study (ROMANS): pragmatic trial for spinal pain in primary care, Fam. Pract. 20 (2003) 662–669.

Wiseman N, Ellis A. Fundamentals of Chinese Medicine, Paradigm Publications, Brookline, MA, 1991.

Wolfe F, et al. The fibromyalgia and myofascial pain syndromes: a preliminary study of tender points and trigger points in persons with fibromyalgia, myofascial pain syndrome and no disease, J. Rheumatol. 19 (1992) 944–951.

World Association for Laser Therapy (WALT), Dosage recommendations, 2005. Zugriff am 5.6.2008 unter http://www.walt.nu/dosage-recommendations.html.

Wurz H. Das Sonnengebet, Herder, Freiburg, 2002.

Yamamoto T. YNSA – Yamamoto New Scalp Acupuncture, Springer, Tokyo, 1997.

Zahnd F. Stretching - Suche nach Erklärungen. Physiotherapie in Sport und Orthopädie, Manuelle Therapie 9 (2005a) 1–8.

Zahnd F. Trainingsmaßnahmen bei schmerzhaften Funktionsstörungen der LWS, Manuelle Therapie 9 (2005b) 161–170.

Zeier H. Biofeedback. Physiologische Grundlagen – Anwendungen in der Psychotherapie, 2. Aufl, Hans Huber, Bern, 1997.

Zenz M, Jurna I. Lehrbuch der Schmerztherapie, Grundlagen, Theorie und Praxis für Aus- und Weiterbildung, 2. Aufl, Wissenschaftliche Verlagsgesellschaft, 2001.

Zhang Y. Bio-Holographic Diagnosis and Therapy, Shandong University Press, 1987.

Zimmermann M, Handwerker HO (Hrsg.), Schmerz, Konzepte und ärztliches Handeln, Springer, Berlin, Heidelberg New York Tokyo, 1984.

Zink W, et al. Myotoxizität von Lokalanästhetika, Der Anästhesist 56 (2007) 118–127.

Zollmann C, Vickers A. What is complementary medicine? BMJ 319 (1999a) 693–696.

Zollmann C, Vickers A. Users and practitioners of complementary medicine, BMJ 319 (1999b) 836–838.

Zorn A. The spring-like function of the lumbar fascia in human walking, in: Findley T, Schleip R (Eds.), Fascia Research – Basic Science and Implications for Conventional and Complementary Health Care, Elsevier, Urban & Fischer, München, 2007.

Index

Note: Page numbers followed by *b* indicate boxes, *f* indicate figures and *t* indicate tables.

Printed in the United States
By Bookmasters